Pediatric Gastroenterology and Nutrition in Clinical Practice

Pediatric Gastroenterology and Nutrition in Clinical Practice

edited by

Carlos H. Lifschitz

USDA/ARS Children's Nutrition Research Center
Baylor College of Medicine and
Texas Children's Hospital
Houston, Texas

MARCEL DEKKER, INC.　　　　　　NEW YORK • BASEL

ISBN: 0-8247-0510-6

This book is printed on acid-free paper.

Headquarters
Marcel Dekker, Inc.
270 Madison Avenue, New York, NY 10016
tel: 212-696-9000; fax: 212-685-4540

Eastern Hemisphere Distribution
Marcel Dekker AG
Hutgasse 4, Postfach 812, CH-4001 Basel, Switzerland
tel: 41-61-261-8482; fax: 41-61-261-8896

World Wide Web
http://www.dekker.com

The publisher offers discounts on this book when ordered in bulk quantities. For more information, write to Special Sales/Professional Marketing at the headquarters address above.

Current printing (last digit):
10 9 8 7 6 5 4 3 2 1

PRINTED IN THE UNITED STATES OF AMERICA

To my daughters Paula and Lucia, my mother Emma, and my brother Eduardo, and to the memory of my father Rafael and my wife Malena

Preface

An increasing amount of information must be acquired by medical students and physicians in training and in practice. With this abundance of information, it can be difficult to keep up to date with all the new developments in pediatric gastroenterology and nutrition, and at the same time determine what is pertinent to the clinical practice of the nonspecialist. This book is intended to meet these needs by presenting a clear and useful summary of the most relevant new facts in molecular biology and genetics, as well as recently acquired clinical information, in conjunction with a practical approach to pediatric gastroenterology and nutrition. The idea is to provide new information that seems to be here to stay, along with a comprehensive update on the management of nutritional and gastrointestinal problems that affect the pediatric population, from the newborn to the adolescent.

We have also provided, when appropriate, a section on ''what can go wrong.'' This section lists common errors, oversights, and complications specific to the topic under discussion.

In assembling all this material, I selected a variety of talented contributors who are regarded as authorities in their fields and who are capable of presenting a general view of the topics addressed. We designed our reference lists to represent a limited number of original and review articles that we believe will best serve the specific interests of our readership.

Carlos H. Lifschitz

Contents

Part II   Gastroenterology

Contributors

Steven A. Abrams, M.D.   Professor, Department of Pediatrics, Baylor College of Medicine and USDA/ARS Children's Nutrition Research Center, Houston, Texas

Carlo Agostini, M.D.   Department of Pediatrics, University of Milan, and San Paolo Hospital, Milan, Italy

Marvin E. Ament, M.D.   Professor, Department of Pediatrics, and Chief, Division of Gastroenterology and Nutrition, Mattel Children's Hospital at UCLA, UCLA School of Medicine, Los Angeles, California

J. Timothy Bricker, M.D.   Professor and Chief of Pediatric Cardiology, Department of Pediatrics, Baylor College of Medicine, and Texas Children's Hospital, Houston, Texas

Kenneth H. Brown, M.D.   Professor, Department of Nutrition, and Director, Program in International Nutrition, University of California, Davis, Davis, California

Hans A. Büller, M.D., Ph.D.   Professor, Department of Pediatrics, Erasmus University Medical Center, and Chief, Department of Pediatrics, Sophia Children's Hospital, Rotterdam, The Netherlands

Douglas G. Burrin, Ph.D.   Research Physiologist, USDA/ARS Children's Nutrition Research Center, Baylor College of Medicine, Houston, Texas

Gisela Chelimsky, M.D.   Assistant Professor, Department of Pediatrics, Case Western Reserve University School of Medicine, and Department of Pediatric Gastroenterology, Rainbow Babies & Children's Hospital, Cleveland, Ohio

Steven J. Czinn, M.D.   Department of Pediatrics, Case Western Reserve University School of Medicine, and Chief, Division of Pediatric Gastroenterology, Hepatology and Nutrition, Rainbow Babies & Children's Hospital, Cleveland, Ohio

Beverly Barrett Dahms, M.D.   Professor, Departments of Pathology and Pediatrics, Case Western Reserve University School of Medicine, and University Hospitals of Cleveland, Cleveland, Ohio

Jan Dekker, Ph.D.   Associate Professor, Department of Pediatric Gastroenterology and Nutrition, Erasmus University Rotterdam, Rotterdam, The Netherlands

Carlo Di Lorenzo, M.D.   Associate Professor, Department of Pediatric Gastroenterology, University of Pittsburgh, and Children's Hospital of Pittsburgh, Pittsburgh, Pennsylvania

Alexandra W. C. Einerhand, Ph.D.   Associate Professor, Department of Pediatric Gastroenterology and Nutrition, Erasmus University Rotterdam, Rotterdam, The Netherlands

Kevin J. Gaskin, M.D., F.R.A.C.P.   Professor, James Fairfax Institute of Pediatric Nutrition, Royal Alexandra Hospital for Children, Sydney, New South Wales, Australia

George Gershman, M.D., Ph.D.   Assistant Professor, Department of Pediatric Gastroenterology, Harbor-UCLA Medical Center, Torrance, California

Angel Gil, Ph.D.   Professor, Department of Biochemistry and Molecular Biology, School of Pharmacy, University of Granada, Granada, Spain

Marcello Giovannini, M.D.   Professor and Chairman, Department of Pediatrics, University of Milan, and San Paolo Hospital, Milan, Italy

Tracy Harpel Laird, M.D.   Fellow, Department of Pediatric Cardiology, Baylor College of Medicine, and Texas Children's Hospital, Houston, Texas

Andrea S. Hiralall, Ph.D. Psychologist, Department of Gastroenterology and Nutrition, The Children's Hospital of Philadelphia, Philadelphia, Pennsylvania

Jeffrey S. Hyams, M.D. Professor, Division of Digestive Diseases and Nutrition, Department of Pediatrics, University of Connecticut School of Medicine, Farmington, and Connecticut Children's Medical Center, Hartford, Connecticut

Deirdre Anne Kelly, M.D., F.R.C.P.CH, F.R.C.P., F.R.C.P.I. Reader in Pediatric Hepatology, The Liver Unit, Birmingham Children's Hospital, Birmingham, England

Berthold Koletzko, M.D. Professor and Head, Division of Metabolic Diseases and Nutrition, Department of Pediatrics, University of Munich, and Dr. von Hauner Children's Hospital, Munich, Germany

Akio Kubota, M.D., Ph.D. Director, Department of Pediatric Surgery, Osaka Medical Center and Research Institute for Maternal and Child Health, Izumi, Osaka, Japan

Carlos H. Lifschitz, M.D. Associate Professor, Section of Nutrition and Gastroenterology, Department of Pediatrics, USDA/ARS Children's Nutrition Research Center, Baylor College of Medicine, and Texas Children's Hospital, Houston, Texas

Fima Lifshitz, M.D. Professor, Department of Pediatrics, State University of New York Health Science Center at Brooklyn, New York, New York, and Chief of Staff and Senior Vice President for Academic Affairs, Miami Children's Hospital, Miami, Florida

Jere Ziffer Lifshitz, M.S., R.N. President, Prime Health Consultants, Inc., Miami, Florida

Vera Loening-Baucke, M.D. Professor, Department of Pediatrics, University of Iowa, Iowa City, Iowa

Jacqueline Madden, M.S., R.N., C.S. Pediatric Nurse Practitioner, Department of Pediatric Gastroenterology and Nutrition, MassGeneral Hospital for Children, Boston, Massachusetts

George Marx, M.D. Fellow, Division of Pediatric Gastroenterology and Nutrition, Department of Pediatrics, University of Montreal, and Ste. Justine Hospital, Montreal, Quebec, Canada

Carmen Mikhail, Ph.D. Assistant Professor, Department of Pediatrics and Department of Psychiatry and Behavioral Science, Baylor College of Medicine, Houston, Texas

Josef Neu, M.D.   Professor, Division of Neonatology, Department of Pediatrics, University of Florida College of Medicine, Gainesville, Florida

Akira Okada, M.D., F.A.C.S.   Professor and Chairman, Department of Pediatric Surgery, Osaka University Medical School, Suita, Osaka, Japan

Sarah Phillips, M.S., R.D., L.D., C.N.S.D.   Department of Pediatrics, Baylor College of Medicine, Houston, Texas

Isabel Polanco, M.D., Ph.D.   Professor, Department of Pediatrics, Universidad Autónoma de Madrid, and Head, Department of Pediatric Gastroenterology and Nutrition, Hospital Infantil Universitario "La Paz," Madrid, Spain

Peter J. Reeds, Ph.D.   Professor, Department of Pediatrics, USDA/ARS Children's Nutrition Research Center, Baylor College of Medicine, Houston, Texas

Enrica Riva, M.D.   Professor and Chairman, Department of Neonatology, University of Milan, and San Paolo Hospital, Milan, Italy

Colin D. Rudolph, M.D., Ph.D.   Professor, Department of Pediatrics, Medical College of Wisconsin, Milwaukee, Wisconsin

Richard J. Schanler, M.D.   Professor, Department of Pediatrics, Baylor College of Medicine, Houston, Texas

Ernest G. Seidman, M.D.   Professor, Departments of Pediatrics and Nutrition, University of Montreal, and Director, Division of Gastroenterology and Nutrition, Ste. Justine Hospital, Montreal, Quebec, Canada

Uzma Shah, M.D.   Instructor, Combined Program in Gastroenterology and Nutrition, Harvard Medical School, and MassGeneral Hospital and Children's Hospital, Boston, Massachusetts

Robert J. Shulman, M.D.   Professor, Department of Pediatrics, Baylor College of Medicine, Houston, Texas

Virginia A. Stallings, M.D.   Professor, Department of Pediatrics, University of Pennsylvania School of Medicine, and Division of Gastroenterology and Nutrition, The Children's Hospital of Philadelphia, Philadelphia, Pennsylvania

Barbara Stoll, Ph.D.   Research Associate, Department of Pediatrics, USDA/ARS Children's Nutrition Research Center, Baylor College of Medicine, Houston, Texas

Andrew M. Tershakovec, M.D.   Associate Professor, Division of Gastroenterology and Nutrition, Department of Medicine, University of Pennsylvania School of Medicine, and The Children's Hospital of Philadelphia, Philadelphia, Pennsylvania

William R. Treem, M.D.   Professor, Department of Pediatrics, Duke University Medical Center, and Chief, Division of Pediatric Gastroenterology and Nutrition, Duke Children's Hospital, Durham, North Carolina

Yvan Vandenplas, M.D., Ph.D.   Chair, Department of Pediatrics, Academic Children's Hospital, Free University of Brussels, Brussels, Belgium

Jon A. Vanderhoof, M.D.   Professor and Director, Joint Section of Pediatric Gastroenterology and Nutrition, Department of Pediatrics, University of Nebraska Medical Center, Omaha, Nebraska

W. A. Walker, M.D.   Conrad Taff Professor of Nutrition and Professor of Pediatrics, Harvard Medical School, and Chief, Combined Program in Pediatric Gastroenterology and Nutrition, MassGeneral Hospital and Children's Hospital

John Angus Walker-Smith, M.D.(Sydney), F.R.C.P., F.R.A.C.P., F.R.C.H.C.H.   Emeritus Professor, Department of Paediatric Gastroenterology, University of London, London, England

Harland S. Winter, M.D.   Associate Professor of Pediatrics, Department of Pediatric Gastroenterology and Nutrition, Harvard Medical School, and MassGeneral Hospital for Children, Boston, Massachusetts

Rosemary J. Young, B.S.N., M.S.   Clinical Nurse Specialist, Pediatric Gastroenterology, Creighton University, Omaha, Nebraska

Donna K. Zeiter, M.D.   Assistant Professor, Division of Pediatric Digestive Diseases and Nutrition, Department of Pediatrics, University of Connecticut School of Medicine, Farmington, and Connecticut Children's Medical Center, Hartford, Connecticut

1

New Knowledge About Protein

Peter J. Reeds
USDA/ARS Children's Nutrition Research Center, Baylor College of Medicine, Houston, Texas

1 INTRODUCTION

Interest in protein nutrition extends back well into the nineteenth century. In some respects, the first phase of research in this area ended in the late 1950s, when Rose completed the identification of the amino acids that are nutritionally indispensable for humans and proceeded to produce the first systematic estimates of the indispensable amino acid requirements of adult men (1). This work was extended to women by Leverton (2) and to infants and children by Holt and Snyderman (3); the data published in these papers were used by the Food Agricultural Organization/World Health Organization/United Nations University (FAO/ WHO/UNU) (1985) consultation to define what remain the most widely accepted recommended dietary allowances (4). In the late 1960s the dynamic nature of protein metabolism, first identified in the pioneering stable isotopic studies of Schoenheimer (5), was, in some respects, rediscovered, and a number of aspects of the regulation of protein turnover and amino acid catabolism were established during the 1970s (6). Since then, the traditional techniques of protein nutrition have been increasingly supported by studies with stable, isotopically labeled amino acids (7,8). The application of these techniques has, in its turn, reopened an active debate on the quantification of dietary amino acid requirements, leading to reappraisals (9,10) of the highly influential 1985 FAO report. Finally, and particularly over the last decade, the exploitation of molecular techniques has increased our understanding of a number of mechanistic aspects of amino acid function as they relate to aspects of physiology not directly related to protein metabolism (11).

This chapter considers nutritional, metabolic, and mechanistic aspects of the subject and concentrates, as far as possible, on the more recent advances. Furthermore, the discussion focuses on those subjects that bear most closely on human nutrition in general and pediatric nutrition in particular.

2 TERMINOLOGY

Despite the longevity of research into protein and amino acid requirements, there is a continuing controversy with regard to their magnitude (12,13). As I believe that the failure to resolve these difficulties stems in part from different uses of a common set of terms, I think it useful to define the following:

2.1 Metabolic Need

This is a direct reflection of the rates of metabolic pathways (e.g., protein deposition) that consume amino acids. The metabolic need is therefore a function of the genotype as well as the developmental, nutritional, and physiological state of the individual. The metabolic needs can usefully be divided into those directly associated with protein deposition, a critical issue in pediatric nutrition, and those associated with the maintenance of body protein balance, the more important portion of adult amino acid requirements.

2.2 Dietary Requirement

This is the quantity of the nutrient that must be supplied in the diet in order to satisfy the metabolic need. It therefore includes factors associated with digestion, absorption, cellular bioavailability, and transport. An important development in the last decade has been the realization of the critical influence of intestinal and hepatic metabolism on the systemic availability of amino acids (14) and the importance of amino acids to the maintenance of gut function (15). Accordingly, recent discussions of the application of isotopically labeled amino acids to the determination of amino acid requirements have stressed the importance of studying tracers that are given by the enteral route (8).

2.3 Recommended Dietary Allowance

This is the practical expression of nutritional recommendations. A recommended dietary allowance (RDA) is primarily designed to be applicable to populations rather than to individuals and thus attempts to account for interindividual variability in need and dietary requirement. This objective is usually accomplished by the addition of two standard deviations (2 SD) to the mean requirement (see Ref. 10 for discussion). It is important to emphasize that the traditional focus of the RDA has been on the prevention of nutrient deficiency, and the RDA is often expressed as a ''safe level,'' defined as the intake that reduces the prevalence of a given nutrient deficiency to some small (usually 5%) proportion of the population. One important conceptual development in recent years has been the switch of thinking away from an emphasis on frank deficiency to a consideration of the levels of nutrient intake that optimize function. This development has become particularly evident in vitamin research, but it is generating interest in other areas of nutritional investigation, including amino acid nutrition.

It is obvious that metabolic need determines dietary requirement, which indicates the recommended dietary allowance. Thus, the daily nitrogen loss of an adult ingesting a protein-free diet, a measure of the metabolic need, is approximately 50 mg N/kg body weight; the mean daily nitrogen intake necessary to maintain nitrogen equilibrium, the equivalent of the dietary requirement, is between 75 and 100 mg N/kg, while the current adult RDA, or ''safe'' level of intake of a high-quality protein, lies between 96 and 125 mgN/kg (600 to 800 mg protein), with the range of the RDA reflecting differences in opinion of expert committees in Europe and the Americas.

2.4 Protein Quality

The use of the term *high-quality protein* in the RDA indicates that dietary proteins differ in their nutritional quality. This reflects the differences in the amino acid compositions of dietary proteins and the fact that the individual's protein need is, in reality, a surrogate for the sum of the needs for each amino acid. In theory, the term *high quality* should reflect a close match between the amino acid composition of the dietary protein and metabolic need. In human nutrition, the term *high quality* is often taken to be synonymous with proteins of animal origin (usually from milk or whole egg). However, the assessment of the quality of a given dietary protein should start with a consideration of the amino acid needs of the individuals to whom it will be fed, so that the equation of ''high quality'' and ''animal origin'' is not necessarily correct for any stage of life other than, perhaps, early infancy. For example, it has been shown that the relative requirements for different amino acids of preschool children are not the same as the relative quantities of amino acids in mixed egg or milk proteins, and that it is possible to prepare mixtures of proteins of plant origin that, for school-aged children, have a higher biological value than mixed egg and milk diets (16).

3 ESSENTIAL, NONESSENTIAL, AND CONDITIONALLY ESSENTIAL AMINO ACIDS

For at least 60 years, it has been the convention to divide amino acids into two categories: indispensable (or essential) and dispensable (or nonessential). This categorization (Table 1) provides a convenient and generally useful way of viewing amino acid nutrition. The original definition (17) of an indispensable (essential) amino acid was strictly nutritional, as follows: "...one which cannot be synthesized by the animal organism out of materials *ordinarily available* to the cells *at a speed* commensurate with the demands for *normal growth*," the italics being part of the original publication. In other words, an indispensable amino acid must be part of the diet, while an dispensable amino acid need not necessarily be present in food.

However, the nutritional terms *indispensable* and *dispensable* become blurred when we consider amino acid metabolism. By definition, an indispensable amino acid cannot be synthesized by the organism in question. In the strictest sense, lysine and perhaps threonine are the only metabolically indispensable amino acids because they are not transaminated to any nutritionally significant extent. This is a crucial point, because lysine and threonine are the first and second limiting amino acids in many dietary proteins, including human milk (18).

It can be argued in reverse that glutamic acid and possibly serine are the only truly dispensable amino acids, because they can be synthesized by mammals via the reductive amination of the appropriate keto acid (α-ketoglutarate and

TABLE 1   Essential, Nonessential, and Conditionally Essential Amino Acids for Humans

Essential	Nonessential	Conditionally essential
Lysine	Glutamate	Arginine
Threonine	Aspartate	Cysteine
Tryptophan	Glutamine	Proline
Leucine	Asparagine	Tyrosine
Isoleucine	Alanine	Glycine (?)
Valine	Serine	
Phenylalanine	Glycine	
Methionine		
Histidine		

hydroxypyruvate, respectively). Other dispensable amino acids (Fig. 1) derive from transamination reactions and require either glutamate or serine as nitrogen and/or carbon donors. Stable isotopic studies of the scale of amino acid synthesis (Table 2) suggest that the contribution of endogenous synthesis to glutamate and serine turnover is greater than the contribution of endogenous synthesis to the metabolism of other "dispensable" amino acids.

There is, however, a third group of amino acids for which the term *conditionally essential* has been coined (19). This group of amino acids is characterized by three features:

1. *Their synthesis uses other amino acids as carbon precursors.* This is an important metabolic distinction from the dispensable amino acids. For some conditionally essential amino acids (e.g., tyrosine), the precursor is an indispensable amino acid (phenylalanine); for others (e.g., arginine and proline), the precursor is a dispensable amino acid (glutamate); while for still others (e.g., cysteine), both essential (methionine as sulfur donor) and nonessential (serine as carbon donor) amino acids are required. It follows that, at the metabolic level, the ability of the organism to synthesize a given conditionally essential amino acid can be constrained by the availability of a suitable amino acid precursor.

2. *Their synthesis may be confined to specific organs.* The best-established example of this phenomenon is the role of the intestine in the synthesis of both proline and arginine (20,21). Moreover, in the case of these two amino acids, the available evidence suggests that dietary, as opposed to systemic, amino

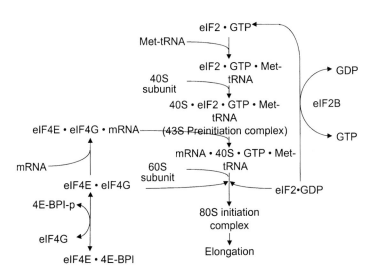

FIGURE 1 Factors involved in translational regulation.

TABLE 2 Contribution of Synthesis De Novo
to Amino Acid Flux in Humans

Amino acid	Percent of flux from synthesis	
	Fed state	Fasted state
Glutamate[a]	98	98
Serine[a]	94	95
Aspartate[a]	76	78
Alanine[a]	45	46
Glycine[a]	35	35
Arginine[b]	14	10
Proline[b]	0	7

[a] Berthold HK, Klein PD, Reeds PJ, unpublished.
[b] From Ref. 25.

acid precursors are critical (22–25). Thus, alterations either in the scale of intestinal metabolism or in the route of nutrition can have a critical bearing on the ability of the organism to synthesize these amino acids. This is shown strikingly by the problems of arginine and ammonia homeostasis that accompany total parenteral nutrition (26).

3. *The maximum rate at which their synthesis can proceed may be limited.* The most extreme example of this is the very low birth weight infant who may have a compromised ability to synthesize cysteine and proline (27,28). Furthermore, because mixed milk proteins have a very low glycine content (18), prematurely delivered infants exclusively fed on unsupplemented human milk may lack the ability to synthesize *adequate* quantities of glycine to support intrauterine rates of protein accretion (29). In addition, studies in adults suggest strongly that the synthesis of proline (30), arginine (31), and cysteine (32) may not only be limited but may fail to be activated to any great extent due to a complete lack of the respective amino acids in the diet (Table 3). This implies that disorders affecting the metabolism of conditionally essential amino acids may impose such

TABLE 3 Relationship Between Conditionally Essential
Amino Acid Intake and Synthesis (mg/kg/day) in Adults

Amino acid	Diet		
	Devoid	Adequate	Surfeit
Cysteine (32)	0.57	0.30	0.34
Arginine (22,31)	2.81	2.78	0.87
Proline (30)	1.95	2.03	0.70

biosynthetic demands that they outstrip the patient's ability to carry out their synthesis. Such appears to be the case for proline nutrition in severely burnt patients (33), and it may well apply to cysteine needs in chronic infection, as by HIV (34).

4   FUNCTIONAL AND METABOLIC BASIS FOR AMINO ACID NEEDS

4.1   Minimal Needs for Growth

At the simplest level, the optimum pattern of amino acids required for protein deposition is the product of the amino acid composition of the proteins deposited and the rate at which they are deposited. That being so, the composition of body protein should provide a firm basis for defining the quantities of individual indispensable amino obligatorily needed for protein deposition (10). The relative "requirements" of different essential amino acids, as measured with nitrogen balance trials, show a commonality among nonprimate species, and these relative needs are similar to the composition of body protein (Table 4). While there is no reason to suppose that the human infant will greatly differ from this general mammalian pattern, all current amino acid RDAs for infants (4,10) use the amino acid pattern of human milk as the standard (Table 5). However, it is important to note that the "safe level" of amino acid intake (as defined by the amino acid composition of milk) may not directly reflect the amino acid needs of the infant, and in fact the mixed proteins of human milk have a biological value of only 0.75. The dissimilarity between the amino acid needs for protein deposition and the amino acid composition of mixed milk protein is not unique to the human (18).

4.2   Minimal Needs for Maintenance of Body Nitrogen Equilibrium

The other major "process" that demands the continual provision of amino acids in the diet is the maintenance of the existing body protein mass. In this context, it is critical to emphasize that because human beings have a remarkably slow rate of postnatal protein deposition, the maintenance amino acid needs of the infant even at 1 month of age account for about 50% of the total need (10). Basal nitrogen loss is a function of body weight and, when normalized to body weight ($kg^{0.75}$), varies little across development. This implies that basal amino acid requirements are a function of overall metabolic activity. However, while there is a consensus regarding the maintenance *protein* requirement, the optimal pattern of amino acids within this protein requirement is currently very controversial.

The pioneering nitrogen balance work of Rose (1) in men and of Leverton (2) in women suggested that the pattern of indispensable amino acids that optimizes protein utilization at body protein equilibrium is substantially different

TABLE 4 Essential Amino Acid Composition (mg/g) of Whole-Body Protein in Newborn Mammals

	Lysine	Phenylalanine	Methionine	Histidine	Valine	Isoleucine	Leucine	Threonine
Rat	77	43	20	30	52	39	85	43
Human	72	41	20	26	47	35	75	41
Pig	75	42	20	28	52	38	72	37
Sheep	75	42	17	23	53	33	79	47
Calf	69	39	18	27	42	30	74	43

Source: Abstracted from Ref. 18.

TABLE 5 "Safe" Levels of Protein and Indispensable Amino Acid Intake for Infants and Children

Age range (years)	Protein intake (g/kg/day)	Amino acid intake (mg/kg/day)								
		Lysine	Phenylalanine + tyrosine	Methionine + cysteine	Histidine	Valine	Isoleucine	Leucine	Threonine	Tryptophan
0–0.1	2.69	191	223	97	62	137	142	280	118	46
0.1–0.25	1.91	136	159	69	44	97	101	199	84	33
0.3–0.5	1.32	94	110	47	31	67	70	137	58	22
0.5–1	1.12	72	82	34	24	46	46	95	44	26
1–2	1.05	61	66	26	21	36	29	69	36	23
2–4	0.91	52	57	23	18	32	26	61	31	23
5–10	0.86	51	55	22	17	31	24	58	2	10

Source: Data from Refs. 4, 9, and 10.

from the mixture that optimizes protein deposition (compare Tables 5 and 6) and quite similar to estimates in other mammals. The specific features of the maintenance amino acid pattern, as defined from measurements of nitrogen balance, are (1) a much lower total essential amino acid contribution (about 20% of the total compared with 40%, or more, for growth), (2) particularly low needs from lysine and the branched-chain amino acids, and (3) relatively high needs for the sulfur amino acids and threonine.

These features were widely accepted as the standard for more than two decades, but in the early 1980s Young and coworkers (summarized in Ref. 35) initiated a stable isotope approach in which they measured the carbon catabolism of specific indispensable amino acids and used this as the basis of the determination of the dietary requirement of adult males. They also measured the intake of a given essential amino acid at which body protein synthesis (measured from the kinetics of the labeled amino acid in plasma) was maximized. This approach represented an important conceptual advance because it was based on a *functional index* of amino acid adequacy—i.e., body protein turnover. More recently (36), the group has extended this work to measure the 24-hr carbon balance of indispensable amino acids. Table 6 compares the recommendations of FAO (4) with the pattern defined from Young's studies (the so-called MIT pattern) (9) and it is quite clear are substantial. If correct, the new values have very important implications for food policy, especially the assessment of the adequacy of amino acid (especially lysine) intakes in populations consuming cereals as their staple. Unfortunately it is still not obvious why the two values differ so greatly and to

TABLE 6   Comparison of Recommendations of the Food Agricultural Organization (1985), FAO (1991, tentative), and Young/El Khoury for Indispensable Amino Acid Intakes for Adults[a]

	FAO/WHO/UNU 1985 (4)	FAO/WHO (9)	Young and El Khoury (35)
Lysine	12	52	39
Phenylalanine + tyrosine	14	57	39
Methionine + cysteine	13	23	15
Histidine	12	16	ND
Valine	10	32	20
Isoleucine	10	26	23
Leucine	14	61	39
Threonine	7	31	15
Tryptophan	4	10	6

[a] mg/kg/day.

this point discussion has centered to a great extent on technical matters (37,38). It should, however, be emphasized that results obtained with a different isotopic approach involving different assumptions largely support Young's findings (39).

4.3 Functional View of Maintenance Amino Acid Needs

The continuing need for the provision of protein in the diet ultimately reflects the continuing catabolism of indispensable amino acids, and, of course, it is this idea that underlies the reasoning behind Young's carbon balance approach to the determination of indispensable amino acid requirements. It is noteworthy that isotopic studies have revealed that there are mechanisms allowing the virtually complete suppression of the catabolism of some indispensable amino acids when they are strongly limiting (40), but values obtained under conditions of single–amino acid limitation are much less than those obtained in individuals who are close to nitrogen equilibrium or who are receiving no dietary protein. One argument to explain this metabolic difference is that the higher rate of oxidation of essential amino acids when protein is limiting reflects the consumption of specific amino acids by metabolic pathways that are not directly linked to protein metabolism. This creates what is, in effect, an internal amino acid imbalance, which then restricts the recycling of all other amino acids back into body protein.

An important current area of amino acid research is the definition and quantification of these pathways. In this context, the maintenance of both host defenses and of neural and muscular function seems likely to be of crucial importance, and a case can be made both for the importance of amino acids in general and specifically for the importance of nonessential or conditionally essential amino acids in the synthesis of compounds that are important for all three aspects of physiology (Table 7).

Two factors would seem to be important to the preservation of the ability of the individual to withstand bacterial and viral invasion: the maintenance of a barrier to prevent the invasion of pathogenic organisms and the maintenance of all the elements of immune protection. An important part of the barrier function at the two most vulnerable surfaces, the lungs and the small intestine, is the continual secretion of mucous glycoproteins. Approximately 90% of the mass of these proteins is carbohydrate, and the complex carbohydrate side chains are attached to an extensively cysteine sulfur cross-linked core protein particle via O-glycosidic linkages to threonine. Threonine contributes 22% of the mass of the core protein. Critically, it appears that the secretion of these proteins continues independently of current protein intake and places a persistent drain on the individual's threonine supplies. Recent measurements of amino acid losses in ileostomy effluents (41) imply that 65% of the maintenance threonine needs of the adult can be ascribed to threonine loss from the small intestine. It is also well established that protein-depleted individuals have impaired immune competence,

TABLE 7 Functional Pathways of Amino Acid Utilization

System	Function	Product	Precursor
Intestine	Energy generation	ATP	Glu, Asp, Glutamine
	Proliferation	Nucleic acids	Glutamine, Gly, Asp
	Protection	Glutathione	Cys, Glu, Gly
		Nitric oxide	Arg
		Mucins	Thr, Cys, Ser, Pro
Skeletal muscle	Energy generation	Creatine	Gly, Arg, Met
	Peroxidative protection	Taurine (?)	Cys
Nervous system	Transmitter synthesis	Adrenergic	Phe
		Serotinergic	Tryp
		Glutaminergic	Glu
		Glycinergic	Gly
		Nitric oxide	Arg
	Peroxidative protection	Taurine (?)	Cys
Immune system	Lymphocyte proliferation	(?)	Glutamine, Arg, Asparagine
	Peroxidative protection	Glutathione	Cys, Glu, Gly
	Macrophage activation	Nitric oxide	Arg
Cardiovascular	Blood pressure regulation	Nitric oxide	Arg
	Peroxidative protection (?)	Red cell glutathione	Cys, Glu, Gly

and part of this impairment can be ascribed to a limited availability of amino acids to support the synthesis of the cellular proteins of the immune system and to support the hepatic acute-phase protein response. The acute-phase response is suboptimal in protein-malnourished laboratory animals (42) and infants (43).

However, amino acids are also involved in other aspects of the defense mechanism. Glutathione, a key free radical scavenger, is synthesized from glutamate (glutamine), glycine, and cysteine. Hepatic and intestinal mucosal glutathione, sites at which glutathione synthesis is particularly high (44), is depleted in protein-restricted animals. It is of particular note that the glutathione concentration is low in the erythrocytes of infants suffering from kwashiorkor (45), of low-birth-weight infants (46) and of patients infected with HIV (34,47). In each case, low levels of glutathione may well be due to a limited supply of cysteine, reflecting either a grossly inadequate intake or an inability of the patient to synthesize cysteine at a rate that can sustain adequate levels of glutathione (34).

Glutamine, an amino acid that is strongly concentrated in the skeletal musculature, also appears to play a specific role in maintaining the function of rapidly proliferating cells, including lymphocytes (48) and the cells of the intestinal mucosa (49). Glutamine may also regulate muscle protein (50), and it is noteworthy that under conditions of infection and trauma, muscle concentrations of glutamine fall. Recent work also suggests that glutamine utilization by the tissues of the splanchnic bed under traumatic conditions plays a specific role in maintaining glutathione synthesis (see Chap. 3).

Other amino acid metabolites may also play important physiological roles in both the immune and neural systems. Taurine, a β-amino sulfonic acid derived from cysteine metabolism, appears to be an effective scavenger of peroxidative products (particularly those containing the oxychloride groups) and acts as a neuromodulatory agent. It is of interest that taurine is specifically concentrated in the skeletal musculature and the central nervous system and has been advanced as an important component of infant feedings (51).

Creatine, a compound that is crucial for energy flow within the skeletal musculature and central nervous system, is synthesized from glycine and arginine and a suitable source of methyl groups. It is also concentrated in skeletal muscle and brain; infection and trauma lead not only to a loss of muscle protein and glutamine but also to a specific loss of creatine and taurine. These conditions are also accompanied by derangements of muscle contractile function. Finally, glutamine, creatine, and taurine are maintained at substantial concentrations in the free amino acid fraction of milk (52), an observation that implies an important role for all three compounds in the support of postnatal development.

A particularly important development, and one that was the subject of the 1998 Nobel Prize for Medicine, has been the identification of nitric oxide, a product of arginine metabolism, as a key regulator of a wide variety of physiological processes (53). These include the regulation of blood vessel tone and hence blood pressure and flow, the development of higher cognitive functions, and the neural regulation of intestinal motility and pancreatic secretion. Arginine appears to play an important role in the immune system, particularly in relation to inflammation and reperfusion injury (54). While the exact mechanism underlying these observations is not known with any certainty, nitric oxide production from arginine appears to be involved in macrophage killer function and in regulating the interactions between macrophages and lymphocyte adhesion and activation. These are crucial new findings, the nutritional significance of which is still a subject of intense investigation. Unfortunately, with the exception of some recent studies (e.g., Ref. 55), neither the quantitative impact of nitric oxide synthesis on the body's need for arginine nor the impact of arginine status on nitric oxide–mediated responses has been studied extensively. Nonetheless, work in animals indicates that arginine deficiency inhibits the expression of nitric oxide synthase (56).

Dispensable or conditionally essential amino acids appear to be of particular nutritional importance in individuals who are close to nitrogen equilibrium; this may reflect their role in these key ''nonprotein'' pathways of disposal. Despite research extending over a number of years, the details of nonessential and conditionally essential amino acid synthesis and metabolism remain an important issue in understanding amino acid requirements in general.

4.4 The Role of the Gut in Amino Acid Nutrition

4.4.1 Digestibility and Intestinal Amino Acid Utilization

Traditionally, the assessment of the availability of dietary proteins and amino acids under practical conditions has been based on ''apparent digestibility''— i.e., the difference between nitrogen intake and fecal nitrogen output. However, for two reasons (discussed in detail in Ref. 14), this method is unsatisfactory for the calculation of the availability of individual amino acids: (1) Fecal nitrogen consists largely of bacterial protein. Thus, because the composition of bacterial protein differs markedly from that of common dietary proteins, it gives very little information on the digestibility of different amino acids. (2) The bacterial nitrogen derived from undigested protein as well as proteins secreted into the intestinal lumen and urea nitrogen that has diffused from the blood; these are now known to be important contributors to colonic nitrogen flow.

Recently, Tomé's group (e.g., Refs. 57 and 58) has given ^{15}N-labeled dietary proteins to adults and, by measuring the flow of ^{15}N from the terminal ileum, has calculated the ''true'' digestibility of the dietary source. There have also been a number of studies in pigs in which ^{15}N-amino acids have been infused intravenously for prolonged periods of time. This labels the host proteins, so that the ^{15}N-labeling of ileal proteins allows the calculation of the endogenous contribution to the luminal protein pool. A similar approach (60) in infants has used prolonged feedings of ^{15}N-glycine for the same purpose. By and large, the results of all these studies lead to the same conclusion, i.e., that most dietary protein exceeds 90% and that the majority of the fecal nitrogen is ultimately derived from the host rather than the diet. Thus, differences in apparent digestibility reflect differences in the endogenous contribution to the luminal nitrogen pool.

Despite the good evidence that favors virtually complete protein digestion in the small bowel, it is quite clear that a considerable amount of amino acid metabolism occurs in the tissues of the splanchnic bed in general and in the intestinal mucosa in particular (14,61–64). Indeed, calculations based on these papers suggest that intestinal amino acid utilization (both from the diet and from the mesenteric arterial circulation) can account for as much as 50% of whole-body amino acid turnover. That being so, it is important to note that the degree to which individual amino acids are utilized by the gut varies markedly among the amino acids (Table 8). Among the essential amino acids, the utilization of threonine is particularly high and virtually all the dietary glutamate and aspartate is utilized within the mucosa. The scale of splanchnic leucine metabolism appears to be at least twofold higher in infants than in adults (65,66).

In considering the nutritional and functional significance of this first-pass "metabolism," it is important to separate protein synthesis and amino acid catabolism (see below); in considering the influence of intestinal metabolism, this distinction is particularly important. It is well known that the rate of protein synthesis in the intestinal mucosa is very high (67), and it seems likely that a considerable proportion of this protein synthesis is destined for export into the intestinal lumen. A critical nutritional issue, and one that has received little attention, concerns the factors that influence the subsequent digestion and reabsorption of these secre-

TABLE 8 Splanchnic and Intestinal First-Pass Utilization of Dietary Amino Acids— Percent of Intake

Amino acid	Splanchnic metabolism (humans)	Intestinal metabolism (pigs)
Leucine	26 ± 7	33
Lysine	32	37
Phenylalanine	39	42
Tyrosine	40	ND
Threonine	ND	57
Glutamine	53	67
Glutamate	88	96

Source: Abstracted from Ref. 61.

tions. Understanding these factors may prove crucial, because amino acids lost in secretions that are not recycled in the small bowel constitute part of the amino acid needs of the individual, and a failure to recycle these secretions could be a crucial part of the increased protein needs of individuals with intestinal disease. In addition, other evidence indicates that a luminal supply of amino acids is necessary for normal mucosal cell function and turnover and the deleterious effects of total parenteral nutrition on mucosal mass and function are well established, at least in animal studies (see Chap. 17).

There is, in addition, evidence extending back into the 1970s (68) to suggest that amino acids also play a critical role in intestinal energy generation. Recent studies in fed pigs (69), using a combination of portal measurements and enteral and intravenous infusions of ^{13}C-amino acids and glucose, show that at least 50% of intestinal CO_2 production arises from the metabolism of glutamate, glutamine, and aspartate and that dietary glucose plays a minor role. Intriguingly, there is also evidence that the intestinal tissues catabolize leucine and, under conditions of high protein feeding, lysine. Finally, in addition to this evidence, it is now established that dietary glutamate plays a critical role in the synthesis of mucosal glutathione (and hence bears on gut-protective mechanisms) and arginine synthesis (with importance to systemic immune function).

4.4.2 Bacterial Metabolism and Amino Acid Supply

It has been known for 50 years that urea nitrogen circulating in the blood can enter the intestinal tract, where it is hydrolyzed by the resident flora and becomes fixed in bacterial protein. The appearance of urea nitrogen in fecal protein has been repeatedly demonstrated, but recent work has developed the provocative argument not only that this host/bacterial urea nitrogen recycling is regulated but also that fixation of urea nitrogen into indispensable amino acids can occur— i.e., true nutritional benefit accrues from this process (70). This idea is, of course, controversial, but recent evidence in humans (71) has provided some direct support by demonstrating that systemic lysine becomes labeled with ^{15}N-when ^{15}N-urea or ^{15}N-ammonium salts are administered into the gut. If confirmed, the observation of the apparent availability, to the host, of an indispensable amino acid synthesized by the intestinal microflora will, of course, have an important bearing on the differences in the estimates of dietary amino acid requirements derived from the nitrogen and carbon balance methods.

5 PROTEIN TURNOVER AND PROTEIN DEPOSITION

5.1 Whole-Body Protein Turnover

Quantitatively, by far the greatest influence on amino acid turnover and metabolism is the ''protein turnover cycle,'' in which proteins are continuously degraded and resynthesized (6). The coregulation of the synthetic and degradative arms of the cycle is crucial to the maintenance of cellular viability, to the regulation of growth and cellular protein mass, and to the control of enzyme levels. It seems likely that at least 20% of basal energy expenditure is used in maintaining whole-body protein synthesis. Because of the critical physiological importance of the processes of protein synthesis and degradation, considerable efforts have been expended in devising methods for their measurement, especially in vivo.

The most frequently applied method for the measurement of whole-body protein turnover relies on the measurement of the dilution of a tracer amino acid in the plasma (or whole blood) free amino acid pool. The tracer can be given as a single injection followed by analysis of the time course of changes in isotopic enrichment (72) or as a constant tracer infusion, with analysis of the isotopic enrichment at isotopic steady state (6). The constant infusion approach is particularly easy to apply and requires only a few blood samples. However, although the method gives no information on different components of the whole, the overall approach has the signal advantage of practicality. This enables its application in a wide variety of subjects studied under many physiological, pathological, and nutritional conditions. Thus recent papers using this approach report results obtained in the critically ill (73), the severely malnourished (74,75) and the extremely young (76).

5.2 Measuring Tissue Protein Synthesis

It is obvious that measurements of whole-body protein turnover represent the summation of the protein metabolic activities of all the components of the body. For many applications—particularly those focusing on the effects of nutrition, stress, and endocrine factors on protein turnover—it is essential to gain more direct information on the relative rates of protein synthesis and degradation in specific organs and tissues.

The measurement of the incorporation of tracer amino acids into tissue protein provides the most direct approach to this problem and has been used extensively to measure plasma (77–79), muscle (80,81), intestinal (67,82), and hepatic (77) protein synthesis in humans.

Over the last 10 years, another method has been developed that is based on the intravenous infusion of a stable, isotopically labeled amino acid followed by repeated measurements of tracer balance (which is proportional to protein synthesis) and tracee balance (which measures the difference between protein synthesis and degradation) across a tissue as defined by its venous outflow. This tracer balance method has some important advantages. First, it is dynamic, so that changes in amino acid uptake and protein turnover can be measured over quite short time intervals. This is a highly significant advantage in the design of studies focusing on acute nutritional or hormonal effects (83,84). Second, provided that the conclusions based on the isotopic data are confined to the tracer alone (for example, by examining changes in the fractional tracer balance), the estimates of changes in protein synthesis can be relatively assumption-free. Third, in principle at least, both protein synthesis and protein degradation within the tissues under investigation can be calculated from the difference between uni-directional tracer uptake and net tracee balance.

A particularly important recent advance in the measurement of tissue pro-tein synthesis has been the combination of this transorgan balance approach with direct measurements of amino acid labeling within the tissue itself. This has been applied to the study of intestinal mucosal and hepatic amino acid utilization in animals (62,85) and to the study of human leg muscle protein metabolism (84).

5.3 Factors Regulating Overall Protein Synthesis and Degradation

The protein mass and the rates of protein gain or loss in a cell are entirely depen-dent on the balance (i.e., the relative rates) of protein synthesis and degradation. However, it is important to recognize that the two processes are mechanistically distinct. Although both processes are influenced (Table 9) by protein and energy status and by the same hormones (insulin, growth factors, growth hormone, and glucocorticoids), the direction and magnitude of a response of either process are not easily predicted. Furthermore, nutritional status, especially amino acid intake, and the response of protein turnover to endocrinological changes interact in a complex way. As a result of these complexities, it has proved difficult to identify a common response, even when the same outcome variable (e.g., increased protein deposition) is achieved. For example, stimulation of proliferative growth involves a simultaneous increase in protein synthesis and a decrease in protein degradation, while hypertrophic growth (e.g., of a muscle in response to increased workload) involves simultaneous increases in both protein synthesis and degradation. Simi-larly, increases in whole-body protein retention brought about by an increased intake of energy, the limiting amino acid or by insulin infusion appear to involve primary changes in whole-body protein degradation. Furthermore, the magnitude of changes in whole-body protein turnover, even in response to a common nutri-tional manipulation, can depend on the prior nutritional status of the indivi-dual.

The rate of protein turnover also varies systematically between tissues, and the relative importance of protein synthesis and degradation to the control of cellular protein mass may be tissue-specific. Failure to recognize tissue-specific effects can readily lead to confusion in interpreting studies of whole-body protein turnover because the failure to find a change in the body as a whole can merely reflect equal but opposite changes at different sites. Such may be the case with respect to the changes in protein turnover accompanying lactation in the human

TABLE 9 Humoral and Nutritional Factors Affecting Protein Turnover in the Human

Factor	Whole-body effects		Tissue effects	
	Synthesis	Degradation	Synthesis	Degradation
Protein	+	+/−	++ (all tissues)	?
Energy	+/−	−	+ (muscle)	?
Insulin	+/−	−	+ (muscle)	− (all tissues)
Insulin-like growth factor I	+/−	−	+ (muscle)	− (intestine)
Growth hormone	variable	−	+	?
Thyroid hormone	+	+	+	+/−
Glucocorticoids	+/−	+	− (muscle)	+ (all tissues)

(86), a circumstance in which it seems that increases in protein turnover in the visceral compartment are balanced by a lower rate of peripheral protein turnover.

There are also major developmental influences on the regulation of protein turnover as it relates to protein deposition. First, as shown in Table 10, protein turnover in general is high in the neonate and falls progressively as the individual approaches maturity. Moreover, changes in protein synthesis appear to be of particular importance to the nutritional regulation of the growth of immature tissues (88), especially skeletal muscle, and the response of protein synthesis to food intake becomes progressively smaller as adulthood is approached. In adults, protein degradation seems to be the critical factor that regulates protein balance in the short term.

5.4 Mechanistic Aspects of Regulation

5.4.1 Protein Synthesis

The regulation of protein synthesis (i.e., mRNA translation) is almost necessarily complex. First, it is important to note that because the enzymes responsible for the synthesis of the amino acyl-tRNA's have very low Km's, under all but the most extreme circumstances of amino acid depletion, amino acid tRNA synthetases are fully saturated with their substrate amino acid. Thus, although severe amino acid deprivation will inhibit protein synthesis via substrate limitation, it is unlikely that amino acid concentrations regulate protein synthesis via a kinetic mechanism. This stands in marked contrast to the regulation of amino acid catabolism. Thus, the translation of mRNA is regulated by "enzyme activity"—i.e., the concentration and translational activity of the ribosomes. Both these aspects are under developmental, nutritional, and hormonal control, and considerable advances in our understanding of the biochemical steps and regulation of translation have been taken in the past decade (89,90). Protein synthesis is regulated in both the short and long term. Long-term regulation, such as that associated with postnatal development and tissue differences in protein synthesis, is largely a function of the concentration of ribosomes—i.e., the capacity for protein synthesis. It is clear that cellular ribosome concentrations are affected by nutrient status, increased functional demand, and a number of hormones including insulin, thyroid hormone, growth hormone, and the glucocorticoid hormones. In this context, it is important to recognize that the ribosome is an extremely complex organelle and contains at least 85 proteins in addition to the rRNA species. Thus, the control of ribosome biosynthesis involves the coregulation of the synthesis of both the RNA and protein moieties. Although there have been considerable advances in understanding rRNA synthesis and processing (91), less is known about the factors that regulate r-protein synthesis (92).

As regards the short-term regulation of translation, most evidence suggests that primary regulation by insulin, glucocorticoids, and amino acids is exerted

TABLE 10 Developmental Changes in Whole-body Protein Turnover (g/kg/day)

	Rat		Pig		Sheep		Human	
Stage		PT[a]	Stage	PT	Stage	PT	Stage	PT
20-day fetus		45 ± 4	2.5 kg	31 ± 1	4.5 kg	32 ± 1	Preterm	11 ± 2
21-day-old		34 ± 1	7.5 kg	24 ± 7	25 kg	8 ± 1	Term	8 ± 1
56-day-old		20 ± 1	30 kg	18 ± 4	45 kg	5 ± 1	18-month-old	6 ± 1
Adult		13 ± 1	90 kg	7 ± 2	60 kg	4 ± 1	Adult	4 ± 1

[a] Protein turnover.
Source: Adapted from Ref. 87.

at the initiation stage (89), although other factors, such as the cellular ATP supply, may act at other steps in addition to the formation of the initiation complex. Activation of initiation, and hence translation as a whole, can occur very rapidly, and it can be argued that the rapidity of this response has a very important effect on the efficiency with which dietary amino acids are stored in protein as opposed to being irrevocably catabolized. Although there is some lack of certainty as to the initiation factors responsible for the short-term regulation of translation in vivo, a picture is emerging suggesting that the EIF-4 family is critical in both insulin and amino acid regulation of translation (Fig. 1).

5.4.2 Proteolysis

Degradation of cellular protein is also an ongoing process; among other functions, the process serves to remove "error" proteins (93) and provides cells with a supply of free amino acids during periods of nutrient deprivation. In understanding protein degradation and its regulation, two major factors have to be taken into account: (1) There is a wide range (at least three orders of magnitude) in the half lives of different proteins even within a given cell, and these protein substrate differences are maintained when there are changes in overall proteolysis. (2) Proteins do not exist in free solution within cells but may be organized either in distinct organelles or in other structures, such as myofilaments and multi-enzyme complexes, which, when formed, appear to protect the complex as a whole from degradation.

Over the last 15 years, there have been considerable advances in our understanding of protein degradation at the mechanistic level. It is now clear not only that there are multiple proteolytic systems but also that these systems have specific protein substrate specificities and may well play different roles within the cell.

1. *The lysosomal/autophagic system* (94). This system involves primarily the cathepsins and is of importance to the degradation of proteins that have entered cells via endocytosis. The system involves the formation of distinct vacuolar structures, which are capable of engulfing and degrading complete organelles. Although most evidence suggests that this pathway of degradation is unselective, there is some evidence for the involvement of specific peptide sequences in targeting proteins to the lysosomal compartment. The system may also be involved in hepatic RNA turnover. It appears to be of specific importance under conditions in which cellular proteolysis is maximally activated—e.g., under conditions of extreme nutrient and anabolic hormonal or growth factor deprivation—and considerable attention has been paid to the role of macroautophagy in the amino acid and insulin regulation of hepatic proteolysis. As a result of this work, leucine and alanine have been identified as key regulatory amino acids that interact with one another and with insulin in the regulation of the pathway. Research is now making significant inroads into identifying cell-surface amino acid receptors that interact with this pathway of proteolysis (95).

2. *The calpain/calpastatin system* (96). This is the major calcium-activated pathway of protein degradation and consists of a complex of a papain-like cysteine protease and a lower-molecular-weight calmodulin-like calcium binding regulatory subunit. At least two main calpain isoforms, the μ-(μmolar) and m-(mmolar) forms, have been identified on the basis of the calcium concentrations at which they are activated. The system is also subject to inhibition by the protein calpastatin. Paradoxically, there appears to be a persistent excess of calpastatic over calpain activity; in some cases coactivation of the expression of the genes for both components has been demonstrated. A characteristic of calpain-catalyzed proteolysis is that it is incomplete, and it is generally held that these proteases play an important role in the proteolytic processing of proteins associated with the membrane and microfilamentous structures of the cell. It seems likely that the calpains play a key role in muscle myofibrillar protein turnover by catalyzing the initial disruption of the structure via proteolysis at the Z disk.

3. *The ubiquitin/proteasome system* (97). Since its identification in the 1980s, this system of proteolysis has received substantial attention; therefore the proteolytic mechanisms and their regulation are, perhaps, better understood than those involved in the other pathways of proteolysis. There are four key features of this pathway. First, it is widely distributed among tissues; second, it has a relatively broad protein specificity; third, it catalyzes the complete hydrolysis of the protein substrates; and finally, it is energy (ATP)-dependent.

The pathway consists of two components: a recognition system, involving the protein ubiquitin, together with multiple polypeptides that are responsible for recognizing and targeting the protein substrates toward degradation, and a high-molecular-weight multifunctional protease now generally termed the *proteasome*. A strong case has been made for the involvement of the proteasomal system in the initial proteolytic steps of antigen processing (98) and in the rapid turnover of oncogenic products (99) and ''abnormal'' (93) proteins.

Even less is known about the regulation of proteolysis than about that of protein synthesis. Nevertheless, it is becoming increasingly clear that long-term changes in proteolysis that are associated with frank catabolic states generally involve an overall increase in the levels of all components of the respective proteolytic systems (100), and there is an increasing literature on the level of expression of the mRNAs for key protein components under a number of different circumstances (101,102).

6 CONCLUSION

Although there has been steady progress in understanding the biological basis of amino acid requirements and very substantial advances in our understanding of the regulation of cellular and tissue protein mass, a number of important aspects of protein nutrition remain. The regulation of tissue amino acid intermediary metabolism still remains a subject about which new information continues to emerge, and recent in vivo data suggest that some long-held hypotheses may require modification. In addition, important questions regarding the role of conditionally essential amino acids, particularly under conditions of disease and trauma, remain unanswered. Finally, new roles for amino acids in the maintenance of physiological function and cellular regulation continue to be identified—observations that reflect the continuing dynamism of this long-standing aspect of nutrition.

REFERENCES

1. Rose WC. The amino acid requirements of adult man. Nutr Abstr Rev 27: Wallingford, UK: Commonwealth Agricultural Bureau, 1957, pp 631–647.
2. Leverton RM. Amino acid requirements of young adults. In: Protein and Amino Acid Nutrition. New York: Academic Press, 1959, pp 477–506.
3. Snyderman SE, Boyer A, Norton PM, Roitman E, Holt LE. The amino acid requirements of infants. Am J Clin Nutr 1964; 15:313–330.
4. Food and Agriculture Organization, World Health Organization, and United Nations University Energy and Protein Requirements. World Health Organization Technical Report Series 724. Geneva, Switzerland: WHO, 1985.
5. Schoenheimer R, Rattner S, Rittenberg D. Studies in protein metabolism: X. The metabolic activity of body proteins investigated with $L(-)$ leucine containing two isotopes. J Biol Chem 1939; 130:709–721.
6. Waterlow JC. Protein turnover with special reference to man. Q J Exp Physiol 1984; 69:409–438.
7. Bier DM. Stable isotopes in biosciences: Their measurement and models for amino acid metabolism. Eur J Pediatr 1997; 156(suppl 1):S2–S8.
8. Young VR, Ajami A. The Rudolf Schoenheimer Centenary Lecture: Isotopes in nutrition research. Proc Nutr Soc 1999; 58:15–32.
9. Food and Agriculture Organization, World Health Organization. Protein Quality Evaluation. Food and Nutrition paper 51. Rome: Food and Agriculture Organization, 1991.
10. Dewey KG, Beaton G, Fjeld C, Lonnerdal B, Reeds P. Protein requirements of infants and children. Eur J Clin Nutr 1996; 50:S119–S150.
11. Reeds PJ, Hutchens TW. Protein requirements: From nitrogen balance to functional impact. J Nutr 1994; 124:1754S–1764S.
12. Millward DJ. Metabolic demands for amino acids and the human dietary requirement: Millward and Rivers (1988) revisited. J Nutr 1998; 128(12 suppl):2563S–2576S.
13. Young VR, Borgonha S. Adult human amino acid requirements. Curr Opin Clin Nutr Metab Care 1999; 2:39–45.
14. Fuller MF, Reeds PJ. Endogenous nitrogen in the gut. Annu Rev Nutr 1998; 18: 385–411.
15. Burrin DG, Reeds PJ. Alternative fuels in the gastrointestinal tract. Curr Opin Gastroenterol 1997; 13:165–170.
16. Gattas V, Barrera GA, Riumallo JS, Uauy R. Protein-energy requirements of boys

12–14 y old determined by using the nitrogen-balance response to a mixed protein diet. Am J Clin Nutr 1992; 56:499–503.

17. Borman A, Wood TR, Balck HC, Anderson EG, Oesterling MJ, Womack M, Rose WC. The role of arginine in growth with some observations on the effects of argininic acid. J Biol Chem. 1946; 166:585–594.

18. Davis TA, Nguyen HV, Garcia-Bravo R, Fiorotto, ML, Jackson EM, Lewis DS, Lee DR, Reeds PJ. Amino acid composition of human milk is not unique. J Nutr 1994; 124:1126–1132.

19. Laidlaw SA, Kopple JD. Newer concepts of the indispensable amino acids. Am J Clin Nutr 1987; 46:593–605.

20. Wakabayashi Y, Yamada E, Yoshida T, Takahashi H. Arginine becomes an essential amino acid after massive resection of the rat small intestine J Biol Chem 1994; 269:32667–32671.

21. Wu G, Davis PK, Flynn NE, Knabe DA, Davidson JT. Endogenous synthesis of arginine plays an important role in maintaining arginine homeostasis in postweaning growing pigs. J Nutr 1997; 127:2342–2349.

22. Beaumier L, Castillo L, Ajami AM, Young VR. Urea cycle intermediate kinetics and nitrate excretion at normal and ''therapeutic'' intakes of arginine in humans. Am J Physiol 1995; 269:E884–E896.

23. Brunton JA, Bertolo RF, Pencharz PB, Ball RO. Proline ameliorates arginine deficiency during enteral but not parenteral feeding in neonatal piglets. Am J Physiol 1999; 277:E223–E231.

24. Murphy JM, Murch SJ, Ball RO. Proline is synthesized from glutamate during intragastric infusion but not during intravenous infusion in neonatal piglets. J Nutr 1996; 126:878–886.

25. Berthold HK, Reeds PJ, Klein PD. Isotopic evidence for the differential regulation of arginine and proline synthesis in man. Metabolism 1995; 44:466–473.

26. Heird WC, Nicholson JF, Driscoll JM Jr, Schullinger JN, Winters RW. Hyperammonemia resulting from intravenous alimentation using a mixture of synthetic I-amino acids: A preliminary report. J Pediatr 1972; 81:162–165.

27. Gaull G, Sturman JA, Raiha NC. Development of mammalian sulfur metabolism: Absence of cystathionase in human fetal tissues. Pediatr Res 1972; 6:538–547.

28. Miller RG, Jahoor F, Reeds PJ, Heird WC, Jaksic T. A new stable isotope tracer technique to assess human neonatal amino acid synthesis. J Pediatr Surg 1995; 30: 1325–1329.

29. Jackson AA, Shaw JC, Barber A, Golden MH. Nitrogen metabolism in preterm infants fed human donor breast milk: The possible essentiality of glycine. Pediatr Res 1981; 15:1454–1461.

30. Jaksic T, Wagner DA, Burke JF, Young VR. Plasma proline kinetics and the regulation of proline synthesis in man. Metabolism 1987; 36(11):1040–1046.

31. Castillo L, Ajami A, Branch S, Chapman TE, Yu YM, Burke JF, Young VR. Plasma arginine kinetics in adult man: Response to an arginine-free diet. Metabolism 1994; 43:114–122.

32. Hiramatsu T, Fukagawa NK, Marchini JS, Cortiella J, Yu YM, Chapman TE, Young VR. Methionine and cysteine kinetics at different intakes of cystine in healthy adult men. Am J Clin Nutr 1994; 60:525–533.

33. Jaksic T, Wagner DA, Burke JF, Young VR. Proline metabolism in adult male burned patients and healthy control subjects. Am J Clin Nutr 1991; 54:408–413.

34. Jahoor F, Jackson A, Gazzard B, Philips G, Sharpstone D, Frazer ME, Heird W. Erythrocyte glutathione deficiency in symptom-free HIV infection is associated with decreased synthesis rate. Am J Physiol 1999; 276:E205–E211.

35. Young VR, Bier DM, Pellett PL. A theoretical basis for increasing current estimates of the amino acids requirements in adult man, with experimental support. Am J Clin Nutr 1989; 50:80–92.

36. Young VR, el-Khoury AE. Can amino acid requirements for nutritional maintenance in adult humans be approximated from the amino acid composition of body mixed proteins? Proc Natl Acad Sci USA 1995; 92:300–304.

37. Fuller MF, Garlick PJ. Human amino acid requirements: Can the controversy be resolved? Annu Rev Nutr 1994; 14:217–241.

38. Waterlow JC. The requirements of adult man for indispensable amino acids. Eur J Clin Nutr 1996; 50(suppl 1):S151–S176.

39. Zello GA, Pencharz PB, Ball RO. Dietary lysine requirement of young adult males determined by oxidation of L-[1-13C]phenylalanine. Am J Physiol 1993; 264: E677–E685.

40. Raguso CA, Pereira P, Young VR. A tracer investigation of obligatory oxidative amino acid losses in healthy, young adults. Am J Clin Nutr 1999; 70:474–483.

41. Fuller MF, Milne A, Harris Cl, Reid TM, Keenan R. Amino acid losses in ileostomy fluid on a protein-free diet. Am J Clin Nutr 1994; 59:70–73.

42. Grimble RF, Jackson AA, Persaud C, Wride MJ, Delers F, Engler R. Cysteine and glycine supplementation modulate the metabolic response to tumor necrosis factor-α in rats fed a low protein diet. J Nutr 1992; 122:2066–2073.

43. Doherty JF, Golden MHN, Rayned JG, Griffin GE, McAdam KPWJ. Acute phase protein response is impaired in severely malnourished children. Clin Sci 1993; 84: 169–175.

44. Jahoor F, Wykes LJ, Reeds PJ, Henry JF, del Rosario MP, Frazer ME. Protein-deficient pigs cannot maintain reduced glutathione homeostasis when subjected to the stress of inflammation. J Nutr 1995; 125:1462–1472.

45. Jackson AA. Blood glutathione in severe malnutrition in childhood. Trans R Soc Trop Med Hyg 1986; 80:911–913.

46. Smith CV, Hansen TN, Martin NE, McMicken HW, Elliott Oxidant stress responses in premature infants during exposure to hyperoxia. Pediatr Res 1993; 34: 360–365.

47. Droge W. Cysteine and glutathione in catabolic conditions and immunological dysfunction. Curr Opin Clin Nutr Metab Care 1999; 2(3):227–233.

48. Newsholme EA, Crabtree B, Ardawi MSM. Glutamine metabolism in lymphocytes: Its biochemical, physiological and clinical importance. Q J Exp Physiol 1985; 70: 473–489.

49. Souba WW, Herskowitz K, Salloum RM, Chen MK, Austgen TR. Gut glutamine metabolism. J Parenter Enter Nutr 1990; 14:456–460.

50. McLennan PA, Brown RA, Rennie MJ. A positive relationship between protein synthetic rate and intracellular glutamine concentration in perfused rat skeletal muscle. FEBS Lett 1987; 215:187–191.

51. Chesney RW, Helms RA, Christensen M, Budreau AM, Han X, Sturman JA. An updated view of the value of taurine in infant nutrition. Adv Pediatr 1998; 45:179–200.
52. Rassin DK, Sturman, JA, Gaull GE. Taurine and other free amino acids in the milk of man and other mammals. Early Hum Dev 1978; 2:1–13.
53. Murad F. Discovery of some of the biological effects of nitric oxide and its role in cell signaling. Biosci Rep 1999; 19:133–154.
54. Efron DT, Barbul A. Modulation of inflammation and immunity by arginine supplements. Curr Opin Clin Nutr Metab Care 1998; 1:531–538.
55. Castillo L, DeRojas-Walker T, Yu YM, Sanchez M, Chapman TE, Shannon D, Tannenbaum S, Burke JF, Young VR: Whole body arginine metabolism and nitric oxide synthesis in newborns with persistent pulmonary hypertension. Pediatr Res 1995; 38:17–24.
56. Wu G, Flynn NE, Flynn SP, Jolly CA, Davis PK. Dietary protein or arginine deficiency impairs constitutive and inducible nitric oxide synthesis by young rats. J Nutr 1999; 129:1347–1354.
57. Gausseres N, Mahe S, Benamouzig R, Luengo C, Ferriere F, Rautureau J, Tome D. [^{15}N]-labeled pea flour protein nitrogen exhibits good ileal digestibility and postprandial retention in humans. J Nutr 1997; 127:1160–1165.
58. Gaudichon C, Mahe S, Benamouzig R, Luengo C, Fouillet H, Dare S, Van Oycke M, Ferriere F, Rautureau J, Tome D. Net postprandial utilization of [15N]-labeled milk protein nitrogen is influenced by diet composition in humans. J Nutr 1999; 129:890–895.
59. de Lange CFM, Souffrant WB, Sauer WC. Real ileal and amino acid digestibilities in feedstuffs for growing pigs as determined with the ^{15}N-isotope dilution technique. J Anim Sci 1990; 68:409–418.
60. Shulman RJ, Gannon N, Reeds PJ. Cereal feeding and its impact on the nitrogen economy of the infant. Am J Clin Nutr 1995; 62:969–972.
61. Reeds PJ, Burrin DG, Stoll B, van Goudoever JB. Consequences and regulation of gut metabolism. In: Lobley GE, White A, MacRae JC (eds). Protein Metabolism and Nutrition. The Netherlands: Wageningen Pers, 1999, pp 127–153.
62. Yu Y-M, Burke JF, Vogt JA, Chambers L, Young VR. Splanchnic and whole body L-[1-^{13}C,^{15}N]leucine kinetics in relation to enteral and parenteral amino acid supply. Am J Physiol. 1992; 262:E687–E694.
63. Stoll B, Burrin DG, Henry J, Jahoor F, Reeds PJ. Intestinal and hepatic phenylalanine utilization in fasted and fed piglets determined with intravenous and intragastric tracers. Am J Physiol 1997; 273:G1208–G1217.
64. Stoll B, Henry J, Reeds PJ, Yu H, Jahoor F, Burrin DG. Catabolism dominates the first-pass intestinal metabolism of dietary essential amino acids in milk protein-fed piglets. J Nutr 1998; 128:606–614.
65. Beaufrere B, Fournier V, Salle B, Putet G. Leucine kinetics in fed low-birth-weight infants: Importance of splanchnic tissues. Am J Physiol 1992; 263:E214–E220.
66. Darmaun D, Roig JC, Auestad N, Sager BK, Neu J. Glutamine metabolism in very low birth weight infants. Pediatr Res 1997; 41:391–396.
67. Bouteloup-Demange C, Boirie Y, Dechelotte P, Gachon P, Beaufrere B. Gut muco-

sal protein synthesis in fed and fasted humans. Am J Physiol 1998; 274:E541–E546.

68. Windmueller H, Spaeth AE. Respiratory fuels and nitrogen metabolism in vivo in small intestine of fed rats: Quantitative importance of glutamine, glutamate, and aspartate. J Biol Chem 1980; 255:107–112.

69. Stoll B, Burrin DG, Henry J, Yu H, Jahoor F, Reeds PJ. Substrate oxidation by the portal drained viscera of fed piglets. Am J Physiol 1999; 277:E168–E175.

70. Jackson AA, Doherty J, de Benoist MH, Hibbert J, Persaud C. The effect of the level of dietary protein, carbohydrate and fat on urea kinetics in young children during rapid catch-up weight gain. Br J Nutr 1990; 64:371–385.

71. Metges CC, El-Khoury AE, Henneman L, Petzke KJ, Grant I, Bedri S, Pereira PP, Ajami AM, Fuller MF, Young VR Availability of intestinal microbial lysine for whole body lysine homeostasis in human subjects. Am J Physiol 1999; 277:E597–E607.

72. Cobelli C, Saccomani MP, Tessari P, Biolo G, Luzi L, Matthews DE. Compartmental model of leucine kinetics in humans. Am J Physiol 1991; 261:E539–E550.

73. Patterson BW, Nguyen T, Pierre E, Herndon DN, Wolfe RR. Urea and protein metabolism in burned children: Effect of dietary protein intake. *Metabolism* 1997; 46:573–578.

74. Manary MJ, Broadhead RL, Yarasheski KE. Whole-body protein kinetics in marasmus and kwashiorkor during acute infection. Am J Clin Nutr 1998; 67:1205–1209.

75. Morlese JF, Forrester T, Badaloo A, Del Rosario M, Frazer M, Jahoor F. Albumin kinetics in edematous and nonedematous protein-energy malnourished children. Am J Clin Nutr 1996; 64:952–959.

76. Battista MA, Price PT, Kalhan SC. Effect of parenteral amino acids on leucine and urea kinetics in preterm infants. J Pediatr 1996; 128:130–134.

77. Barle H, Nyberg B, Essen P, Andersson K, McNurlan MA, Wernerman J, Garlick PJ. The synthesis rate of total liver protein and plasma albumin determined simultaneously in vivo in humans. Hepatology 1997; 25:154–158.

78. Fearon KCH, Falconer S, Slater C, McMillan DC, Ross JA, Preston T. Albumin synthesis rates are not decreased in hypoalbuminemic cachetic cancer patients with an ongoing acute-phase protein response. Ann Surg 1998; 227:249–254.

79. Morlese JF, Forrester T, Del Rosario M, Frazer M, Jahoor F. Repletion of the plasma pool of nutrient transport proteins occurs at different rates during the nutritional rehabilitation of severely malnourished children. J Nutr 1998; 128:214–219.

80. Balagopal P, Ljungqvist O, Nair KS. Skeletal muscle myosin heavy-chain synthesis rate in healthy humans. Am Physiol 1997; 272:E45–E50.

81. Tjader I, Essen P, Thorne A, Garlick PJ, Wernerman J, McNurlan MA. Muscle protein synthesis rate decreases 24 h after abdominal surgery irrespective of total parenteral nutrition. 1996; 20:135–138.

82. O'Keefe SJ, Lemmer ER, Ogden JM, Winter T. The influence of intravenous infusions of glucose and amino acids of pancreatic enzyme and mucosal protein synthesis in human subjects. J Parenter Enter Nutr 1998; 22:253–258.

83. Fryburg DA, Jahn LA, Hill SA, Oliveras DM, Barrett EJ. Insulin and insulin-like growth factor I enhance human skeletal muscle protein metabolism during hyperaminoacidemia by different mechanisms. J Clin Invest 1995; 96:1722–1729.

84. Biolo G, Tipton KD, Klein S, Wolfe RR. An abundant supply of amino acids enhances the metabolic effect of exercise on muscle protein. Am J Physiol 1997; 273: E122–E129.

85. Halseth AE, Flakoll PJ, Reed EK, Messina AB, Krishna MG, Lacy DB, Williams PE, Wasserman DH. Effect of physical activity and fasting on gut and liver proteolysis in the dog. Am J Physiol 1997; 273:E1073–E1082.

86. Thomas MR, Irving CS, Reeds PJ, Malphus EW, Wong WW, Boutton TW, Klein PD. Lysine and protein metabolism in the young lactating woman. Eur J Clin Nutr 1991; 45:227–242.

87. Reeds PJ, Burrin DG, Davis TA, Fiorotto ML, Stoll B, van Goudoever JB. Protein nutrition of the neonate Proc Nutr Soc. In press.

88. Davis TA, Burrin DG, Fiorotto ML, Nguyen HV. Protein synthesis in skeletal muscle and jejunum is more responsive to feeding in 7- than in 26-day-old pigs. Am J Physiol 1996; 270:E802–E809.

89. Kimball SR, Vary TC, Jefferson LS. Regulation of protein synthesis by insulin. Annu Rev Physiol 1994; 56:321–348.

90. Pain VM. Initiation of protein synthesis in eukaryotic cells. Eur J Biochem 1996; 236:747–771.

91. Eichler DC, Craig N Processing of eukaryotic ribosomal RNA Prog Nucleic Acid Res Mol Biol 1994; 49:197–239.

92. Larson DE, Zahradka P, Sells BH. Control points in eukaryotic ribosome biogenesis. Biochem Cell Biol 1994; 69:5–22.

93. Schubert U, Anton LC, Gibbs J, Norbury CC, Yewdell JW, Bennink JR. Rapid degradation of a large fraction of newly synthesized proteins by proteasomes. Nature 2000; 404:770–744.

94. Lardeux BR, Mortimore GE. Amino acid and hormonal control of macromolecular turnover in perfused rat liver: Evidence for selective autophagy. J Biol Chem 1987; 262(30):14514–14519.

95. Miotto G, Venerado R, Khurana KK, Siliprandi N, Mortimore GE. Control of hepatic proteolysis by leucine and isovaleryl-L-carnitine through a common locus: Evidence for a possible mechanism of recognition at the plasma membrane. J Biol Chem 1992; 267:22066–22072.

96. Melloni E, Pontremoli S. The calpain-calpastatin system: Structural and functional properties J Nutr Biochem 1991; 2:467–476.

97. Schwartz AL, Ciechanover A. The ubiquitin-proteasome pathway and pathogenesis of human diseases. Annu Rev Med 1999; 50:57–74.

98. Goldberg AL, Rock KL. Proteolysis, proteasomes and antigen presentation. Nature 1992; 357:375–359.

99. Ciechanover A, DiGiuseppe JA, Barcovich B, Orian A, Richter JD, Schwartz AL, Brodeur GM. Degradation of nuclear oncogenes by the ubiquitin system in vitro. Proc Natl Acad Sci USA 1991; 88:139–143.

100. Mansoor O, Beaufrere B, Boirie Y, Ralliere C, Taillandier D, Aurousseau E, Schoeffler P, Arnal M, Attaix D. Increased mRNA levels for components of the lysosomal, Ca^{2+}-activated, and ATP-ubiquitin-dependent proteolytic pathways in skeletal muscle from head trauma patients. Proc Natl Acad Sci USA 1996; 93: 2714–2718.

101. Lecker SH, Solomon V, Mitch WE, Goldberg AL. Muscle protein breakdown and
      the critical role of the ubiquitin-proteasome pathway in normal and disease states.
      J Nutr 1999; 129:227S–237S.
102. Attaix D, Aurousseau E, Combaret L, Kee A, Larbaud D, Ralliere C, Souweine B,
      Taillandier D, Tilignac T. Ubiquitin-proteasome-dependent proteolysis in skeletal
      muscle. Reprod Nutr Dev 1998; 38:153–165.

2

Lipids

Berthold Koletzko
University of Munich and Dr. von Hauner Children's Hospital,
Munich, Germany

1 INTRODUCTION

Fats provide the major portion of the dietary energy required by infants and young children and of the energy stored in the organism. Therefore, the supply, digestion, absorption, and metabolic utilization of lipids are of great importance for growth, body composition, health, and well-being. The assimilation and metabolic utilization of lipids can be markedly altered in children with gastrointestinal, hepatic and pancreatic disorders, when specific requirements need to be considered (1).

The role of fats in the diet has created an important area of research because of the major impact of lipid intake on energy balance and on the quality of body growth, biological functions, and long-term health. Lipid intake and metabolism in childhood are related to the development of early vascular lesions and long-term risk of cardiovascular disease (see Chap. 11). Infants and young children need relatively large amounts of polyunsaturated fatty acids (PUFA), which are indispensable components of structural lipids in the cell membranes of tissues; thereby, they modulate membrane functions such as membrane fluidity, activity of membrane-bound enzymes and receptors, metabolite exchange, and signal transduction. The availability of polyunsaturated lipids has been shown to affect the functional development of the central nervous system during the phase of rapid brain growth in infancy. Some long-chain polyunsaturated fatty acids are also precursors of bioactive lipid mediators, including prostaglandins, thromboxanes, and leukotrienes. During the last two decades, evidence has accumulated indicating that dietary lipid intake affects the immune response and may have an impact on the activity of inflammatory diseases and possibly the manifestation of atopic diseases.

2 COMPOSITION OF LIPIDS

Fatty acids are the predominant component of lipids in the diet and in the body. Fatty acids are conventionally classified according to their chain length as short- (chain length <8 carbon atoms), medium-(8 to 11), intermediate-(12 to 15), and long-chain fatty acids (≥16). Short formulas are used to describe fatty acids, which indicate the number of carbon atoms and double bonds as well as the position of the terminal double bond (Table 1). The carbon atom chain length of a fatty acid is the major determinant of melting point, energy content (kJ/g), degree of solubility in polar (e.g., water) and nonpolar liquids (e.g., hexane), and hence the efficacy of absorption in relation to the availability of conjugated bile salts in the intestinal lumen as well as metabolic properties such as effects on lipoprotein metabolism, oxidative degradation, and tissue fat deposition. Moreover, fatty acid properties are also modulated by the number, type, and position of double bonds, ranging from none (saturated fatty acids) to one (monounsaturated) or more (polyunsaturated) (Fig. 1).

The position of the double bonds is described by their distance from the terminal methyl group—i.e., the omega end of the fatty acid (Fig. 1). This terminal part of the fatty acid molecule is minimally changed in human metabolism, because fatty acids are activated by reacting with coenzyme A at the carboxyl end. Therefore, enzyme-mediated biochemical reactions such as chain elongation, chain shortening by β-oxidation, or the introduction of new double bonds occur at the carboxyl end of the molecule. In contrast, the omega end of a fatty acid is usually unchanged in intermediary metabolism unless the fatty acid is completely oxidized to carbon dioxide. Since humans and other higher organisms cannot introduce double bonds in the n-6 or n-3 positions, n-6 PUFA (e.g., linoleic acid) and n-3 PUFA (e.g., α-linolenic acid) are essential nutrients that must be provided with the enteral or parenteral substrate supply (2).

There are two isomeric forms of double bonds, *cis* and *trans*. Plants and mammalian cells introduce almost entirely *cis*-configured double bonds into fatty acids, in which both parts of the adjoining carbon chain point in the same direction as the double bond; therefore, the molecule is bent and becomes more flexible and fluid. *Trans* isomeric fatty acids are formed primarily by rumen bacteria (in

TABLE 1 Nutritionally Important Fatty Acids[a]

Name	Short formula
Saturated fatty acids	
Acetic acid	C2:0
Propionic acid	C3:0
Butyric acid	C4:0
Caproic acid	C6:0
Caprylic acid	C8:0
Capric acid	C10:0
Lauric acid	C12:0
Myristic acid	C14:0
Pentadecanoic acid	C15:0
Palmitic acid	C16:0
Margaric acid	C17:0
Stearic acid	C18:0
Arachidic acid	C20:0
Behenic acid	C22:0
Lignoceric acid	C24:0
Cis-monounsaturated fatty acids	
Palmitoleic acid	C16:1n-7
Oleic acid	C18:1n-9
Vaccenic acid	C18:1n-7
Essential fatty acids	
Linoleic acid (LA)	C18:2n-6
α-Linolenic acid (ALA)	C18:3n-3
γ-Linolenic acid	C18:3n-6
Dihomo-γ-linolenic acid	C20:3n-6
Arachidonic acid (AA)	C20:4n-6
Eicosapentaenoic acid	C20:5n-3
Docosahexaenoic acid (DHA), Cervonic acid	C22:6n-3
Trans-fatty acids	
Elaidic acid	C18:1n-9t
Trans-vaccenic acid	C18:1n-7t
Linolelaidic acid	C18:2n-6t
Conjugated linoleic acid (CLA)	C18:2n-6t
Other nonessential unsaturated fatty acids	
Mead acid	C20:3n-9

[a] Short formulas are conventionally used to describe the number of carbon (C) atoms, the number of double bonds, the omega-position of the last double bond (n-x) and the double bond configuration in cis (c) or trans (t) position.
Source: Modified from Ref. 1.

Saturated

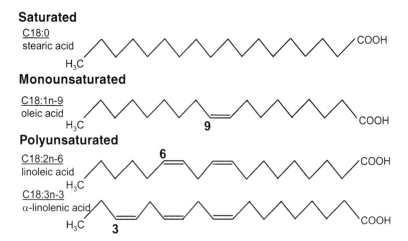

Monounsaturated

Polyunsaturated

FIGURE 1 Structure of the saturated fatty acid stearic acid (C18.0), the *cis*-monounsaturated fatty acid oleic acid (C18:1n-9, one double bond located 9 carbon atoms from the methyl end of the molecule), the n-6 polyunsaturated fatty acid linoleic acid (C18:2n-6; n-6 fatty acid with the terminal double bond located 6 carbon atoms from the methyl end of the molecule), and the n-3 polyunsaturated fatty acid α-linolenic acid (18:3n-3; n-3 fatty acid with the terminal double bond 3 carbon atoms from the methyl end).

the forestomach of cows, goats, and sheep) and by technical fat hydrogenation (3). *Trans* fatty acids have a straight carbon chain, with a tertiary structure similar to that of saturated fatty acids, and have lower melting points and less fluidity at body temperature than their respective *cis* isomers. *Trans* fatty acids may exert adverse effects on lipoprotein and essential fatty acid metabolism as well on fetal growth (4–9).

Positional and *trans* isomers of linoleic acid in which the double bonds are conjugated are called conjugated linoleic acids (CLAs). CLAs are formed primarily by biohydrogenation in ruminants. CLAs in the western diet are predominantly supplied by cow's milk and cheeses. The CLA content in bovine milk is on the order of about 1 to 2% of total fatty acids, with higher amounts resulting from barn feeding in winter than from pasture feeding in summer (10). Human milk contains about 0.4% CLAs, originating from the maternal intake of dietary fat (11). CLA was found to be a high-affinity ligand and activator of the peroxisome proliferator–activated receptor alpha (PPARα) (12) and thereby appears to have marked effects on lipid and energy metabolism. In experimental animals, an obesity-preventing action of CLA with a reduced energy intake, increased metabolic rate, and decreased body fat content has been reported (13,14). Other experimental studies have reported that CLAs may reduce plasma lipoprotein levels and early aortic atherosclerosis (15) and can inhibit the development of mammary (16,17), skin (18), and prostatic (19) cancers. Potential health-promoting effects of dietary CLA intake in humans remain to be further elucidated.

Three fatty acids esterified with glycerol form a triglyceride molecule, whereas di- and monoglycerides contain two and one fatty acid per molecule, respectively. In water and other polar fluids, triglycerides and other nonpolar lipids, such as nonesterified cholesterol, form a separate phase (e.g., lipid droplets on a clear soup) or an emulsion (e.g., milk, lipid droplets in an intravenous emulsion, lipoproteins in plasma). Lipids with polar components that can enhance the emulsification include phospholipids, nonesterified cholesterol, and monoglycerides.

3 INTESTINAL LIPID ASSIMILATION

The major part of the dietary lipid intake in breast- or formula-fed infants as well as in children and adults comprises triglycerides with long-chain fatty acids, while usually less than 2% of the dietary fat intake is contributed by lecithin and other phospholipids (20,21). A greater part of the lecithin found in the intestinal lumen, however, stems from the biliary tract (10 to 20 g of phospholipids per day in adults); some lecithin is also contributed by the membrane lipids of desquamated epithelial cells. Dietary cholesterol intake varies widely, depending on dietary habits, and ranges from about 150 mg/day in an exclusively breast-fed baby to about 250 to 500 mg in adolescents and adults consuming western-type diets. Vegetable oils and other plant lipids provide considerable amounts of plant sterols (phytosterols), such as β-sitosterol, campesterol, and stigmasterol, which can effectively inhibit cholesterol absorption and thereby lower plasma cholesterol levels (22).

Lecithin and, to a smaller extent, cholesterol enable the effective dispersion of dietary triglycerides into a stable emulsion with a large surface area. This dispersion, which is already initiated in the esophagus and stomach and is enhanced by the shearing action of peristaltic motility, is of great importance for exposing the dietary lipids to lipases. In the intestine, the dispersion of lipids is further enhanced by conjugated bile salts.

Lipolytic enzymes adsorb sequentially to the emulsified lipid droplets and enable the lipolytic cleavage of esterified fatty acids. Lipolysis is initiated prior to the small intestine by the action of lingual lipase (pregastric lipase) and gastric lipase (Table 2) (23). Preduodenal lipase, which is active over a broad pH range with a pH optimum of about 3 to 5.5, cleaves predominantly triglyceride fatty acids in the sn-3 position. Preduodenal lipolysis may contribute some 20 to 30% of lipid digestion in healthy individuals and 90% or more in patients with pancreatic insufficiency, as in cystic fibrosis (24–27). After transitioning into the duode-

TABLE 2   Major Lipolytic Enzymes Contributing to the Digestion
of Dietary Lipids

Lipase	Source	Functional characteristics
Lingual lipase (pregastric lipase)	Ebner's glands (beneath the circumvallate papillae of the tongue)	Contributes to initiation of lipolysis.
Gastric lipase	Gastric fundus	Contributes to initiation of lipolysis.
Pancreatic lipase	Pancreatic acini	Cleaves primarily triglyceride fatty acids in sn-1 and sn-3 positions to form two fatty acids and a sn-2 monoglyceride. Little hydrolysis of monoglycerides, phospholipids and sterol esters. The lipolytic activity of pancreatic lipase is enhanced by 40–50% by the presence of pancreatic colipase.
Pancreatic colipase	Pancreatic acini	After colipase adsorption to emulsified lipids, lipase binds to colipase in a configuration exposing the active site.
Human milk bile salt stimulated lipase = pancreatic cholesterol ester hydrolase	Mammary alveolar epithelium, pancreatic acini	Enzyme activity requires the presence of bile salts. Cleaves triglycerides, sterol esters, and esterified vitamins, important for vitamin and sterol assimilation.
Pancreatic phospholipase A_2	Pancreatic acini	Enzyme activity requires the presence of ionized calcium. Cleaves phospholipids at the sn-2 position to form a nonesterified fatty acid and a lysophospholipid, enhances the activity of colipase.
Various bacterial lipases	Colonic microflora	Cleave nonabsorbed lipids in the colon. Future therapeutic application?

num, preduodenal lipolytic activity is inactivated in the presence of an intact exocrine pancreatic and biliary function by bile salts and an alkaline pH and is rapidly degraded by pancreatic proteases (28,29).

In healthy individuals, the major part of lipolysis occurs in the small intestine. At the alkaline pH of 6.0 to 7.5 typically found in the duodenum, free fatty acids liberated by preduodenal lipolysis become ionized and hence migrate to the surface of emulsified particles and enhance emulsification (29). Moreover, the ionized fatty acids strengthen anchoring of pancreatic colipase at the surface of the lipid particles. Bile acids further enhance lipid emulsification, form mixed micelles, and clear proteins from the particle surface. Pancreatic lipase, which is secreted from pancreatic acini together with colipase in equimolar amounts, binds to colipase anchored at the surface of the lipid particle, resulting in a lipase configuration that exposes its active site. Pancreatic phospholipase A2 activity requires the presence of bile salts and ionized calcium. Phospholipase A2 hydrolyzes phospholipids on the surface of the lipid particle and thereby strengthens the exposure of the particle triglycerides to the colipase-lipase complex. The enzyme pancreatic cholesterol ester hydrolase, which is identical to the bile salt–stimulated lipase found in human milk (Table 2) (30), requires bile salts for its activation and is responsible for the cleavage of vitamin esters (tocopherol and retinol esters) and esters of cholesterol and other sterols. A recombinant enzyme has become available (31).

The fatty acids and monoglycerides liberated by the lipolytic cascade are absorbed by the intestinal mucosa and, in the case of short- and medium-chain fatty acids, also the gastric mucosa (32). Bile salts are required not only for enhancement of lipolysis but also, together with lecithin, for the effective solubilization of lipolysis products in mixed micelles, which aid in overcoming the diffusional barrier at the mucosal brush-border membrane and hence in mucosal uptake of lipolytic products (29). The solubility and efficacy of absorption is greater for unsaturated than for saturated fatty acids and decreases with increasing fatty acid chain length (33). The absorption of long-chain saturated fatty acids appears to be enhanced if they are esterified primarily in the β or sn-2 position of the triglyceride molecule (Fig. 2), as is found in palmitic acid in human milk triglycerides and in some animal fats or in structured triglycerides that have recently become available (2,34). The use of lipids with preferential esterification of long-chain saturated fatty acids in the sn-2 position might be of advantage in patients with fat malabsorption with respect to both fat and calcium assimilation, but results from a systematic evaluation in various gastrointestinal diseases are not yet available.

Unabsorbed lipids that reach the colon can be hydrolyzed by bacterial lipases, which have also been considered for therapeutic use in purified form (35–38). Colonic bacteria also metabolize long-chain fatty acids and form hydroxylation products. Short-chain fatty acids, such as butyric and propionic acids,

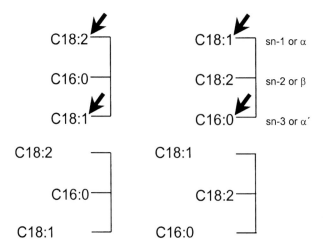

FIGURE 2   Lipases hydrolyze triglyceride fatty acids preferentially at the sn-1 and sn-3 positions. Human milk lipids, lard, and some specifically structured lipids contain the saturated palmitic acid (C16:0) predominantly in the sn-2 position (left panel). Thus, lipolysis of these substrates produces C16:0 preferentially as a monoglyceride which is very water-soluble and, therefore, well absorbed. In contrast, saturated fatty acids in vegetable oils are more or less randomly esterified to the different positions of the molecule. Here a greater proportion of C16:0 is liberated as a hydrophobic free fatty acid, which may associate with cations and hence lead to poorer absorption both of the saturated fats and of calcium (formation of calcium soaps). Beneficial effects of structured lipids with saturated fatty acids in the sn-2 position both on fat and mineral absorption have been documented in preterm and term infants.

are primarily formed from nondigestible carbohydrates and other polysaccharides.

3.1   Lipid Flux in the Intestinal Mucosa

Uptake of long-chain fatty acids across the intestinal microvillous membrane appears to be facilitated by a concentration gradient between the lumen and the intracellular space, but recent evidence indicates that it is mediated by a specific carrier. The microvillous membrane fatty acid–binding protein (FABP) is localized on the apical portions of jejunal villi and represents a carrier for long-chain fatty acid uptake that is saturable, heat-sensitive, and inactivated by trypsin (39). FABPs also direct the intracellular trafficking of fatty acids. In the intestinal mucosa, the principal FABPs are I-FABP (intestinal FABP), found only in the enterocyte of the small intestine, and L-FABP (liver FABP), found not only in the small intestine but also in liver, stomach, and colon cells (40,41). It is thought that these two cytosolic FABPs, which are regulated independently from each other, serve to transport absorbed fatty acids to specific intracellular compartments for the resynthesis of triglycerides, phospholipids, sterol, and vitamin esters, thereby regulating mucosal lipid metabolism.

Cholesterol uptake into the cell is considered a concentration gradient– driven passive diffusion. After its uptake, cholesterol is bound in a 1:1 molar ratio to the sterol carrier protein 2 (SCP 2), which channels the intracellular trafficking of cholesterol (42,43).

In the intestinal mucosa, about 75% of the absorbed triglyceride fatty acids are resynthesized to triglycerides and secreted as lipoproteins (21). The major part of absorbed sn-2 monoglycerides is used for this resynthesis of triglycerides. However, if the intraepithelial availability of monoglycerides is limited, as in the postabsorptive state, the glycerol-3-phosphate pathway is activated (44). Glycerol-3-phosphate is derived from glucose and lysolecithin from degradation of biliary and dietary phospholipids. Phospholipids, which are indispensable components both of cellular membranes and of lipoproteins, can be formed by reacylation of absorbed lysolecithin or by phophatidic acid-phosphorylcholine pathway (21).

4   LIPID METABOLISM

Within a few minutes after the appearance of dietary lipids in the intestinal lumen, lipid droplets accumulate within the intestinal epithelium and lipoprotein formation is activated. Lipids are resynthesized at the smooth endoplasmatic reticulum, whereas apoprotein formation occurs in the rough endoplasmatic reticulum. Lipids and apoproteins are assembled in Golgi organelles, which are thought to be precursors of secretory vesicles that fuse with the basolateral cell membrane to discharge the newly formed lipoproteins into the extracellular space and lymph (45).

Chylomicrons are large, triglyceride-rich particles that also contain phospholipids, cholesterol, cholesterol esters, lipid-soluble vitamins, and apoproteins A and B48 (Table 3). Most of their triglyceride content is hydrolyzed by endothelial-bound lipoprotein lipase, and the liberated fatty acids and lipid-soluble vitamins are taken up by peripheral tissues (e.g., muscle, adipose tissue). The activity of lipoprotein lipase is enhanced by apoprotein CII and in most tissues by insulin, while it is inhibited by apoprotein CIII. The production of apoprotein CIII is regulated by nuclear receptors acting as gene transcription factors, such as apoprotein AI regulatory protein. Dietary fat intake modulates chylomicron clearance, with unsaturated fatty acids forming larger chylomicrons that are cleared more effectively by lipoprotein lipase, because it has a higher affinity to unsaturated fatty acids. Therefore, diets rich in n-6 and n-3 polyunsaturated fatty acids

TABLE 3 Major Characteristics of Plasma Lipoproteins

Lipoprotein	Size (nm)	Origin	Major lipid classes	Major apoproteins
Chylomicrons	>100	Intestine	Triglycerides	Apo A1, A2, A4, B48 (acquires E and C in the circulation)
Chylomicron remnants	about 100	Circulation	Cholesterol, phospholipids	Apo E, B48
Very low density lipoproteins (VLDL)	30–90	Liver	Triglycerides	Apo B100, E, C
Intermediate-density lipoproteins (IDL)	30–60	Circulation	Cholesterol, phospholipids	Apo B100, E
Low-density lipoproteins (LDL)	about 20	Circulation	Cholesterol, phospholipids	Apo B100
High-density lipoproteins (HDL)	8–12	Intestine, liver, circulation	Cholesterol, phospholipids	Apo A1, A2, A4, E

Source: Modified from Ref. 162.

can markedly lower postprandial chylomicron concentrations (2). Chylomicron remnants are formed as a result of triglyceride clearance. Chylomicron remnants are taken up primarily by hepatocytes via low-density-lipoprotein (LDL) receptors (apoprotein B/E receptors) or apoprotein E–mediated chylomicron remnant receptors.

Very low density lipoproteins (VLDLs) secreted by the liver are rich in triglycerides and contain apoproteins B100 and E; they are also catabolized by lipoprotein lipase. The balance between fatty acid uptake and oxidation determines hepatic triglyceride synthesis, because de novo lipacidogenesis seems to be very limited in humans. A high intake of saturated fatty acids increases plasma VLDL, whereas VLDL is reduced by unsaturated fatty acids, particularly by long-chain n-3 polyunsaturated fatty acids (fish oils) that enhance lipolysis and decrease hepatic VLDL synthesis. Dietary cholesterol intake modulates VLDL cholesterol content to some extent, but hepatic cholesterol synthesis usually exceeds dietary intake by far.

The hydrolysis of VLDL triglycerides in the circulation results in the formation of intermediate density lipoproteins (IDLs), which can be taken up via LDL receptors in liver cells or be converted further in the circulation to LDLs, again influenced by the type of dietary fat. Mediated by binding of apoprotein B100 to the LDL receptor, LDL is taken up by hepatocytes and peripheral tissues. The major regulator of LDL receptor synthesis, and hence of LDL uptake, is the intracellular cholesterol pool size. In addition, dietary saturated fatty acids suppress LDL receptor activity and LDL removal. LDL may be modified by peroxidation, which is enhanced by prooxidants (e.g., unbound iron) and polyunsaturated fatty acids and inhibited by antioxidants (e.g., α-tocopherol). Modified LDL is rapidly removed from the plasma by scavenger cells in various tissues, including the vascular intima. Thus, vascular lipid deposition is enhanced by high plasma concentrations of LDL (increased by dietary saturated fat, particularly by the saturated fatty acids lauric, myristic and palmitic acids with 12 to 16 carbons atoms), by *trans*-monounsaturated fatty acids, and by peroxidative LDL modification (enhanced by an excess of prooxidants and polyunsaturates and a low dietary intake of antioxidants).

Dietary cholesterol intakes also modulate the cholesterol pool in plasma and tissues, but the major portion of plasma and tissue cholesterol is derived from endogenous synthesis primarily in the liver (46–50). The activity of endogenous cholesterol synthesis is modulated by the size of the intracellular cholesterol pool and affects gene expression (51). Cholesterol represses the expression of genes involved either in the synthesis of cholesterol (cytoplasmic hydroxymethylglutaryl-CoA synthase) or in its uptake from external sources, the LDL receptor (LDL are lipoproteins rich in cholesterol) (52). In the absence of cholesterol, the transcription of these genes is activated by a transcription factor called sterol regulatory element binding protein (SREBP). SREBP is usually bound to the

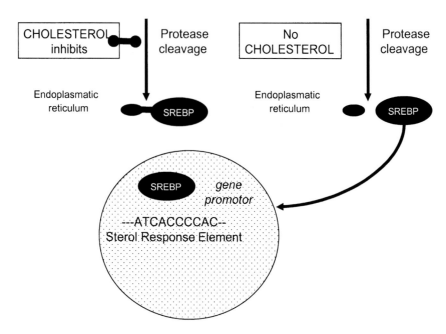

FIGURE 3 Cholesterol modulates the expression of genes involved in the synthesis of cholesterol (cytoplasmic hydroxymethylglutaryl-CoA synthase) and its uptake from external sources, the LDL receptor (LDL are lipoproteins rich in cholesterol). In the absence of cholesterol, the transcription of these genes is activated by a transcription factor called sterol regulatory element binding protein (SREBP). SREBP is usually bound to the endoplasmic reticulum where it can be cleaved by a protease. SREBP can then be transferred into the nucleus and activates the transcription of relevant genes. In the presence of cholesterol, however, the protease is inhibited and SREBP can no longer enter into the nucleus and stimulate gene transcription. (Modified from Ref. 52.)

endoplasmic reticulum, where it can be cleaved by a protease (Fig. 3). SREBP can then be transferred into the nucleus and activates the transcription of relevant genes. In the presence of cholesterol, however, the protease is inhibited and SREBP can no longer enter into the nucleus and stimulate gene transcription.

Although excessive plasma cholesterol levels are deleterious for cardiovascular health and increase the long-term risk for occurrence of myocardial infarction (53), cholesterol is indispensable for the formation of cell membranes and steroid hormones. An inborn defect of endogenous cholesterol synthesis in children with Smith-Lemli-Optiz syndrome causes severe mental retardation (54,55).

TABLE 4   Effects of Dietary Lipids on Plasma Lipoprotein Cholesterol

	LDL cholesterol	HDL cholesterol
Saturated fatty acids (lauric acid, 12:0, myristic acid, 14:0, and palmitic acid 16:0)	↑↑↑	↑
Trans-monounsaturated fatty acids	↑↑	↓
Cis-monounsaturated fatty acids	↓↓	↑
n-6 polyunsaturated fatty acids	↓↓	↓
n-3 polyunsaturated fatty acids	↑	≈
Cholesterol	↑	≈

Source: Adapted from Ref. 2.

Disk-shaped nascent high-density lipoproteins (HDLs) contain apoproteins AI and AII and are secreted by the liver and the gut, or they are formed in the circulation during lipolysis of triglyceride-rich lipoproteins (chylomicrons and VLDLs). Cholesterol from peripheral tissues is taken up by HDL esterified by the action of lecithin cholesterol acyl transferase (LCAT), and thereby transformed from nascent HDL to HDL$_3$ and HDL$_2$, which can be taken up in the liver by specific binding proteins. High HDL levels have a strong protective effect against vascular cholesterol deposition and the development of atherosclerosis. Diet affects HDL levels. Polyunsaturated fatty acids both of the n-6 and the n-3 series reduce LCAT activity; therefore high intakes of dietary PUFA have the untoward effect of lowering the protective HDL. Diet also modulates the activity of cholesterol ester transfer protein (CETP), which mediates redistribution of newly formed cholesterol esters from HDL to VLDL and LDL. Dietary cholesterol, saturated fats and *trans* monounsaturated fats increase plasma CETP and LDL (46,56). A schematic summary of the effects of dietary lipid intake on plasma LDL and HDL cholesterol levels is shown in Table 4.

4.1   Lipids and Energy Balance

Triglycerides serve as the major form of energy supply and storage for the body. Long-chain triglycerides have a metabolizable energy content of about 9 kcal/g, which is 2.25-fold higher than that of carbohydrates and protein. In growing infants and young children, the biological energy value of lipids —i.e., the capacity to generate adenosine triphosphate (ATP) and deposit tissue lipids during growth—appears to differ even more from that of nonlipid calories. During the first half year of life, lipids contribute about 35% of the weight gain or about 90% of the energy retained in newly formed tissue of normally growing full-term infants (57). Although lipids for tissue deposition might be synthesized de novo from other substrates such as carbohydrates, the activity of this endogenous de novo lipacidogenesis appears to be very limited (58). Endogenous lipacidogenesis would also require more energy, because a substantial amount of the energy from dietary carbohydrates would be lost in energetically futile use of ATP for the synthesis of molecules for storage as metabolic fuel or tissue components. For example, the synthesis of fat from glucose requires about 25% of the glucose energy invested for the cost of synthesis, whereas the synthesis of fat from fat requires only about 1 to 4% of the energy invested (59). The extent of energy loss in vivo is difficult to determine, but a higher thermogenic effect of dietary carbohydrates and proteins as compared with that of long-chain lipids has been well documented (60). Some studies supplying isoenergetic diets with different fat contents actually found a higher body weight and fat gain and a lower energy expenditure on the higher-fat diets (60–62).

Medium-chain triglycerides (MCTs) are successfully used in patients with chronic fat malassimilation, since they have a high water solubility, are rapidly cleaved by lipases, and are readily absorbed even without intraluminal bile salts and pancreatic lipases (63). However, MCTs do not provide the same energy supply as long-chain triglycerides (LCT). MCTs contain saturated fatty acids primarily with 8 and 10 carbon atoms (octanoic and decanoic acids). Due to the shorter fatty acid chain length, their energy content per gram of fat is about 16% lower than that of long-chain triglycerides (LCT) (Fig. 4). Moreover, MCTs are

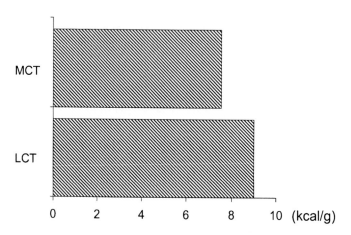

FIGURE 4   Medium-chain triglycerides (MCTs) provide approximately 16% less energy per gram than long-chain triglycerides (LCTs). Therefore, the therapeutic use of MCT oils will improve the metabolizable energy intake of the patient only if the increase in fat absorption achieved with MCT is greater than the difference in energy content (i.e., >16%).

very rapidly oxidized and have a high thermogenic effect, because they can reach the liver directly without prior incorporation into chylomicrons and quickly enter the mitochondria for β-oxidation, in large part without the need for binding to coenzyme A and for carnitine-regulated transport (63,64). Larger amounts of dietary MCTs are metabolized in several tissues by carnitine-dependent mechanisms and may increase the need for carnitine (65,66). About one-half of the dietary MCTs are not oxidized and not deposited to any appreciable extent in human tissues but are chain-elongated in another energy-consuming process (67,68). In some studies, dietary MCTs induced a greater thermogenic effect than LCTs (69) but had no advantage with respect to energy balance or weight gain in premature infants (70,71). Hence, the therapeutic use of MCT oils should be restricted to patients in whom the increase in fat absorption achieved with MCTs can be expected to be greater than the difference in energy content (about 16%), which may be the case in patients with severe cholestasis or other forms of severe steatorrhea.

4.2 Low-Fat Diets

For preventive purposes, a low dietary fat intake (≤30% of energy intake) has been recommended for adults and children, particularly in the United States (72), with the aim of reducing the risk for cardiovascular disease, obesity, type II diabetes, and certain forms of cancer. However, with respect to coronary heart disease it is not a low total fat intake but rather a low intake of saturated and *trans* fatty acids that appears to be of preventive value (53,73) (see Chap. 11). Epidemiological and biochemical studies indicate a much more marked benefit of the so-called Mediterranen diet, with its relatively high fat content, as compared with low fat diets (74,75). In fact, higher intakes of unsaturated fats may be beneficial by reducing LDL cholesterol and also, in the case of monounsaturated fats, by increasing the protective HDL cholesterol (Table 4). Also, total fat intake is associated with the intake of lipid-soluble antioxidants such as vitamin E, considered to reduce LDL oxidation and cardiovascular risk (53).

Moreover, it has been questioned whether low fat intakes are safe for growing infants and young children, with their high energy requirements. Indeed, high dietary fat intakes appear to have important practical advantages for providing ample energy to young children and to patients who are underweight or suffer from malabsorption (73,76). High-fat diets usually have a high energy density, and fat contributes greatly to the palatability and taste of foods, thereby helping to increase total energy intake. Failure to thrive was reported in school-aged children on very low fat diets (<20% of energy) (77), while high dietary fat intakes are associated high total body weight and body fat mass in children and adolescents (78–80) (Fig. 5). The clinical relevance of fat intake in chronic malabsorption is illustrated by the reported association between fat intake, body

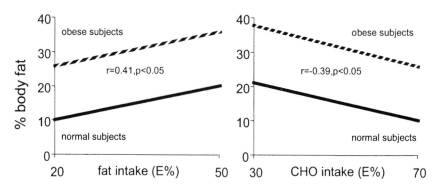

FIGURE 5 The percentage of dietary energy contributed by fat is positively correlated to body fat content in both obese and normal children aged 9 to 11 years ($n = 48$), whereas there is an inverse relationship to the percentage contribution of carbohydrates (CHO) to energy intake. (From Ref. 80.)

weight, and clinical course of disease in patients with cystic fibrosis (CF) who suffer both from fat malabsorption (primarily due to exocrine pancreatic insufficiency) and from high energy expenditure (81). Corey and coworkers (82) reported that CF patient populations on high as opposed to low-fat diets had markedly higher body weights and a significantly longer life expectancy (Table 5).

In spite of these data, many young families consider low-fat diets important or very important, even for infants (83). The effects of a low fat intake from 7 months of age onward were studied by Simell and coworkers in Finnish infants. The authors reported that low dietary fat intakes of about 29% at 8 months and 26% at 13 months were not associated with subnormal height, weight, weight for height, and head circumference up to the age of 36 months in this carefully supervised group of infants and young children from an affluent society (84,85). However, it appears conceivable that these effects might have been associated with adaptive mechanisms, such as a change in physical activity, and it is not known whether a similar fat intake is safe in less affluent populations stressed by high rates of infection or diarrhea or in children with chronic health problems.

It has been proposed that low-fat diets in young children may be a cause of chronic nonspecific diarrhea, toddler's diarrhea, or "pea and carrot diarrhea" (see Chap. 28) (86). Chronic nonspecific diarrhea is considered a motility disorder, and improvement was reported after an increase in fat intake, which slows gastric emptying and small-intestinal motility.

As there is no conclusive evidence for a benefit of total fat restriction in early childhood versus other options of a healthy dietary composition, neither the European nor the Canadian pediatric nutrition committees have supported restrictive low-fat diets for young children (53,87) (see Chap. 11).

TABLE 5 Body Weight and Outcome in Cystic Fibrosis
Patients Is Related to Dietary Fat Intake

	CF Patients in	
	Boston	Toronto
Number	499	534
Female	43%	42%
Age (years, M ± SD)	15.9 ± 9.6	15.2 ± 8.3
Dietary fat intake	Low	Normal
Weight (mean percentile)	35th	43rd
Median life expectancy	21 years	30 years

[a] Patients in Boston used to be advised to follow a low-fat diet
to reduce abdominal discomfort, while in Toronto a high-fat diet
with a somewhat more generous use of pancreatic enzyme preparations had been used since the 1970s. The higher fat intake of
the Canadian patients was associated with a higher body weight
as well as a 9-year-higher median life expectancy.
Source: Adapted from Ref. 82.

4.3 Essential Polyunsaturated Fatty Acids

Linoleic acid (C18:2n-6) and α-linolenic acid (C18:3n-3, ALA) (Fig. 1) are essential fatty acids because humans, like other higher mammals, cannot insert
double bonds in the ω-6 and ω-3 position of a fatty acid (i.e., at 6 or 3 carbon
atoms from the methyl end of the molecule). Linoleic and α-linolenic acids are
the precursors of ω-6 and ω-3 LC-PUFA (i.e., polyunsaturated fatty acids) with
20 and 22 carbon atoms (Fig. 6). The biologically most important LC-PUFA are
dihomo-γ-linolenic acid (C20:3n-6) and arachidonic acid (C20:4n-6) of the ω-6
and eicosapentaenoic acid (C20:5n-3) series and docosahexaenoic acid (C22:6n-
3, DHA) of the ω-3 series. Enzymatic conversion of linoleic and α-linolenic acids
to arachidonic acid is a relatively short metabolic pathway consisting of one chain
elongation and two desaturation steps (Fig. 6). In contrast, DHA is synthesized
from α-linolenic acid via several consecutive desaturation and elongation steps
also involving indirect steps via fatty acids with 24 carbon atoms (88,89).

Arachidonic acid and DHA are indispensable components of plasma membranes and are incorporated in relatively large amounts in membrane-rich tissues,
such as the brain and retina, during early human growth (90–92). Phospholipids
of membranes with high fluidity, such as synaptosomal membranes and retinal
photoreceptors, contain particularly high LC-PUFA concentrations. Moreover,
dihomo-γ-linolenic acid, arachidonic acid, and eicosapentaenoic acid serve as
precursors for the formation of prostaglandins, prostacyclins, thromboxanes, leu-

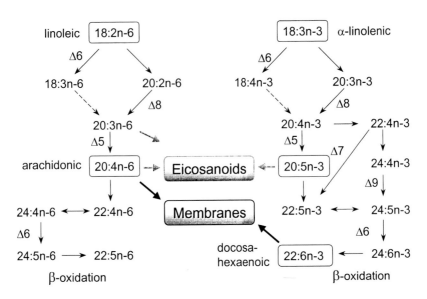

FIGURE 6 Conversion of the parent essential fatty acids linoleic acid (18:2*n*-6) and α-linolenic acid (18:3*n*-3) to their long-chain polyunsaturated metabolites (LC-PUFA).

kotrienes, and other lipid mediators that are powerful regulators of various cell and tissue processes, like thrombocyte aggregation, leukocyte function, and in-flammation (2).

4.4 Intrauterine PUFA Supply

Intrauterine growth during the latter part of pregnancy is characterized by a very rapid deposition of fat, which exceeds by far that of any other nutrient and accounts for about 75% of the energy retained in the newly formed tissues (93). The analysis of tissue composition from deceased infants and fetuses of different gestational ages has demonstrated a very rapid incorporation of long-chain poly-unsaturated fatty acids (LC-PUFA), especially arachidonic acid and DHA, into structural lipids of the brain, retina, and other tissues during the latter part of pregnancy (90,91). Particularly high LC-PUFA concentrations are found in the phospholipids of membranes with high fluidity, such as synaptosomal membranes and retinal photoreceptors.

Intrauterine supply of PUFA to the fetus depends entirely on placental transfer. If one compares the fatty acid composition of plasma lipids in pairs of mothers and their healthy full-term infants (Table 6), one finds markedly lower

TABLE 6 Total Fatty Acid Concentration (mg/dL) and Percentage Contributions of Major Essential Fatty Acids (% wt/wt) in Plasma Lipids in 41 Pairs of Mothers and Their Term Infants at the Time of Birth[a]

	Triglycerides		Phospholipids	
	Maternal	Cord	Maternal	Cord
Total (mg/dL)	143.31 (63.73)	24.27 (12.43)*	172.22 (37.63)	62.55 (18.08)*
C18:2n-6	11.91 (5.48)	10.05 (3.45)*	20.99 (3.38)	7.42 (1.37)*
C20:3n-6	0.22 (0.07)	0.81 (0.43)*	3.37 (0.82)	4.82 (0.83)*
C20:4n-6	0.75 (0.29)	2.92 (1.11)*	7.68 (1.90)	16.14 (2.49)*
Total n-6-LC-PUFA	1.54 (0.41)	5.74 (2.20)*	12.37 (2.16)	22.55 (2.56)*
C18:3n-3	0.52 (0.19)	0.20 (0.27)*	0.20 (0.10)	0.00 (0.03)*
C20:5n-3	0.06 (0.04)	0.00 (0.17)	0.35 (0.15)	0.20 (0.16)*
C22:6n-3	0.32 (0.22)	1.33 (1.27)*	2.89 (0.99)	4.76 (1.70)*
Total n-3-LC-PUFA	0.51 (0.28)	1.59 (1.66)*	3.72 (1.24)	5.44 (2.12)*

	Cholesterol esters		Nonesterified fatty acids	
	Maternal	Cord	Maternal	Cord
Total (mg/dL)	120.13 (48.99)	33.57 (17.85)*	25.21 (13.04)	9.60 (6.95)*
C18:2n-6	48.75 (8.19)	15.28 (4.04)*	7.69 (4.28)	4.13 (2.94)*
C20:3n-6	0.78 (0.30)	1.28 (0.39)*	0.33 (0.34)	0.41 (0.73)
C20:4n-6	5.66 (1.70)	11.39 (3.36)*	0.74 (0.56)	1.04 (1.27)*
Total n-6-LC-PUFA	6.69 (1.48)	14.75 (3.39)*	2.35 (3.47)	6.30 (7.22)*
C18:3n-3	0.56 (0.31)	0.08 (0.15)*	0.15 (0.30)	0.00 (0.06)*
C20:5n-3	0.33 (0.20)	0.22 (0.34)*	0.00 (0.11)	0.00 (0.00)
C22:6n-3	0.52 (0.38)	0.92 (0.52)*	0.18 (0.31)	0.00 (0.49)
Total n-3-LC-PUFA	0.93 (0.57)	1.26 (0.72)	0.29 (0.60)	0.00 (0.63)

[a] Median (interquartile range); * = $p < 0.05$.
Source: Modified from Ref. 163.

levels of linoleic and α-linolenic acids in cord than in maternal plasma lipids (94,95). In contrast, percentage values for arachidonic acid, DHA, and other LC-PUFAs are significantly higher in infants than in their mothers (94,95), which indicates a preferential and selective materno–fetal LC-PUFA transfer in utero. Since no activity of the two key enzymes for LC-PUFA synthesis, Δ-6- and Δ-5-desaturase, has been detected in human placental tissue, LC-PUFA in the fetal circulation must be derived either from synthesis in fetal tissues or from the mother by preferential placental transfer. The contribution of preferential maternal–fetal LC-PUFA transfer by the placenta is supported by experimental studies in the perfused human placenta (96). In these experiments, the major portion of radioactively labeled arachidonic acid from the maternal perfusate was incorporated into fetal phospholipids, in contrast to only small amounts of α-linolenic and linoleic acids.

4.5 PUFA Supply with Human Milk

Human milk is considered the ideal form of feeding for healthy babies and the best way to meet substrate requirements for the first four to six months of life (97) (see Chap. 6). Human milk lipids provide not only linoleic and α-linolenic acids but also considerable amounts of preformed LC-PUFA, the concentration of which changes with the duration of lactation. Human milk from mothers of term and preterm infants is similar with respect to AA and DHA content and the decrease in the percentage of LC-PUFA during the first month of lactation (98) (Fig. 7). Obviously, the presumed higher LC-PUFA requirements of preterm infants are not met any better by the milk of their own mothers than by mature milk.

The medians and ranges for the percentage contents of PUFA in human milk were calculated from the results of 14 European and 10 African studies on the fatty acid composition of mature human milk (99). Median contents of linoleic acid (11% wt/wt and 12%), α-linolenic acid (0.9% and 0.8%), arachidonic acid (0.5% and 0.6%), and DHA (0.3% and 0.3%) were surprisingly similar in European and in African human milk samples, respectively, in spite of very different dietary habits and living conditions. However, the overall ranges of reported values were wide (linoleic acid 5.7% to 17.2%, α-linolenic acid 0.1% to 1.44%, arachidonic acid 0.2% to 1.2%, DHA: 0.1% to 0.9%), which appear to reflect not only biological variation but also great differences in methodology used in the various studies. To exclude some of this methodological bias, we calculated data from eight relatively recently published studies that determined the fatty acid composition of mature human milk with modern methods such as capillary gas-liquid chromatography (100–107). This review shows the variation of linoleic and arachidonic acids to be within a rather narrow range (Table 7). In contrast, there were more than fourfold differences between the lowest and highest α-linolenic acid and DHA values, respectively. Thus, the relative variability of

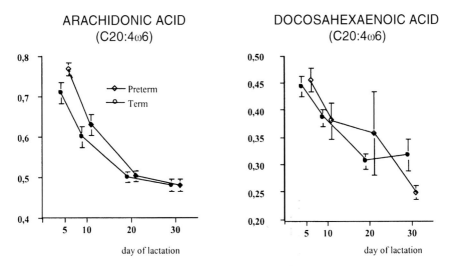

FIGURE 7 Arachidonic and docosahexaenoic acid percentage contribution to human milk lipids (% wt/wt) decrease during the first month of lactation in parallel to an increasing total milk lipid secretion. LC-PUFA contents of human milk from mothers of term and preterm infants do not differ in LC-PUFA contents during the first month of lactation, hence, the milk of mothers of preterm infants is not better suited to meet the higher LC-PUFA requirements of their infants than mature human milk. (From Ref. 98.)

ω-3 fatty acid contents in human milk seems to be larger than that of ω-6 fatty acids.

The observed variability of the fatty acid composition of human milk questions the approach to delineate the requirements of essential nutrients in young infants from human milk composition. Moreover, breast-milk volumes, even in well-nourished populations, vary considerably, ranging from 550 to 1100 mL per day (108); thus it is rather difficult to define a standard intake for breast-fed babies. Moreover, the bioavailability and metabolism of nutrients may differ considerably between breast- and formula-fed infants. However, the considerable uncertainties in defining the LC-PUFA content characteristic of mature human milk should not mask the fact that all lactating women provide some amount of preformed dietary LC-PUFA to their infants.

Although the LC-PUFA content of milk is influenced to a certain extent by maternal dietary composition, compositional studies have given indications for some metabolic control of PUFA contents (99,109). The sources of essential fatty acids in human milk can be studied with stable isotope techniques that are safe and free of adverse effects (110). We supplied U-^{13}C-labeled linoleic acid

TABLE 7 Contribution of Linoleic Acid (C18:2ω-6), Arachidonic Acid (C20:4ω-6), α-Linolenic Acid (C18:3ω-3), and Docosahexaenoic Acid (C22:6ω-3) to the Fatty Acid Composition of Mature Human Milk[a]

Reference	Australia (100)	Canada (101)	Congo (102)	France (103)	Germany (104)	Italy (105)	Norway (106)	Spain (107)
Linoleic acid	14.06	11.8	13.65	13.23	11.33	9.79	11.60	12.02
Arachidonic acid	0.41	0.4	0.44	0.50	0.45	0.47	0.40	0.50
α-Linolenic acid	0.97	1.5	1.19	0.57	0.90	0.36	0.93	0.78
Docosahexaenoic acid	0.21	0.3	0.55	0.38	0.23	0.12	0.46	0.34

[a] Data from nonintervention arms of the studies only. Data are % weight/weight, medians or means from recently published studies using high-resolution capillary gas-liquid chromatography.
Source: Modified from Ref. 164.

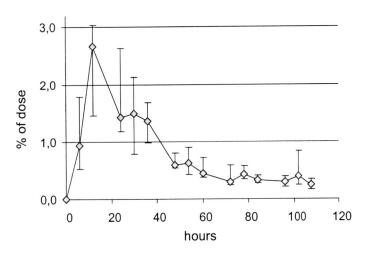

FIGURE 8 Time course of the transition of U-^{13}C–labeled linoleic acid from the diet of lactating women into their breast milk. (Modified from Refs. 165 and 111.)

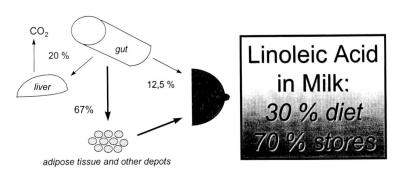

FIGURE 9 Schematic depiction of linoleic acid flux in breast-feeding women, based on results of turnover of a stable isotope after oral administration of U-^{13}C–labeled linoleic acid and measurements of its oxidation from breath gas analyses and its transfer into milk by analysis of milk samples collected over 5 days (111). About 30% of milk linoleic acid is directly transferred from the diet, whereas about 11% of dihomo-γ-linolenic acid and 1.2% of arachidonic acid from milk originate from direct endogenous conversion of dietary linoleic acid. The major portion of polyunsaturated fatty acids in human milk lipids is derived from maternal body stores and not directly from the maternal diet. Thus, the influence of maternal diet on milk composition is moderated by the quantitatively larger contribution of fatty acids from maternal body pools, resulting in a relatively constant milk PUFA supply to the recipient infant.

to breast-feeding women and estimated its oxidation from analysis of breath gas enrichment and its transfer into milk by analysis of milk samples collected over 5 days (111). The transition of dietary fat into milk is rapid, with the peak of milk linoleic enrichment occurring at about 12 hr after oral intake (Fig. 8). We estimated that only about 30% of milk linoleic acid is directly transferred from the diet, whereas about 11% of milk dihomo-γ-linolenic acid and 1.2% of milk arachidonic acid originates from direct endogenous conversion of dietary linoleic acid (Fig. 9). In contrast, the major portion of polyunsaturated fatty acids in human milk lipids is derived from maternal body stores and not directly from the maternal diet. Thus, short-term changes of maternal dietary intake have only relatively moderate effects on milk composition, resulting in a relatively constant milk PUFA supply to the recipient infant, which might be of biological benefit.

4.6 PUFA Sources for Infants Fed Infant Formula Milk: Diet, Body Stores, and Endogenous Synthesis

Infant formulas based on vegetable oils contain linoleic and α-linolenic acids, usually in amounts similar to those found in breast milk; but conventional infant formulas based on vegetable oils do not contain appreciable amounts of LC-PUFA (112,113). More recently, formulas that do contain LC-PUFA have become available in most countries (114). Infants fed formulas without preformed LC-PUFA depend on utilization of body stores accreted during intrauterine growth, endogenous synthesis from the precursor PUFA, or a combination thereof to obtain the LC-PUFA deposited in structural lipids of newly formed cell membrane systems.

It has previously been questioned whether infants can synthesize LC-PUFA endogenously. Recent refinements of isotope techniques rendered it possible to investigate fatty acid turnover in vivo even in infants (115). The availability of uniformly ^{13}C-labeled, highly enriched tracer fatty acids and the high sensitivity and precision of gas chromatography isotope ratio mass spectrometry have made it possible to perform accurate measurements on ^{13}C-enrichment in precursor and product fatty acids from very small volumes of blood. Endogenous arachidonic acid synthesis could be demonstrated in full-term infants given a diet providing linoleic acid with an increased content of the stable isotope ^{13}C (116). Using a simplified isotope balance equation, we estimated that the contribution of arachidonic acid synthesis to the total renewal of the plasma arachidonic acid pool is only in the order of about 6% per day. More recent results indicate that endogenous AA synthesis already occurs in the first week of life, but again the contribution of LA conversion to the total plasma pool is very small (117) (Fig. 10). Similar results are obtained in enterally fed preterm infants given oral bolus doses

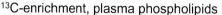

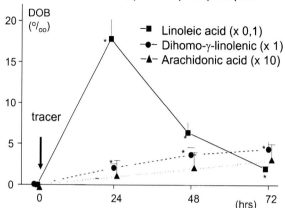

FIGURE 10   Change of ^{13}C-enrichment (δ^{13}C over baseline, DOB) in plasma phospholipid fatty acids of 10 full-term breast-fed infants given a tracer dose of U-^{13}C–labeled linoleic acid on the second day of life. The rapid increase of ^{13}C-content in the plasma linoleic acid indicates the uptake from the gut. The much lower enrichment in the metabolites dihomo-γ-linolenic acid (10-fold smaller scale) and arachidonic acid (100-fold smaller scale) reflects a limited conversion of linoleic acid to these LC-PUFA. (From Ref. 117.)

of U-^{13}C-labeled linoleic and α-linolenic acids (93,118). It appears that the activity of endogenous LC-PUFA synthesis may not always suffice to provide the amounts of LC-PUFA required for tissue incorporation during phases of rapid growth.

4.7   Functional Effects of LC-PUFA for Infant Growth and Development

Although it has been demonstrated that infants are capable of synthesizing LC-PUFA, preterm and term infants fed formulas with precursor EFA but lacking LC-PUFA develop a pronounced decline in LC-PUFA status relative to infants receiving human milk or formula enriched with LC-PUFA (119–123). Obviously LC-PUFA utilization for deposition, oxidation and metabolic conversion to eicosanoids exceeds the infant's capability of synthesizing n-6 and n-3 LC-PUFA from the precursors LA and ALA. Not only plasma but also tissue LC-PUFA contents are affected. On autopsy studies of infants who died suddenly, higher brain and retinal DHA contents were found if these infants had been fed human milk that provides preformed LC-PUFA than in those fed formula without LC-PUFA (124,125).

Studies that evaluated the supplementation of infant formulas with DHA and partly also AA have reported normalization of LC-PUFA status in infants who were supplemented relative to reference groups fed human milk (119,121, 122,123,126,127). Some double-blind randomized trials found an LC-PUFA associated improved performance in tests of visual and cognitive functions in both preterm (93,123,126,128) and term infants (129). Two studies in term infants showed lasting effects of early LC-PUFA supplementation on functional development toward the end of the first year of life. Birch et al. (130) compared the visual devepment of infants fed a formula in which 0.35% of the total fatty acids were DHA—either alone or combined with arachidonic acid—with a control group that did not receive preformed DHA. DHA-supplementation resulted in significantly better visual acuity as determined by visual evoked potentials at the ages of 6, 17, and 52 weeks. Thus, the provision of dietary preformed DHA improved visual function up to 1 year of age in healthy term babies.

Willats and coworkers (131) assessed cognitive behavior with sophisticated problem-solving tests at the age of 10 months in infants who had been assigned in a double blind randomized study to early feeding with formulas with or without 0.15 to 0.25% DHA and 0.30 to 0.40% arachidonic acid, respectively. The test used evaluated the intentional execution of a sequence of steps in order to find a hidden toy and is considered to be specially apt for studying early development of complex cognitive functions, since tests results at the age of 9 months were reported to correlate closely with intelligence quotients and vocabulary scores at the age of 3 years. At the age of 10 months, the tested infants who had received preformed dietary LC-PUFA during early infancy had significantly more intentional solutions and better intention scores than infants whose formula was devoid of LC-PUFA (Fig. 11).

Although these results are impressive and point to an important role of the early dietary supply of LC-PUFA, some other studies did not find significant advantages associated with different LC-PUFA additions to infant formulas (132). These discrepancies between different studies (133) might be related to differences in the methods and interventions used as well as the populations investigated.

Some formulas with apparently unbalanced lipid composition have even been associated with potential adverse effects. Formulas supplemented with oils comprising high amounts of eicosapentaenoic acid (EPA, C20:5n-3) relative to DHA, but no n-6 LC-PUFA, were associated with a prolonged decrease of serum arachidonic acid levels throughout the first year of life as well as with poor growth (134,135). Reduced levels of arachidonic acid have also been related to poor intrauterine growth (136,137). Recently, enhanced growth of premature infants receiving a preterm infant formula with both DHA and arachidonic acid compared

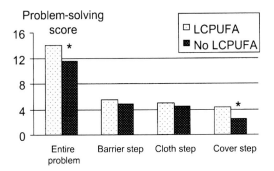

FIGURE 11 The ability to solve a complex, three-step problem (recovery of a hidden toy) by healthy, term infants at the age of 10 months is related to early LC-PUFA supply. Infants were randomized to formula feeding with or without LC-PUFA (0.3 to 0.4% AA, 0.15 to 0.25% DHA) for the first 4 months. * = significantly different, $p < 0.05$. (From Ref. 131.)

to infants fed formulas containing no LC-PUFA, or only DHA, has been reported in abstract form. In view of the benefit reported in several studies and the absence of adverse effects with a balanced supply of both arachidonic acid and DHA, a recent expert consensus conference recommended that both preterm and term infants should be preferentially fed human milk, which provides LC-PUFA, or that formula-fed infants should receive formulas enriched with LC-PUFA at levels matching at least the lower range of LC-PUFA content reported for human milk (138).

4.8 Effects of PUFA on the Immune System

There is accumulating evidence that lipids and in particular some fatty acids can influence the immune response. The balance between n-6 and n-3 fatty acids modulates the formation of different eicosanoids. For example, 5-lipoxygenase products derived from the n-6 fatty acid arachidonic acid are proinflammatory, whereas those synthesized from the n-3 fatty acid eicosapentaenoic acid are inactive (Fig. 12); hence supplementation with n-3 fatty acids may suppress inflammatory processes (139). Also the production of NO and of cytokines such as interleukins-1α and β, interleukin-2, and tumor necrosis factor-α are strongly modulated by n-3 fatty acids (140). Many of the effects of n-3 fatty acids are not eicosanoid-mediated but follow other mechanisms, such as the modulation of signal transduction pathways and the direct modulation of gene expression by regulating several transcription factors, including the nuclear factor κB and the peroxisome proliferator-activated receptor (141). Clinical studies have evaluated

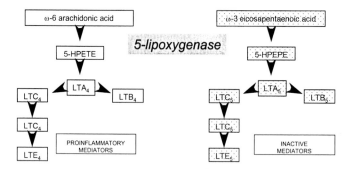

FIGURE 12   The n-6 and n-3 fatty acids are precurors of eicosanoids with different biological functions. Both arachidonic acid and eicosapentaenoic acid are substrates for 5-lipoxygenase. The 5-lipoxygenase products of arachidonic acid, such as leukotriene B4, are potent proinflammatory mediators, whereas 5-lipoxygenase products of eicosapentaenoic acid are inactive. Supplementation with n-3 fatty acids, resulting in an increase of the n-3/n-6 balance, may thus suppress inflammatory processes.

the use of n-3 fatty acids in chronic inflammatory disorders such as inflammatory bowel disease, rheumatoid arthritis, cystic fibrosis, and critical injury (139,142–146). Although beneficial effects have been reported, results are inconsistent, probably due in part to very different study protocols.

In premature infants, dietary intake of preformed n-6 and n-3 LC-PUFA was shown to markedly affect immune phenotypes (147). Peripheral blood cells were identified by monoclonal antibodies and IL-10 production after mitogen stimulation of peripheral lymphocytes was measured by ELISA. Immune phenotypes at age 42 days were significantly different in infants fed formula without LC-PUFA than in infants who got preformed arachidonic and docosahexaenoic acids from either formula or human milk (Table 8). Recently it has been proposed that the supply of polyunsaturated fatty acids and the balance between n-6 and n-3 fatty acids may be linked to the risk of manifestation of atopic disease (148,149).

4.9   Essential Fatty Acid Metabolism in Children with Chronic Cholestasis

Children with chronic cholestasis suffer from fat malabsorption and disturbed hepatic lipid metabolism. In these patients, essential fatty acid status is often very poor, as their bile acid secretion is impaired. Bile acids facilitate PUFA absorption from the gut, while LC-PUFA are synthesized from their precursors mainly in the liver. PUFA depletion of plasma lipid fractions was reported in adult cirrhotic

TABLE 8 Immune Phenotypes of Premature Infants Aged 42 Days After Random Assignment to Formula with or Without the LC-PUFA Arachidonic and Docosahexaenoic Acids, or with Human Milk Providing LC-PUFA[a]

	Preterm formula without LC-PUFA	Preterm formula with LC-PUFA	Human milk with LC-PUFA
CD4/CD8 ratio	4.1 ± 0.5	2.9 ± 0.2	2.9 ± 0.2
CD4 + CD45RO + (% total)	5.6 ± 0.4	7.1 ± 1.0	7.0 ± 0.7
CD4 + CD45RA + (% total)	85 ± 2	77 ± 4	72 ± 3
IL10 (pg/mL)	11 ± 32	167 ± 38	296 ± 44

[a] Immune phenotypes of infants fed formula without LC-PUFA differ significantly from those of infants receiving LC-PUFA from formula or from human milk.
Source: Modified from Ref. 147.

patients in association with protein energy malnutrition and encephalopathy (150,151). Information on cholestatic children has been limited.

Data on the essential fatty acid metabolism in children with chronic intra- and extrahepatic cholestasis show markedly lower plasma phospholipid linoleic and arachidonic acid values than in healthy children (152) (Table 9). Levels of the nonessential fatty acids oleic acid (18:1n-9), mead acid (20:3n-9), and palmitoleic acid (16:1n-7) are high, which is indicative of essential fatty acid deficiency. Serum bilirubin levels were unrelated to the essential fatty acid precursors linoleic acid and α-linolenic acid but correlated inversely with the long-chain metabolites dihomo-γ-linolenic (20:3n-6), arachidonic (20:4n-6), docosapentaenoic (22:5n-3), and docosahexaenoic acids (22:6n-3) (152). Both arachidonic and

TABLE 9 Linoleic Acid, α-Linolenic Acid, and LC-PUFA Contents of Plasma Phospholipids in Children with Chronic Cholestasis and Age-Matched Healthy Controls[a]

Fatty acids	Cholestatic patients	Age-matched healthy controls	p
Linoleic (C18:2n-6)	14.04 (12.63–18.75)	18.18 (16.13–20.23)	0.04
Total n-6 LC-PUFA	8.87 (6.27–11.28)	13.97 (12.48–14.32)	0.0004
α-Linolenic (C18:3n-3)	0.23 (0.19–0.34)	0.15 (0.12–0.21)	0.01
Total n-3 LC-PUFA	2.34 (1.68–4.23)	3.5 (3.18–4.03)	0.09

[a] Median (Q_1-Q_3), % wt/wt.
Source: From Ref. 152.

docosahexaenoic acids reached very low levels in children with bilirubin concentrations over 100 μmol/L. These results, together with increased levels of palmitoleic and mead acids, indicate the regular occurrence of essential fatty acid deficiency in cholestatic children.

Reduced availability of arachidonic acid in these patients may contribute to a disturbed eicosanoid balance and be one factor in the pathogenesis of altered coagulation, immunological response, and renal function. It is conceivable that poor arachidonic acid status might contribute to the growth disturbances observed in cholestatic children. In addition to vitamin E deficiency (153), poor LC-PUFA status might also contribute to the neurological impairment observed as a frequent complication in children with severe cholestatis. Supplementation of cholestatic infants and children with LC-PUFA might be beneficial and is currently under evaluation.

5 PARENTERAL LIPID INFUSION

Full parenteral feeding of infants and young children requires the use of lipid emulsions to meet their high energy needs for maintenance and growth and to supply essential fatty acids (see Chap. 17). Lipid emulsions consist of different oils (Table 10), egg yolk phospholipids, and glycerol. The fat particles in the emulsions resemble endogenously produced chylomicrons in size, physicochemical properties, and metabolism and are hydrolyzed by lipoprotein lipase. Hepatic lipase contributes to the removal of the triglyceride-depleted remnant particles (154). Lipolysis of infused triglycerides is usually very efficient in mature neonates, even after surgery (155), but prematurity may alter lipoprotein metabolism (156). In contrast, phospholipids from the infusion tend to accumulate in the recipient patient's plasma. The extent of the resulting hyperphospholipidemia and hypercholesterolemia depends on the amount of excess phospholipid infused (157). Therefore emulsions with a low phospholipid/triglyceride ratio (such as the usual 20% emulsions) are preferred for use in infants and young children.

Prospective and retrospective studies in very low birth weight neonates have reported an association of very early lipid infusion during the first days of life with a poor outcome, such as increased rates of chronic lung disease and retinopathy of prematurity, while other observations do not confirm such an association. The limited data available from clinical studies might point to a possible risk of very early lipid infusion for very immature and sick infants with extremely low birth weight, but a recent metanalysis of all available studies (158) did not indicate any increased risk with early introduction of lipid infusion in premature infants (Table 11). One hypothesis raised regarding possible mechanisms of potential risks for subgroups of susceptible children, such as immature infants with very low birth weight, is that infusion of highly unsaturated fats to sick and very immature infants during the first days of life will expose them to enhanced oxida-

TABLE 10 Commercial Intravenous Lipid Emulsions Used for Pediatric Patients

Oils used	Soybean	Soybean/MCT	Olive/soybean	Soybean/fish
Product names	Intralipid, Ivelip, Lipofundin, Lipovenous, Liposyn III	Lipofundin MCT	ClinOleic	Lipovenous + Omegavenous, 9 + 1 parts mix
Fat contents				
Triglycerides (%)	10, 20, and 30%	20%	20%	10%
Ratio phospholipids/triglycerides (mg/g)	120, 60, and 40	60	60	66
Glycerol (%)	2.5	2.5	2.25	2.5
kcal/mL	1.1–2.0	1.9	2.0	
Fatty acid composition (% wt/wt)				
Medium chain (8:0 + 10:0)	n.d.	50	n.d.	n.d.
Palmitic (16:0)	9–11.2	5	13.5	10.8
Stearic (18:0)	4–4.2	2	2.9	3.7
Oleic (18:1n9)	20.4–26	12	59.5	19.9
Linoleic (18:2n6)	52.4–54.5	27	18.5	49.7
α-Linolenic (18:3n3)	8–8.5	4	2	6.5
γ-Linolenic (18:3n6)				
Arachidonic (20:4n6)	n.d.–0.2	n.d.	0.2	0.2
Eicosapentaenoic (20:5n3)	n.d.	n.d.	n.d.	2.4
Docosahexaenoic (22:6n3)	n.d.–0.1	n.d.	0.1	2.3

Source: Modified from Ref. 2.

TABLE 11 Metanalyses of the Effects of Early or Late Introduction of Intravenous Lipids to Preterm Infants on Mortality and Chronic Lung Disease[a]

Outcome	Early lipid infusion	Late lipid infusion	Relative risk (95% confidence interval)
Death	53/265	50/257	1.01 (0.7–1.4)
Chronic lung disease at 28 days	104/265	99/257	1.03 (0.8–1.3)
Chronic lung disease at 36 weeks	23/96	22/93	1.02 (0.6–1.7)

[a] The results show no increased risk with early introduction of lipid infusion.
Source: Modified from Ref. 158.

tive stress, which might contribute to adverse outcomes (159). Although this hypothesis remains to be tested further, it appears prudent to provide infants and children receiving lipid emulsions with an adequate supply of antioxidants such as vitamin E.

Of the different emulsions available (Table 10), those based on soybean oil have been most extensively evaluated, and they are widely used in pediatric patients. Soybean oil emulsions provide both precursor essential fatty acids of the n-6 and the n-3 series, whereas safflower oil emulsions did not contain appreciable amounts of n-3 fatty acids and are inadequate for the parenteral nutrition of children over more than just a few days. New products with metabolites of the classical essential fatty acids, such as long-chain n-3 fatty acids, have been developed with the aim of improving the fatty acid supply to the infant (Table 10). Also, emulsions with a reduced content of the precursor essential fatty acids achieved by a mixture of soybean oil with MCT or with olive oil may have beneficial effects on infantile essential fatty acid metabolism. An emulsion containing a mixture of soybean oil, providing long-chain fatty acids, and MCT oil was reported to have advantages in adult intensive care patients and in infants.

Advisable for the parenteral nutrition of infants and children are lipid emulsions with a low phospholipid/triglyceride ratio and continuous infusion over about 20 to 24 h/day if that is practically feasible. Initially the daily dose may be increased stepwise from 1 g/kg body weight to 2 to 3 g/kg (see Chap. 17). Dosages above 3 g/kg should be used only in selected cases, with repeated monitoring of serum triglyceride and cholesterol concentrations. The mixture of lipid emulsions, heparin, and high concentrations of calcium may lead to aggregation of the lipid particles (creaming of the emulsion) and should be avoided (160).

Similarly, the serum of children with high concentrations of C-reactive protein (CRP) mixed ex vivo with lipid emulsion induces creaming (161). Since the in vivo effects are not known, it appears prudent to lower the dose of infused lipids to about 0.5 g triglyceride per kilogram of bodyweight per day in patients with a transient rise of CRP to>2 mg/100 mL.

6 OUTLOOK

The provision of lipids and their metabolism are of major importance for growth, body composition, development, and long-term health both of healthy children and of children with gastrointestinal and hepatic disorders. For a long time lipids had been viewed as a largely exchangeable source of energy only. In contrast, today the quantity and particularly the quality of the lipid supply is known to have clinically relevant effects for the outcome of both healthy and sick children. Improved understanding of the basic physiological mechanisms and good clinical research may help us in providing even better patient care in the years to come.

ACKNOWLEDGMENTS

The author is deeply grateful for the fruitful collaboration and stimulating discussions with many fine colleagues, including Thomas Berghaus, Uta Clausen, Hans Demmelmair, Ulrike Diener, Natasa Fidler, Maria Fink, Yvonne Göbel, Martha del Prado, Maria Rodriguez-Palmero, Thorsten Sauerwald, Piotr Socha and Peter Szitanyi, who contributed greatly to the development of the thoughts laid down in this chapter. The author's work is supported in part by Deutsche Forschungsgemeinschaft, Bonn, Germany (Ko 912/5-2) and the 5th Framework Research Program of the European Union, Brussels, Belgium (QLK1-CT-1999-00888).

REFERENCES

1. Koletzko B, Demmelmair H, Socha P. Nutritional support of infants and children: supply and metabolism of lipids. Ballieres Clin Gastroenterol 1998; 12:671–696.
2. Importance of dietary lipids. In: Koletzko B, Tsang R, Zlotkin SH, Nichols B, Hansen JW, eds. Nutrition During Infancy: Principles and Practice. Cincinnati, OH: Digital Educational Publishing, 1997, pp 123–153.
3. Koletzko B. Potential adverse effects of trans fatty acids in infants and children. Eur J Med Res 1995; 1(2):123–125.
4. Koletzko B. Trans fatty acids may impair biosynthesis of long-chain polyunsaturates and growth in man. Acta Paediatr Scand 1992; 81:302–306.
5. Jendryczko A, Gruszczynski J, Tomala J, Szpyrka G. Unsaturated fatty acids of trans isomers in plasma of pregnant women and birth weight. Ginekol Pol 1993; 64(3):113–116.

6. Koletzko B, Decsi T. Metabolic aspects of trans fatty acids. Clin Nutr 1998; 17: 229–237.

7. Innis SM, King DJ. Trans fatty acids in human milk are inversely associated with concentrations of essential all-cis n-6 and n-3 fatty acids and determine trans, but not n-6 and n-3, fatty acids in plasma lipids of breast-fed infants. Am J Clin Nutr 1999; 70(3):383–390.

8. Stender S, Dyerberg J, Holmer G, Ovesen L, Sandstrom B. The influence of trans fatty acids on health: a report from the Danish Nutrition Council (see comments). Clin Sci Colch 1995; 88(4):375–392.

9. Carlson SE, Clandinin MT, Cook HW, Emken EA, Filer LJJ. Trans fatty acids: infant and fetal development. Am J Clin Nutr 1997; 66(3):715S–736S.

10. Precht D, Molkentin J. Effect of feeding on conjugated cis delta 9, trans delta 11-octadecadienoic acid and other isomers of linoleic acid in bovine milk fats. Nahrung 1997; 41(6):330–335.

11. Precht D, Molkentin J. C18:1, C18:2 and C18:3 trans and cis fatty acid isomers including conjugated cis delta 9, trans delta 11 linoleic acid (CLA) as well as total fat composition of German human milk lipids. Nahrung 1999; 43(4):233–244.

12. Moya CS, Vanden HJ, Blanchard SG, Leesnitzer LA, Belury MA. Conjugated linoleic acid is a potent naturally occurring ligand and activator of PPARalpha. J Lipid Res 1999; 40(8):1426–1433.

13. Yamasaki M, Mansho K, Mishima H, Kasai M, Sugano M, Tachibana H, Yamada K. Dietary effect of conjugated linoleic acid on lipid levels in white adipose tissue of Sprague-Dawley rats. Biosci Biotechnol Biochem 1999; 63(6):1104–1106.

14. West DB, Delany JP, Camet PM, Blohm F, Truett AA, Scimeca J. Effects of conjugated linoleic acid on body fat and energy metabolism in the mouse. Am J Physiol 1998; 275(3 pt 2):R667–R672.

15. Nicolosi RJ, Rogers EJ, Kritchevsky D, Scimeca JA, Huth PJ. Dietary conjugated linoleic acid reduces plasma lipoproteins and early aortic atherosclerosis in hypercholesterolemic hamsters. Artery 1997; 22(5):266–277.

16. Ip C, Briggs SP, Haegele AD, Thompson HJ, Storkson J, Scimeca JA. The efficacy of conjugated linoleic acid in mammary cancer prevention is independent of the level or type of fat in the diet. Carcinogenesis 1996; 17(5):1045–1050.

17. Ip C, Scimeca JA. Conjugated linoleic acid and linoleic acid are distinctive modulators of mammary carcinogenesis. Nutr Cancer 1997; 27(2):131–135.

18. Belury MA, Nickel KP, Bird CE, Wu Y. Dietary conjugated linoleic acid modulation of phorbol ester skin tumor promotion. Nutr Cancer 1996; 26(2):149–157.

19. Cesano A, Visonneau S, Scimeca JA, Kritchevsky D, Santoli D. Opposite effects of linoleic acid and conjugated linoleic acid on human prostatic cancer in SCID mice. Anticancer Res 1998; 18(3A):1429–1434.

20. Rodriguez PM, Koletzko B, Kunz C, Jensen R. Nutritional and biochemical properties of human milk: II. Lipids, micronutrients, and bioactive factors. Clin Perinatol 1999; 26(2):335–359.

21. Intestinal lipid absorption. In: Davidson NO, Magun AM, Yamada T, Alpers DH, Owyang C, Powell DW, Silverstein FE, eds. Textbook of Gastroenterology. Philadelphia: Lippincott, 1995, pp 428–455.

22. Jones PJ, MacDougall DE, Ntanios F, Vanstone CA. Dietary phytosterols as choles-

terol-lowering agents in humans. Can J Physiol Pharmacol 1997; 75(3):217–227.

23. Bernback S, Blackberg L, Hernell O. The complete digestion of human milk triacylglycerol in vitro requires gastric lipase, pancreatic co-lipase-dependent lipase, and bile salt stimulated lipase. J Clin Invest 1990; 85:1221–1226.

24. Sbarra V, Mas E, Henderson TR, Hamosh M, Lombardo D, Hamosh P. Digestive lipases of the newborn ferret: compensatory role of milk bile salt-dependent lipase. Pediatr Res 1996; 40(2):263–268.

25. Hamosh M. Digestion in the newborn. Clin Perinatol 1996; 23(2): 191–209.

26. Roberts IM, Jaffe R. Lingual lipase: immunocytochemical localization in the rat von Ebner gland. Gastroenterology 1986; 90(5 pt 1):1170–1175.

27. Fredrikzon B, Hernell O, Blackberg L. Lingual lipase. Its role in lipid digestion in infants with low birthweight and/or pancreatic insufficiency. Acta Paediatr Scand Suppl 1982; 296:75–80.

28. Roberts IM, Hanel SI. Stability of lingual lipase in vivo: studies of the iodinated enzyme in the rat stomach and duodenum. Biochim Biophys Acta 1988; 960(1): 107–110.

29. Blackberg L, Hernell O, Olivecrona T. Hydrolysis of human milk fat globules by pancreatic lipase: role of colipase, phospholipase A2, and bile salts. J Clin Invest 1981; 67(6):1748–1752.

30. Stromqvist M, Hernell O, Hansson L, Lindgren K, Skytt A, Lundberg L, Lidmer AS, Blackberg L. Naturally occurring variants of human milk bile salt–stimulated lipase. Arch Biochem Biophys 1997; 347(1):30–36.

31. Hansson L, Blackberg L, Edlund M, Lundberg L, Stromqvist M, Hernell O. Recombinant human milk bile salt-stimulated lipase: catalytic activity is retained in the absence of glycosylation and the unique proline-rich repeats. J Biol Chem 1993; 268(35):26692–26698.

32. Hamosh M, Bitman J, Liao TH, Mehta NR, Buczek RJ, Wood DL, Grylack LJ, Hamosh P. Gastric lipolysis and fat absorption in preterm infants: effects of medium-chain triglyceride or long-chain triglyceride-containing formulas. Pediatrics 1989; 83:86–92.

33. Chappell JE, Clandinin MT, Kearney-Volpe C, Reichmann B, Swyer PW. Fatty acid balance studies in premature infants fed human milk or formula: effect of calcium supplementation. J Pediatr 1986; 108:439–447.

34. Carnielli VP, Luijendijk IH, Van GJ, Sulkers EJ, Boerlage AA, Degenhart HJ, Sauer PJ. Structural position and amount of palmitic acid in infant formulas: effects on fat, fatty acid, and mineral balance. J Pediatr Gastroenterol Nutr 1996; 23(5): 553–560.

35. Ghosh PK, Saxena RK, Gupta R, Yadav RP, Davidson S. Microbial lipases: production and applications. Sci Prog 1996; 79(pt 2):119–157.

36. Kovac A, Stadler P, Haalck L, Spener F, Paltauf F. Hydrolysis and esterification of acylglycerols and analogs in aqueous medium catalyzed by microbial lipases. Biochim Biophys Acta 1996; 1301(1–2):57–66.

37. Pabai F, Kermasha S, Morin A. Use of continuous culture to screen for lipase-producing microorganisms and interesterification of butter fat by lipase isolates. Can J Microbiol 1996; 42(5):446–452.

38. Greenough RJ, Perry CJ, Stavnsbjerg M. Safety evaluation of a lipase expressed in Aspergillus oryzae. Food Chem Toxicol 1996; 34(2):161–166.
39. Stremmel W, Lotz G, Strohmeyer G, Berk PD. Identification, isolation, and partial characterization of a fatty acid binding protein from rat jejunal microvillous membranes. J Clin Invest 1985; 75(3):1068–1076.
40. Luxon BA, Milliano MT. Cytoplasmic transport of fatty acids in rat enterocytes: role of binding to fatty acid-binding protein. Am J Physiol 1999; 277(2 pt 1):G361–G366.
41. Richieri GV, Ogata RT, Kleinfeld AM. Kinetics of fatty acid interactions with fatty acid binding proteins from adipocyte, heart, and intestine. J Biol Chem 1996; 271(19):11291–11300.
42. Frolov A, Cho TH, Billheimer JT, Schroeder F. Sterol carrier protein-2, a new fatty acyl coenzyme A-binding protein. J Biol Chem 1996; 271(50):31878–31884.
43. Puglielli L, Rigotti A, Amigo L, Nunez L, Greco AV, Santos MJ, Nervi F. Modulation of intrahepatic cholesterol trafficking: evidence by in vivo antisense treatment for the involvement of sterol carrier protein-2 in newly synthesized cholesterol transport into rat bile. Biochem J 1996; 317(pt 3):681–687.
44. Polheim D, David JS, Schultz FM, Wylie MB, Johnston JM. Regulation of triglyceride biosynthesis in adipose and intestinal tissue. J Lipid Res 1973; 14(4):415–421.
45. Shiau YF. Mechanisms of intestinal fat absorption. Am J Physiol 1981; 240(1):G1–G9.
46. Koletzko B. Classification and therapy of hyperlipidaemias. Int Semin Paediatr Gastroenterol Nutr 1996; 5:10–15.
47. Russell DW. Cholesterol biosynthesis and metabolism. Cardiovasc Drugs Ther 1992; 6:103–110.
48. Rudney H, Panini SR. Cholesterol biosynthesis. Curr Opin Lipido 1993; 4:230–237.
49. Wong WW, Hachey DL, Insull W, Opekun AR, Klein PD. Effect of dietary cholesterol on cholesterol synthesis in breast-fed and formula-fed infants. J Lipid Res 1993; 34:1403–1411.
50. Wong WW, Hachey DL, Clarke LL, Zhang S. Cholesterol synthesis and absorption by 2H2O and 18O-cholesterol and hypocholesterolemic effect of soy protein. J Nutr 1995; 125:612S–618S.
51. Wang X, Zelenski NG, Yang J, Sakai J, Brown MS, Goldstein JL. Cleavage of sterol regulatory element binding proteins (SREBPs) by CPP32 during apoptosis. EMBO J 1996; 15(5):1012–1020.
52. Koletzko B, Aggett PJ, Bindels JG, Bung P, Ferre P, Gil A, Lentze MJ, Roberfroid M, Strobel S. Growth, development and differentiation: a functional food science approach. Br J Nutr 1998; 80(suppl 1):S5–S45.
53. Aggett PJ, Haschke F, Heine W, Hernell O, Koletzko B, Lafeber H, Ormisson A, Rey J, Tormo R. ESPGAN Committee on Nutrition Report: childhood diet and prevention of coronary heart disease. J Pediatr Gastroenterol Nutr 1994; 19:261–269.
54. Tint GS, Salen G, Batta AK, Shefer S, Irons M, Elias ER, Abuelo DN, Johnson VP, Lambert M, Lutz R. Correlation of severity and outcome with plasma sterol

levels in variants of the Smith-Lemli-Opitz syndrome. J Pediatr 1995; 127:82–87.

55. Abuelo DN, Tint GS, Kelley R, Batta AK, Shefer S, Salen G. Prenatal detection of the cholesterol biosynthetic defect in the Smith-Lemli-Opitz syndrome by the analysis of amniotic fluid sterols. Am J Med Genet 1995; 56:281–285.

56. Quinet EM, Agellon LB, Kroon PA, et al. Atherogenic diet increases cholesteryl ester transfer protein messenger RNA levels in rabbit liver. J Clin Invest 1990; 85: 357–363.

57. Fomon SJ, Haschke F, Ziegler EE, Nelson SE. Body composition of reference children from birth to age 10 years. Am J Clin Nutr 1982; 35(suppl):1169–1175.

58. Flatt JP. The difference in the storage capacities for carbohydrate and for fat, and its implications in the regulation of body weight. Ann NY Acad Sci 1987;499:104–123.

59. Flatt JP, Ravussin E, Acheson KJ, Jéquier E. Effects of dietary fat on postprandial substrate oxidation and on carbohydrate and fat balances. J Clin Invest 1985; 76: 1019–1024.

60. Lean MEJ, James PT. Metabolic effects of isoenergetic nutrient exchange over 24 hours in relation to obesity in women. Int J Obesity 1988; 12:15–27.

61. Wood JD, Reid JT. The influence of dietary fat on fat metabolism and body fat deposition in meal-feeding and nibbling rats. Br J Nutr 1975; 34:15–24.

62. van Aerde JE, Sauer PJ, Pencharz PB, Smith JM, Heim T, Swyer PR. Metabolic consequences of increasing energy intake by adding lipid to parenteral nutrition in full term infants. Am J Clin Nutr 1994; 59:659–662.

63. Bach AC, Babayan V. Medium-chain triglycerides: an update. Am J Clin Nutr 1982; 36:950–962.

64. Baba N, Bracco EF, Hashim SA. Enhanced thermogenesis and diminished deposition of fat in response to overfeeding with diet containing medium chain triglyceride. Am J Clin Nutr 1982; 35:678–682.

65. Borum PR. Medium-chain triglycerides in formula for preterm neonates: implications for hepatic and extrahepatic metabolism. J Pediatr 1992; 120:S139–S145.

66. Rebouche CJ, Panagides DD, Nelson SE. Role of carnitine in utilization of dietary medium-chain triglycerides by term infants. Am J Clin Nutr 1990; 52:820–824.

67. Sarda P, Lepage G, Roy CC, Chessex P. Storage of medium-chain triglycerides in adipose tissue of orally fed infants. Am J Clin Nutr 1987; 45:399–405.

68. Carnielli V, Sulkers EJ, Moretti C, Wattimena JL, van Goudoever JB, Degenhart HJ, Zachello F, Sauer PJ. Conversion of octanoic acid into long-chain saturated fatty acids in premature infants fed a formula containing medium-chain triglycerides. Metabolism 1994; 43:1287–1292.

69. Seaton TB, Welle SL, Warenko MK, Campbell RG. Thermic effect of medium-chain and long-chain triglycerides in man. Am J Clin Nutr 1986; 44:630–634.

70. Brooke OG. Energy balance and metabolic rate in preterm infants fed standard and high-energy formulas. Br J Nutr 1980; 44:13–23.

71. Whyte RK, Campbell D, Stanhope R, Bayley HS, Sinclair JC. Energy balance in low birth weight infants fed formula of high or low medium-chain triglyceride content. J Pediatr 1986; 108:964–971.

72. American Academy of Pediatrics. National Cholesterol Education Program. Report

of the expert panel on blood cholesterol levels in children and adolescents. Pediatrics 1992; 89:525–584.

73. Koletzko B. Response to and range of acceptable fat intakes in infants and children. Eur J Clin Nutr 1999; 53 (suppl 1):S78–S83.

74. Galli C, Visioli F. Antioxidant and other activities of phenolics in olives/olive oil, typical components of the Mediterranean diet. Lipids 1999;34(suppl):S23–S26.

75. de-la-Torre BM. Scientific basis for the health benefits of the Mediterranean diet. Drugs Exp Clin Res 1999; 25(2–3):155–161.

76. Koletzko B, Dokoupil K, Reitmayr S, Weimert-Harendza B, Keller E. Dietary fat intake in infants and primary school children in Germany. Am J Clin Nutr 2000; 72:13925–13985.

77. Lifshitz F, Moses N. Growth failure. A complication of dietary treatment of hypercholesterolemia. Am J Dis Child 1989; 143:537–542.

78. Ortega RM, Requejo AM, Andres P, Lopez SA, Redondo R, Gonzalez FM. Relationship between diet composition and body mass index in a group of Spanish adolescents. Br J Nutr 1995; 74(6):765–773.

79. Tucker LA, Seljaas GT, Hager RL. Body fat percentage of children varies according to their diet composition. J Am Diet Assoc 1997; 97(9):981–986.

80. Gazzaniga JM, Burns TL. Relationship between diet composition and body fatness, with adjustment for resting energy expenditure and physical activity, in preadolescent children. Am J Clin Nutr 1993; 58(1):21–28.

81. Koletzko S, Koletzko B, Reinhardt D. Aktuelle Aspekte der Ernährungstherapie bei zystischer Fibrose. Monatsschr Kinderheilkd 1994;142:432–445.

82. Corey M, McLaughlin FJ, Williams M, Levison H. A comparison of survival, growth, and pulmonary function in patients with cystic fibrosis in Boston and Toronto. J Clin Epidemiol 1988; 41:583–591.

83. Morgan JB, Kimber AC, Redfern AM, Stordy BJ. Healthy eating for infants—mothers' attitudes. Acta Paediatr 1995; 84(5):512–515.

84. Niinikoski H, Viikari J, Ronnemaa T, Helenius H, Jokinen E, Lapinleimu H, Routi T, Lagstrom H, Seppanen R, Valimaki I, et al. Regulation of growth of 7- to 36-month-old children by energy and fat intake in the prospective, randomized STRIP baby trial. Pediatrics 1997; 100(5):810–816.

85. Niinikoski H, Lapinleimu H, Viikari J, Ronnemaa T, Jokinen E, Seppanen R, Terho P, Tuominen J, Valimaki I, Simell O. Growth until 3 years of age in a prospective, randomized trial of a diet with reduced saturated fat and cholesterol. Pediatrics 1997; 99(5):687–694.

86. Cohen SA, Hendricks KM, Eastham EJ, Mathis RK, Walker WA. Chronic nonspecific diarrhea: a complication of dietary fat restriction. Am J Dis Child 1979; 133:490–492.

87. Canadian Pediatric Society and Health Canada Working Group Nutrition Recommendations Update: Dietary Fat and Children. Ottawa: Health Canada, 1993.

88. Voss A, Reinhart M, Sankarappa S, Sprecher H. The metabolism of 7,10,13,16,19-docosapentaenoic acid to 4,7,10,13,16,19-docosahexaenoic acid in rat liver is independent of a 4-desaturase. J Biol Chem 1991; 266:19995–20000.

89. Sauerwald T, Hachey DL, Jensen CL, Chen H, Anderson RE, Heird WC. Intermedi-

ates in endogenous synthesis of C22:6w3 and C20:4w6 by term and preterm infants. Pediatr Res 1997; 41:183–187.

90. Clandinin MT, Chappell JE, Leong S, Heim T, Swyer PR, Chance GW. Intrauterine fatty acid accretion in human brain: implications for fatty acid requirements. Early Hum Dev 1980; 4:121–129.

91. Martinez M. Tissue levels of polyunsaturated fatty acids during early human development. J Pediatr 1992; 120:S129–S138.

92. Innis SM. n-3 Fatty acid requirements of the newborn. Lipids 1992; 27(11):879–885.

93. Supply and biological effects of long-chain polyunsaturated fatty acids (LCPUFA) in premature infants. In: Koletzko B, Diener U, Fink M, et al. Ziegler E, Lucas A, Moro G, editors. Nutrition of the Extremely Low Birthweight Infant. Philadelphia: Lippincott-Raven, 1999; pp. 33–52.

94. Koletzko B, Müller L. Cis- and trans-isomeric fatty acids in plasma lipids of newborn infants and their mothers. Biol Neonate 1990; 57:172–178.

95. Berghaus TM, Demmelmair H, Koletzko B. Fatty acid composition of lipid classes in maternal and cord plasma at birth. Eur J Pediatr 1998; 157(9):763–768.

96. Kuhn DC, Crawford MA, Stevens P. Transport and metabolism of essential fatty acids by the human placenta. Contr Gynecol Obstet 1985; 13:139–140.

97. Kunz C, Rodriguez PM, Koletzko B, Jensen R. Nutritional and biochemical properties of human milk: Part I. General aspects, proteins, and carbohydrates. Clin Perinatol 1999; 26(2):307–333.

98. Genzel-Boroviczeny O, Wahle J, Koletzko B. Fatty acid composition of human milk during the first month after term and preterm delivery. Eur J Pediatr 1997; 156:142–147.

99. Koletzko B, Thiel I, Abiodun PO. The fatty acid composition of human milk in Europe and Africa. J Pediatr 1992; 120:S62–S70.

100. Makrides M, Neumann MA, Gibson RA. Effect of maternal docosahexaenoic acid (DHA) supplementation on breast milk composition. Eur J Clin Nutr 1996; 50(6):352–357.

101. Cherian G, Sim JS. Changes in the breast milk fatty acids and plasma lipids of nursing mothers following consumption of n-3 polyunsaturated fatty acid enriched eggs. Nutrition 1996; 12(1):8–12.

102. Rocquelin G, Tapsoba S, Dop MC, Mbemba F, Traissac P, Martin PY. Lipid content and essential fatty acid (EFA) composition of mature Congolese breast milk are influenced by mothers' nutritional status: impact on infants' EFA supply. Eur J Clin Nutr 1998; 52(3):164–171.

103. Guesnet P, Antoine JM, Rochette-de LJ, Galent A, Durand G. Polyunsaturated fatty acid composition of human milk in France: changes during the course of lactation and regional differences. Eur J Clin Nutr 1993; 47(10):700–710.

104. Genzel BO, Wahle J, Koletzko B. Fatty acid composition of human milk during the 1st month after term and preterm delivery. Eur J Pediatr 1997; 156(2):142–147.

105. Serra G, Marletta A, Bonacci W, Campone F, Bertini I, Lantieri PB, Risso D, Ciangherotti S. Fatty acid composition of human milk in Italy. Biol Neonate 1997; 72(1):1–8.

106. Helland IB, Saarem K, Saugstad OD, Drevon CA. Fatty acid composition in maternal milk and plasma during supplementation with cod liver oil. Eur J Clin Nutr 1998; 52:839–845.
107. de-la-Presa OS, Lopez SM, Rivero UM. Fatty acid composition of human milk in Spain. J Pediatr Gastroenterol Nutr 1996; 22(2):180–185.
108. Can infant formula be made more similar to human milk? In: Koletzko B, Fitzpatrick DW, L'Abbe ML, eds. Proceedings of the 16th International Congress on Nutrition—Nutrition Montreal 97. Ottawa, Ontario: Canadian Federation of Biological Societies, 1998, pp 97–100.
109. Koletzko B, Thiel I, Abiodun PO. Fatty acid composition of mature human milk in Nigeria. Z Ernährungwiss 1991; 30:289–297.
110. Koletzko B, Sauerwald T, Demmelmair H. Safety of stable isotope use. Eur J Pediatr 1997; 156(Suppl 1):S12–S17.
111. Demmelmair H, Baumheuer M, Koletzko B, Dokoupil K, Kratl G. Metabolism of U13C-labelled linoleic acid in lactating women. J Lipid Res 1998; 39:1389–1396.
112. Koletzko B, Bremer HJ. Fat content and fatty acid composition of infant formulas. Acta Pediatr Scand 1989; 78:513–521.
113. Decsi T, Behrendt E, Koletzko B. Fatty acid composition of Hungarian infant formulae revisited. Acta Paediatr Hung 1994; 34:107–116.
114. Koletzko B. Lipid supply for infants with special needs. Eur J Med Res 1997; 2(2): 69–73.
115. Demmelmair H, Sauerwald T, Koletzko B, Richter T. New insights into lipid and fatty acid metabolism via stable isotopes. Eur J Pediatr 1997; 156(suppl 1):S70–S74.
116. Demmelmair H, von Schenck U, Behrendt E, Sauerwald T, Koletzko B. Estimation of arachidonic acid synthesis in full term neonates using natural variation of 13C content. J Pediatr Gastroenterol Nutr 1995; 21(1):31–36.
117. Szitanyi P, Koletzko B, Mydlilova A, Demmelmair H. Metabolism of 13C-labeled linoleic acid in newborn infants during the first week of life. Pediatr Res 1999; 45(5 pt 1):669–673.
118. Sauerwald T, Hachey DL, Jensen CL, Chen H, Anderson RE, Heird WC. Effect of dietary α-linolenic acid intake on incorporation of docosahexaenoic and arachidonic acids into plasma phospholipids of term infants. Lipids 1996; 31:S131–S135.
119. Koletzko B, Schmidt E, Bremer HJ, Haug M, Harzer G. Effects of dietary long-chain polyunsaturated fatty acids on the essential fatty acid status of premature infants. Eur J Pediatr 1989; 148:669–675.
120. Carlson SE, Wilson WW. Docosahexaenoic acid (DHA) supplementation of preterm (PT) infants: effect on the 12-month Bayley mental developmental index (MDI) (abstr). Pediatr Res 1994; 35:20A.
121. Koletzko B, Edenhofer S, Lipowsky G, Reinhardt D. Effects of a low birthweight infant formula containing docosahexaenoic and arachidonic acids at human milk levels. J Pediatr Gastroenterol Nutr 1995; 21:200–208.
122. Decsi T, Thiel I, Koletzko B. Essential fatty acid status in full-term infants fed breast milk or formula. Arch Dis Child 1995; 72:F23–F28.
123. Carlson SE, Ford AJ, Werkman SH, Peeples JM, Koo WK. Visual acuity and fatty acid status of term infants fed human milk and formulas with and without docosa-

hexaenoate and arachidonate from egg yolk lecithin. Pediatr Res 1996; 39:882–888.

124. Makrides M, Neumann MA, Byard RW, Simmer K, Gibson RA. Fatty acid composition of brain, retina, and erythrocytes in breast- and formula-fed infants. Am J Clin Nutr 1994; 60:189–194.

125. Farquharson J, Cockburn F, Patrick WA, Jamieson EC, Logan RW. Infant cerebral cortex phospholipid fatty-acid composition and diet. Lancet 1992; 340:810–813.

126. Carlson SE, Werkman SH. A randomized trial of visual attention of preterm infants fed docosahexaenoic acid until two months. Lipids 1996; 31(1):85–90.

127. Decsi T, Koletzko B. Growth, fatty acid composition of plasma lipid classes, and plasma retinol and tocopherol concentrations in fullterm infants fed formula enriched with long-chain polyunsaturated fatty acids. Acta Paediatr 1995; 84:725–732.

128. Uauy R, Birch DG, Birch EE, Tyson JE, Hoffman DR. Effect of dietary omega-3 fatty acids on retinal function of very-low-birth-weight neonates. Pediatr Res 1990; 28:485–492.

129. Agostoni C, Trojan S, Bellu R, Riva E, Giovannini M. Neurodevelopmental quotient of healthy term infants at 4 months and feeding practice: the role of long-chain polyunsaturated fatty acids. Pediatr Res 1995; 38:262–266.

130. Birch EE, Hoffman DR, Uauy R, Birch DG, Prestidge C. Visual acuity and the essentiality of docosahexaenoic acid and arachidonic acid in the diet of term infants. Pediatr Res 1998; 44(2):201–209.

131. Willatts P, Forsyth JS, DiModugno MK, Varma S, Colvin M. Effect of long-chain polyunsaturated fatty acids in infant formula on problem solving at 10 months of age. Lancet 1998; 352(9129):688–691.

132. Scott DT, Janowsky JS, Carroll RE, Taylor JA, Auestad N, Montalto MB. Formula supplementation with long-chain polyunsaturated fatty acids: are there developmental benefits? Pediatrics 1998; 102(5):E59.

133. Lucas A, Morley R. Efficacy and safety of long-chain polyunsaturated fatty acid supplementation of infant-formula milk: a randomised trial. Lancet 2000; 352:1703–1705.

134. Carlson SE, Cooke RJ, Werkman SH, Tolley EA. First year growth of preterm infants fed standard compared to marine oil n-3 supplemented formula. Lipids 1992; 27:901–907.

135. Carlson SE, Werkman SH, Peeples JM, et al. Growth and development of premature infants in relation to n-3 and n-6 fatty acid status. In: Galli C, Simopoulos AP, Tremoli E, eds. Fatty Acids and Lipids: Biological Aspects. Basel, Karger, 1994; pp 63–69.

136. Koletzko B, Braun M. Arachidonic acid and early human growth: is there a relation? Ann Nutr Metab 1991; 35:128–131.

137. Leaf AA, Leighfield MJ, Costeloe KL, Crawford MA. Long chain polyunsaturated fatty acids and fetal growth. Early Hum Dev 1992; 30:183–191.

138. Koletzko B, Agostoni C, Carlson SE, Clandinin MT, Hornstra G, Neuringer M, Uauy R, Yamashiro Y, Willatts P. Long chain polyunsaturated fatty acids (LC-PUFA) and perinatal development. Acta Paediatr. In press.

139. Keicher U, Koletzko B, Reinhardt D. Omega-3 fatty acids suppress the enhanced

production of 5-lipoxygenase products from polymorph neutrophil granulocytes in cystic fibrosis. Eur J Clin Invest 1995; 25:915–919.

140. Endres S, Ghorbani R, Kelley VE, Georgilis K, Lonnemann G, Van der Meer JWM, Cannon JG, Rogers TS, Klempner MS, Weber PC, et al. The effect of dietary supplementation with n-3 polyunsaturated fatty acids on the synthesis of interleukin-1 and tumor necrosis factor by mononuclear cells. N Engl J Med 1989; 320:265–271.

141. Miles EA, Calder PC. Modulation of immune function by dietary fatty acids. Proc Nutr Soc 1998; 57(2):277–292.

142. Lorenz R, Weber PC, Szimnau P, Heldwein W, Strasser T, Loeschke K. Supplementation with n-3 fatty acids from fish oil in chronic inflammatory bowel disease—a randomized, placebo-controlled, double-blind cross-over trial. J Intern Med Suppl 1989; 225(731):225–232.

143. Campbell JM, Fahey-GC J, Lichtensteiger CA, Demichele SJ, Garleb KA. An enteral formula containing fish oil, indigestible oligosaccharides, gum arabic and antioxidants affects plasma and colonic phospholipid fatty acid and prostaglandin profiles in pigs. J Nutr 1997; 127(1):137–145.

144. James MJ, Cleland LG. Dietary n-3 fatty acids and therapy for rheumatoid arthritis. Semin Arthritis Rheum 1997; 27(2):85–97.

145. Katz DP, Manner T, Furst P, Askanazi J. The use of an intravenous fish oil emulsion enriched with omega-3 fatty acids in patients with cystic fibrosis. Nutrition 1996; 12(5):334–339.

146. Wachtler P, Konig W, Senkal M, Kemen M, Koller M. Influence of a total parenteral nutrition enriched with omega-3 fatty acids on leukotriene synthesis of peripheral leukocytes and systemic cytokine levels in patients with major surgery. J Trauma 1997; 42(2):191–198.

147. Field CJ, Thomson C, van Aerde J, et al. The effects of supplementing preterm formula with long-chain unsaturated fatty acids on immune phenotypes and cytokine production (abstr). J Pediatr Gastroenterol Nutr 1998; 26:590.

148. Yu G, Bjorksten B. Serum levels of phospholipid fatty acids in mothers and their babies in relation to allergic disease. Eur J Pediatr 1998; 157(4):298–303.

149. Yu G, Kjellman NI, Bjorksten B. Phospholipid fatty acids in cord blood: family history and development of allergy. Acta Paediatr 1996; 85(6):679–683.

150. Cabre E, Periago JL, Abad-Lacruz A, Gil A, Gonzales-Huix F, Sanchez de Medina F, Gassull MA. Polyunsaturated fatty acid deficiency in liver cirrhosis: its relation to associated protein-energy malnutrition (preliminary report). Am J Gastroenterol 1988; 83:712–717.

151. Gonzales J, Periago JL, Gil A, Cabre E, Abad-Lacruz A, Gassull MA, Sanchez de Medina F. Malnutrition-related polyunsaturated fatty acid changes in plasma lipid fractions of cirrhotic patients. Metabolism 1992; 41:954–960.

152. Socha P, Koletzko B, Pawlowska J, Socha J. Essential fatty acid status in children with cholestasis, in relation to serum bilirubin concentration. J Pediatr 1997; 131(5): 700–706.

153. Socha P, Koletzko B, Pawlowska J, Proszynska K, Socha J. Treatment of cholestatic children with water-soluble vitamin E (alpha-tocopheryl polyethylene glycol succinate): effects on serum vitamin E, lipid peroxides, and polyunsaturated fatty acids. J Pediatr Gastroenterol Nutr 1997; 24(2):189–193.

154. Die Bedeutung der Fettapplikation in der Ernährungstherapie von Säuglingen und Kleinkindern. In: Koletzko B. Grünert A, Reinauer H, eds. Fettemulsionen: Betrachtungen zur Pathophysiologie, Toxikologie und klinischen Anwendung. München: Zuckschwerdt Verlag, 1993, pp 116–121.

155. Stoffwechsel einer Lipidemulsion bei parenteral ernährten Neugeborenen: Analyse der Plasma-Lipoproteine. In: Koletzko B. Grünert A, Reinauer H, eds. Fettemulsionen: Betrachtungen zur Pathophysiologie, Toxikologie und klinischen Anwendung. München: Zuckschwerdt Verlag, 1993, pp 122–128.

156. Koletzko B, Filler RM, Heim T. Immaturity alters plasma lipoprotein composition of intravenously alimented newborn infants. Eur J Med Res 1998; 3:89–94.

157. Haumont D, Deckelbaum RJ, Richelle M, Dahlan W, Coussaert E, Bihain BE, Carpentier YA. Plasma lipid and plasma lipoprotein concentrations in low birth weight infants given parenteral nutrition with twenty or ten percent lipid emulsion. J Pediatr 1989; 115:787–793.

158. Wilson DC, Fox GF, Ohlsson A. Meta-analyses of effects of early or late introduction of intravenous lipid to preterm infants on mortality and chronic lung disease (abstr). J Pediatr Gastroenterol Nutr 1998; 26:597.

159. Neuzil J, Darlow BA, Inder TE, Sluis KB, Winterbourn CC, Stocker R. Oxidation of parenteral lipid emulsion by ambient and phototherapy lights: potential toxicity of routine parenteral feeding. J Pediatr 1995; 126:785–790.

160. Raupp P, von Kries R, Schmidt E, Pfahl HG, Günther O. Incompatibility between fat emulsion and calcium plus heparin in parenteral nutrition of premature babies. Lancet 1988; 1:700.

161. Lindh A, Johansson B, Lindholm M, Rössner S. Agglutinate formation in serum samples mixed with intravenous fat emulsions. Crit Care Med 1985; 13:151–154.

162. Störungen des Lipidstoffwechsels. In: Koletzko B. Reinhardt D, eds. Therapie der Krankheiten im Kindes- und Jugendalter, 6th ed. Berlin: Springer, 1997, pp 127–135.

163. Berghaus T, Demmelmair H, Koletzko B. Fatty acid composition of lipid classes in maternal and cord plasma at birth. Eur J Pediatr 1998; 157:763–768.

164. The role of long-chain polyunsaturated fatty acids for infant growth and development. In: Koletzko B, Decsi T, Bendich A, Deckelbaum R, eds. Preventive Nutrition: Primary and Secondary Prevention. Totowa, NJ: Humana Press, 2000. In press.

165. Sauerwald TU, Demmelmair H, Fidler N, Koletzko B. Polyunsaturated fatty acid supply with human milk. In: Koletzko B, Hernell O, Michaelsen KF, eds. Short and Long Term Effects of Breast Feeding on Child Health. Advances in Experimental Medicine and Biology, Vol. 248. New York, Kluwer Academic/Plenum Publishers 2000:261–270.

3

Modulators of Gut Growth and Intestinal Well-Being

Barbara Stoll and Douglas G. Burrin
USDA/ARS Children's Nutrition Research Center, Baylor College
of Medicine, Houston, Texas

1 NUTRIENTS AS GROWTH MODULATORS

1.1 Overview

Gut growth is affected by numerous nutritional and nonnutritional factors. A number of important observations over the past decade led to the general conclusion that the trophic effects of these factors are mediated by changes in both cellular metabolism and gene expression. However, the diet is the most potent stimulus of gastrointestinal mucosal growth. The diet stimulates gut growth directly by providing nutrients locally to the mucosal cells, but also indirectly by triggering the release of humoral substances (e.g., gut hormones) and activating neural pathways. Moreover, the intestinal trophic effects of nutrition are highly dependent on the route of administration, rate of input, and, to a lesser extent, dietary composition. Given that the cells within the gut are continually replaced, it is generally held that cell proliferation is a key regulatory point influenced by nutrition. However, it is now widely recognized that the processes of differentiation, cell migration, and programmed cell death (i.e., apoptosis) are also affected by nutrition. It is also critical to recognize that maintaining intestinal structure and morphology with proper nutrition has an important bearing on intestinal functions, such as immune surveillance and host defense, as well as digestion and absorption of the diet.

1.2   Route of Nutrient Delivery and Dietary Composition

The gut is dependent on nutrition not only to maintain structure and function but also to sustain the renewal of epithelial cells and overall growth. Fasting or starvation results in marked loss of gut tissue mass, blunted villi, and generalized increased catabolism; these catabolic effects are proportionally greater at earlier stages of development (1–3). However, when nutrition is provided to the gut, it is critical that it be provided enterally, in order to sustain normal mucosal growth and function. The importance of enteral nutrition for intestinal development starts during fetal life, when ingestion of amniotic fluid stimulates gut growth (4). Then at birth, the route of nutrition shifts exclusively to the enteral route, in the form of breast milk or formula, which further provides a potent stimulus for intestinal growth and functional development (5,6). However, in many infants, especially those born preterm, who either cannot tolerate enteral feeding or suffer from compromised intestinal function, nutritional support is provided exclusively via the parenteral route (i.e., total parenteral nutrition, or TPN), thereby depriving the intestine of luminal nutrients. Studies in neonatal animals (7–11) and adult humans (12) have shown that TPN results in gut atrophy, net loss of protein, decreased cell proliferation, decreased activity of some brush-border disaccharidases, and increased intestinal permeability. To counteract the adverse impact of TPN and prime the gut, neonatologists often provide small volumes of enteral nutrition to TPN-fed infants, referred to as *minimal enteral feeding*; this has been shown to enhance gastrointestinal motility and function (13,14) (see Chap. 8). However, while these clinical studies indicated a stimulatory effect of relatively low levels of enteral nutrition, recent studies in neonatal piglets have shown that an enteral intake of 20% of the total is necessary to prevent gut protein loss, while an intake of at least 40% is needed to significantly increase growth (7,8).

Additional considerations regarding enteral nutrition are whether it is provided orally, intragastrically, as a bolus, or continuously (15). Studies in piglets (16) demonstrated that gut growth was similar regardless of whether animals were either orally fed cow's milk formula or intragastrically fed an isocaloric, isonitrogenous elemental diet. However, a rat study showed that feeding the same diet intragastrically versus orally depressed weight gain (17). Further studies in piglets suggest that bolus feeding is more trophic to the gut than continuous feeding (18).

Nutrient composition is another important factor that influences the impact of enteral nutrition on gut growth and function. Elemental diets, which usually do not contain fiber, maintain the growth and morphological structure of the proximal gut, but the effect is progressively diminished, such that the distal small intestine and colon become atrophied, as with TPN (19). Moreover, feeding elemental diets is associated with disruption of the microflora and bacterial translocation in the distal gut (20–23), but this can be reversed by adding fiber to the diet. Several studies indicate that restriction of dietary protein, energy, or both generally suppress gut growth and immune function (24–26). However, because the gut can utilize dietary amino acids as they are absorbed, growth of the gut is maintained to a much greater extent than skeletal muscle during protein restriction (27). Much less is known about the relative intestinal trophic effects of macronutrients (e.g., carbohydrate, amino acids, and lipid) in infants and young animals. Studies in rats suggest that nonmetabolizable substrates are trophic and that complex forms of nutrients—such as disaccharides, long-chain triglycerides, and intact proteins—are more trophic than their simple forms (glucose, fatty acids, and amino acids) (2). However, active transport does not seem to be required to produce a trophic stimulus. Recent studies in neonatal piglets suggest that the stimulatory effects of carbohydrate, amino acids, and lipid are not markedly different. Interestingly, enteral amino acids, but not carbohydrate or lipid, stimulated intestinal protein synthesis, whereas each of these stimulated gut protein accretion, suggesting that carbohydrate and lipid suppressed gut proteolysis (28). In contrast, other studies have shown that enteral amino acids rapidly decrease intestinal protein synthesis and proteolysis in young pigs (29). Studies in rats that were refed after a 72-hr fast demonstrated that when casein, starch, or lipid was provided at isocaloric intakes, lipid most effectively restored normal intestinal growth (30). Consistent with this finding, parenteral infusion of lipid was shown to stimulate intestinal protein synthesis more than either glucose or glutamine (31).

1.3 Amino Acids and Polyamines

Of the specific nutrients examined for their intestinal trophic actions, glutamine has been studied most extensively. Glutamine and glutamate are two of the most important nonessential amino acids. Glutamate, the center of transamination reactions in the body (Fig. 1), is synthesized and catabolized via transamination of α-ketoglutarate. Glutamine is synthesized from amidation of glutamate via glutamine synthetase and catabolized via deamidation back to glutamate via glutaminase (Fig. 2). Glutamine is also the most abundant amino acid in the blood (500 to 900 µM), and it makes up more than 60% of the free intracellular amino acid pool (32). From a metabolic standpoint, glutamine is unique in that it functions not only as a key respiratory fuel for rapidly proliferating cells such as enterocytes and lymphocytes but also as an important precursor of nucleic acids, nucleotides, amino sugars, amino acids, and glutathione in intestinal health and disease

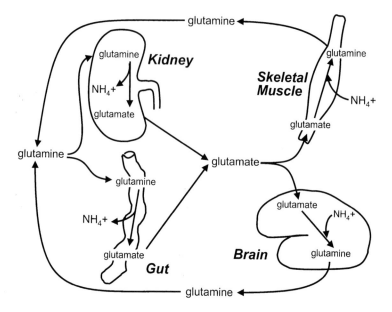

FIGURE 1   Transport of ammonia (NH_3) from peripheral tissues to visceral organs via glutamine-glutamate cycles.

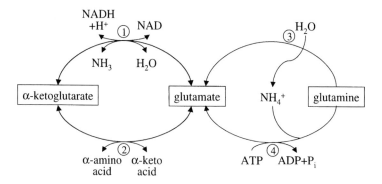

FIGURE 2   Synthesis and degradation of glutamine and glutamate. (1) Glutamate dehydrogenase; (2) alanine aminotransferase, aspartate aminotransferase, or branched-chain amino acid aminotransferase; (3) glutaminase; (4) glutamine synthetase.

(33–37). From a clinical perspective, glutamine is considered to be a critical metabolic fuel because it is rapidly mobilized (via de novo synthesis and proteolysis) and released from peripheral tissues, mainly skeletal muscle, during catabolic stress, sepsis, and injury (38–40).

The importance of glutamine to the gut stems from the seminal studies of Windmueller and others (see review in Ref. 41), which demonstrated that there is substantial utilization and oxidation of arterial and luminal glutamine by the intestine. Based on these observations, glutamine has been postulated as the preferred respiratory fuel for the gut (42). After surgery or injury, the intestinal tract increases its rate of glutamine consumption, and this appears to be regulated in part by corticosteroids. Intestinal glutamine uptake increases by >50% after laparotomy, a response which can be reproduced by the administration of exogenous glucocorticoids (43). During stress states, the requirement for glutamine by other tissues, especially the gut, may outstrip the synthetic capacity of skeletal muscle. Thus glutamine, a nonessential amino acid under conditions of health, may become ''conditionally essential'' in catabolic or stressed states (44).

Numerous studies demonstrate that glutamine supplementation improves the structural integrity and growth of the intestine during catabolic conditions associated with gastrointestinal disease and TPN. In rats, glutamine-supplemented TPN prevented increases in TPN-induced intestinal permeability and atrophy (45), improved gut recovery following starvation atrophy (46), and enhanced structure and function of transplanted small intestine (47). In humans, glutamine-supplemented TPN attenuated TPN-related increased intestinal permeability, preserved intestinal mucosal morphology, improved nitrogen balance, lowered the rate of clinical infection and microbial colonization, and shortened hospital stays after bone marrow transplantation (48,49).

In rats, enterally administered glutamine increased growth and absorptive capacity of intestinal mucosa after malnutrition (50) and reduced bacterial translocation after small bowel transplantation (47). TPN-fed low-birth-weight infants who were given minimal enteral feedings supplemented with glutamine experienced less hospital-acquired sepsis, an improved tolerance of enteral feeding, and an altered amino acid profile consistent with decreased metabolism; they also incurred decreased hospital costs (51) (see also Chap. 8). The mechanism whereby glutamine decreases bacterial translocation may be that it functions as precursor for glucosamines, which are involved in the formation of mucus and intercellular junctional complexes, both of which are critical for mucosal integrity. In vitro models (Caco2 cells, IEC-6 cells) have shown that inhibition of endogenous glutamine synthesis or deprivation of exogenous glutamine from the apical rather than the basolateral side reduces expression of disaccharidases, glucoamylase, ATPase, decreases cell proliferation and differentiation, and increases bacterial translocation (52–54).

In contrast to the studies demonstrating a stimulatory effect of glutamine, some studies have shown no effect of glutamine on gut growth and function. In healthy infant pigs, glutamine supplementation, either parenterally (55) or enterally (56), did not confer any trophic effects on the intestinal mucosa. Similarly, studies with rats have shown that supplementing either an elemental or chow diet with glutamine did not enhance gut growth after small bowel resection (57,58). Thus, the trophic effects of glutamine may be more evident in compromised states such as TPN, sepsis, and diarrhea, whereas in healthy animals, glutamine provides limited benefit. Additional clinical studies are necessary to confirm the beneficial effects of glutamine supplementation on gut growth and function in humans.

Since the original studies of Windmueller and others, there has been considerable research that has focused primarily on glutamine as the preferred fuel for intestinal mucosal cells. However, it is interesting to note that early studies (see review in Ref. 41) indicated that the intestinal metabolism of glutamine and glutamate is essentially identical and that approximately 60% of the carbon of both precursors is oxidized to CO_2. A study in rats (59) showed that adding 4% glutamate to an elemental diet deficient in both glutamine and glutamate significantly increased intestinal growth, crypt cell mitosis, and lactase activity without affecting body weight gain. Taken together, these studies suggest a perhaps equally important metabolic role for glutamate, contradicting the widely held belief that glutamine is the major or preferred fuel for intestinal growth (60). Indeed, studies in humans have shown that the splanchnic extraction of enteral glutamate exceeds that of glutamine (61), while in piglets, dietary glutamate is almost completely metabolized by the small intestine (62) and represents the single most important contributor to mucosal oxidative energy generation (63).

The importance of glutamine to gut metabolism appears to go beyond its role as an oxidative fuel. Studies using isolated perfused rat small intestine (64) demonstrated that inhibition of glutaminase/amidotransferase reactions, but not glutamine synthetase, decreased glutamine gut consumption and deteriorated tissue function. The authors concluded that although glutamine is dispensable as a metabolic fuel for the intestinal mucosa, it is necessary for the provision of nitrogen precursors for mucosal anabolic pathways, an optimal substrate mix for the liver, and citrulline, which is a key precursor for arginine synthesis for the whole organism. A number of studies with adult rats, neonatal pigs, and porcine enterocytes demonstrated that glutamine/glutamate are precursors for synthesis of several nonessential amino acids, including alanine, aspartate, proline, citrulline, and arginine (63,65–68). In addition, Reeds et al. (69) reported that luminal glutamate, rather than glutamine-derived glutamate, is the preferential source of glutathione synthesis (Fig. 3) in the intestinal mucosa of the infant pig, suggesting a highly compartmentalized catabolism of intestinal glutamate and glutamine. Furthermore, a study in burned rats (70) showed that despite increased glutamine

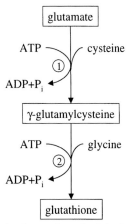

(γ-glutamylcysteinylglycine)

FIGURE 3 Glutathione synthesis from glutamate, cysteine, and glycine. (1) γ-Glutamylcysteine synthetase, (2) glutathione synthetase.

utilization by the intestine after burn injury, intestinal glutathione levels were higher in rats fed a glutamate-supplemented diet than in rats given a glutamine-supplemented or isonitrogenous control diet. In both glutamate- and glutamine-supplemented groups, mucosal protein synthesis was higher (glutamate > glutamine) than in the control group. These results suggest that enteral supplementation of glutamate may be as effective as glutamine in enhancing gut mucosal function during stress states.

Studies with cultured enterocytes demonstrate that glutamine stimulates cell proliferation, expression of ornithine decarboxylase (ODC) and immediate early genes (c-*jun*), and polyamine synthesis (71,72). Glutamine also suppresses enterocyte apoptosis, suggesting that it may be an important survival factor (73). In a recent review, Rhoads (74) postulated that glutamine stimulates cell proliferation by a signaling mechanism that involves the activation of two related but distinct classes of mitogen-activated protein kinases. Although the mitogenic effects of glutamine appear to be dependent on its metabolism, they cannot, interestingly, be reproduced with glutamate. This apparent specificity of glutamine as a crypt cell mitogen may be explained by the fact that the crypt cell lines used in these studies had a limited capacity to transport glutamate across the cell membrane. Yet this contradicts the findings of extensive intestinal glutamate metabolism documented in vivo (41,62). On the other hand, it may be that crypt cells are capable of basolateral transport of blood-borne glutamine (but not glutamate) for proliferative processes, but as they differentiate and mature, they acquire the ability to transport luminal glutamate for use as a metabolic fuel and as a biosynthetic precursor. This idea is supported by evidence showing that glutamine transport was high in undifferentiated Caco-2 cells, but in confluent differentiated cells, glutamine transport was decreased, whereas glutamate transport was substantially increased (75).

Studies in infant pigs have shown that the small intestine is an important site of proline and arginine synthesis (Fig. 4) (63,76,77). Similarly, in adult rats and weaning pigs (65,78), intestinal citrulline synthesis from glutamine, glutamate, and proline is the main source for circulating citrulline, which plays a critical role in arginine homeostasis. In many adult animals and humans, arginine is synthesized by the kidney from intestinally derived citrulline at rates that are inadequate to support growth in neonatal animals. As the milk of humans, pigs, rats, and many other mammals is deficient in arginine (79), it is considered to be an essential amino acid for growing animals. However, studies with enterocytes from newborn pigs (67,68) and developing mouse and rat small intestine (80,81) have shown developmental changes and metabolic zonation along the crypt-villus axis of arginine-metabolizing enzymes. At birth, the enterocytes of

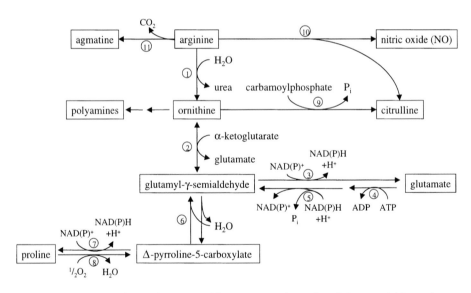

FIGURE 4 Metabolic pathways and interconversion of arginine, ornithine, glutamate, and proline. (1) Arginase, (2) ornithine aminotransferase, (3) glutamate-γ-semialdehyde dehydrogenase, (4) γ-glutamyl kinase, (5) γ-glutamyl dehydrogenase, (6) spontaneous, (7) pyrroline-5-carboxylate reductase, (8) proline oxidase, (9) ornithine transcarbamoylase, (10) NO synthase, (11) arginine decarboxylase.

the upper villus (81) are the major sites of arginine synthesis, but they gradually become the major sites of net citrulline production as intestinal arginase expression increases via a glucocorticoid-dependent mechanism. This transition is compensated by the gradually increasing capacity of the kidney to use citrulline for arginine synthesis. Thus, following the transition from suckling to weaning, the intestine becomes a site of arginine degradation rather than synthesis (see review in Ref. 82).

The limited arginine degradation by enterocytes from newborn pigs ensures a maximum output of arginine (synthesized from glutamine or derived from milk) into the portal circulation for utilization by extraintestinal tissues. Type II arginase, a mitochondrial enzyme is expressed at lower levels in kidney, brain, small intestine, mammary gland, and macrophages, but not in liver; it is distinct from type I arginase, a cytosolic enzyme, which is highly expressed in liver as a component of the urea cycle. The induction of type II arginase in enterocytes after weaning possibly regulates the availability of arginine for the synthesis of nitric oxide (NO), ornithine, and thus, polyamines, agmatine, proline, and glutamate; it may also regulate ureagenesis in the small intestinal mucosa (Fig. 4). Although considerably less than in the liver, gut ureagenesis may be a first-line defense in detoxification of ammonia derived from tissue metabolism and luminal microorganisms (see review in Ref. 82). However, the major end products of arginine metabolism by intestinal enterocytes from weaned pigs are proline and ornithine. Proline, required for collagen synthesis, is one of the most abundant amino acids in human milk (79). Arginine-derived proline is not detectable in enterocytes of newborn or suckling pigs. However, providing proline in the diet can ameliorate the hyperammonemia associated with dietary arginine deficiency in neonatal pigs (83). Thus, while proline is not considered an absolute dietary essential nutrient, it may be conditionally essential for maintaining arginine synthesis in neonates. It is apparent from a number of studies that a normally functioning gut is important for maintenance of whole-body arginine and proline status, especially in neonates. Furthermore, any situation that markedly reduces gut mass or compromises function could render these amino acids conditionally essential.

Recent studies in cultured intestinal cells (84) have shown that ornithine derived from arginine metabolism is converted to polyamines (Figs. 4 and 5). Polyamines (putrescine, spermidine, spermine, cadaverine) are ubiquitous cationic amines, and although many of their functions and mechanisms of action are as yet poorly understood, it is well established that polyamines are involved in cell proliferation and differentiation in many tissues, including the gastrointestinal tract (see review in Ref. 85). Ornithine decarboxylase (ODC) and S-adenosyl-methionine decarboxylase (SAMDC), converting ornithine to putrescine and putrescine to spermine, respectively, are the rate-limiting enzymes in polyamine synthesis (Fig. 5). The synthesis of polyamines from arginine is negligible in enterocytes of newborn and suckling animals (86,87) but increases in

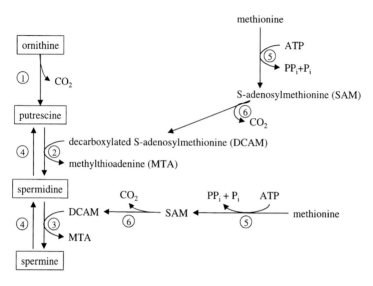

FIGURE 5   Polyamine synthesis. (1) Ornithine decarboxylase, (2) spermidine synthase (propylamine transferase), (3) spermidine synthase (propylamine transferase), (4) polyamine oxidase, (5) methionine adenosyl transferase, (6) S-adenosylmethionine decarboxylase.

enterocytes of postweaning animals, concurrent with the induction of both arginase and ODC (82). Luminal administration of polyamines increases intestinal growth in adult rats (88) and has been shown to enhance intestinal maturation (89) and cell proliferation in developing rats (90). Polyamines are present in human milk in micromolar concentrations for up to 4 months of lactation (91,92). Polyamine concentrations in infant formulas are dependent on the method of preparation. Semielemental diets prepared by hydrolytic procedures using crude extracts of pancreatic enzymes are major sources of polyamines, with a profile similar to that of human milk (92). Results of a recent study in cultured intestinal cells suggested that both human and rat milk—but neither bovine milk nor infant formula—contain sufficient amounts of polyamines to sustain cell growth during inhibition of polyamine synthesis with difluoromethylornithine (DFMO), a specific and irreversible inhibitor of ODC (93). Thus, when the ingestion of milk-borne polyamines by the neonate ceases after weaning, the induction of intestinal polyamine synthesis from arginine, and other dietary amino acids that can be converted to ornithine, may be of physiological significance for the maintenance of normal intestinal growth and function. In the mature intestine, intraluminal polyamines are derived from the diet, pancreaticobiliary secretions, microbial flora, and mature cells that are shed into the lumen (85).

1.4 Nucleotides

Nucleotides (NT) are ubiquitous, low-molecular-weight, intracellular compounds
that are integral to numerous biochemical processes, especially as precursors for
nucleic acid synthesis (94). Nucleotides consist of a purine or pyrimidine base,
a pentose sugar (ribose or deoxyribose), and one or more phosphate groups. Nucleosides can be viewed as subsets of nucleotides, inasmuch as they are lacking
the phosphate groups. Nucleotides and nucleic acids are constantly being formed
and degraded (Fig. 6). Purine and pyrimidine bases can be synthesized within
cells de novo from glutamine, aspartic acid, glycine, formate, and carbon dioxide
as precursors or they can be salvaged from the degradation of nucleic acids and
nucleotides. Nucleotides appear to be important in supporting cellular metabolism, particularly in rapidly dividing tissues such as lymphoid cells and the intestine. These tissues seem to lack significant capacity for de novo synthesis of
nucleotides and therefore require exogenous sources of purine and pyrimidine
bases. Numerous reports demonstrate that the provision of extracellular (dietary
or systemic) nucleosides, nucleotides, or nucleic acids support small intestinal
mucosal function and morphology in vivo and in vitro (60,95–97), most likely
by providing substrates for the salvage pathway of the nucleotide synthesis and by
decreasing the need for precursors, especially glutamine, in the de novo synthesis.
Human milk is the exclusive source of dietary nucleotides for infants during the

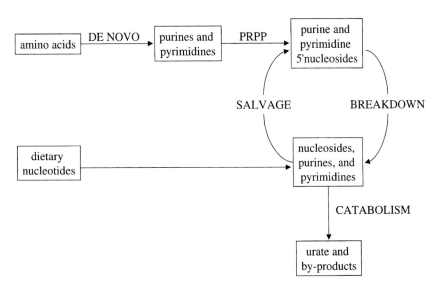

FIGURE 6 Synthesis, salvage, and catabolism of nucleotides. PRPP = phos-
phoribosylpyrophosphate.

first months of life, and its nucleotide profile differs markedly from that of cow's milk and most infant formulas. More detailed information regarding the beneficial effects of nucleotides on the infant gastrointestinal tract can be found in Chapter 4.

1.5   Short-Chain Fatty Acids and Oligosaccharides

Short-chain fatty acids (SCFAs), formerly known as volatile fatty acids, are the C_{1-6} organic fatty acids, primarily formed together with gases such as carbon dioxide (CO_2), hydrogen (H_2), and methane (CH_4) in the mammalian rumen, cecum, and colon by microbial fermentation of carbohydrates (98). Carbohydrates—such as nonstarch polysaccharides (dietary fiber), resistant starch, and sometimes simple carbohydrates—escape digestion or absorption in the small intestine and end up fermented in the large intestine and colon (Fig. 7) (99,100). The primary function of the human colon microbiota is to salvage energy from these carbohydrates. This is achieved through fermentation and absorption of the major products, SCFAs, which represent 40 to 50% of the available energy of the carbohydrate. The colonic epithelium derives 60 to 70% of its energy from SCFAs; depending on the diet, the amount of SCFA produced by the human colon microbiota (300 to 800 mmol/day) (101) theoretically represents 5 to 10%

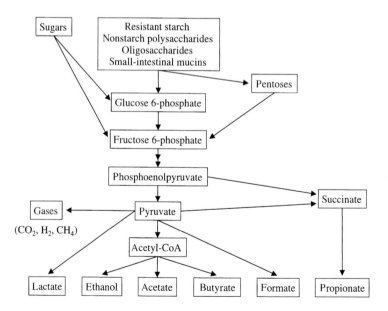

Figure 7   Carbohydrate metabolism in the large intestine and the principal fermentation products.

of the host's total energy requirements. Protein fermentation, although in smaller proportions, also leads to SCFAs, H_2, and CO_2, as well as the generation of branched-chain fatty acids (BCFAs) such as isobutyrate, isovalerate, and α-methylbutyrate from valine, leucine, and isoleucine, respectively (102). The principal SCFAs—acetate, propionate, and butyrate—account for approximately 85% of formed SCFAs and are produced in a nearly constant molar ratio 60:25:15. These SCFAs are metabolized by the colonic epithelium (butyrate), liver (propionate), and muscle (acetate); very little propionate or butyrate normally reaches the peripheral circulation (103,104).

Butyrate is the preferred oxidative fuel for colonocytes, compared to glucose, glutamine, or ketone bodies (105–108). Butyrate is absorbed by colonocytes in the proximal colon via passive diffusion and by active transport mechanisms linked to various ion-exchange transporters. In the distal colon, the main mechanism of absorption is passive diffusion of the lipid-soluble form. Butyrate and other SCFAs are important for the absorption of electrolytes by the large intestine and may play a role in preventing certain types of diarrhea, including starvation and refeeding diarrhea (109–115).

The trophic effects of ingested fiber or resistant starch on the colonic mucosa are, at least partially, mediated by SCFAs released from luminal fermentation (103,112,114). Conversely, a fiber-free diet or TPN induces atrophy in the intestinal mucosa. Butyrate, apart from being oxidized to CO_2, also provides the main source of acetylcoenzyme A for lipid synthesis and cell-membrane assembly in epithelial cells (116). Intraluminal infusions of SCFAs have a stimulatory effect on colonic mucosal proliferation under various experimental conditions in rats and patients. The effects of SCFAs are dose-dependent and vary among the acids (butyrate > propionate > acetate) (117). Deficient production of SCFAs has been associated with diversion colitis, ulcerative colitis (112,114), and colitis resulting from severe starvation or caloric malnutrition, such as kwashiorkor, which is reversible on refeeding (115).

Although SCFAs are undoubtedly metabolized by the colonic mucosa, many of the trophic effects of SCFAs, such as the increase of mucosal blood flow (118), cannot be explained solely by direct luminal effects of the SCFAs absorbed. The release of SCFAs may also have indirect actions on gastrointestinal motility mediated by the autonomic nervous system (119) and activation of enteroendocrine cells to release gut hormones (120,121). Studies show that both dietary fiber (122) and systemic SCFAs (120,121) increase the abundance of proglucagon in the small intestine and plasma glucagon-like peptide 2 (GLP-2) concentration. Moreover, luminal SCFAs and fiber in the isolated vascularly perfused rat colon are potent stimulants of peptide YY release (123). Both systemic and intracolonic SCFAs exert trophic effects on the small intestine. Studies in rats have demonstrated that both intravenous and intracolonic infusions of SCFAs significantly reduce the mucosal atrophy associated with long-term TPN (124).

Furthermore, systemic SCFAs administered during TPN (120,121) increase ileal proglucagon and ornithine decarboxylase mRNA, expression of the glucose transporter GLUT2 and immediate early genes (c-*myc*, c-*jun*, c-*fos*). Enteral butyrate supplements have also been shown to increase amino acid absorptive capacity in pigs following massive small bowel resection (125).

Studies in animals and humans suggest that diets rich in fiber reduce the risk of colon cancer, whereas diets high in fat and protein may promote colon cancer (126–129). Of the SCFAs produced by fiber fermentation, butyrate seems to play a key role in colon cancer. Studies in animals demonstrate that diets rich in insoluble fibers (wheat bran), which serve as a substrate precursor for colonic butyrate, protect the large bowel against tumor growth. On the other hand, diets rich in soluble fiber (pectin, guar gum), which do not increase colonic butyrate levels, were less effective. However, there is an ongoing debate as to whether butyrate stimulates or inhibits tumorigenesis (130). Numerous in vivo and in vitro studies show that butyrate is a major metabolic fuel and stimulates proliferation of colonocytes. However, evidence largely based on studies with cultured colonic tumor cell lines indicates that butyrate induces differentiation and apoptosis, thereby suppressing neoplasia (60,103,112–114,131). Specific and nonspecific effects of butyrate on gene expression and regulatory mechanisms of gene expression have been described (60,103,112–114,131). However, it is of great interest to understand the molecular mechanisms that explain the differential effect of butyrate on normal and neoplastic colon cells. It has been postulated that the shift from aerobic to anaerobic metabolism that takes place with neoplastic transformation might lead to the inability to oxidize butyrate (132). The resulting accumulation of butyrate in the cytoplasm of the neoplastic colonocyte, plus the altered affinity of certain mutated proteins, may be the cause of increased sensitivity to butyrate and the paradoxical effect of butyrate on neoplastic versus normal cells.

There is a limited microflora in the large bowel of newborn infants, which explains the very low level (10% of adult level) of SCFAs in the meconium of neonates (133). At the first stage of development, differences in gestational age, type of delivery, and type of feeding are associated with significantly different colonization patterns of anaerobic and aerobic bacteria during the first week after birth (134). Furthermore, differences in the fecal flora of breast- and formula-fed infants appear to be related to the type of ingested protein (135), the availability of iron (136), the presence of oligosaccharides (137), and the pH (138). The development of the intestinal flora provides the basis for a barrier that prevents pathogenic bacteria from invading the gastrointestinal tract. The composition of the intestinal microflora together with the gut immune system allow resident bacteria to exert a protective function. Thus, modification of the flora by dietary means offers one of the most effective opportunities for development of functional foods.

Compared with milk from other species, human milk is unique with regard to its content of complex oligosaccharides (137,139–141). After lactose and fat, the oligosaccharide fraction is the third-largest solute in human milk (approximately 22 g/L in colostrum, and over 12 g/L in mature milk) and is present in higher amounts than protein. For many years, oligosaccharides have been considered only as "soluble fiber," serving as a substrate in the development of normal gut flora in breast-fed infants. However, today there is increasing evidence that free oligosaccharides as well as glycoproteins are potent inhibitors of bacterial adhesion to epithelial surfaces. Bacterial adhesion in general is a ligand-receptor interaction between structures on the bacterial surface and complementary structures on the mucosal surface of the host. Cell surfaces contain a large number of oligosaccharide moieties, primarily in the form of glycoproteins and glycolipids, that function in intercellular communication. As there are similarities between oligosaccharides in human milk and the receptors for pathogenic microorganisms on the mucosal surface, the specificity for certain ligands of microorganisms—like *Escherichia coli* strains; influenza viruses A, B, and C; and *Vibrio cholerae*—could explain the differences in colonization and prevention of infection in breast-versus formula-fed newborns. The free oligosaccharides or the carbohydrate moiety of glycoproteins or glycolipids in human milk might prevent intestinal attachment of microorganisms by acting as receptor analogues competing with epithelial ligands for bacterial binding. However, very little is known about the persistence or modification of oligosaccharides during transit through the infant's gastrointestinal tract. Additional studies are needed to investigate how far oligosaccharides are degraded by intestinal enzymes and further processed in intestinal cells.

2   GROWTH FACTORS

2.1   Overview

In addition to the nutrients consumed in the diet, numerous molecules produced in the body affect gut growth and function (Table 1). In general, most of these are polypeptides, such as tissue growth factors and gut hormones; yet others, like cortisol and prostaglandins, can be classified chemically as either steroids or phospholipids. Thus, while the term *gut growth factor* usually refers to polypeptides, it is frequently used in a more generic context to describe any compound that stimulates gut growth. Most of the polypeptide growth factors and their receptors are expressed not only in the gut but also in tissues throughout the body. Furthermore, within the gut, many of these growth factors are expressed by non-epithelial cells, such as fibroblasts and lymphocytes, that reside in the lamina propria in close proximity to the epithelial layer yet have receptors that are expressed in epithelial cells (Fig. 8). As a consequence, many of these factors act

TABLE 1   Nonnutritional Factors That
Affect Gastrointestinal Growth

Growth factors
  Epidermal growth factor
  Transforming growth factor-α
  Insulin-like growth factors I and II
  Hepatocyte growth factor
  Keratinocyte growth factor
  Fibroblast growth factor
  Vascular endothelial growth factor
Cytokines
  Transforming growth factor-β
  Tumor necrosis factor-α
  Interleukins (IL-1, IL-6, IL-10, IL-12)
Gastrointestinal hormones
  Glucagon-like peptide 2
  Gastrin
  Peptide YY
  Neurotensin
  Bombesin
Pituitary-adrenal-thyroid
  Growth hormone
  Corticosterone
  Thyroid hormone
Phospholipid mediators
  Platelet-activating factor
  Prostaglandins

locally through paracrine, autocrine, and juxtacrine cellular mechanisms. Some growth factors, namely epidermal growth factor (EGF), are present in digestive secretions and also act on the epithelial cells via the luminal surface; this may explain part of the trophic effect of pancreaticobiliary secretions on the gut (2). Most of these factors also are found in milk and have been suggested to play a functional role in the growth and development of the neonatal gut (142).

The expression and secretion of intestinal growth factors are regulated by numerous variables, including nutrition, stage of development and differentiation, and immune status. Many of the growth factors are categorized into different "families" based on the structural characteristics of the ligand (i.e., the growth factor) and its particular receptor. The biological actions of most growth factors are initiated by binding to specific cellular receptor domains present either on the cell surface or within the cell (Fig. 9). Growth factor receptors are coupled to various intracellular signaling cascades mediated by intrinsic receptor tyrosine

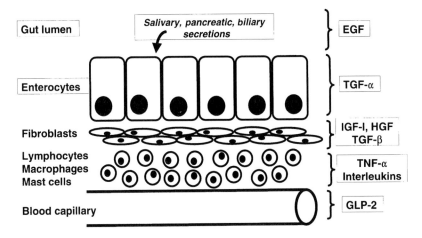

FIGURE 8 Schematic view of the spatial organization of different cell types within the intestinal mucosa. Growth factor and cytokine expression are localized in different mucosal regions and cell types. Growth factors are also presented to the apical and basolateral mucosal surfaces via the digestive secretions and the arterial circulation.

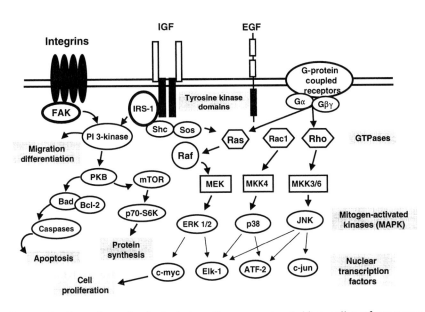

FIGURE 9 Overview of selected signaling cascades linking cell-surface receptors with intracellular proteins involved in regulation of numerous cell functions. (Adapted from Refs. 233–237.)

kinase activity or G-protein linkage to adenylate cyclase, phosphatidylinositol turnover, or activation of calcium ion channels. These cascades are further coupled to an increasingly complex network of docking and scaffolding proteins that are activated by phosphorylation on serine, threonine, and tyrosine residues and transmit the signal from the receptor to target proteins and genes that mediate the biological effects within the cell. Although our understanding of these signaling networks has increased tremendously in recent years, information regarding their role in mediating growth factor actions specific for gut tissues has lagged behind.

2.2 Epidermal Growth Factor

The EGF family of peptides includes EGF, transforming growth factor alpha (TGF-α), amphiregulin, heparin-binding EGF, epiregulin (EPR), betacellulin (BTC), neuregulin (NRG), and neuregulin 2 (NRG2) (143). These factors bind to the membrane-bound EGF-receptor and other EGF-related (ErbB family) receptors and activate a complex network of intracellular signaling pathways that lead to cell proliferation and differentiation. EGF is the most extensively characterized of these peptides and is widely distributed in most body fluids (notably mammary, salivary, biliary, and pancreatic secretions), but it is not produced in the epithelial cells, in contrast to its homologue, TGF-α, which is expressed in enterocytes. Based on these observations, one would expect that enteral nutrition and stimulation of gastrointestinal secretion would increase the release of EGF into the lumen. Indeed, some have suggested that EGF secreted into the lumen acts as a protective/surveillance peptide under conditions of mucosal injury, whereas TGF-α functions in the maintenance of epithelial cell proliferation and migration in the healthy gut (144). However, evidence from several studies suggests that EGF is more trophic to the gut when it is given intravenously than when given enterally. This is perhaps due to the fact that the EGF receptor is predominantly localized to the basolateral rather than the apical membrane of the epithelium. In contrast, many studies with neonatal animals have shown that oral administration of EGF augments gut growth and functional development. These findings, combined with the fact that EGF and TGF-α concentrations are relatively high in colostrum and milk, have led many to postulate that these factors play a physiological role in neonatal gut growth and development; however, this remains to be clearly established (142).

   In general, most of the EGF family peptides are trophic to the gut, stimulating cell proliferation and suppressing apoptosis; however, they also modulate a number of other physiological functions, including enhanced tooth eruption, decreased gastric acid secretion, increased mucus secretion and gastric blood flow, reduced gastric emptying, and increased sodium and glucose transport (145–148). Furthermore, EGF serves to increase mucosal growth and functional adaptation following intestinal resection, diarrhea, TPN, and ulcerative conditions. Most of the reported effects of EGF and TGF-α have been shown in animals; however, there is one reported case where EGF given intravenously restored intestinal integrity in an infant with necrotizing enterocolitis (144). Although most of the other EGF family peptides, besides EGF and TGF-α, appear to stimulate cell proliferation, their effect on other gut functions remains to be determined.

2.3   Insulin-like Growth Factors

The insulin-like growth factor (IGF) family of peptides includes insulin, IGF-I, and IGF-II (149–151). These peptides and their receptors are structurally related and their specificity is based largely on the relative binding affinities for their respective ligands. The biological actions of insulin are mediated via the insulin receptor, whereas the actions of both IGF-I and IGF-II are largely mediated through the type I IGF receptor. The insulin and type I IGF receptors are present in epithelial cells; they are more abundant on the basolateral than the apical membrane and more abundant in proliferating crypt cells than in differentiated enterocytes. Although insulin secretion is confined to the pancreas, both IGF-I and IGF-II are expressed throughout the body, including the gut. However, within the intestinal mucosa, expression of both IGF-I and IGF-II appears to be localized to mesenchymal cells in the lamina propria, although epithelial cells may also produce IGF-II. The expression of IGF-I and II in the gut is highest in the fetal and neonatal periods and declines with age. In addition, insulin, IGF-I, and IGF-II are present in milk, and IGF-I is found in salivary, biliary, and pancreatic secretions. As is the case with EGF, there is conflicting evidence as to whether milk-borne insulin or IGFs play a physiological role in neonatal gut growth and development. Some studies with neonatal animals given pharmacological oral doses of insulin and IGF-I have demonstrated a stimulation of gut growth, disaccharidase activity, and glucose transport, while others have shown only limited effects of oral IGF on the gut (152–155). In contrast, numerous studies have shown that either administering IGF systemically or increasing its expression locally (as in transgenic mice) stimulates intestinal growth and function in normal animals as well as under conditions of TPN, gut resection, dexamethasone treatment, sepsis, and radiation therapy (150,156–158). The IGF-binding proteins (IGFBPs 1 to 6) are present in the circulation and also expressed locally in gut tissues. Considerable evidence indicates that the IGFBPs inhibit the biological functions of IGFs. This is based on evidence that the IGF analogue des(1-3)IGF-I, which does not bind to IGF binding proteins, is more potent than the native IGF-I (157,159). Thus, factors that increase intestinal IGFBP expression would inhibit gut growth, as has been shown with IGFBP-4 (158). The IGFs have also been implicated in the development of colon cancer, based on evidence that the expression of both IGF-II and the type I receptor is increased in tumors (160).

2.4   Other Growth Factors

Hepatocyte growth factor (HGF), vascular endothelial growth factor (VEGF), fibroblast growth factor (FGF), and keratinocyte growth factor (KGF) are expressed in the gut tissues and may play a role in mucosal growth and repair. Hepatocyte growth factor is expressed by mesenchymal, but not epithelial cells, whereas the HGF receptor (c-*met*) is found in epithelial cells; the c-*met* receptor is localized on the basolateral membrane. Studies with cultured intestinal epithelial cells demonstrate that HGF stimulates cell proliferation and wound closure proliferation but decreases transepithelial resistance (161,162). Hepatocyte growth factor is found in human milk mononuclear cells and partially accounts for the stimulatory effect of human milk on intestinal cell proliferation (163). Studies in rats have shown that HGF, given either systemically or orally, increased gut growth and nutrient transport after massive small bowel resection (164).

VEGF is expressed in the small intestine, predominantly in the lamina propria mast cells (165). A recent report indicates that the receptor (flt-1) for the VEGF 165 amino acid isoform is present in intestinal epithelial cells; however, VEGF did not stimulate cell proliferation of these cells (166). A recent report in mice demonstrated that VEGF and FGF-2 reduce the rate of crypt cell apoptosis following total-body irradiation (167). Although FGF and the FGF receptors have been found in intestinal tissues, their physiological function is unknown (168). However, it has been suggested that VEGF and FGF-2 are involved in stimulating angiogenesis during intestinal repair (169). Increased local expression of KGF has been found in patients with inflammatory bowel disease, and administration of KGF enhanced mucosal healing in rats following induction of colitis (170,171).

2.5   Gastrointestinal Hormones

2.5.1   Gastrin

Gastrin is secreted from the G cells within the antrum of the stomach and acts primarily to stimulate proliferation of parietal and enterochromaffin-like cells within the gastric mucosa (172,173). There is structural homology between gastrin and cholecystokinin (CCK) with respect to both the peptide sequence and receptor function. Both gastrin and CCK bind with similar affinities to the CCK-B receptor, a G protein–linked membrane protein, whereas the CCK-A receptor binds CCK but not gastrin. Studies have shown that hypogastrinemia, produced by antrectomy and targeted disruption of the gastrin gene, leads to atrophy of the gastric mucosal cells (174). Likewise, hypergastrinemia resulting from either exogenous gastrin administration or as observed in patients with Zollinger-Ellison syndrome results in increased gastric mucosal growth. The neonate exhibits hypergastrinemia, and this has been linked to the development of gastric growth and function. However, the evidence that gastrin stimulates mucosal growth in the small intestine and colon remains controversial. Concern about the carcinogenic effects of gastrin was raised by the evidence that gastrin stimulated colonic cell growth and carcinoid tumors related to enterochromaffin-like cell (ECL) proliferation. However, additional direct and indirect evidence was put forth that refuted the role of gastrin in colon carcinogenesis (175). Further debate has revolved around issues such as whether both the carboxyamidated and glycine-extended gastrin peptides are trophic and if there are as yet unidentified receptors for gastrin, because the CCK-B receptor does not bind glycine-extended gastrin and it has not been found in either the small intestine or colon (176).

2.5.2 Cholecystokinin

Cholecystokinin is expressed in endocrine cells of the gut and in neurons within the gut and brain, while its primary receptor (CCK-A) is found in the pancreas, gallbladder, esophagus, ileum, and colon (172). CCK stimulates pancreatic growth and cell proliferation, and these trophic effects have been attributed exclusively to interaction via the CCK-A receptor (177,178). Moreover, the pancreatic growth associated with feeding high-protein diets and soybean lectins has been linked to induction of CCK secretion and its trophic action via the CCK-A receptor (179,180). Increased expression of the CCK-A receptor has also been demonstrated in pancreatic adenocarcinomas (181,182).

2.5.3 Somatostatin

Somatostatin is secreted by the endocrine D cells present throughout the gut and pancreas, whereas there are multiple isoforms of the somatostatin receptor, which are also found throughout the gut (172). Somatostatin has a generalized inhibitory effect on numerous gut functions and thus has been used in the treatment of several endocrine and malabsorptive disorders of the gut, including short-bowel syndrome. Direct inhibitory effects of somatostatin have been difficult to establish in vivo because somatostatin suppresses the secretion of several other trophic hormones. However, studies with cultured epithelial cells have demonstrated inhibitory effects of somatostatin on cell proliferation which are consistent with its antiproliferative actions on intestinal growth and regeneration in vivo (183). In support of this, recent evidence from human pancreatic and colon cancer patients indicates significantly reduced expression of the receptor isoforms that mediate the antiproliferative effects of somatostatin, namely sst2 and sst5 (184). Somatostatin also is found in milk; however, its effects on neonatal gut growth have not been established.

2.5.4 Glucagon-like Peptide 2

Glucagon-like peptide 2 (GLP-2), like GLP-1, oxyntomodulin, and glicentin, is a product of the intestinal proglucagon gene expressed in the enteroendocrine ''L'' cells located predominantly in the distal intestine (185,186). GLP-2 has recently been found to have significant trophic effects on the gut (187). These effects are mediated by both increased cell proliferation and decreased apoptosis, but GLP-2 also stimulates epithelial glucose transport (188). It would appear that many of the gut trophic stimuli previously associated with increased circulating enteroglucagon can be ascribed specifically to increased GLP-2 secretion. Recent studies have shown that GLP-2 is secreted in response to feeding, especially carbohydrate (189); it is directly correlated with enteral intake and small intestinal growth (7); and its secretion is significantly blunted in ileal resected short-bowel patients (190). Furthermore, GLP-2 administration stimulates gut growth under several conditions of compromised intestinal function and integrity. The biologically active form of GLP-2 is a 33–amino acid peptide that has a short half-life because it is highly sensitive to rapid proteolytic inactivation by dipeptidylpeptidase IV (DPP IV). Studies have shown that DPP IV inhibitors and DPP IV–resistant GLP-2 analogues can increase the biological potency of GLP-2.

2.5.5 Neurotensin

Neurotensin (NT) is a 13–amino acid peptide secreted from the enteroendocrine "N" cells located exclusively in the gut within the distal small intestine; however, NT expression is also found in the brain (191). Neurotensin expression is markedly increased during the neonatal period, and secretion is stimulated specifically by ingestion of fat (172). Administration of NT stimulates gut growth in animals following small bowel resection (192) and reverses the intestinal atrophic effect of an elemental diet (193); the trophic effects occur in the absence of enteral nutrients (194). A recent report also demonstrated that an NT antagonist significantly reduced the growth of transplanted colonic tumors in nude mice, implicating NT in colon carcinogenesis (195).

2.5.6 Peptide YY

Peptide YY (PYY) is a 36–amino acid peptide produced by the enteroendocrine "L" cells in the distal intestine and colon (196). Although synthesized from a separate gene, PYY is secreted from the same enteroendocrine cell as the glucagon-like peptides GLP-1 and 2 in response to the ingestion of fat and has been implicated along with these peptides as factors responsible for the "ileal brake" phenomenon. Consistent with this notion is the fact that administration of PYY and GLPs have similar physiological effects on gastric secretion and motility (197,198). Likewise, both circulating PYY and GLP concentrations are markedly increased following small bowel resection and in malabsorption syndromes; thus they have been implicated as humoral mediators of the intestinal trophic response. However, PYY has been shown to stimulate gut growth in some (196) but not all cases (199) and does not stimulate proliferation of cultured epithelial cells. As a result, the direct trophic effects of PYY on epithelial cells have been questioned; instead, the effects of PYY may be mediated indirectly via interaction with heterotypic cells within the mucosa.

2.5.7   Gastrin-Releasing Peptide (Bombesin)

Gastrin-releasing peptide (GRP) is a 27–amino acid peptide with a C-terminus region that is structurally related to bombesin, a 14–amino acid neuropeptide found in amphibian skin (200). Gastrin-releasing peptide is secreted from neurons located throughout the gastrointestinal tract in response to vagal stimulation. The primary function of GRP is to mediate the neural-activated gastrin release; however, it has also been shown to stimulate other gut-derived peptides. A number of studies have demonstrated that exogenous administration of bombesin stimulates growth of the normal and damaged intestine (201,202); the effects are independent of luminal nutrients and pancreaticobiliary secretions (203). Despite evidence of a GRP receptor in the gut, it is unknown whether the effects of bombesin are direct; indeed, one report suggests that the trophic effects could be mediated indirectly by increased enteroglucagon secretion (204). However, bombesin does stimulate cell proliferation and has been shown to enhance experimentally induced carcinogenesis (205). Bombesin is also found in milk (142), and both oral and systemic administration to suckling animals stimulates intestinal growth (206).

2.6   Growth Hormone

There is conflicting evidence as to whether growth hormone has trophic effects on the gut, despite recent clinical interest in its use for treatment of short-bowel syndrome. Studies in rodents indicate that hypophysectomy results in gut atrophy (207), whereas transgenic overexpression of GH in mice increases gut growth (208). However, in both animals and humans, GH treatment after massive small bowel resection has been shown in some (209–211), but not all studies to increase intestinal growth (57,212). Other recent studies in rats demonstrate that GH treatment does not prevent the intestinal atrophy associated with TPN, even though it increases circulating IGF-I concentrations (213,214). This finding, coupled with evidence that administration of IGF-I alone does prevent TPN-associated gut atrophy, implies that GH treatment may affect the intestinal responsiveness to endogenous IGF-I. Given evidence of the presence of GH receptors within the gut, it is conceivable that GH could act locally in the gut independent of IGF-I; however, this has not been shown.

2.7   Glucocorticoids and Thyroid Hormones

There is an extensive literature describing how both glucocorticoids and thyroid hormones stimulate intestinal development and maturation, especially with regard to disaccharidase expression (215). However, there are conflicting reports as to whether these hormones stimulate cell proliferation and mucosal growth. In weaned, adult animals, evidence suggests that they suppress growth and proliferation (216,217). A recent report demonstrates that dexamethasone induces growth arrest in cultured intestinal epithelial cell lines (218). Likewise, triiodothyronine (T3) was shown to induce apoptosis in primary intestinal cultures (219). Studies in vivo also show that dexamethasone treatment suppresses intestinal growth both in healthy neonatal pigs (220) and in weaned rats following massive small bowel resection (221). In contrast, some studies in fetal and neonatal animals suggest that increased glucocorticoid levels may stimulate intestinal growth (222,223).

3 CYTOKINES

3.1 Transforming Growth Factor Beta

Transforming growth factor beta (TGF-β) is structurally unrelated to TGF-α and is found in three major forms (TGF-β 1 to 3) in mammalian tissues (224). Expression of TGF-β has been found throughout the small intestine in both lamina propria and epithelial cells. Expression of TGF-β-1 in the lamina propria is low in neonatal rats and increases with age (225). In contrast, the levels of TGF-β-2 are high in early milk and decline as lactation progresses. At least five receptors (types I to V) have been found to bind one or more of the various TGF-β ligands, although the type I and II receptors appear to mediate the effects on cell proliferation. TGF-β is a potent inhibitor of epithelial cell proliferation and may also induce differentiation. It has been implicated as an intermediate signal whereby butyrate suppresses proliferation and induces differentiation of colonic epithelial cells (226). TGF-β also stimulates epithelial cell migration and production of extracellular matrix proteins such as collagen via induction of connective tissue growth factor, thus making it a critical factor in the process of restitution of the epithelium following mucosal damage (227). This latter function of TGF-β may play an important role in the intestinal inflammatory response, as evident by the fact that its expression is upregulated in inflammatory bowel disease and that transgenic mice deficient in TGF-β develop inflammatory disease.

3.2 Interleukins and Interferon-γ

It has become increasingly apparent that cytokines are critical signaling molecules involved in the normal homeostatic communication among luminal microbes, epithelial cells, and the immune system (228). Moreover, it is evident that the production of cytokines plays a central regulatory role in the development of inflammatory bowel disease (229). The optimum balance between proinflammatory (interleukins-1, -6, -8, and -12 and TNF-α) and immunoregulatory (TGF-β, INF-γ, and interleukins-2, -4, and -10) cytokines is essential for normal intestinal function. However, in addition to their role in inflammatory bowel disease, the proinflammatory cytokines may be involved in other enteropathies associated with suppressed gut growth, such as diarrhea, chemotherapy, radiation therapy, and TPN. Although some of the proinflammatory cytokines have been shown to stimulate the proliferation of crypt cells (230), they markedly reduced villus height. Recent evidence suggests that TNF-α causes villus atrophy by rapidly inducing apoptosis and shedding of villus enterocytes (231), which may constitute an initial step in the proinflammatory processes subsequent to bacterial invasion (232).

REFERENCES

1. Raul F, Schleiffer R. Intestinal adaptation to nutritional stress. Proc Nutr Soc 1996; 55:279–289.
2. Jenkins AP, Thompson RPH. Mechanisms of small intestinal adaptation. Dig Dis 1994; 12:15–27.
3. Burrin DG, Davis TA, Fiorotto ML, Reeds PJ. Stage of development and fasting affect protein synthetic activity in the gastrointestinal tissues of suckling rats. J Nutr 1991; 121:1099–1108.
4. Trahair JF, Sangild PT. Systemic and luminal influences on the perinatal development of the gut. Equine Vet J Suppl 1997; 24:40–50.
5. Widdowson EM. Development of the digestive system: Comparative animal studies. Am J Clin Nutr 1985; 41:384–390.
6. Burrin DG, Davis TA, Ebner S, Schoknecht PA, Fiorotto ML, Reeds PJ, McAvoy S. Nutrient-independent and nutrient-dependent factors stimulate protein synthesis in colostrum-fed newborn pigs. Pediatr Res 1995; 37:593–599.
7. Burrin DG, Stoll B, Jiang R, Chang X, Hartmann B, Holst JJ, Greeley GH Jr, Reeds PJ. Minimal entral nutrient requirements for intestinal growth in neonatal piglets: How much is enough? Am J Clin Nutr 2000; 71:1603–1610.
8. Stoll B, Chang X, Fan MZ, Reeds PJ, and Burrin DG. Enteral nutrient intake level determines intestinal protein synthesis and accretion in neonatal pigs. Am J Physiol 2000; 279:G288–G294.
9. Shulman RJ. Effect of different total parenteral nutrition fuel mixes on small intestinal growth and differentiation in the infant miniature pig. Gastroenterology 1988; 95:85–92.
10. Morgan W 3d, Yardley J, Luk G, Niemiec P, Dudgeon D. Total parenteral nutrition and intestinal development: A neonatal model. J Pediatr Surg 1987; 22:541–545.
11. Goldstein RM, Hebiguchi T, Luk GD, Taqi F, Guilarte TR, Franklin FA Jr, Niemiec PW, Dudgeon DL. The effects of total parenteral nutrition on gastrointestinal growth and development. J Pediatr Surg 1985; 20:785–791.
12. Buchman AL, Moukarzel AA, Bhuta S, Belle M, Ament ME, Eckhert CD, Hollander D, Gornbein J, Kopple JD, Vijayaroghavan SR. Parenteral nutrition is associated with intestinal morphologic and functional changes in humans. J Parenter Enter Nutr 1995; 19:453–460.
13. Berseth CL. Minimal enteral feedings. Clin Perinatol 1995; 22:195–205.
14. Lucas A, Bloom SR, Aynsley-Green A. Gut hormones and minimal enteral feeding. Acta Paediatr Scand 1986; 75:719–723.
15. Bragg LE, Thompson JS, Rikkers LF. Influence of nutrient delivery on gut structure and function. Nutrition 1991; 7:237–243.

16. Stoll B, Price P, Reeds PJ, Henry J, Burrin DG. Feeding an elemental diet versus a milk-based formula does not decrease intestinal mucosal growth in infant pigs. J Pediatr Gastroenterol Nutr 2000; 31:S169.
17. Young EA, Cioletti LA, Traylor JB, Balderas V. Gastrointestinal response to oral versus gastric feeding of defined formula diets. Am J Clin Nutr 1982; 35:715–726.
18. Shulman RJ, Redel CA, Stathos TH. Bolus versus continuous feedings stimulate small-intestinal growth and development in the newborn pig. J Pediatr Gastroenterol Nutr 1994; 18:350–354.
19. Morin CL, Ling V, Bourassa D. Small intestinal and colonic changes induced by a chemically defined diet. Dig Dis Sci 1980; 25:123–128.
20. Kayama S, Mitsuyama M, Sato N, Hatakeyama K. Overgrowth and translocation of Escherichia coli from intestine during prolonged enteral feeding of rats. J Gastroenterol 2000; 35:15–19.
21. Frankel W, Zhang W, Singh A, Bain A, Satchithanandam S, Klurfeld D, Rombeau J. Fiber: Effect on bacterial translocation and intestinal mucin content. World J Surg 1995; 19:144–148.
22. Deitch EA. Bacterial translocation: The influence of dietary variables. Gut 1994; 25:S23–S27.
23. Mainous M, Xu DZ, Lu Q, Berg RD, Deitch EA. Oral-TPN-induced bacterial translocation and impaired immune defenses are reversed by refeeding. Surgery 1991; 110:277–283.
24. Wykes LJ, Fiorotto ML, Burrin DG, Del Rosario M, Frazer ME, Pond WG, Jahoor F. Chronic low protein intake reduces tissue protein synthesis in a pig model of protein malnutrition. J Nutr 1996; 126:1481–1488.
25. Firmansyah A, Suwandito L, Penn D, Lebenthal E. Biochemical and morphological changes in the digestive tract of rats after prenatal and postnatal malnutrition. Am J Clin Nutr 1989; 50:261–268.
26. Buts JP, Nyakabasa M. Role of dietary protein adaptation at weaning in the development of the rat gastrointestinal tract. Pediatr Res 1985; 19:857–862.
27. Ebner S, Schoknecht PA, Reeds PJ, Burrin DG. Growth and metabolism of gastrointestinal and skeletal muscle tissues in protein-malnourished neonatal pigs. Am J Physiol 1994; 266:R1736–R1743.
28. Stoll B, Chang X, Jiang R, Van Goudoever JB, Reeds PJ, Burrin DG. Enteral carbohydrate and lipid inhibit small intestinal proteolysis in neonatal pigs. FASEB J 2000; 14:A558.
29. Adegoke OA, McBurney MI, Samuels SE, Baracos VE. Luminal amino acids acutely decrease intestinal mucosal protein synthesis and protease mRNA in piglets. J Nutr 1999; 129:1871–1878.
30. Buts JP, Vijverman V, Barudi C, De Keyser N, Maldague P, Dive C. Refeeding after starvation in the rat: Comparative effects of lipids, proteins and carbohydrates on jejunal and ileal mucosal adaptation. Eur J Clin Invest 1990; 20:441–452.
31. Stein TP, Yoshida S, Schluter MD, Drews D, Assimon SA, Leskiw MD. Comparison of intravenous nutrients on gut mucosal protein synthesis. J Parenter Enter Nutr 1994; 18:447–452.
32. Bergström J, Fürst P, Noree LO, Vinnars E. Intracellular free amino acid concentration in human muscle tissue. J Appl Physiol 1974; 36:693–697.

33. Smith RJ. Glutamine metabolism and its physiologic importance. J Parenter Enter Nutr 1990; 14:40S–44S.
34. Souba WW. Interorgan ammonia metabolism in health and disease: A surgeon's view. J Parenter Enter Nutr Suppl 1987; 11:569–579.
35. Souba WW, Klimberg VS, Plumley DA, Salloum RM, Flynn TC, Bland KI, Copeland EM III. The role of glutamine in maintaining a healthy gut and supporting the metabolic response to injury and infection. J Surg Res 1990; 48:383–391.
36. Rouse K, Nwokedi E, Woodliff JE, Epstein J, Klimberg VS. Glutamine enhances selectivity of chemotherapy through changes in glutathione metabolism. Ann Surg 1995; 221:420–426.
37. Klimberg VS. Glutamine, cancer, and its therapy. Am J Surg 1996; 172:418–424.
38. Souba WW, Scott TE, Wilmore DW. Intestinal consumption of intravenously administered fuels. J Parenter Enter Nutr 1985; 9:18–22.
39. Muhlbacher F, Kapadia CR, Colpoys MF, Smith RJ, Wilmore DW. Effects of glucocorticoids on glutamine metabolism in skeletal muscle. Am J Physiol 1984; 247: E75–E83.
40. Wilmore DW. Alterations in protein, carbohydrate, and fat metabolism in injured and septic patients. J Am Coll Nutr 1983; 2:3–13.
41. Windmueller HG. Glutamine utilization by the small intestine. Adv Enzymol Relat Areas Mol Biol 1982; 53:201–237.
42. Souba WW. Glutamine: A key substrate for the splanchnic bed. Annu Rev Nutr 1991; 11:285–308.
43. Souba WW, Smith RJ, Wilmore DW. Effects of glucocorticoids on glutamine metabolism in visceral organs. Metabolism 1985; 34:450–456.
44. Lacey JM, Wilmore WW. Is glutamine a conditionally essential amino acid? Nutr Rev 1990; 48:297–309.
45. Platell C, McCauley R, McCulloch R, Hall J. The influence of parenteral glutamine and branched-chain amino acids on total parenteral nutrition-induced atrophy of the gut. J Parenter Enter Nutr 1993; 17:348–354.
46. Inoue Y, Grant JP, Snyder PJ. Effect of glutamine-supplemented total parenteral nutrition on recovery of the small intestine after starvation atrophy. J Parenter Enter Nutr 1993; 17:165–170.
47. Frankel WL, Zhang W, Afonso J, Klurfeld DM, Don SH, Laitin E, Deaton D, Furth EE, Pietra GG, Naji A, Rombeau JL. Glutamine enhancement of structure and function in transplanted small intestine in the rat. J Parenter Enter Nutr 1993; 17:47–55.
48. van der Hulst RR, van Kreel BK, von Meyenfeldt MF, Brummer RJ, Arends JW, Deutz NE, Soeters PB. Glutamine and the preservation of gut integrity. Lancet 1993; 341:1363–1365.
49. Ziegler TR, Young LS, Benfell K, Scheltinga M, Hortos K, Bye R, Morrow FD, Jacobs DO, Smith RJ, Antin JH, Wilmore DW. Clinical and metabolic efficacy of glutamine-supplemented parenteral nutrition after bone marrow transplantation: A randomized, double-blind, controlled study. Ann Intern Med 1992; 116:821–828.
50. Wiren M, Magnusson KE, Larsson J. Enteral glutamine increases growth and absorptive capacity of intestinal mucosa in the malnourished rat. Scand J Gastroenterol 1995; 30:146–152.

51. Neu J, DeMarco V, Weiss M. Glutamine supplementation in low-birth-weight infants: Mechanisms of action. J Parenter Enter Nutr 1999; 23:S49–S51.
52. Panigrahi P, Gewolb IH, Bamford P, Horvath K. Role of glutamine in bacterial transcytosis and epithelial cell injury. J Parenter Enter Nutr 1997; 21:75–80.
53. DeMarco V, Dyess K, Strauss D, West CM, Neu J. Inhibition of glutamine synthetase decreases proliferation of cultured rat intestinal epithelial cells. J Nutr 1999; 129:57–62.
54. Weiss MD, DeMarco V, Strauss DM, Samuelson DA, Lane ME, Neu J. Glutamine synthetase: A key enzyme for intestinal epithelial differentiation? J Parenter Enter Nutr 1999; 23:140–146.
55. Burrin DG, Shulman RJ, Langston C, Storm MC. Supplemental alanylglutamine, organ growth and nitrogen metabolism in neonatal pigs fed by total parenteral nutrition. J Parenter Enter Nutr 1994; 18:313–319.
56. Bertolo RFP, Pencharz PB, Ball RO. A comparison of parenteral and enteral feeding in neonatal piglets, including an assessment of the utilization of a glutamine-rich, pediatric elemental diet. J Parenter Enter Nutr 1999; 23:47–55.
57. Vanderhoof JA, Kollman KA, Griffin S, Adrian TE. Growth hormone and glutamine do not stimulate intestinal adaptation following massive small bowel resection in the rat. J Pediatr Gastroenterol Nutr 1997; 25:327–331.
58. Michail S, Mohammadpour H, Park JH, Vanderhoof JA. Effect of glutamine-supplemented elemental diet on mucosal adaptation following bowel resection in rats. J Pediatr Gastroenterol Nutr 1995; 21:394–398.
59. Horvath K, Jami M, Hill ID, Papadimitriou JC, Magder LS, Chanasongcram S. Isocaloric glutamine-free diet and the morphology and function of rat small intestine. J Parenter Enter Nutr 1996; 20:128–134.
60. Burrin DG, Reeds PJ. Alternative fuels in the gastrointestinal tract. Curr Opin Gastroenterol 1997; 13:165–170.
61. Matthews DE, Marano MA, Campbell RG. Splanchnic bed utilization of glutamine and glutamic acid in humans. Am J Physiol 1993; 264:E848–E854.
62. Reeds PJ, Burrin DG, Jahoor F, Wykes L, Henry J, Frazer EM. Enteral glutamate is almost completely metabolized in first pass by the gastrointestinal tract of infant pigs. Am J Physiol 1996; 270:E413–E418.
63. Stoll B, Burrin DG, Henry J, Yu H, Jahoor F, Reeds PJ. Substrate oxidation by the portal drained viscera of fed piglets. Am J Physiol 1999; 277:E168–E175.
64. Plauth M, Raible A, Vieillard-Baron D, Bauder-Gross D, Hartmann F. Is glutamine essential for the maintenance of intestinal function? A study in the isolated perfused rat small intestine. Int J Colorectal Dis 1999; 14:86–94.
65. Windmueller HG, Spaeth AE. Respiratory fuels and nitrogen metabolism in vivo in small intestine of fed rats: Quantitative importance of glutamine, glutamate, and aspartate. J Biol Chem 1980; 255:107–112.
66. Wu G, Knabe DA, Yan W, Flynn NE. Glutamine and glucose metabolism in enterocytes of the neonatal pig. Am J Physiol 1995; 268:R334–R342.
67. Wu G, Knabe DA. Arginine synthesis in enterocytes of neonatal pigs. Am J Physiol 1995; 269:R621–R629.
68. Blachier F, M'Rabet-Touil H, Posho L, Darcy-Vrillon B, Duee PH. Intestinal argi-

nine metabolism during development: Evidence for de novo synthesis of L-arginine in newborn pig enterocytes. Eur J Biochem 1993; 216:109–117.

69. Reeds PJ, Burrin DG, Stoll B, Jahoor F, Wykes L, Henry J, Frazer ME. Enteral glutamate is the preferential source for mucosal glutathione synthesis in fed piglets. Am J Physiol 1997; 273:E408–E415.

70. Hasebe M, Suzuki H, Mori E, Furukawa J, Kobayashi K, Ueda Y. Glutamate in enteral nutrition: Can glutamate replace glutamine in supplementation to enteral nutrition in burned rats? J Parenter Enter Nutr 1999; 23:S78–S82.

71. Wang J-Y, Viar MJ, Blanner PM, Johnson LR. Expression of the ornithine decarboxylase gene in response to asparagine in intestinal epithelial cells. Am J Physiol 1996; 271:G164–G171.

72. Kandil HM, Argenzio RA, Chen W, Berschneider HM, Stiles AD, Westwick JK, Rippe RA, Brenner DA, Rhoads JM. L-glutamine and L-asparagine stimulate ODC activity and proliferation in a porcine jejunal enterocyte line. Am J Physiol 1995; 269:G591–G599.

73. Papaconstantinou HT, Hwang KO, Rajaraman S, Hellmich MR, Townsend CM Jr, Ko TC. Glutamine deprivation induces apoptosis in intestinal epithelial cells. Surgery 1998; 124:152–159.

74. Rhoads M. Glutamine signaling in intestinal cells. J Parenter Enter Nutr 1999; 23: S38–S40.

75. Mordrelle A, Jullian E, Costa C, Cormet-Boyaka E, Benamouzig R, Tome D, Huneau JF. EAAT1 is involved in transport of L-glutamate during differentiation of the Caco-2 cell line. Am J Physiol 2000; 279:G366–G373.

76. Murphy JM, Murch SJ, Ball RO. Proline is synthesized from glutamate during intragastric infusion but not during intravenous infusion in neonatal piglets. J Nutr 1996; 126:878–886.

77. Wu G. Intestinal mucosal amino acid catabolism. J Nutr 1998; 128:1249–1252.

78. Dugan MER, Knabe DA, Wu G. The induction of citrulline synthesis from glutamine in enterocytes of weaned pigs is not due primarily to age or change in diet. J Nutr 1995; 125:2388–2393.

79. Davis TA, Nguyen HV, Garcia-Bravo R, Fiorotto ML, Jackson EM, Lewis DS, Lee DR, Reeds PJ. Amino acid composition of human milk is not unique. J Nutr 1994; 124:1126–1132.

80. Hurwitz R, Kretchmer N. Development of arginine-synthesizing enzymes in mouse intestine. Am J Physiol 1986; 251:G103–G110.

81. De Jonge WJ, Dingemanse MA, de Boer PA, Lamers WH, Moorman AF. Argininemetabolizing enzymes in the developing rat small intestine. Pediatr Res 1998; 43: 442–451.

82. Wu G, Morris SM Jr. Arginine metabolism: Nitric oxide and beyond. Biochem J 1998; 336:1–17.

83. Brunton JA, Bertolo RF, Pencharz PB, Ball RO. Proline ameliorates arginine deficiency during enteral but not parenteral feeding in neonatal piglets. Am J Physiol 1999; 277:E223–E231.

84. Blachier F, Selamnia M, Robert V, M'Rabet-Touil H, Duee PH. Metabolism of L-arginine through polyamine and nitric oxide synthase pathways in proliferative or

differentiated human colon carcinoma cells. Biochim Biophys Acta 1995; 1268: 255–262.

85. McCormack SA, Johnson LR. Role of polyamines in gastrointestinal mucosal growth. Am J Physiol 1991; 260:G795–G806.
86. Blachier F, Darcy-Vrillon B, Sener A, Duee PH, Malaisse WJ. Arginine metabolism in rat enterocytes. Biochim Biophys Acta 1991; 1092:304–310.
87. Blachier F, M'Rabet-Touil H, Posho L, Morel MT, Bernard F, Darcy-Vrillon B, Duee PH. Polyamine metabolism in enterocytes isolated from newborn pigs. Biochim Biophys Acta 1992; 1175:21–26.
88. Seidel ER, Haddox MK, Johnson LR. Ileal mucosal growth during intraluminal infusion of ethylamine or putrescine. Am J Physiol 1985; 249:G434–G438.
89. Grant AL, Thomas JW, King KJ, Liesman JS. Effects of dietary amines on small intestinal variables in neonatal pigs fed soy protein isolate. J Anim Sci 1990; 68: 363–371.
90. Dufour C, Dandrifosse G, Forget P, Vermesse F, Romain N, Lepoint P. Spermine and spermidine induce intestinal maturation in the rat. Gastroenterology 1988; 95: 112–116.
91. Pollack PF, Koldovsky O, Nishioka K. Polyamines in human and rat milk and in infant formulas. Am J Clin Nutr 1992; 56:371–375.
92. Buts JP, De Keyser N, De Raedemaeker L, Collette E, Sokal EM. Polyamine profiles in human milk, infant artificial formulas, and semi-elemental diets. J Pediatr Gastroenterol Nutr 1995; 21:44–49.
93. Capano G, Bloch KJ, Carter EA, Dascoli JA, Schoenfeld D, Harmatz PR. Polyamines in human and rat milk influence intestinal cell growth in vitro. J Pediatr Gastroenterol Nutr 1998; 27:281–286.
94. Cosgrove M. Perinatal and infant nutrition: Nucleotides. Nutrition 1998; 14:748–751.
95. Koletzko B, Aggett PJ, Bindels JG, Bung P, Ferre P, Gil A, Lentze MJ, Roberfroid M, Strobel S. Growth, development and differentiation: A functional food science approach. Br J Nutr 1998; 80(suppl 1):S5–S45.
96. Carver JD, Barness LA. Trophic factors for the gastrointestinal tract. Clin Perinatol 1996; 23:265–285.
97. Uauy R, Quan R, Gil A. Role of nucleotides in intestinal development and repair: Implications for infant nutrition. J Nutr 1994; 124(suppl 8):1436S–1441S.
98. Cummings JH. Colonic absorption: the importance of short chain fatty acids in man. Scand J Gastroenterol 1984; 93(suppl):89–99.
99. Englyst HN, Trowell H, Southgate DA, Cummings JH. Dietary fiber and resistant starch. Am J Clin Nutr 1987; 46:873–874.
100. Ravich WJ, Bayless TM, Thomas M. Fructose: Incomplete intestinal absorption in humans. Gastroenterology 1983; 84:26–29.
101. Royall D, Wolever TM, Jeejeebhoy KN. Clinical significance of colonic fermentation. Am J Gastroenterol 1990; 85:1307–1312.
102. Cummings JH, Macfarlane GT. Role of intestinal bacteria in nutrient metabolism. J Parenter Enter Nutr 1997; 21:357–365.
103. Bugaut M, Bentejac M. Biological effects of short-chain fatty acids in nonruminant mammals. Annu Rev Nutr 1993; 13:217–241.

104. Cummings JH. Short chain fatty acids in the human colon. Gut 1981; 22:763–779.

105. Roediger WEW. Role of anaerobic bacteria in the metabolic welfare of the colonic mucosa in man. Gut 1980; 21:793–798.

106. Roediger WEW. Utilization of nutrients by isolated epithelial cells of the rat colon. Gastroenterology 1982; 83:424–429.

107. Clausen MR, Mortensen PB. Kinetic studies on colonocyte metabolism of short chain fatty acids and glucose in ulcerative colitis. Gut 1995; 37:684–689.

108. Chapman MA, Grahn MF, Hutton M, Williams NS. Butyrate metabolism in the terminal ileal mucosa of patients with ulcerative colitis. Br J Surg 1995; 82:36–38.

109. Ruppin H, Bar-Meir S, Soergel KH, Wood CM, Schmitt MG Jr. Absorption of short-chain fatty acids by the colon. Gastroenterology 1980; 78:1500–1507.

110. Binder HJ, Mehta P. Short-chain fatty acids stimulate active sodium and chloride absorption in vitro in the rat distal colon. Gastroenterology 1989; 96:989–996.

111. Bowling TE, Raimundo AH, Grimble GK, Silk DBA. Reversal by short-chain fatty acids of colonic fluid secretion induced by enteral feeding. Lancet 1993; 342:1266–1268.

112. Velazquez OC, Seto RW, Rombeau JL. The scientific rationale and clinical application of short-chain fatty acids and medium-chain triacylglycerols. Proc Nutr Soc 1996; 55:49–78.

113. Velazquez OC, Lederer HM, Rombeau JL. Butyrate and the colonocyte: Production, absorption, metabolism, and therapeutic implications. Adv Exp Med Biol 1997; 427:123–134.

114. Kien CL. Digestion, absorption, and fermentation of carbohydrates in the newborn. Clin Perinatol 1996; 23:211–228.

115. Roediger WEW. Famine, fiber, fatty acids, and failed colonic absorption: Does fiber fermentation ameliorate diarrhea? J Parenter Enter Nutr 1994; 18:4–8.

116. Roediger WE, Kapaniris O, Millard S. Lipogenesis from n-butyrate in colonocytes: Action of reducing agent and 5-aminosalicylic acid with relevance to ulcerative colitis. Mol Cell Biochem 1992; 118:113–118.

117. Sakata T. Stimulatory effect of short-chain fatty acids on epithelial cell proliferation in the rat intestine: A possible explanation for trophic effects of fermentable fibre, gut microbes and luminal trophic factors. Br J Nutr 1987; 58:95–103.

118. Mortensen FV, Hessov I, Birke H, Korsgaard N, Nielsen H. Microcirculatory and trophic effects of short chain fatty acids in the human rectum after Hartmann's procedure. Br J Surg 1991; 78:1208–1211.

119. Cherbut C, Aube AC, Blottiere HM, Galmiche JP. Effects of short-chain fatty acids on gastrointestinal motility. Scand J Gastroenterol 1997; 222(suppl):58–61.

120. Tappenden KA, Thomson AB, Wild GE, McBurney MI. Short-chain fatty acids increase proglucagon and ornithine decarboxylase messenger RNAs after intestinal resection in rats. J Parenter Enter Nutr 1996; 20:357–362.

121. Tappenden KA, McBurney MI. Systemic short-chain fatty acids rapidly alter gastrointestinal structure, function, and expression of early response genes. Dig Dis Sci 1998; 43:1526–1536.

122. Reimer RA, McBurney MI. Dietary fiber modulates intestinal proglucagon messen-

ger ribonucleic acid and postprandial secretion of glucagon-like peptide-1 and insulin in rats. Endocrinology 1996; 137:3948–3956.

123. Plaisancie P, Dumoulin V, Chayvialle JA, Cuber JC. Luminal peptide YY-releasing factors in the isolated vascularly perfused rat colon. J Endocrinol 1996; 151:421–429.

124. Koruda MJ, Rolandelli RH, Bliss DZ, Hastings J, Rombeau JL, Settle RG. Parenteral nutrition supplemented with short-chain fatty acids: effect on the small-bowel mucosa in normal rats. Am J Clin Nutr 1990; 51:685–689.

125. Reilly KJ, Frankel WL, Bain AM, Rombeau JL. Colonic short chain fatty acids mediate jejunal growth by increasing gastrin. Gut 1995; 37:81–86.

126. Hague A, Butt AJ, Paraskeva C. The role of butyrate in human colonic epithelial cells: An energy source or inducer of differentiation and apoptosis? Proc Nutr Soc 1996; 55:937–943.

127. Jacobs LR. Relationship between dietary fiber and cancer: Metabolic, physiologic, and cellular mechanisms. Proc Soc Exp Biol Med 1986; 183:299–310.

128. McIntyre A, Gibson PR, Young GP. Butyrate production from dietary fibre and protection against large bowel cancer in a rat model. Gut 1993; 34:386–391.

129. Howe GR, Benito E, Castelleto R, Cornee J, Esteve J, Gallagher RP, Iscovich JM, Deng-ao J, Kaaks R, Kune GA, Kune S, L'Abbé KA, Lee HP, Lee M, Miller AB, Peters RK, Potter JD, Riboli E, Slattery ML, Trichopoulos D, Tuyns A, Tzonou A, Whittemore AS, Wu-Williams AH, Shu Z. Dietary intake of fiber and decreased risk of cancers of the colon and rectum: Evidence from the combined analysis of 13 case-control studies. J Natl Cancer Inst 1992; 84:1887–1896.

130. Hague A, Singh B, Paraskeva C. Butyrate acts as a survival factor for colonic epithelial cells: Further fuel for the in vivo versus in vitro debate. Gastroenterology 1997; 112:1036–1040.

131. Scheppach W, Bartram HP, Richter F. Role of short-chain fatty acids in the prevention of colorectal cancer. Eur J Cancer 1995; 31A:1077–1080.

132. Jass JR. Diet, butyric acid and differentiation of gastrointestinal tract tumours. Med Hypotheses 1985; 18:113–118.

133. Rasmussen HS, Holtug K, Ynggard C, Mortensen PB. Faecal concentrations and production rates of short chain fatty acids in normal neonates. Acta Paediatr Scand 1988; 77:365–368.

134. Long SS, Swenson RM. Development of anaerobic fecal flora in healthy newborn infants. J Pediatr 1977; 91:298–301.

135. Kleessen B, Bunke H, Tovar K, Noack J, Sawatzki G. Influence of two infant formulas and human milk on the development of the faecal flora in newborn infants. Acta Paediatr 1995; 84:1347–1356.

136. Roberts AK, Chierici R, Sawatzki G, Hill MJ, Volpato S, Vigi V. Supplementation of an adapted formula with bovine lactoferrin: 1. Effect on the infant faecal flora. Acta Paediatr 1992; 81:119–124.

137. Kunz C, Rudloff S. Biological functions of oligosaccharides in human milk. Acta Paediatr 1993; 82:903–912.

138. Bullen CL, Willis AT. Resistance of the breast-fed infant to gastroenteritis. Br Med J 1971; 3:338–343.

139. Kunz C, Rodriguez-Palmero M, Koletzko B, Jensen R. Nutritional and biochemical

properties of human milk: Part I. General aspects, proteins, and carbohydrates. Clin Perinatol 1999; 26:307–333.

140. Newburg DS. Do the binding properties of oligosaccharides in milk protect human infants from gastrointestinal bacteria? J Nutr 1997; 127:980S–984S.

141. Newburg DS. Human milk glycoconjugates that inhibit pathogens. Curr Med Chem 1999; 6:117–127.

142. Koldovsky O. Hormonally active peptides in human milk. Acta Paediatr Suppl 1994; 402:89–93.

143. Barnard JA, Beauchamp RD, Russell WE, Dubois RN, Coffey RJ. Epidermal growth factor–related peptides and their relevance to gastrointestinal pathophysiology. Gastroenterology 1995; 108:564–580.

144. Searle NJ, Playford RJ. Growth factors and gut function. Proc Nutr Soc 1998; 57: 403–408.

145. Thompson JS. Epidermal growth factor inhibits somatostatin-induced apoptosis. J Surg Res 1999; 81:95–100.

146. Thompson JS. Epidermal growth factor and the short bowel syndrome. J Parenter Enter Nutr 1999b; 23:S113–S116.

147. Wong W-M, Wright NA. Epidermal growth factor, epidermal growth factor receptors, intestinal growth, and adaptation. J Parenter Enter Nutr 1999; 23:S83–S88.

148. Uribe JM, Barrett KE. Nonmitogenic actions of growth factors: An integrated view of their role in intestinal physiology and pathophysiology. Gastroenterology 1997; 112:255–268.

149. Donovan SM, Odle J. Growth factors in milk as mediators of infant development. Annu Rev Nutr 1994; 14:147–167.

150. Lund PK. Molecular basis of intestinal adaptation: the role of the insulin-like growth factor system. Ann NY Acad Sci 1998; 859:18–36.

151. MacDonald RS. The role of insulin-like growth factors in small intestinal cell growth and development. Horm Metab Res 1999; 31:103–113.

152. Shulman RJ. Oral insulin increases small intestinal mass and disaccharidase activity in the newborn miniature pig. Pediatr Res 1990; 28:171–175.

153. Park YK, Monaco MH, Donovan SM. Enteral insulin-like growth factor-I augments intestinal disaccharidase activity in piglets receiving total parenteral nutrition. J Parenter Enter Nutr 1999; 29:198–206.

154. Burrin DG, Fiorotto ML, Hadsell DL. Transgenic hypersecretion of des(1-3) human insulin-like growth factor I in mouse milk has limited effects on the gastrointestinal tract in suckling pups. J Nutr 1999; 129:51–56.

155. Alexander AN, Carey HV. Oral IGF-I enhances nutrient and electrolyte absorption in neonatal piglet intestine. Am J Physiol 1999; 277:G619–G625.

156. Ney DM, Huss DJ, Gillingham MB, Kritsch KR, Dahly EM, Talamantez JL, Adamo ML. Investigation of insulin-like growth factor (IGF)-I and insulin receptor binding and expression in jejunum of parenterally fed rats treated with IGF-I or growth hormone. Endocrinology 1999; 140:4850–4860.

157. Read LC, Tomas FM, Howarth GS, Martin AA, Edson KJ, Gillespie CM, Owens PC, Ballard FJ. Insulin-like growth factor-I and its N-terminal modified analogues induce marked gut growth in dexamethasone-treated rats. J Endocrinol 1992; 133: 421–431.

158. Wang J, Niu W, Nikiforov Y, Naito S, Chernausek S, Witte D, LeRoith D, Strauch A, Fagin JA. Targeted overexpression of IGF-I evokes distinct patterns of organ remodeling in smooth muscle cell tissue beds of transgenic mice. J Clin Invest 1997; 100:1425–1439.

159. Steeb CB, Shoubridge CA, Tivey DR, Read LC. Systemic infusion of IGF-I or LR(3)IGF-I stimulates visceral organ growth and proliferation of gut tissues in suckling rats. Am J Physiol 1997; 272:G522–G533.

160. Singh P, Rubin N. Insulinlike growth factor and binding proteins in colon cancer. Gastroenterology 1993; 105:1218–1237.

161. Nusrat A, Parkos CA, Bacarra AE, Godowski PJ, Delp-Archer C, Rosen EM, Madara JL. Hepatocyte growth factor/scatter factor effects on epeithelia. J Clin Invest 1994; 93:2056–2065.

162. Göke M, Kanai M, Podolsky DK. Intestinal fibroblasts regulate intestinal epithelial cell proliferation via hepatocyte growth factor. Am J Physiol 1998; 274:G809–G818.

163. Yamada Y, Saito S, Morikawa H. Hepatocyte growth factor in human breast milk. Am J Reprod Immunol 1998; 40:112–120.

164. Kato Y, Yu D, Schwartz MZ. Enhancement of intestinal adaptation by hepatocyte growth factor. J Pediatr Surg 1998; 33:235–239.

165. Fan L, Iseki S. Immunohistochemical localization of vascular endothelial growth factor in the globule leukocyte/mucosal mast cell of the rat respiratory and digestive tracts. Histochem Cell Biol 1999; 111:13–21.

166. Siafakas CG, Anatolitou F, Fusunyan RD, Walker WA, Sanderson IR. Vascular endothelial growth factor (VEGF) is present in human breast milk and its receptor is present on intestinal epithelial cells. Pediatr Res 1999; 45:652–657.

167. Okunieff P, Mester M, Wang J, Maddox T, Gong X, Tang D, Coffee M, Ding I. In vivo radioprotective effects of angiogenic growth factors on the small bowel of C3H mice. Radiat Res 1998; 150:204–211.

168. Poldovsky DK. Regulation of intestinal epithelial proliferation: A few answers, many questions. Am J Physiol 1993; 264:G179–G186.

169. Jones MK, Tomikawa M, Mohajer B, Tarnawski AS. Gastrointestinal mucosal regeneration: Role of growth factors. Front Biosci 1999; 4:d303–d309.

170. Ziegler TR, Estivariz CF, Jonas CR, Gu LH, Jones DP, Leader LM. Interactions between nutrients and peptide growth factors in intestinal growth, repair, and function. J Parenter Enter Nutr 1999; 23:S174–S183.

171. Playford RJ, Marchbank T, Mandir N, Higham A, Meeran K, Ghatei MA, Bloom SR, Goodlad RA. Effects of keratinocyte growth factor (KGF) on gut growth and repair. J Pathol 1998; 184:316–322.

172. Walsh JH. Gastrointestinal hormones. In: Johnson LR, Alpers DH, Christensen J, Jacobson ED, Walsh JH, eds. Physiology of the Gastrointestinal Tract. New York: Raven, 1994, pp 1–128.

173. Johnson LR, McCormick SA. Regulation of gastrointestinal mucosal growth. In: Johnson LR, Alpers DH, Christensen J, Jacobson ED, Walsh JH, eds. Physiology of the Gastrointestinal Tract. New York: Raven, 1994, pp 611–641.

174. Koh TJ, Goldenring JR, Ito S, Mashimo H, Kopin AS, Varro A, Dockray GJ, Wang

TC. Gastrin deficiency results in altered gastric differentiation. Gastroenterology 1997; 113:1015–1025.

175. Pinson DM, Hvu N, Sztgern MI, Mattsson H, Looney GA, Kimler BF, Hurwitz A. Drug-induced hypergastrinemia: Absence of trophic effects on colonic carcinoma in rats. Gastroenterology 1995; 108:1068–1074.

176. Rehfeld JF. Gastrin and colorectal cancer: a never-ending dispute? Gastroenterology 1995; 108:1307–1310.

177. Varga G, Kisfalvi K, Pelosini I, D'Amato M, Scarpignato C. Different actions of CCK on pancreatic and gastric growth in the rat: effect of CCK(A) receptor blockade. Br J Pharmacol 1998; 124:435–440.

178. Miyasaka K, Shinozaki H, Suzuki S, Sato Y, Kanai S, Masuda M, Jimi A, Nagata A, Matsui T, Noda T, Kono A, Funakoshi A. Disruption of cholecystokinin (CCK)-B receptor gene did not modify bile or pancreatic secretion or pancreatic growth: A study in CCK-B receptor gene knockout mice. Pancreas 1999; 19:114–118.

179. Konturek SJ, Dembinski A, Warzecha Z, Jaworek J, Konturek PK, Cai R-Z, Schally AV. Antagonism of receptors for bombesin, gastrin and cholecystokinin in pancreatic secretion and growth. Digestion 1991; 48:89–97.

180. Lacourse KA, Swanberg LJ, Gillespie PJ, Rehfeld JF, Saunders TL, Samuelson LC. Pancreatic function in CCK-deficient mice: Adaptation to dietary protein does not require CCK. Am J Physiol 1999; 276:G1302–G1309.

181. Weinberg DS, Ruggeri B, Barber MT, Biswas S, Miknyocki S, Waldman SA. Cholecystokinin A and B receptors are differentially expressed in normal pancreas and pancreatic adenocarcinoma. J Clin Invest 1997; 100:597–603.

182. Andren-Sandberg A, Hoem D, Backman PL. Other risk factors for pancreatic cancer: Hormonal aspects. Ann Oncol 1999; 10:131–135.

183. Thompson JS, Nguyen B-L T, Harty RF. Somatostatin analogue inhibits intestinal regeneration. Arch Surg 1993; 128:385–389.

184. Buscail L, Saint-Laurent N, Castre E, Vaillant JC, Gespach C, Capella G, Kalthoff H, Lluis F, Vaysse N, Susini C. Loss of sst2 somatostatin receptor gene expression in human pancreatic and colorectal cancer. Cancer Res 1996; 56:1823–1827.

185. Holst JJ, Enteroglucagon. Annu Rev Physiol 1997; 59:257–271.

186. Drucker DJ. Glucagon-like peptides. Diabetes 1998; 47:159–169.

187. Drucker DJ. Glucagon-like peptide 2. Trends Endocrinol Metabol 1999; 10:153–156.

188. Cheeseman CI. Upregulation of SGLT-1 transport activity in rat jejunum induced by GLP-2 infusion in vivo. Am J Physiol 1997; 273:R1965–R1971.

189. Xiao Q, Boushey RP, Drucker DJ, Brubaker PL. Secretion of the intestinotropic hormone glucagon-like peptide 2 is differentially regulated by nutrients in humans. Gastroenterology 1999; 117:99–105.

190. Jeppesen PB, Hartmann B, Hansen BS, Thulesen J, Holst JJ, Mortensen PB. Impaired meal stimulated glucagon-like peptide 2 response in ileal resected short bowel patients with intestinal failure. Gut 1999; 45:559–563.

191. Evers BM. Expression of the neurotensin/neuromedin N gene in the gut. In: Greeley GH Jr, ed. Gastrointestinal Endocrinology. Totowa, NJ: Humana, 1999, pp 425–438.

192. Izukura M, Evers BM, Parekh D, Yoshinaga K, Uchida T, Townsend CM Jr, Thompson JC. Neurotensin augments intestinal regeneration after small bowel resection in rats. Ann Surg 1992; 215:520–526.

193. Evers BM, Izukura M, Townsend CM Jr, Uchida T, Thompson JC. Differential effects of gut hormones on pancreatic and intestinal growth during administration of an elemental diet. Ann Surg 1990; 21:630–636.

194. Chung DH, Evers BM, Shimoda I, Townsend CM Jr, Rajaraman S, Thompson JC. Effect of neurotensin on gut mucosal growth in rats with jejunal and ileal Thiry-Vella fistulas. Gastroenterology 1992; 103:1254–1259.

195. Maoret JJ, Anini Y, Rouyer-Fessard C, Gully D, Laburthe M. Neurotensin and nonpeptide neurotensin receptor antagonist control human colon cancer cell growth in cell culture and in cells xenografted into nude mice. Int J Cancer 1999; 80:448–454.

196. Gomez G, Udupi V, Greeley GH Jr. Peptide YY. In: Greeley GH Jr, ed. Gastrointestinal Endocrinology. Totowa, NJ: Humana, 1999, pp 551–576.

197. Wøjdemann M, Wettergren A, Hartmann B, Holst JJ. Glucagon-like peptide-2 inhibits centrally induced antral motility in pigs. Scand J Gastroenterol 1998; 33: 828–832.

198. Wøjdemann M, Wettergren A, Hartmann B, Hilsted L, Holst JJ. Inhibition of sham feeding-stimulated human gastric acid secretion by glucagon-like peptide-2. J Clin Endocrinol Metab 1999; 84:2513–2517.

199. Goodlad RA, Ghatei MA, Domin J, Bloom SR, Wright NA. Is peptide YY trophic to the intestinal epithelium of parenterally fed rats? Digestion 1990; 46:177–181.

200. Dockray GJ. Physiology of enteric neuropeptides. In: Johnson LR, Alpers DH, Christensen J, Jacobson ED, Walsh JH, eds. Physiology of the Gastrointestinal Tract. New York: Raven, 1994, pp 169–209.

201. Chu KU, Evers BM, Ishizuka J, Townsend CM Jr, Thompson JC. Role of bombesin on gut mucosal growth. Ann Surg 1995; 222:94–100.

202. Gulluoglu BM, Kurtel H, Gulluoglu MG, Aktan AO, Yegen BC, Dizdaroglu F, Yalin R, Yegen BC. Bombesin ameliorates colonic damage in experimental colitis. Dig Dis Sci 1999; 44:1531–1538.

203. Chu KU, Higashide S, Evers BM, Ishizuka J, Townsend CM Jr, Thompson JC. Bombesin stimulates mucosal growth in jejunal and ileal Thiry-Vella fistulas. Ann Surg 1995; 221:602–609.

204. Sagor GR, Ghatei MA, O'Shaughnessy DJ, Al-Mukhtar MY, Wright NA, Bloom SR. Influence of somatostatin and bombesin on plasma enteroglucagon and cell proliferation after intestinal resection in the rat. Gut 1985; 26:89–94.

205. Ide A, Yoshinaga K, Iwama T, Mishima Y. Bombesin enhances experimental carcinogenesis induced in rat colon by 1,2-dimethylhydrazine. Carcinogenesis 1994; 15: 2095–2098.

206. Puccio F, Lehy T. Bombesin ingestion stimulates epithelial digestive cell proliferation in suckling rats. Am J Physiol 1989; 256:G328–G334.

207. Yeh KY, Moog F. Hormonal influences on the growth and enzymic differentiation of the small intestine of the hypophysectomized rat. Growth 1978; 42:495–504.

208. Ulshen MH, Dowling RH, Fuller CR, Zimmermann EM, Lund PK. Enhanced

growth of small bowel in transgenic mice overexpressing bovine growth hormone. Gastroenterology 1993; 104:973–980.

209. Byrne TA, Morrissey TB, Nattakom TV, Ziegler TR, Wilmore DW. Growth hormone, glutamine, and modified diet enhance nutrient absorption in patients with severe short bowel syndrome. J Parenter Enter Nutr 1995; 19:296–302.

210. Velasco B, Lassaletta L, Garcia R, Tovar JA. Intestinal lengthening and growth hormone in extreme short bowel syndrome: A case report. J Pediatr Surg 1999; 34:1423–1424.

211. Benhamou PH, Canarelli JP, Richard S, Cordonnier C, Postel IJP, Grenier E, Leke A, Dupont C. Human recombinant growth hormone increases small bowel lengthening after massive small bowel resection in piglets. J Pediatr Surg 1997; 32:1332–1336.

212. Scolapio JS, Camilleri M, Fleming CR, Oenning LV, Burton DD, Sebo TJ, Batts KP, Kelly DG. Effect of growth hormone, glutamine,and diet on adaptation in short-bowel syndrome: A randomized, controlled study. Gastroenterology 1997; 113: 1074–1081.

213. Ney DM. Effects of insulin-like growth factor-I and growth hormone in models of parenteral nutrition. J Parenter Enter Nutr 1999; 23:S184–S189.

214. Peterson CA, Carey HV, Hinton PL, Lo HC, Ney DM. GH elevates serum IGF-I levels but does not alter mucosal atrophy in parenterally fed rats. Am J Physiol 1997; 272:G1100–G1108.

215. Henning SJ, Rubin DC, Shulman RJ. Ontogeny of the intestinal mucosa. In: Johnson LR, Alpers DH, Christensen J, Jacobson ED, Walsh JH, eds. Physiology of the Gastrointestinal Tract. New York: Raven, 1994, pp 571–610.

216. Scott J, Batt RM, Maddison YE, Peters TJ. Differential effect of glucocorticoids on structure and function of adult rat jejunum. Am J Physiol 1981; 241:G306–G312.

217. Wright NA, Al-Dewachi HS, Appleton DR, Watson AJ. The effect of single and of multiple doses of prednisolone tertiary butyl acetate on cell population kinetics in the small bowel mucosa of the rat. Virchows Arch B Cell Pathol 1978; 28:339–350.

218. Quaroni A, Tian JQ, Goke M, Podolsky DK. Glucocorticoids have pleiotropic effects on small intestinal crypt cells. Am J Physiol 1999; 277:G1027–G1040.

219. Su Y, Shi Y, Stolow MA, Shi YB. Thyroid hormone induces apoptosis in primary cell cultures of tadpole intestine: Cell type specificity and effects of extracellular matrix. J Cell Biol 1997; 139:1533–1543.

220. Burrin DG, Wester TJ, Davis TA, Fiorotto ML, Chang X. Dexamethasone inhibits small intestinal growth via increased protein catabolism in neonatal pigs. Am J Physiol 1999; 276:E269–E277.

221. Park JH, McCusker RH, Mohammadpour H, Blackwood DJ, Hrbek M, Vanderhoof JA. Dexamethasone inhibits mucosal adaptation after snmall bowel resection. Am J Physiol 1994; 266:G497–G503.

222. Trahair JF, Perry RA, Silver M, Robinson PM. Studies on the maturation of the small intestine in the fetal sheep: II. The effects of exogenous cortisol. Q J Exp Physiol 1987; 72:71–79.

223. Chapple RP, Cuaron JA, Easter RA. Effect of glucocorticoids and limiting nursing

on the carbohydrate digestive capacity and growth rate of piglets. J Anim Sci 1989; 67:2956–2973.

224. Poldovsky DK. Peptide growth factors in the gastrointestinal tract. In: Johnson LR, Alpers DH, Christensen J, Jacobson ED, Walsh JH, eds. Physiology of the Gastrointestinal Tract. New York: Raven, 1994, pp 129–167.

225. Penttila IA, van Spriel AB, Zhang MF, Xian CJ, Steeb CB, Cummins AG, Zola H, Read LC. Transforming growth factor-beta levels in maternal milk and expression in postnatal rat duodenum and ileum. Pediatr Res 1998; 44:524–531.

226. Schroder O, Hess S, Caspary WF, Stein J. Mediation of differentiating effects of butyrate on the intestinal cell line Caco-2 by transforming growth factor-beta 1. Eur J Nutr 1999; 38:45–50.

227. Poldovsky DK. Mucosal immunity and inflammation: V. Innate mechanisms of mucosal defense and repair: The best offense is a good defense. Am J Physiol 1999; 277:G495–G499.

228. Kagnoff MF, Eckmann L. Epithelial cells as sensors for microbial infection. J Clin Invest 1997; 100:6–10.

229. Fiocchi C. Inflammatory bowel disease: Etiology and pathogenesis. Gastroenterology 1998; 115:182–205.

230. Rafferty JF, Noguishi Y, Fischer JE, Hasselgren P-O. Sepsis in rats stimulates cellular proliferation in the mucosa of the small intestine. Gastroenterology 1994; 107: 121–127.

231. Piguet PF, Vesin C, Donati Y, Barazzone C. TNF-induced enterocyte apoptosis and detachment in mice: Induction of caspases and prevention by a caspase inhibitor ZVAD-fmk. Lab Invest 1999; 79:495–500.

232. Kim JM, Eckmann L, Savidge TC, Lowe DC, Witthöft T, Kagnoff MF. Apoptosis of human intestinal epithelial cells after bacterial invasion. J Clin Invest 1998; 102: 1815–1823.

233. Garrington TP, Johnson GL. Organization and regulation of mitogen-activated protein kinase signaling pathways. Curr Opin Cell Biol 1999; 11:211–218.

234. Butler AA, Yakar S, Gewolb IH, Karas M, Okubo Y, LeRoith D. Insulin-like growth factor-I receptor signal transduction: At the interface between physiology and cell biology. Comp Biochem Physiol B Biochem Mol Biol 1998; 121:19–26.

235. Knall C, Johnson GL. G-protein regulatory pathways: rocketing into the twenty-first century. J Cell Biochem Suppl 1998; 30–31:137–146.

236. Cary LA, Guan J-L. Focal adhesion kinase in integrin-mediated signaling. Front Biosci 1999; 4:102–113.

237. Denhardt DT. Signal-transducing protein phosphorylation cascades mediated by RAS/Rho proteins in the mammalian cell: The potential for multiplex signalling. Biochem J 1996; 318:729–747.

4

New Additions to Infant Formulas

Angel Gil
University of Granada, Granada, Spain

1   INTRODUCTION

Recommended daily nutrient intakes to support adequate growth of the human infant have been established. However, there is a lack of information about how semiessential nutrients can affect growth in early life and in particular situations, including disease. Human milk provides all necessary nutrients for growth of the term infant. Furthermore, in addition to universally recognized nutrients, human milk contains a number of nonnutritive components—such as enzymes, hormones, and growth factors—that are likely to play a role in supporting infant growth (1).

In the last few years, owing to their potential or proven benefits in infancy, new additions of nonnutritive components and semiessential nutrients to infant formulas have been implemented by a number of milk formula manufacturers. Nucleotides and long-chain polyunsaturated fatty acids are the most relevant recent additions to infant formulas, and these have been approved by a number of international agencies. Other nutrients—namely, amino acids, aminosugars, and glycolipids—a few of them with prebiotic functions, are under consideration to be added in the near future (2). Moreover, selected strains of bacteria with probiotic functions have recently been added to follow-on infant formulas in the European Union and other countries.

The aim of this chapter is to summarize the scientific rationale for the addition of those components to infant formulas and provide a practical guide of current formulas containing those substances in the European Union and the United States. Specific information about polyunsaturated fat and probiotics are found in Chapters 2 and 5, respectively.

2 NONPROTEIN NITROGEN COMPOUNDS OF HUMAN MILK AND FORMULAS

Up to 30% of the total nitrogen in human milk is nonprotein nitrogen, whereas this fraction represents about 5% in cow's milk. The nonprotein fraction of human milk has been partially characterized and includes ammonia, urea, free amino acids, amino alcohols, amino sugars, some syaloconjugated lipids, creatine, creatinine, carnitine, polyamines, peptides, nucleic acids, nucleotides, and uric acid (see Chap. 6). In recent years, a number of these nitrogen-containing compounds have been recognized as modulators of important physiologic functions in the neonate. The significance of these compounds is not proportional to their contribution to the nitrogen supply of human milk, as they may play regulatory roles in neonatal development rather than serving as precursors for the synthesis of biomolecules (2,3).

The contribution of the nonprotein nitrogen fraction to the total nitrogen content of milk is at least three times greater in human milk than in formula. In the last decade, manufacturers of infant formula have supplemented both cow's milk–and soy-based formulas with various amounts of nonprotein nitrogen constituents present in human milk; some of such products are taurine and carnitine. Nucleotides, currently considered as semiessential nutrients for the neonate, are now being added in many countries to some infant formulas. Likewise, some amino acids and derivatives—namely, arginine, glutamine, and choline as well as other miscellaneous substances such as myoinositol—are now being added to infant formulas to levels found in human milk. Other compounds exhibiting prebiotic functions and found in relatively high levels in human milk, such as polyamines, are also candidates to be added to infant formulas.

2.1 Nucleotides and Nucleic Acids

2.1.1 Biological Roles of Nucleotides

Nucleotides are low-molecular-weight intracellular compounds that play a key role in nearly all biochemical processes. They contain three characteristic components: a nitrogenous base [cytosine (C), thymine (T), uracil (U), adenine (A), guanine (G), hypoxanthine (H), xanthine (X), and orotate (O)], a pentose (ribose or deoxyribose), and one or more phosphate groups. A nucleoside is formed from a glycosidic linkage of a pentose to a nitrogenous base. A nucleotide is a phosphate ester of a nucleoside. The most common site of esterification is carbon No. 5 of the pentose, and this is referred to as a $5'$ nucleotide.

Nucleotides are the activated precursors of nucleic acids (DNA and RNA); adenosine triphosphate (ATP) is the universal currency of energy in biological systems; guanosine triphosphate (GTP) powers many movements of macromolecules, such as translocation of nascent polypeptides and the activation of signal-coupling proteins in the hormonal responses. Adenine nucleotides are components of the major coenzymes NAD^+, $NADP^+$, and coenzyme A; nucleotide derivatives (i.e., UDP-glucose, CDP-choline, and CDP-diacylglycerol) are precursors of glycogen and phosphoglycerides; while S-adenosylmethionine is an important methyl donor in some biosynthetic processes. Cyclic nucleotides are important regulators of many pathways and mediators of the action of many hormones (4).

Soluble nucleotides are present in milk from various mammals, contributing up to 20% of the nonprotein nitrogen. Although nucleotide deficiency has not been related to any particular disease, dietary nucleotides have reportedly been beneficial to infants, since they positively influence lipid metabolism, immunity, and tissue growth for both development and repair (5–10).

2.1.2 Nucleotides and Nucleic Acids in Foods

Nucleotides are naturally present in all foods of animal and vegetable origin as free nucleotides and nucleic acids. Concentrations of RNA and DNA in foods depend mainly on the food's cell density, whereas the content of free nucleotides is species-specific. Thus, beef, fish, and seeds have a high content of nucleic acids, while milk, eggs, and fruits have relatively lower levels. The total content of RNA varies between 50 and 400 mg/100 g for animal viscera, 80 and 350 mg/100 g for marine foods, and 140 and 490 mg/100 g for dry legumes (7,8).

Meat and fish have unusually high levels of free inosine monophosphate (IMP) derived from adenosine monophosphate (AMP) deamination (about 200 mg/100 g) and low levels of free AMP (about 10 mg/100 g). However, the main nucleotides in vegetable foodstuffs are AMP and uridine monophosphate (UMP), except for mushrooms, which contain large amounts of guanosine monophosphate (GMP). Both IMP and GMP contribute to meat and fish flavor, and those nucleotides are widely used in foods as flavor enhancers (8).

2.1.3 Nucleotides and Nucleic Acids in Human Milk and Formulas

Nucleotides were first isolated from human milk about 30 years ago. Since then, a number of investigators have identified at least 13 acid-soluble nucleotides in human milk, of which cytidine, adenosine, and uridine phosphates are in relatively high concentration whereas orotate, a pyrimidine nucleotide precursor, is absent or only minimally detected. On the contrary, cow's milk is known to contain relatively high concentrations of orotate and low levels of cytidine and adenine derivatives (5). Milk also contains nucleic acids; the total DNA and RNA in milk varies according to the particular species and the number of lymphocytes and other immune cells present (5,11).

A number of authors have demonstrated both qualitative and quantitative differences in the nucleotide composition of milk from different species. Wide ranges and differences between authors are due to variability in stage of lactation at which the milk was sampled and to methods used to collect and assay samples. Table 1 gives a summary of the nucleotide and nucleic acid contents in human and cow's milk.

Milk has a specific free nucleotide profile for each species. The nucleotide content of colostrum is qualitatively similar but quantitatively distinct in human and ruminants. In general, total colostrum nucleotide content increases immediately after parturition, reaches maximum levels from 24 to 48 hr after birth, and decreases thereafter with advancing lactation (5,6,11).

Differences in nucleotide patterns between species are more pronounced in mature milk than in colostrum. Free nucleosides, monophosphate and diphosphate nucleosides, and nucleotide adducts of purine and pyrimidine have been reported in human milk, with values being highest at earlier stages of lactation (about 200 µmol/L) (1–6). Cytidine and uridine nucleotides make up the first and second largest free nucleotide fractions. CMP, CDP-choline, UMP, and UDP adduct of glucose, galactose, N-acetyl-glucosamine, and N-acetyl-galactosamine remain high throughout lactation in human milk, whereas in cow's milk, cytidine and uridine derivatives rapidly decrease from colostrum to mature milk. Values

TABLE 1 Comparison of Human and Cow's Milk Nucleotides by Different Authors[a]

Reference	Milk	RNA	NT	NS	NT Adducts	Total
Gil and Uauy (5)	Human	36.7–200	70.8	52.6[a]	50.7	121.5[c]
Leach et al. (11)	Human	89.8	67.4	15.0	16.8	189
Thorell et al. (13)	Human	68	84.2	10.3	N.A	163
Gil and Uauy (5)	Cow	26.7–63.3	13.3	9.2[b]	15.9	29.2[c]

[a] All data expressed in micromoles per liter. RNA data in Gil and Uauy (5) were obtained by RNA isolation and UV quantitation.
[b] Nucleoside values were obtained by Schlimme et al. (1986) as specified in Gil and Uauy (5).
[c] Included only acid-soluble nucleotides but not polymeric forms.

for AMP are the most variable, and GMP and guanosine derivatives are found in lesser amounts. IMP may appear in human milk, but its presence is apparently due to enzymatic deamination of AMP after sample collection. Minor fluctuating amounts of the cyclic derivatives of adenosine and guanosine are also present in human milk (5).

Nucleic acids in human milk have been found in concentrations ranging from 100 to 5600 mg of RNA per liter milk and from 10 to 120 mg of DNA per liter of milk (3). The wide ranges reported reflect differences attributed to both stages of lactation and socioeconomic groups. However, the methods used to measure nucleic acids were unreliable and had low specificity. In recent years, a new enzymatic method capable of quantifying free nucleosides, free nucleotides, nucleotide adducts, and RNA in milk has been used to determine the total potentially available nucleosides (TPAN) in human milk (11). The mean TPAN concentration ranged from 49 mg/L in colostrum to 87 mg/L in mature milk, with an overall mean of 67 mg/L. Data from a pooled sample collected from American women had a mean of 72 mg/L, and nucleotides were predominantly present in the monomeric (36%) and polymeric (48%) forms. These concentrations are two to three times higher than those previously reported for acid-soluble nucleotides.

Most of the milk formulas currently marketed over the world contain minor amounts of nucleosides and nucleotides and have a wide range for orotate. This is caused by differences in the raw materials used in their manufacture—namely, cow's milk and its by-products (milk protein isolates, whey protein concentrates, casein, caseinates, etc.). The variability in the orotate content is mainly due to whey protein concentrates utilized in the manufacture of infant formulas; the ultrafiltration of the whey considerably reduces the content of orotate and other relatively low-molecular-weight compounds.

The first term-infant formula supplemented with 10.2 mg/L nucleotides appeared in Spain in 1983; this was followed by a number of special formulas, including lactose-free, preterm, and extensively hydrolyzed formulas. In 1989, an infant formula containing 33 mg/L nucleotides was launched in a few European countries. Infant formula with 72 mg/L has been marketed since 1996. In the design of formulas with high levels of nucleotides, it has been considered that human milk contains not only free nucleotides but also RNA, which helps to increase the infant's TPAN.

The European Union has recently regulated the use of nucleotides in infant formulas based exclusively on the acid-soluble nucleotide composition of human milk (12). However, nucleotides derived from RNA and DNA present in human milk were not taken into consideration. This is the reason why nucleotide levels in European formulas are lower than those of formulas used in the United States and other countries. Table 2 offers a comparison of U.S. and European infant formulas containing nucleotides.

TABLE 2 Nucleotide Content in American and European Nucleotide-Supplemented Formulas[a]

	Total	CMP	UMP	AMP	GMP	IMP
American formulas						
Similac With Iron (low iron)	72	30	16	11	15	0
Carnation Good Start	31.1					
Enfamil With Iron (low iron)	14					
European formulas						
Similac-1	30.6	14.5	7.8	5.3	3	
SMA	29.5	16.5	5	4	2	2
Puleva-1	10.3	1.5	4.5	1.7	2	0.6

[a] Data expressed in milligrams per liter. Similac, Similac-1, and Puleva-1 are registered trademarks of Abbott Laboratories; Carnation and Good Start are registered trademarks of Nestlé; Enfamil is a trademark of Mead Johnson & Company.

2.1.4 Bioavailability of Dietary Nucleotides

Most dietary nucleotides are ingested in the form of nucleoproteins, from which the nucleic acids are liberated in the intestinal tract by the action of proteolytic enzymes. Pancreatic nucleases degrade nucleic acids into a mixture of mono-, di-, tri-, and polynucleotides. The nucleases are specific for the major types of nucleic acids and are appropriately termed ribonucleases or deoxyribonucleases (6,8).

In response to enterokinin, intestinal Brunner's glands and Lieberkuhn's glands secrete phosphoesterases, which supplement the action of pancreatic nucleases in producing mononucleotides. Hydrolysis of nucleotides to nucleosides is, for the most part, a function of intestinal alkaline phosphatase. In addition to the actions of this enzyme, intestinal nucleotidases and nucleosidases act to render a mix of nucleosides and free purine and pyrimidine bases (6,10). Digestion of nucleic acids and nucleotides clearly occurs in humans and animals. Using an intestinal homogenate from a 22-week-old fetus, hydrolysis of human milk RNA was demonstrated (13). More recently, it has been observed that cultured intestinal pig explants are able to hydrolyze RNA and DNA when present in the culture medium in similar concentrations to those found in human milk (14). Figure 1 shows a scheme of the nucleotide digestion process.

Mechanisms of nucleotide digestion and absorption have been studied primarily in animal everted gut models. The few studies on this topic in humans specifically addressed the effect of dietary purines on serum uric acid levels in individuals with gout. Earlier studies in rat and hamster intestine demonstrated that purine nucleosides and bases readily penetrated everted sacs but

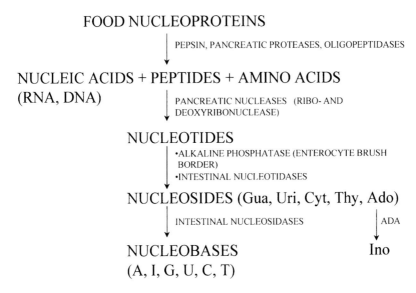

FIGURE 1 Digestion of dietary nucleotides.

were not concentrated within the sacs and did not enter the serosal solution. Subsequent experiments suggested that ATP was able to penetrate epithelial cells of rat small intestine, with a net increase in sodium flux. Further studies demonstrated that exogenous ATP increased the intracellular concentration of this nucleotide (6).

The permeation of nucleosides across the plasma membrane of mammalian cells is complex, and two major classes of transport systems have been identified: 1) equilibrative facilitated diffusion transport with a broad substrate specificity and present in practically all mammalian cells with a few exceptions and 2) concentrative, Na^+-dependent transport. The equilibrative system has two distinct forms of the carrier that differ in their sensitivity to inhibition by nitrobenzyl-thioinosine. The concentrative nucleoside transporters are particularly prevalent in intestinal and kidney epithelial cells, and there are at least three major classes, designated as N1 or cif, N2 or cit, and N3 or cib. The genes termed *cNT1* and *SNST1*, encoding the N1 and N2 nucleoside transporters, have been cloned. As in the case for nucleosides, both facilitated diffusion and active transport systems for nucleobases have been characterized, although the molecular properties of these nucleobase carriers are almost unknown (8). Figure 2 shows the different carriers involved in the transport of nucleobases and nucleosides into the enterocyte.

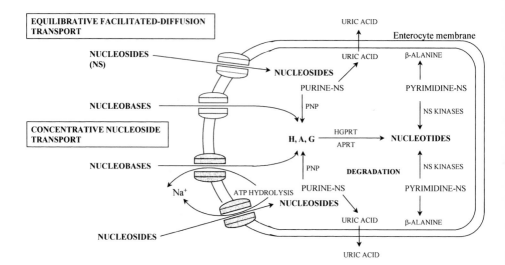

FIGURE 2 Absorption and metabolic fate of dietary nucleotides.

2.1.5 Metabolic Fate of Digested Nucleotides

Both purine and pyrimidine nucleotides are synthesized from simple compounds (de novo synthesis) or by the recycling of preformed bases (salvage pathway). The de novo synthesis of nucleotides requires some specific amino acids (glutamine, aspartate, glycine), tetrahydrofolate derivatives as methyl donors, NH_4^+, and CO_2. The ribose moiety of ribonucleotides comes from 5-phosphoribosyl-1-pyrophosphate. Deoxyribonucleotides are synthesized by a reduction of ribonucleotides catalyzed by a complex enzyme termed *ribonucleotide reductase* (4).

Purine bases and pyrimidine nucleosides can be reutilized after being liberated from nucleic acid catabolism via the salvage pathway. After absorption, dietary nucleosides and bases may also be utilized for the synthesis of nucleotides. Purine bases are efficiently salvaged by hypoxanthine-guanine-phosphoribosyl-transferase (HGPRT), and pyrimidine nucleosides are converted to nucleotides by specific nucleoside kinases (4). Figure 3 summarizes the main steps of the nucleotide salvage pathway.

The general belief that cellular nucleotide tissue needs can be met by the de novo synthesis from nonessential precursors explains why only a limited number of studies have addressed the evaluation of the biological roles of dietary nucleotides in infancy. Studies conducted in experimental animals over the last 20 years have demonstrated that preformed nucleotides, including those present in the diet, may be of special importance for the development and growth of

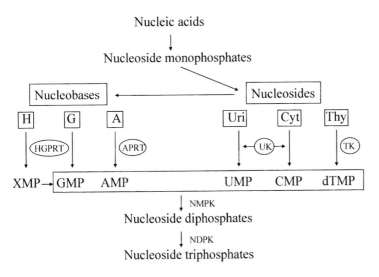

FIGURE 3   Salvage pathway of nucleobases and nucleosides.

tissues with a rapid turnover (7–10). Bone marrow, leukocytes, and the intestinal mucosa preferentially utilize the nucleotide salvage pathway to fulfil their purine and pyrimidine nucleotide requirements (15–17).

Purine and pyrimidine bases in mice fed nucleic acids are utilized and degraded in the small intestine and liver before entry into the systemic circulation. About 1 to 5% of radiolabeled ingested nucleic acids are apparently utilized for tissue nucleic acid synthesis. Similar studies with purines in the rat demonstrated that practically all of the exogenous purines were absorbed and quickly catabolized. Only 5% of ingested purines, especially adenine, were incorporated into tissue nucleic acids; fasted animals tended to retain more dietary purines than fed ones (6,17). Because of the high catabolic enzyme activities in the small intestine, the degradation affects mainly purine nucleosides (18). Dietary nucleosides are also incorporated into other tissues, such as the liver, skeletal muscle, brain, and bone marrow (8). New studies using nucleotides uniformly labeled with stable isotopes have shown that pyrimidines but not purines are readily incorporated into hepatic RNA (19).

The liver has a high capability for nucleotide synthesis; in fact, it is believed that the liver is the supplier of nucleosides for other tissues. Studies in cell lines deficient in amidophosphoribosyltransferase, a key enzyme for the de novo synthesis, and transfected with the human gene have demonstrated that purine nucleosides are synthesized preferentially by the salvage pathway when hypoxanthine, the most important source of purine salvage, is present (20). In vivo studies in rats fed a nucleotide-free diet have shown a transient decrease in liver nucleotide pools, which return to control values after a few days, indicating the preferential use of exogenous nucleosides by the salvage pathway (21). The incorporation of nucleotides by the liver may spare the energetic cost of the de novo synthesis. In short, dietary nucleosides appear to contribute to the overall homeostasis of nucleotides in the body.

Erythrocytes and lymphocytes, enterocytes, and glial cells have in common their limited ability to synthesize nucleotides by the de novo pathway (10). Thus, an external supply of nucleosides seems to be needed for optimal functioning. Several investigations support the hypothesis that the enterocyte is not fully capable of developing the de novo purine synthesis and that this metabolic pathway may be inactive unless it is induced by a purine-deficient diet. The purine salvage pathway, as measured by the activity of its rate-limiting enzyme HGPRT, is highest in the small intestine relative to liver and colon; moreover, a purine-free diet lowers HGPRT activity (17).

Different results are obtained if nucleotides are administered parenterally. Subcutaneous injection of labeled pyrimidine nucleotides in the rat shows direct incorporation of the labeled base into RNA and DNA. Injected thymidine is incorporated unchanged into DNA (22). This latter observation provides the basis for the commonly used technique of labeling newly produced DNA in a variety of in vitro and in vivo experiments.

2.1.6 Roles of Dietary Nucleotides in Infant Nutrition

Dietary nucleotides appear to modulate lipoprotein and fatty acid metabolism in early human life (6–8,23); they affect growth, development, and repair of the small intestine and liver in experimental animals (7,8,10). Moreover, dietary nucleotides modify the intestinal ecology of newborn infants, enhancing the growth of bifidobacteria and limiting that of enterobacteria (6,7), and they have a role in the maintenance of the immune response both in animals and in human neonates (7–10,24–28). Table 3 demonstrates the effects of dietary nucleotides in humans and animals.

Lipid Metabolism. A number of studies using infant formulas that contained relatively high levels of linoleic acid have shown that dietary nucleotides may contribute to increase the proportions of long-chain polyunsaturated fatty acids of the n-6 and n-3 series in plasma and red blood cell membranes of both term and preterm infants (6–8). There are some hypotheses to explain those results; the first considers that dietary nucleotides could modulate the inhibition of the hepatic fatty acid Δ-6 desaturase, reversing the effects of substrate excess inhibition. The second hypothesis establishes that nucleotides may result in an increased hepatic secretion of phospholipids owing to an increased pool of CDP-

TABLE 3 Reported Effects of Dietary Nucleotides in Infant Nutrition

Lipid metabolism
  Increased plasma high-density lipoproteins
  Enhanced lecithin cholesterol acyltransferase (LCAT) activity
  Increased levels of Apo-AI and Apo-AIV
  Increased plasma and erythrocyte levels of long-chain polyunsaturated
    fatty acids
Tissue growth, development, and repair
  Increased small intestinal disaccharidase activities in young animals
  Enhanced repair of small intestine damaged by chronic diarrhea or
    severe starvation in rats at weaning and neonatal pigs
  Enhanced repair of liver damaged by oral intake of thioacetamide or
    carbon tetrachloride
  Enhanced liver protein synthesis
Immune response
  Enhanced cellular immunity
  Increased plasma levels of IgG to polio and Hib vaccines in term infants
  Increased plasma levels of total IgM and IgA in preterm infants
  Increased plasma levels of anticasein and antilactoglobulin antibodies in
    preterm infants
Stool flora
  Increased levels of bifidobacteria and decreased levels of enterobacteria
Protection against disease
  Decreased incidence and duration of acute diarrhea
  Fewer upper-respiratory episodes in mildly malnourished children

choline. The third hypothesis considers that dietary nucleotides enhance the hepatic synthesis of proteins and that, as a consequence, the total activity of the hepatic fatty acid Δ-6 desaturase might increase. Liver fatty acid Δ-6 desaturase activity increases in rats with experimental hepatic cirrhosis fed a nucleotide-supplemented diet, while plasma phospholipids also rise (29). In addition, nucleotide-deprived rats show a low hepatic protein synthesis and hepatocytes present a less dense endoplasmic reticulum (30).

It has been reported that infant formulas supplemented with low levels of nucleotides (equivalent to the free nucleotide concentration present in human milk) increase the levels of high-density lipoprotein (HDL) in term and low-birth-weight infants (6–8). Further studies on the characteristics of isolated HDL revealed that HDL from infants fed nucleotide-supplemented formula contained higher amounts of Apo A-I and Apo A-IV, especially in infants that were small for gestational age, and had a higher cholesterol ester content (8,23). Since dietary nucleotides have been shown to affect the genetic expression of enzymes involved in the salvage pathway of purines (17), a direct effect on exogenous nucleotides of the genetic expression of Apo A-I at the intestinal level cannot be excluded.

Tissue Growth, Development, and Repair. Growing evidence indicates that nucleotides can modulate cell proliferation and differentiation. This is most clearly visible in situations of rapid cell proliferation, either in the normal tissue renewal, such as the intestine and lymphoid tissues, or in the repair of damaged tissues, such as the intestine and liver (7,8). Also, nucleotides affect vital tissues, such as liver or brain, in normal growth and functioning (10).

It has been demonstrated that dietary nucleotides mediate the growth, development, and repair of the small intestine in young animals (10,15,31,32). The administration of a nucleotide-free diet reduced protein and DNA concentrations as well as maltase activity in the intestine of weanling rats. Likewise, starved animals fed with a nucleotide-supplemented diet showed a faster normalization of the differentiation markers in the jejunum. In a clinical trial conduced on small-for-gestational-age newborns whose intestinal mucosa was shown to be functionally impaired by intrauterine malnutrition, babies fed a formula supplemented with nucleotides gained more weight and length and had a greater head circumference than those fed a nucleotide-free formula (9).

The brush-border enzymes sucrase, lactase, and alkaline phosphatase, used as markers of differentiation, have been found to be modulated by dietary nucleotides in both enterocytes and in embryonic cell lines (7,10,33). A decrease in the enzymatic activity of enterocytes isolated along the villus crypt to tip in rats fed a nucleotide-free diet has been reported (39). Similarly, intestinal epithelial cells (IEC-6) and colon carcinoma cells (Caco-2), when cultured in the absence of nucleotides, had lower enzymatic activity than when nucleotides were present (7,33).

Nucleosides and nucleotides also reportedly attenuate atrophy of the intestinal mucosa caused by standard parenteral nutrition and improve intestinal cell turnover in animals with 80% bowel resection (7,8,10). In addition, tight and intermediate mucosal junctions are significantly narrower in rats that receive a parenteral solution containing a nucleotide/nucleoside mixture compared with those of unsupplemented animals, although they are wider than in the group of animals fed orally. The activities of mucosal intracellular proteases (lysosomal cathepsins) increased with total parenteral nutrition, and all activities were normalized by nucleotides, suggesting that these compounds may have a role in the maintenance of the mucosal barrier.

Ample evidence indicates that dietary nucleotides also promote tissue repair. In the intestine, reparative effects by exogenous nucleotides have been reported in different pathologies, such as diarrhea, enterocolitis, and bowel resection. Quicker repair of injured mucosa in the small intestine has been described in weanling rats fed a nucleotide-supplemented diet after lactose-induced chronic diarrhea; dietary nucleotide supplement also enhanced the intestinal DNA content and the activities of disaccharidases (32). It has been reported that nucleotide and nucleoside supplementation reduced the death rate and the incidence of bacterial translocation in protein-deficient mice (34).

Although most studies on dietary nucleotides demonstrate beneficial effects of these compounds in the repair of the intestine, there is some controversy in the case of inflammatory diseases. For example, is has been shown that the administration of a nucleoside- and nucleotide-supplemented parenteral solution aggravated macroscopic and microscopic damage scores as well as signs of inflammation of the colon of rats with trinitrobenzene-sulfonic acid - induced colitis. Other researchers, however, have proposed that nucleotides may diminish the inflammatory response to ischemia reperfusion in the intestine of piglets. In rats with indomethacin-induced ulcerative ileitis, administration of nucleosides and nucleotides either intravenously or as a supplement in the diet significantly decreased the number and size of bowel ulcers (11). These results suggest that dietary nucleotides may have a positive or negative impact, depending on the pathology.

Control of Gene Expression by Dietary Nucleotides. The first report of a direct interaction of dietary nucleotides on gene expression appeared in 1987 (17). Because mRNA of α-actin was not affected, the effect was considered specific for the enzyme. This specific response makes sense in terms of cellular economy, because when nucleotides are absent in the intestinal lumen, the salvage of nucleotides is not required.

A number of studies have demonstrated that dietary nucleotides regulate, in part, gene expression in the intestine. Intestinal mRNA levels of the enzymes HGPRT and APRT declined in response to dietary nucleotide restriction in the diet. Nuclear "run-on" assays both in nuclei isolated from the small intestine and from an intestinal epithelial cell line (IEC-18) demonstrated that dietary nucleotide restriction significantly altered the transcription rate (58). A 35-bp region (HCRE) in the promoter of the *HGPRT* gene has been identified as the element necessary for this response, and the protein that interacts with this region has been identified and purified (10,17).

In cultures of human fetal small intestine, the addition of AMP suppressed crypt-cell proliferation, followed by the restoration of differentiation and the induction of apoptosis; a specific increase in the expression of the *Bax* gene (an apoptosis inducer gene) has also been demonstrated (35). These findings indicate that nucleotides may control the intestinal turnover by shifting from proliferation to full differentiation of the stem cells.

Dietary nucleotides also affect liver growth and functioning (7,8,10). Weanling mice that received a nucleotide-deprived diet exhibited lower liver weight and glycogen content and higher cholesterol and lipid phosphorus contents than did mice that received nucleotides. Lack of an adequate supply of dietary nucleotides impairs liver structure and function, causing both nuclear and cytosolic alterations. The administration of a nucleotide-free diet for 7 days to adult rats reduced hepatic intracellular nucleotide pools and RNA concentration as well (21). In contrast, when rats were fed the same diet for 21 days, the nucleotide pool remained unchanged. This transient effect signifies that the liver can maintain the nucleotide pool by enhancing nucleotide synthesis when exogenous nucleotides are not available. In fact, it has been demonstrated that the administration of a diet lacking nucleotides slowed the protein synthesis rate of the liver and small intestine. In addition, deprivation of nucleotides decreased the RNA concentration and number of ribosomes in the liver (30).

The de novo and salvage pathways of nucleotide synthesis have been assayed in cultures both of primary hepatocytes and of a hepatoma cell line. Treatment with nucleosides and nucleotides (OG-VI mixture) enhanced DNA and RNA synthesis in primary hepatocytes, but high concentrations of nucleosides and nucleotides had an inhibitory effect (7,8,10).

As in the case of the intestine, reparative and preventive effects by dietary nucleotides have been described in models of liver injury with various agents. In rats with cirrhosis induced by thioacetamide (TAA), dietary nucleotides raised the percentage of binucleated hepatocytes and diminished steatosis and fibrosis (36). Other researchers in rats with CCl_4-induced cirrhosis have described beneficial effects of adenosine. Likewise, in a model of hepatitis by intraperitoneal injection of D-galactosamine, nucleotides administered parenterally have been shown to improve both the function and appearance of the liver (8,10).

The reparative effects of dietary nucleotides have also been demonstrated in models of liver regeneration. Rats submitted to 70% hepatectomy and subsequently fed parenteral nutrition supplemented with nucleotides showed an earlier restoration of the nitrogen balance than animals that did not receive nucleotides. Protein synthesis rose in the animals receiving nucleotides, suggesting that the improved nitrogen balance could be due to the higher rate of protein synthesis. It has been reported, in partially hepatectomized rats, that both a nucleotide-free diet and a diet deficient in choline and methionine depress mitosis and delay the S phase of the hepatocyte cell cycle. Supplementation of the diets with yeast RNA partially reversed these effects (8,10).

Other situations in which the activity of nucleotides has been evaluated include cold ischemia. The depletion of the cellular ATP content that occurs in rat livers subjected to cold ischemia is reversed by infusion of adenosine and, to a lesser extent, of adenine. These results indicate that adenine and adenosine are efficiently salvaged by the injured liver to enhance ATP restoration, helping to maintain the cellular energy state (10). In another study, the addition of deoxycytidine and uridine to the culture medium of human NHIK 3025 cells partially reversed the cell-cycle inhibition induced by moderate hypoxia (10).

Adenosine, guanosine, and their mono-, di-, and triphosphates have been reported to stimulate the proliferation of chick astrocytes and human astrocytoma cell lines. The effect appears to be mediated through interaction with purinergic P2y receptors, as the effect is abolished with specific antagonists. Guanosine, GTP, and UTP stimulate neurite outgrowth, and the effects are similar to those induced by neuron growth factor (NGF), although the mechanism involved appears to be different. Guanosine and GTP also stimulate the release of immunoreactive NGF in cultures of neonatal mouse cortical astrocytes. These effects on differentiation appear to be mediated through interaction with P1 receptors, or, in the case of ATP, with P2x receptors (10).

These studies suggest that nucleosides and nucleosites might act as trophic factors in both the central and peripheral nervous systems. Proliferation of brain astrocytes as a result of cell death has been documented; therefore, these findings might have physiological implications in recovery after neuronal injury, including trauma and ischemia associated neurodegeneration, demyelination, and age-related cognitive disorders.

Immune Response.   The activity of nucleotides in intestinal and immune tissues has been traditionally considered as two separate issues. However, today the two tissues are known to be closely related, not only because a large percentage of the intestinal cells are of immune origin but also because the intestinal epithelial cells can produce immunomodulatory molecules, such as cytokines. Both the immune system and the intestine may not be able to fulfil the needs of nucleotides exclusively by de novo synthesis, and exogenous supply of these compounds through the diet could be essential to sustain their growth and functioning. This exogenous supply gains particular importance in situations of metabolic stress, such as malnutrition or infection, in which the rate of cell proliferation in the above-mentioned tissues is increased.

According to these considerations, the regulatory activity of dietary nucleotides on the immune system should be considered together with some of their effects on the intestine. Likewise, different aspects of the immune response, such as cellular and humoral immunity, are intimately linked; for example, B cells require the collaboration of T cells in the process of activation and differentiation. Thus, it is difficult to divorce the effect of nucleotides in one particular aspect from other aspects of the immune response. Nucleotides influence lymphocyte maturation, activation, and proliferation; they also have effects on lymphocyte subpopulations, modulation of the phagocytic capacity of macrophages, modulation of delayed hypersensitivity as well as allograft and tumor responses, immunoglobulin production, and response against infection (6–10,24–28).

Exogenous nucleotides are required to maintain the activity of helper T lymphocytes and to promote the proliferation of T cells but not B cells in response to alloantigens and mitogens. The terminal deoxynucleotidyl transferase (TdT) enzyme has been regarded as an index of the immaturity in lymphocytes. Mice fed on a nucleotide-free diet have shown a higher percentage of TdT-positive cells from the thymus and spleen than those fed a diet supplemented with RNA, adenine, or uracil, suggesting that dietary nucleotides could stimulate the maturation of lymphoid cells (7,8,10,26).

The effects of dietary nucleotides on lymphocyte subset populations in preterm infants have been reported (28,37). No major differences were detected between the nucleotide-supplemented and control groups; however, at 10 days of life, CD4 cells in children fed the nucleotide formula were seen in a significantly higher percentage than in those fed the standard formula. These results appear to confirm those previously detected in mice. In term infants, the activity of natural killer (NK) cells has been reported to be significantly higher in breast-fed and nucleotide supplemented infants compared to controls (7). However, other investigators have not corroborated these observations (38).

In experimental animals, dietary nucleotide restriction results in a decreased delayed cutaneous hypersensitivity, prolonged cardiac graft survival, and decreased resistance to staphylococcal sepsis and *Candida* infection (7,8,11,26). Moreover, dietary nucleotides reverse malnutrition and starvation-induced immunosuppression, prevent the immune function loss that results from protein starvation, enhance the NK-cell activity in mice and newborn infants, and have an effect in macrophage activation in mice (7,8,11,26).

There is a lack of information on the influence of dietary nucleotides on in vivo B-cell function. However, in the last years, new and relevant information is being accumulated. Studies using murine spleen cells and adult peripheral mononuclear cells have demonstrated that yeast RNA preparations markedly increased in vitro antibody production in response to T cell–dependent antigens (39). It has been reported that yeast RNA preparations enhance in vitro IgM and IgG production to T-dependent antigens in normal B6 mice and human lymphocytes and IgM in cord blood mononuclear cells (24). Moreover, the number of plaque-forming cells against sheep red blood cells in mice fed a nucleotide-free diet was significantly decreased as compared to those fed the nucleotide-supplemented diet; UMP and AMP were the responsible nucleotides for the increase of IgG plaque-forming cells (39).

The influence of nucleotide supplementation to an infant formula on total plasma IgG levels and on specific levels of anti–β-casein and anti–β-lactoglobulin in preterm infants has been evaluated (25,37,40). Preterm infants fed a nucleotide-supplemented formula showed significantly higher levels of serum IgM and IgA at 3 months of age that infants fed the standard formula (25,37). Higher concentrations of specific IgG against β-casein and β-lactoglobulin for the first month of life in newborns fed a low-birth-weight-infant nucleotide-supplemented formula were also found (40). In a third study, dietary nucleotide supplementation was evaluated in relation to the recovery of infected and malnourished children;

refeeding after malnutrition did not alter either total serum or specific immuno-globulins against β-casein and β-lactoglobulin or saliva IgA levels (8,25).

More recently, it has been reported that addition of nucleotide to formula (72 mg/L) increases the response to both *Haemophilus influenzae* type b (Hib) and diptheria toxoid vaccines at 7 months. The difference between groups in Hib response, but not diptheria response, persisted at 12 months of age. No effect of nucleotides was observed on antibody response to either oral poliovirus or tetanus vaccines (28,38).

It is difficult to establish whether an increase in immunoglobulins mediated by dietary nucleotides may result in a significant protection of infants. It has been reported that dietary nucleotide supplementation reduces the incidence and duration of acute diarrheal disease in infants in a relatively contaminated environment (41). This fact might be due to an improvement of the small intestine immune function, although a direct effect of nucleotides on intestinal microflora cannot be excluded. Another recent multicenter study carried out in Spain, which involved more than 3000 infants, has confirmed that the incidence of acute diarrhea is significantly reduced in artificially fed infants when they are given a nucleotide supplemented formula (42). Moreover, a significant reduction in the incidence of upper respiratory diseases has been demonstrated in moderately malnourished children fed a nucleotide-supplemented formula for 3 months (8,25).

In conclusion, dietary nucleotides have a number of biological roles in early infancy, particularly on tissue growth and maturation of the immune system. This last effect may be relevant to enhancing the defense system of the young infant against infection and disease.

3   FREE AMINO ACIDS

The free amino acid pool of human milk is small compared to the total amount of milk amino acids in protein. Free amino acids contribute to only 10% of the total nonprotein nitrogen in human milk (3). Glutamine and taurine are the free amino acids found in higher concentrations in human milk. However, other amino acids with special functions, such as arginine and ornithine, are also present in significant amounts (43). Although clinical effects of low dietary intakes of taurine have not been demonstrated even in the preterm infant, there is a concern about the possibility of subclinical deficiency, particularly in premature infants, since their ability to synthesize taurine is known to be limited. Supplementation with taurine to infant formulas increases blood levels of taurine to similar concentrations as those obtained by breast-fed infants while maintaining the rate of taurine to glycine-conjugated bile acids in bile fluid. This is the reason why practically all infant formulas marketed worldwide contain taurine in similar concentrations to those of human milk.

N-acetyl derivatives of amino acids are preferred in some cases to the amino acids themselves, because they prevent bitter taste and unpleasant flavors and give more stability against Maillard browning reactions during food processing. In addition, α-keto acid derivatives of amino acids are more stable during heat treatment and in aqueous solutions than the amino acids. However, those compounds have not been accepted in the European Union for use in FSMPs owing to limited information about bioavailability in humans, hydrolysis, metabolism, and safety (44).

3.1 Glutamine

Free glutamine accounts for about 20% of the total glutamine pool in human milk (3). Glutamine is currently the focus of extensive investigation because of its importance in cell and tissue culture and because it serves as a preferred respiratory fuel for rapidly proliferating and growing cells, such as enterocytes and lymphocytes (see Chap. 3). Moreover, it is a regulator of acid-base balance through the production of urinary ammonia, a carrier or nitrogen between tissues and an important precursor of nucleotides, amino sugars, and proteins (45,46). There is increasing evidence that glutamine may become a conditionally essential amino acid in critically ill patients, and glutamine appears to be important for the maintenance of the structure and function of the small intestine (46). Further research should focus on the effects of free glutamine on infant nutrition in health and disease and the potential roles of this amino acid in the modulation of the immune system in early life.

The Scientific Committee on Foods of the European Union has recently considered glutamine as a substance intended to be added to foodstuffs for special medical purposes (FSMPs), including those intended for very young infants and children. However, glutamine is not allowed for standard infant formulas and other foods for particular nutritional uses (FPNUs) (44).

3.2 Arginine and Ornithine

Arginine and ornithine are also present in human milk as free amino acids, although the first is found in higher concentrations in milk protein (3). Arginine has multiple biological properties, including the ability to stimulate anabolic hormone secretion: intravenous and enteral administration of arginine increases both insulin and human growth hormone (hGH) secretion (47). Several studies show that arginine, when given to patients as well as to various experimental stress models, acts by improving nitrogen balance, accelerating wound healing, and restoring depressed immunity (43). Dietary supplements of arginine have been shown to inhibit tumor growth in animals, probably by activating the immune system. However, in cancer patients, arginine stimulated tumor protein synthesis, suggesting that arginine might have separate stimulatory effects on the tumor and on the immune system; the potential benefit would depend on which effect prevails. Arginine has also been demonstrated to enhance the growth hormone releasing hormone (GHRH) induced hGH rise in patients with anorexia nervosa. Moreover, oral administration of arginine enhances the hGH response to GHRH in short children (43).

Ornithine shares with arginine the ability to stimulate hGH secretion. In addition, ornithine as its α-ketoglutarate salt (OKG) generates various molecules (i.e., glutamine). OKG has been shown to improve nitrogen balance in various acute and chronic malnutrition states. OKG increases muscle protein anabolism in moderate catabolic states and reduces protein catabolism in hypercatabolic states (43,47).

Arginine and ornithine are precursors of nitric oxide and polyamines, respectively. These metabolites intimately participate in permeability and adaptive responses of the gut. Animal studies have shown improved morphology after OKG administration, perhaps through increased polyamine synthesis. The question is whether exogenous arginine can be a relevant precursor of polyamines.

To date, only two infant formulas in Europe have been supplemented with arginine, but its potential clinical benefits have not yet been demonstrated.

4 POLYAMINES

Polyamines are detectable in relatively high quantities in human and rat milk. Artificial infant formula does not contain appreciable amounts of polyamines, specifically putrescine and spermidine, whereas spermine is undetectable (43). Therefore formula-fed infants are not exposed to polyamines or to any of the potential effects that these compounds may have on the developing intestine. It is noteworthy that food contains polyamines and that polyamines are produced by the gastrointestinal microflora. Thus, the direct uptake by enterocytes of preformed polyamines could contribute to the polyamine cellular pool. Indeed, putrescine and spermidine uptake has been shown to occur in isolated rat enterocytes (47).

Until now no formula containing polyamines has been marketed in the United States or the European Union. Moreover, polyamines have not yet been proposed and accepted by international committees for use in the manufacture of FPNUs and particularly infant formulas (44).

5 OLIGOSACCHARIDES AND GLYCOSPHINGOLIPIDS

In addition to lactose, the carbohydrates of human milk include nucleotide sugars, glycolipids, glycoproteins, and oligosaccharides (see Chap. 6). Three main oligosaccharide fractions representing 13 to 18 g/L have been isolated; the concentration varied with the mother's genetic ability to synthesize specific fucosyl linkages. More than 80 neutral and sialic acidic oligosaccharides have been isolated and identified (48).

Human milk oligosaccharides appear to be synthesized by some of the same glycosyltransferases that participate in the synthesis of glycoprotein and glyco-lipid cell-surface components. Thus, it is reasonable to postulate that some of those compounds can act as analogues to host-cell surface receptors for patho-gens. It has been reported that specific oligosaccharides can inhibit binding of *Streptococcus pneumoniae* and *H. influenzae* to their receptors, and an oligosac-charide that inhibits adherence of enteropathogenic *Escherichia coli* to their re-ceptors has been described. Other authors have reported that specific fucosylated oligosaccharides inhibit binding of invasive strains of *Campylobacter jejuni* and the toxicity of *E.coli* in vivo (43,48).

Gangliosides are glycosphingolipids that contain syalic acid (*N*-acetylneur-aminic acid) as part of their carbohydrate moiety. GM_1, a milk ganglioside present in human milk, binds to *E. coli* and *Vibrio cholerae* toxins, which may contribute to infant protection against infection by those enteropathogens (43). More re-cently, it has been found that infant milk formula supplemented with gangliosides helps to decrease fecal enterobacteria and increase bifidobacteria in preterm in-fants (49).

As lactating mothers differ genetically in their ability to produce protective oligosaccharides, this may influence the susceptibility of breast-fed infants to enteric disease. This hypothesis is currently under investigation. Moreover, the influence of supplementing oligosaccharides to infant milk formulas on the sus-ceptibility of infants to gastrointestinal diseases—namely, acute diarrhea—is one of the current fields of intense investigation. However, to date, no infant formula marketed in the United States or the European Union has been supplemented with either oligosaccharides or gangliosides.

REFERENCES

1. Koldovsky O, Strbak V Hormones and growth factors in human milk. In: Jensen RG, ed. Handbook of Milk Composition. San Diego, CA. Academic Press, 1995, pp 428–436.
2. Belliste F, Diplock AT, Hornstra G, Koletzko B, Roberfroid M, Salminen S, Saris WHM. Functional Food Science in Europe. Br J Nutr 1998; 80(suppl 1):S1–S193.
3. Atkinson SA, Lönnerdal B. Nonprotein nitrogen fractions of human milk. In: Jensen RG, ed. Handbook of Milk Composition. San Diego, CA: Academic Press, 1995, pp 369–387.
4. Stryer L. Biochemistry, 4th ed. New York: Freeman, 1995.
5. Gil A, Uauy R. Nucleotides and Related Compounds in Human and Bovine Milks. San Diego, CA: Academic Press, 1995, pp 436–467.
6. Gil A, Uauy R. Dietary nucleotides in infant nutrition. J Clin Nutr Gastroenterol 1989; 4:145–153.

7. Carver JD, Walker WA. The role of nucleotides in human nutrition. J Nutr Biochem 1995; 6:58–72.

8. Gil A, Uauy R, eds. Nutritional and Biological Significance of Dietary Nucleotides and Nucleic Acids: Abbott Laboratories. Barcelona: Limpergraf, 1996.

9. Cosgrove M, Davies DP, Jenkins HR. Nucleotide supplementation and the growth of term small gestational age infants. Arch Dis Child 1996; 74:F122–F125.

10. Sánchez-Pozo A, Rueda R, Fontana L, Gil A. Dietary nucleotides and cell growth. Trends Comp Biochem Physiol 1998; 5:99–111.

11. Leach JL, Baxter JH, Molitor B, Ramstack MB, Masor M. Total potentially available nucleosides of human milk by stage of lactation. Am J Clin Nutr 1995; 61:1224–1230.

12. European Union Directive 96/4 relative to infant and follow-on formulas. 28.2.96, 1996: No. L 49/12–L 49/13.

13. Thorell L, Sjoberg LB, Hernell O. Nucleotides in human milk: Sources and metabolism by the newborn infant. Pediatr Res 1996; 21:892–897.

14. Gómez-León C, Rueda R, Romera JM, Gil A. Ribonucleic acid hydrolysis by intestinal explants of neonatal piglets (abstr). XXII International Congress of Pediatrics, Amsterdam, 1998.

15. Uauy R, Quan R, Gil A. Role of nucleotides in intestinal development and repair: Implications for infant nutrition. J Nutr 1994; 124:1436S–1441S.

16. Cohen A, Barankiewicz J, Gelfand EW. Roles of alternative synthetic and catabolic purine pathways in T lymphocyte differentiation. Proc Natl Acad Sci USA 1984; 81:26–33.

17. LeLeiko NS, Walsh MJ, Abraham S. Gene expression in the intestine: The effect of dietary nucleotides. Adv Pediatr 1995; 42:145–169.

18. Witte DP, Wiginton DA, Hutton JJ, Aronow BJ. Coordinate development regulation of purine catabolic enzyme expression in gastrointestinal and postimplantation reproductive tracts J Cell Biol 1991; 115:179–190.

19. Berthold HK, Crain PF, Gouni I, Reeds PJ, Klein PD. Evidence for incorporation of intact dietary pyrimidine (but not purine) nucleosides into hepatic RNA. Proc Natl Acad Sci USA 1995; 92:10123–10127.

20. Yamaoka T, Kondo M, Honda S, Iwahana H, Moritani M, Ii S, Yoshimoto K, Itakura, M. Amidophosphoribosyltransferase limits the rate of cell growth-linked de novo purine biosynthesis in the presence of constant capacity of salvage purine biosynthesis. J Biol Chem 1997; 272:17719–17725.

21. López-Navarro AT, Gil A, Sánchez-Pozo A. Deprivation of dietary nucleotides results in a transient decrease in acid soluble nucleotides and RNA content in rat liver. J Nutr 1995; 125:2090–2095.

22. Savaiano DA, Ho CY, Chu V, Clifford AJ. Metabolism of orally and intravenously administered purines in rats. J Nutr 1980; 110:1793–1804.

23. Sánchez-Pozo A, Ramírez M, Gil A, Maldonado J, Rosseneu M. Dietary nucleotides enhance plasma lecithin-cholesterol acyl transferase and apolipoprotein A-IV concentration in preterm newborn infants. Pediatr Res 1995; 37:328–333.

24. Jyonouchi H. Nucleotide actions on humoral immune responses. J Nutr 1994; 124:144S–148S.

25. Gil A, Martínez-Augustín O, Navarro J. Role of dietary nucleotides in the modula-

tion of the immune response. In: Bellanti JA, Bracci R, Prindull G, Xanthou M, eds. Neonatal Hematology and Immunology III. Amsterdam: Elsevier Science, 1997, pp 139–144.

26. Rudolph RB, Kulkarni AD, Fanslow WC, Pizzini RP, Kumar S, Van Buren CT. Role of RNA as a dietary source of pyrimidines and purines in immune function. Nutrition 1990; 6:45–52.

27. Walker WA. Exogenous nucleotides and gastrointestinal immunity. Transplant Proc 1996; 28:2438–2441.

28. Kuchan M, Winship T, Masor M. Nucleotides in infant nutrition: effects on immune function. In: Reifen R, Lerner A, Branski D, Heymans HSA, eds. Pediatric Nutrition. Pediatr Adolesc Med Basel: Karger, 1998; 8:80–94.

29. Fontana L, Moreira E, Sánchez de Medina F, Gil A. Effects of dietary polyunsaturated fatty acids and nucleotides on tissue fatty acid profiles of rats with carbon tetrachloride-induced liver damage. Clin Nutr 1999; 18:93–101.

30. López-Navarro AT, Ortega MA, Peragón J, Bueno JD, Gil A, Sánchez-Pozo A. Deprivation of dietary nucleotides decreases protein synthesis in the liver and small intestine in the rats. Gastroenterology 1996; 110:1760–1769.

31. Uauy R, Stringel G, Thomas R, Quan R. Effect of dietary nucleosides on growth and maturation of the developing gut in the rat. J Pediatr Gastroenterol Nutr 1990; 10:497–503.

32. Núñez MC, Ayudarte MV, Morales D, Suárez MD, Gil A. Effect of dietary nucleotides on intestinal repair in rats with experimental chronic diarrhea. JPEN 1990; 14: 598–604.

33. Sanderson IR, He Y. Nucleotide uptake and metabolism by intestinal epithelial cells. J Nutr 1994; 124:131S–137S.

34. Adjei AA, Yamamoto S. A dietary nucleoside-nucleotide mixture inhibits endotoxin-induced bacterial translocation in mice fed protein-free diet. J Nutr 1995; 125: 42–48.

35. Tanaka M, Lee K, Martínez-Augustín O, He Y, Sanderson IA, Walker W. Exogenous nucleotides alter the proliferation, differentiation and apoptosis of human small intestinal epithelium. J Nutr 1996; 126:424–433.

36. Torres M, Fernández I, Gil A, Ríos A. Influence of dietary nucleotides on liver structural recovery and hepatocyte binuclearity in cirrhosis induced by thioacetamide. Gut 1996; 38:260–264.

37. Navarro J, Maldonado J, Narbona E, Ruiz-Bravo A, García-Salmerón JL, Molina JA, Gil A. Influence of dietary nucleotides on plasma immunoglobulins and lymphocyte subsets of preterm infants. Biofactors 1999; 10:67–76.

38. Pickering LK, Granoff DM, Ericson JR, Masor ML, Cordle CT, Schaller JP, Winship TR, Paule CL, Hilty MD. Modulation of the immune system by human milk and infant formula containing nucleotides. Pediatrics 1998; 101:242–249.

39. Navarro J, Ruiz-Bravo A, Jiménez-Valera M, Gil A. Modulation of antibody-forming cell and mitogen-driven lymphoproliferative responses by dietary nucleotides in mice. Immunol Lett 1996; 53:141–145.

40. Martínez-Augustín O, Boza JJ, Del Pino JI, Lucena J, Martínez-Valverde A, Gil A. Dietary nucleotides might influence the humoral immune response against cow's milk proteins in preterm neonates. Biol Neonate 1997; 71:215–223.

41. Brunser O, Espinoza J, Araya M, Cruchet S, Gil A. Effect of dietary nucleotide supplementation on diarrhoeal disease in infants. Acta Paediatr 1994; 83:188–191.
42. Lama RA, Gil-Alberdi B. Effect of nucleotides as dietary supplement on diarrhea in healthy infants. Anal Esp Pediatr 1998; 48:371–375.
43. Koletzko B, Aggett P, Bindels JG, Bung P, Ferré P, Gil A, Lentze MJ, Roberfroid M, Strobel S. Growth, development and differentiation: A functional science approach. Br J Nutr 1998; 1(suppl):S5–S45.
44. Scientific Committee on Food, European Commission. Directorate General XXIV. Consumer Policy and Health Protection. Opinion on substances for nutritional purposes which have been proposed for use in the manufacture of foods for particular nutritional purposes (PARNUTS). 12/05/99, Brussels, 1999:1–19.
45. Lacey JM, Wilmore DW. Is glutamine a conditionally essential amino acid? Nutr Rev 1990; 48:297–309.
46. Newsholme EA, Carrié AL. Quantitative aspects of glucose and glutamine metabolism by intestinal cells. Gut 1994; 1(suppl):S13–S17.
47. Cynober L. Can arginine and ornithine support gut functions? Gut 1994; 1(suppl):S42–S45.
48. Newburg DS, Neubauer SH. Carbohydrates in milks: Analysis, quantities and significance. In: Jensen RG, ed. Handbook of Milk Composition. San Diego, CA: Academic Press, 1995, pp 273–349.
49. Rueda R, Maldonado J, Narbona E, Gil A. Neonatal dietary gangliosides. Early Hum Dev 1998; 53(suppl):S135–S148.

5

Microorganisms Administered for the Benefit of the Host: Facts and Myths

Yvan Vandenplas
Academic Children's Hospital, Free University of Brussels, Brussels, Belgium

1 INTRODUCTION

Since antiquity, humans worldwide have, on a daily basis, used crude mixtures of microorganisms such as fermented milk to improve the digestibility of some food ingredients and to prevent and treat infections. It was the Russian Metchnikoff who provided the first scientific evidence of the therapeutic efficacy of microorganisms when he demonstrated that certain bacteria were able to enhance the proliferation of *Vibrio cholerae* while others inhibited its growth (1).

Simon and Gorbach demonstrated that the human normal or indigenous intestinal microflora consists of two fractions: one a rather static resident (autochthonous) and the other transient (2). Approximately 400 different species of bacteria have been identified in the human intestine, a number that is 10 times greater than the variety of human cells (3). The dominant flora is characterized by the presence of more than 10^8 predominantly anaerobic bacteria (*Bacteroides, Eubacterium, Bifidobacterium, Peptostreptococcus*, etc.) per gram of feces. The turnover of the transient fraction of the flora depends on the composition of the autochthonous fraction, the ingestion of microorganisms, and the antibiotic-related destruction of part of the microflora. One way to affect the flora is by minimizing the intake of (pathogenic) bacteria, which is done by improving hygienic conditions and decreasing the degree of contamination of foods and beverages. Antimicrobial drugs are detrimental to the balance of the intestinal microflora. Indeed, while antibiotics will destroy the sensitive microflora, they will, at the same time, offer a breeding ground for the (multi)resistant flora. The problems due to the multiple resistance of microorganisms are worldwide (4).

The intestinal microflora has many functions (5). It offers protection against intestinal colonization with pathogenic microorganisms and regulates intestinal transit. The intestinal wall is thickened in the presence of intestinal microbes, and cell kinetics is more rapid. Migrating motor complexes as well as production and sensitivity to peptides are dependent on the microflora. The size of the cecum is enlarged in germ-free animals. Other functions of the intestinal flora include deconjugation of bile acids and promotion of the enterohepatic circulation; degradation and digestion of a certain amount of undigested carbohydrates—which, for example, results in improved lactose tolerance; limitation of bacterial translocation and thus dissemination of bacteria to the peripheral organs; production of vitamins and growth factors for host intestinal cells and maturation; and stimulation of the gut immune system. The flora also has some metabolic functions: cholesterol is converted to coprostanol, and mucin, produced by various kinds of cells, is degraded by different bacterial strains. Short-chain fatty acids are intermediate and end products of microbial degradation of endogenously and exogenously derived carbohydrates. As part of the fermentation process, intestinal gases are produced.

Although the autochthonous intestinal microflora is a surprisingly stable bacterial ecosystem, there is evidence that alterations in the transient intestinal microflora (as occur in infections and during antibiotic treatment) are clinically relevant. As a consequence, interest in this transient microflora has bloomed and many attempts have been made to affect this transient microflora in a way that may be beneficial to the host.

2 DEFINITIONS

The term *novel food* is used for each newly developed food. Examples of novel foods are genetically manipulated foods (e.g., soy), functional foods, or a new combination of two existing foods or food preparations.

A *functional food* is a food (preparation) that exerts a positive influence on one or more functions of the human organism, over and above its intrinsic nutritional properties. There are at least four different ways to prepare a functional food:

- By eliminating a component known to cause deleterious effects to the consumer, such as an allergenic protein, as in the case of gluten for the celiac patient
- By increasing the concentration of a component naturally present in food in order to achieve a daily requirement, such as fortification with a micronutrient or by increasing the concentration of either a nutritive component, such as nondigestible oligosaccharides, or a nonnutritive component, such as plant polyphenols, for which data are available to show beneficial effects for the host
- By adding a component normally not present in a given food at a concentration likely to meet recommended daily requirements, such as nonvitamin antioxidants, probiotics, and/or prebiotics
- By replacing a component, usually a macronutrient, the intake of which is commonly excessive and therefore likely to cause deleterious effects, such as fats, with another component with demonstrated beneficial effects, such as cholesterol-lowering margarine

A *prebiotic* is a nondigestible food ingredient that affects the host by selectively targeting the growth and/or activity of one or a limited number of bacteria in the colon and thus has the potential to preserve or improve health. Lactulose, a disaccharide, is a well-known example of a prebiotic (6). Inulin, fructo-oligosaccharides, and galacto-oligosaccharides are other examples. Prebiotics also occur in nature and are present in chicory, onion, artichoke, asparagus, and banana (7). However, despite the fact that prebiotics can be found in some vegetables and fruits, the amount may not be large enough to exert a beneficial effect on the host.

A *probiotic* is a live, nonpathogenic microbial food or food supplement that normally is part of the human intestinal microflora of the host and exerts a beneficial effect on the host by improving the intestinal microbial balance (8). One of the areas of discussion regards the target organ of the probiotic. If a naturally occurring microorganism affects the skin, the respiratory tract, or the mucosa (e.g., the vagina) beneficially, it can be questioned if it should also be considered a probiotic.

Fermented milk products such as yogurt, kefir, and buttermilk contain *natural probiotics*: most frequently *Bifidobacterium bifidum*, *Lactobacillus acidophilus* and *Lactobacillus bulgaricus*, *Streptococcus lactis*, and *Streptococcus cremoris* (8). Kimchi is an example of another naturally fermented food. Fermented milk products are difficult to use in a therapeutic setting because of the need for cold storage and their limited shelf life. It would also be difficult to persuade sick patients (especially the elderly or children) to consume sufficiently large quantities (on the order of *liters*) of yogurt or fermented milk to make any significant therapeutic effect likely. The resistance of most yogurt bacteria to gastric acid and bile is poor, although differences between strains have been observed (9,10). *L. acidophilus* survives gastric acidity better if added to milk rather than to yogurt or buttermilk (10,11). Even if antibiotics such as beta-lactams, tetracyclines, and quinolones are administered intravenously, the hepato-enteric cycle rapidly inactivates many of these natural probiotics.

Some probiotics are registered as medicinal products (see Sec. 3 below), while others are registered as *commercialized food supplements containing probiotics*. If registered as food supplements, products are not subjected to the same testing as medical products, and medical terminology cannot be used to describe the claimed effect(s). For instance, *L. acidophilus*, *L. bulgaricus*, *Streptococcus thermophilus*, and *Streptococcus faecium* SF 68 can be purchased in health food stores as viable bacteria in dried form as granules or capsules and do not require a medical prescription. Probiotic food supplements must fulfill the criteria of food legislation, not the medical drug legislation. Labeling of probiotic foods may be misleading in terms of both their microbiological content and their claimed beneficial effects (12,13). Brewer's yeast (*Saccharomyces cerevisiae*) is sold as a food supplement for the treatment of constipation, but it is not viable. The regulations on probiotic preparations and the marketing of dairy foods that contain probiotic bacteria should give the consumer better guarantees on the quality of these expensive products (13). A *bifidogene* is a pre- or probiotic that stimulates the growth of bifidi. Inulin is an example of a bifidogene.

A *synbiotic* is a combination or mixture of pro- and prebiotics—therefore of viable microorganisms and nondigestible ingredients—that beneficially affect the host by improving the survival and implantation of live microbial dietary supplements in the gastrointestinal tract. An example of a synbiotic is the combination of fructo-oligosaccharides and bifidobacteria or a combination of lactilol and lactobacilli. Hard scientific evidence of the effectiveness of these combinations, however, is still missing.

A *biotherapeutic agent* is a microorganism that has a demonstrated medical effect and therefore is considered to be a drug. By definition, these microorganisms must be prepared, preserved, and administered in a viable form, and must be safe even if administered in very large amounts. Biotherapeutic agents survive the intestinal ecosystem and thus must be resistant to gastric acid, bile, and pancreatic secretions. A biotherapeutic agent must be resistant to the vast majority of commonly used antibiotics. The beneficial effects of a biotherapeutic agent must be multifactorial—it must be capable, for example, of 1) inhibition of adhesion of pathogens by adhering to the intestinal mucosa or producing antimicrobial substances; 2) immunomodulation, by exerting a change in toxins or toxin receptors; or 3) competition for nutrients (14,15). The benefits of a biotherapeutic agent can be preventive, therapeutic, or both. It is important that the existence of the benefits claimed be demonstrated by prospective, double-blind, randomized studies. The importance of double-blind studies is illustrated by the contradictory results found in a randomized open study in which the beneficial effects of *S. faecium* SF 68 in the prevention of antibiotic-associated diarrhea was demonstrated (16) but contradicted in a randomized placebo-controlled study with the same microorganism in a similar patient population (17). Examples of biotherapeutic agents include some of the probiotic strains, such as *Lactobacillus casei* strain GG or *Saccharomyces boulardii*, a yeast that is not part of the autochthonous microflora.

3 BIOTHERAPEUTIC AGENTS

Biotherapeutic agents, in contrast to probiotics, can but do not necessarily have to belong to the natural human intestinal microflora. Therefore, biotherapeutic agents can be separated into two groups: a first group of bacterial biotherapeutic agents that belong to the normal human microflora and a second group of nonbacterial biotherapeutic agents that do not belong to the normal flora.

3.1 Bacterial Biotherapeutic Agents (Group 1)

There are numerous potential benefits that can result from lactobacilli (5). They maintain and restore normal intestinal balance by reducing the intestinal pH and destroying toxic substances by producing antimicrobial molecules, by preventing or reducing traveler's diarrhea, and by minimizing the incidence of antibiotic-associated diarrhea. Some lactic acid bacterial cultures have exogenous lactase activity that reduces abdominal pain, flatulence, or diarrhea caused by undigested lactose. Improvement of the digestibility of milk products may be another beneficial effect of lactobacilli, although it has also been demonstrated that viable *L. acidophilus* does not improve the digestion of lactose (18,19). By inactivation of dietary and intestinally generated mutagenic compounds, such as azo dyes and nitrosamines, and reduction of fecal bacterial enzymes, lactobacilli may enhance resistance to cancerogenic degeneration. Some lactobacilli strains do enhance nonspecific anti-infective defense mechanisms, such as phagocytic activity in peripheral blood. Indeed, children with rotavirus diarrhea secrete significantly more rotavirus-specific IgA cells during the convalescence period if they received a live rather than a heat-killed *L. casei* strain GG (20). During the diarrhea period itself, however, rotavirus-specific antibodies were similar and very low in both groups, and there was no difference in the duration of the diarrhea (20). The increased specific antibody production occurred at a later stage, and this could be relevant for the prevention of reinfection (20).

L. casei strain GG has the potential to increase the gut IgA immune response and enhance the gut immunological barrier in patients with Crohn's disease (21). The beneficial effects of *L. casei* strain GG have also been demonstrated in a small number of patients with juvenile rheumatoid arthritis (22). The addition of *L. casei* strain GG to patients undergoing an elimination diet further contributes to the treatment and prevention of atopic dermatitis (23). Lymphocyte proliferation by bovine casein is suppressed in vitro by enzymes derived from *L. casei* strain GG (24). As a consequence, it has been hypothesized that the increase of atopic disease in modern industrialized societies is related to a "too clean" environment, as the addition of microorganisms decreases atopic disease (25). However, early respiratory infections do not seem to protect for later atopic disease (26), suggesting that future interest should focus on the impact of autochthonous microorganisms on later atopic disease (23,25,26).

It is known that high serum cholesterol is a risk factor for ischemic heart disease. Some epidemiological studies suggest that consumption of fermented milk products can have a hypocholesterolemic effect (5). The mechanisms by which this effect is mediated are unknown but may include cholesterol assimilation by the microorganisms and subsequent removal from the gut. It has also been proposed that bacterial deconjugation of bile salts and their resultant inefficient absorption from the gastrointestinal tract may have hypocholesterolemic effects. Lactobacilli enhance the absorption of calcium, while bifidobacteria are capable of synthesizing some B vitamins and digestive enzymes, such as casein phosphatase and lysozyme. However, because only 1.5 and 37.5% of ingested *L. acidophilus* and bifidobacteria, respectively, reach the ileum (27), all of the above-listed benefits of bacterial probiotics must be considered "potential" because they have not, as of yet, been proven. Table 1 summarizes all the published prospective, randomized, placebo-controlled clinical trials with bacterial probiotics in the treatment or prevention of gastrointestinal disease (28). Many bacterial probiotics have been tested in clinical settings. However, except for *L. casei* strain GG, the vast majority of these prospective randomized trials show disappointing results. At the present time, the only probiotic with demonstrated efficacy in prevention and therapy and that therefore can be considered as a biotherapeutic agent is *L. casei* strain GG.

For a bacterial biotherapeutic agent to be considered as such, it is essential to demonstrate that its natural resistance to antibiotics cannot be transferred to the natural colonic flora or to pathogens present in the gastrointestinal tract of the host (8). Biotherapeutic agents should not be able to acquire the resistance of commensal or pathogenic microorganisms and subsequently transfer it to other commensal or pathogenic microorganisms (8). Colonization resistance is the property of the normal colonic flora to protect the host against colonization by pathogens and is achieved via a complex interaction between the various strains. At this moment, no single bacterium or combination of bacteria is capable of inducing colonization resistance to pathogens in a way similar to that of the natural colonic microflora (8). It is not clear whether the antibacterial substances secreted in vitro by bacterial biotherapeutic agents are also effective in vivo. In vitro, yogurt with *Strep. thermophilus* and *L. bulgaricus* is bactericidal for

Clostridium difficile within 2 hr (63). However, in vivo, hamsters are not protected from death by *C. difficile*–induced colitis, even when very large amounts of the yogurt are administered (63). A competitive inhibition of the bacterial biotherapeutic agents at the level of the adhesion sites of the pathogenic flora has also been reported. However, if *E. coli* is administered before the *L. acidophilus*, as occurs when patients with acute gastroenteritis are treated with a biotherapeutic agent, the protection by the *Lactobacillus* strain is severely reduced because of a nonspecific steric hindrance of the receptor sites (64). As a consequence, the relevance of competitive inhibition for adhesion sites is restricted to prevention, because once the adhesion of the pathogen has taken place, the *Lactobacillus* cannot displace the pathogenic bacteria. *Lactobacillus salivarius* inhibits colonization of the stomach with *Helicobacter pylori* in gnotobiotic BALB/c and germ-free mice (65). This finding, however, cannot immediately be extrapolated to an immunocompetent host.

Different studies have been performed with *Strep. (Enterococcus) faecium* SF 68; the majority of which, however, do not demonstrate therapeutic benefits. *L. casei* strain GG, which belongs to the natural human intestinal microflora, has been shown to (1) grow in bile and acid even at a pH of 3.0, (2) survive and grow in the gut, (3) adhere to the intestinal mucosa in vitro, and (4) produce antimicrobial components. *L. casei* is resistant to penicillin, ceftriaxone, and trimethoprim-sulfamethoxazole but sensitive to most of the other antibiotics (66). *L. casei* strain GG was evaluated and found to be effective in many prospective, randomized, placebo-controlled trials: for the prevention of traveler's diarrhea (42), in the recovery from acute rotavirus diarrhea in children (43,46), in the recovery from nonbloody diarrhea of undetermined etiology (47), in the clinical outcome of premature infants that were enterally fed (44), when added to oral rehydration (46,50), and in the duration of antibiotic-associated diarrhea (48). *L. casei* strain GG has also been reported to be effective in the treatment of *C. difficile* colitis (49). The addition of *L. casei* strain GG to a cow's milk elimination diet in children with atopic dermatitis and food allergy promotes endogenous barrier mechanisms that alleviate intestinal inflammation, resulting in a significant additional improvement of the eczema (23). A locally prepared infant formula with *Strep. thermophilus* and *Bifidobacterium bifidum* was shown to have a statistically significant effect on the prevention of diarrhea occurring in a ward with chronically ill children 5 to 24 months old (60). The incidence of rotavirus diarrhea also tended to be reduced (60). However, in a similarly designed study including only *B. bifidum* as probiotic, there was no difference in the number of infants with diarrhea or in the number of diarrheal episodes (61). In that study, the duration of diarrhea was shorter in the group that received the probiotic (1.2 versus 2.3 days) (61). *Lactobacillus plantarium* 299 V given daily in a fermented oatmeal powder failed to reduced the incidence of diarrhea in a day-care facility (62).

Table 1 Outcome of Double-Blind, Randomized, Prospective Studies with Biotherapeutic Agents

Reference	Study population	Indication	Probiotic	Clinical outcome
29	48	Diarrhea in ETEC Infected volunteers	L. bulgaricus L. acidophilus	NS
30	50	Traveler's diarrhea	L. bulgaricus L. acidophilus	NS
31	38	Amoxicillin-associated diarrhea	L. bulgaricus L. acidophilus	NS
32	79	Ampicillin-associated diarrhea	L. bulgaricus L. acidophilus	NS
33	35	Enteral feeding–associated diarrhea	L. bulgaricus L. acidophilus	NS
34	319	Traveler's diarrhea	L. acidophilus	NS
35	202	Traveler's diarrhea	L. acidophilus	NS
	181	Traveler's diarrhea	L. fermentum	NS
36	71	Acute diarrhea in children	Heat-killed L. acidophilus	NS
37	10	Healthy volunteers	Bifidobacterium longum	<0.05
38	120	Stable ulcerative colitis	E. coli (vs. mesalazine)	NS
39	116	Stable ulcerative colitis	E. coli (vs. mesalazine)	NS
40	57	Bedridden patients with constipation	Bifidus yogurt	<0.05
41	126	Non-ulcer dyspepsia	L. helveticus, E. coli, L. acidophilus	NS
42	820	Traveler's diarrhea	L. casei strain GG	NS
43	71	Acute diarrhea	L. casei strain GG	<0.001
44	20	Enteral feeding in prematures	L. casei strain GG	NS
45	24	Irritable bowel syndrome	L. casei strain GG	NS
46	287	Duration of diarrhea in children	L. casei strain GG	NS
	101	Duration of diarrhea if rotavirus-positive	L. casei strain GG	<0.05
	186	Duration of diarrhea if rotavirus-negative	L. casei strain GG	NS

47	Nonbloody acute diarrhea	L. casei strain GG	<0.01
48	Erythromycin-associated diarrhea	L. casei strain GG	<0.05
49	Clostridium difficile colitis	L. casei strain GG	<0.001
23	Atopic dermatitis with elimination diet	L. casei strain GG	<0.05
50	Acute diarrhea in children, two OR solutions	L. casei strain GG	0.03
51	Bacterial overgrowth	L. fermentum	NS
52	Antibiotic-associated diarrhea	S. (Enterococcus) faecium SF 68	<0.01
78	Acute diarrhea	S. (Enterococcus) faecium SF 68	NS
53	Duration of Vibrio cholerae diarrhea	S. (Enterococcus) faecium SF 68	NS
39	Duration of E. coli diarrhea	S. (Enterococcus) faecium SF 68	NS
54	Acute diarrhea in adults	S. (Enterococcus) faecium SF 68	<0.01
16	Antibiotic-associated diarrhea in tuberculosis	S. (Enterococcus) faecium SF 68	NS
55	Duration of rotavirus diarrhea	Lactobacillus reuteri	NS
56	Duration of rotavirus diarrhea	Lactobacillus reuteri	<0.05
57	Infants with nonbacterial diarrhea	S. lactis, L. bulgaricus, L. Acidophilus L. bulgaricus	NS
58	Diarrhea in children	S. thermophilus, L. acidophilus, L. bulgaricus	NS
59	Traveler's diarrhea	L. acidophilus, L. bulgaricus, B. bifidum, S. thermophilus	0.02
60	Prevention of diarrhea	S. thermophilus B. bifidum	0.035
61	Prevention of diarrhea	B. bifidum	NS
62	Prevention of diarrhea	L. plantarum 299 V	NS

OR, oral rehydration; NS, not significant.

3.1.1   Side Effects of Pharmaceutical Bacterial Probiotics

It is unclear whether viable *L. acidophilus* improves the digestion of lactose
(5,18,19). Disturbances in the subtle balance between gram-positive and gram-
negative bacteria in the natural colonic flora may be induced by the administration
of gram-positive bacteria such as lactobacilli and bifidobacteria, which have a
more rapid growth than gram-negative bacteria. This imbalance may result in
metabolic D-lactate acidosis as a consequence of bacterial carbohydrate metabolism (66). A gram-positive overgrowth may occur in many situations, including
anatomic or functional short bowel, antibiotic treatment, exclusive feeding with
dairy products, excessive amounts of dietary carbohydrates, and/or the use of
oral *L. acidophilus* tablets (67–70).

Endocarditis, meningitis, pneumonia, and sepsis have been reported with
lactobacilli (71–73). In Finland, among 3317 blood culture isolates, lactobacilli
were identified in 8 patients (74), although none were of the *L. casei* strain GG
(74,75). Case reports suggest, however, that *L. casei* strain GG can cause bacteremia (76,77). The pathogenic potential of bacterial probiotics is low but does
exist (74). Enterococci are a known cause of sepsis in premature infants (78).
Nosocomial epidemics with vancomycin-resistant *E. faecium* have been reported
in oncologic patients (79,80), resulting in a mortality of 73% because of the
absence of response to antibiotics (79). *B. subtilis* bacteremia occurred in 4 of
20 oncologic patients but was also reported in other severely sick patients (81,82).
Although the incidence of infections remains extremely low, it is possible that
lactic acid bacteria may become pathogenic under certain circumstances (83).

Transfer of genetic material from multiresistant probiotics or biotherapeutic
agents to the commensal or pathogenic flora could have catastrophic consequences (8), as, for example, many *E. faecium* strains have plasmids that are
resistant to multiple antibiotics, including vancomycin (8). Gene transfer has been
reported between enterococci in the gastrointestinal tract of experimental rats
(84). Vancomycin resistance of *lactobacilli* is chromosomal and not plasmid-
mediated; therefore the risk of transmission to other organisms is small (85). The
induction of beta-lactamase production in anaerobic bacteria was reported as a
complication of the prevention of diarrhea associated with the administration of
ceftriaxone; in other words, the production of beta-lactamase of the antibiotic
was acquired by the anaerobic bacteria (86). A transfer of macrolide-lincosamide-
streptogramin B resistance between *C. difficile* and *B. subtilis*, and vice versa,
has been described without plasmid DNA being found (87). An epidemic of
multiresistant *E. faecium* with transferable vancomycin resistance has been published (80). The increase in vancomycin-resistant enterococci may be associated
with the possible use of vancomycin-resistant probiotics. The safety and the long-
term effects of biotherapeutic agents on antibiotic resistance must be thoroughly
investigated before their large-scale use can be recommended (8).

Cell membranes of streptococci and lactobacilli may cause chronic polyarthritis in men (88). A gram-positive intestinal flora, including bifidobacteria, *L. casei* and *L. acidophilus*, aggravates the consequences of such an induced arthritis in rats (89). This is presumably due to peptidoglycan, an essential component of the gram-positive bacterial cell wall that may cause an immunopathological process (88,89). Peptidoglycan contains D-glutamine and D-alanine, amino acids that do not exist naturally. Mammals do not have proteases that can break down polypeptides containing D-amino acids. This can cause an irreversible B-cell inactivation because of saturation of the membrane receptors. Reactive arthritis (Reiter's syndrome) has been described in *Shigella*, *Salmonella*, and *Campylobacter* infections and is caused by an indirect mechanism (90). Lipopolysaccharides of *Salmonella* spp. were detected in the joints of patients with reactive arthritis after a *Salmonella* infection (91). This finding may possibly limit the use of gram-positive biotherapeutic agents in the treatment of diarrhea caused by bacteria that increase the permeability of the intestinal wall such as salmonellae. Administration of heat-killed *L. acidophilus* is contraindicated in salmonellosis.

3.2 Nonbacterial Biotherapeutic Agents (Group 2)

As of today, there is only one known nonbacterial biotherapeutic agent—the yeast *Saccharomyces boulardii*. This nonpathogenic yeast was isolated from lychees in Indochina and grows at the unusually high temperature of 37°C (92). It is commercially available in a freeze-dried, viable preparation and is the only yeast with which double-blind studies have been carried out. *S. boulardii* differs from baker's yeast (*S. cerevisiae*) in a number of taxonomic, metabolic, and molecular parameters (92). *S. boulardii* survives gastric acid and bile and can be detected alive throughout the entire digestive system when given daily in its freeze-dried form. However, 2 to 5 days after administration the yeast becomes undetectable in the feces (8). *S. boulardii* is intrinsically resistant to antibacterial antibiotics (93,94). Nystatin completely eliminates *S. boulardii* from the gastrointestinal tract, although *S. boulardii* can be administered 4 to 6 hr after fluconazole without any effect on its viability in the intestine (95).

The pharmacodynamics of *S. boulardii* involves three different aspects: 1) a direct antagonistic effect; 2) an antisecretory effect, by acting specifically on the binding of toxins to intestinal receptors; and 3) a trophic effect, by stimulating enzymatic activities and intestinal defense mechanisms (for a detailed review, see Ref. 96). A direct antagonistic effect to several pathogens [such as *Candida albicans*, *Escherichia coli*, *Shigella* species, *Salmonella typhi* (97), *Pseudomonas aeruginosa*, *Staphylococcus aureus* (98), *Entamoeba histolytica* (99)] has been demonstrated both, in vitro and in vivo. Two different antisecretory mechanisms acting specifically on the binding of bacterial toxins have been discovered. *S. boulardii* produces two proteins, one of 54 kDa and another of 120 kDa. The

120-kDa protein has no proteolytic activity and specifically competes with the hypersecretion induced by *Vibrio cholerae* and enterotoxigenic *E. coli* by reducing the formation of cyclic AMP in the intestinal cells (100–102). The second protein produced is a 54-kDa protease, which acts on toxin A of *Clostridium difficile* (102). *S. boulardii* significantly reduces the liquid secretion and permeability caused by toxin A in rat ileum (102). In vivo, *S. boulardii* decreases the amount of toxin A produced, the intestinal lesions, and the mortality rate caused by *C. difficile* (103,104).

Polyamines, such as spermine and spermidine, cause a significant increase in length and weight of the intestine, an accelerated maturation of the microvillous enzymes (lactase, sucrase, maltase, and aminopeptidase), and an increase in the immunoglobulin A secretion in villi and crypt cells of young laboratory animals (105–107). Polyamines increase the number of glucose carriers in the membrane of the enterocyte and are essential for the purpose of achieving maximal glucose absorption in the enterocyte (108). *S. boulardii* contains polyamines (spermine and spermidine), which, when given to laboratory animals, exert similar trophic effects on the intestinal mucosa (increase in disaccharidase activity) as equivalent amounts of spermine and spermidine (109). Whether there is a stimulating effect on intestinal adaptation in short bowel syndrome is not clear, as contradictory results have been reported (110,111). However, there is recent evidence that oral administration of *S. boulardii* soon after proximal enterectomy improves functional adaptation of the remnant ileum in rats (112).

S. boulardii has been studied in many placebo-controlled, prospective, randomized clinical trials (Table 2). Results indicate almost consistently a significant benefit in prevention of each of the following situations: antibiotic-associated diarrhea (113–116), diarrhea associated with enteral feedings (117–119), and traveler's diarrhea (34,120). The addition of *S. boulardii* for 1 month to standard antibiotic therapy (vancomycin and/or metronidazole) for *C. difficile* infection significantly reduced the number of relapses (121). The efficacy of *S. boulardii* was demonstrated in randomized, double-blind studies in 92 adults with acute diarrhea (122,123) and in children with chronic diarrhea caused by *Giardia lamblia* (124). In the latter study, 35 of 40 children improved. In a randomized double-blind study in 35 AIDS patients with chronic diarrhea, 61% were found to be diarrhea-free after 1 week of treatment with *S. boulardii*, compared to 12% in the placebo group (125).

3.2.1 Side Effects of *S. boulardii*

The safety of *S. boulardii* has been investigated in animal models and in randomized double-blind studies. In mice given 5% *S. boulardii* for 70 days in their drinking water, no translocation from the gastrointestinal tract was observed. *S. boulardii* could not be detected in the organs (liver, kidneys, lungs, and heart) or in the mesenteric lymph glands (92). In an immunodepressed animal model

TABLE 2 Outcome of Double-Blind Randomized Prospective Studies with *S. boulardii*

Reference	Study population	Indication	Clinical outcome
113	388	Prevention of antibiotic-associated diarrhea	<0.001
114	180	Prevention of antibiotic-associated diarrhea	0.038
115	193	Prevention of antibiotic-associated diarrhea	0.03
116	69	Prevention of antibiotic-associated diarrhea	NS
117	40	Prevention of enteral feeding–associated diarrhea	<0.001
118	128	Prevention of enteral feeding–associated diarrhea	0.002
119	20	Prevention of enteral feeding–associated diarrhea in patients with severe burns	<0.001
34	1231	Prevention of traveler's diarrhea	<0.001
120	3000	Prevention of traveler's diarrhea	NS
121	124	Recurrence of *C. difficile* colitis	0.04
122	92	Treatment of acute diarrhea in adults	<0.05
123	130	Treatment of acute diarrhea in children	<0.01
124	30	Treatment of acute diarrhea in children	<0.01
125	40	Treatment of chronic diarrhea in children (35/40: *Giardia lamblia*)	<0.001
126	35	Treatment of chronic diarrhea in AIDS patients	<0.002
127	17	Stable Crohn's disease (reduction in diarrhea)	<0.05
128	10	Small bowel overgrowth	NS

(prednisolone and antibiotic decontamination), *S. boulardii* could be detected only at very low concentrations in the mesenteric lymph glands; *S. boulardii* could not be detected in the liver, spleen, or kidneys (129). It was, however, detected in the gastrointestinal mucosal tissue in rotavirus-infected intestine of BALB/c seronegative mice (130). *S. boulardii* was given to more than 40 AIDS patients without any serious side effects (126,131).

Over a period of 10 years during which millions of *S. boulardii* treatments were prescribed, only a few cases of *S. boulardii* fungemia were reported (132–139). All the patients reported with *S. boulardii* fungemia had venous indwelling catheters, most of which were central lines, suggesting that the infection source in fungemia is exogenous. The majority of the contaminated patients had received high doses of *S. boulardii*. Patients recovered after antimycotic treatment without further problems. Careful deployment of *S. boulardii* in patients with (central) venous lines is recommended. In one study, constipation and increased thirst were reported (121). Other side effects have not been reported (85).

4 CONCLUSIONS

Food and feed supplements enriched with microorganisms are part of a recent trend directed toward stimulating healthy eating habits. Although, in principle, there is nothing against this "ecological" trend, one should consider the following: 1) many of these microorganisms do not survive contact with gastric acid, bile, and antibiotics and 2) if they are resistant to antibiotics, their safety must be seriously evaluated because of the danger of transfer of their intrinsic resistance to the autochthonous microflora and/or pathogens. A critical evaluation of the efficacy of biotherapeutic agents is a continuous challenge because many different microorganisms have been tested in different indications, study designs, drug compositions, and combinations. Most studies can be criticized for methodological weaknesses (open, controlled without a placebo, few enrolled patients, etc.). Although some in vitro studies provide very interesting results, the clinical benefits of many bacterial probiotics frequently cannot be demonstrated. Whenever microorganisms are used in prevention, it seems logical to first evaluate the effect of microorganisms that are normally present in the human gastrointestinal microflora. There is, however, no scientific evidence for this rationale. The timing of administration and vehicles (type of feeding) used for the administration of the microorganisms may determine the success of treatment (140,141). Results of clinical trials with one of the bacterial probiotics, *L. casei* strain GG, and with the yeast *S. boulardii* show, almost systematically, a clinical benefit of the microorganisms. In that regard, only those two microorganisms seem to fit the definition of a biotherapeutic agent. The efficacy of each microorganism should be demonstrated in well-designed, randomized, double-blind studies for each of the indications for which a claim is made.

REFERENCES

1. Metchnikoff E. The Prolongation of Life. New York: Putnam, 1907.
2. Simon GL, Gorbach SL. Intestinal flora in health and disease. Gastroenterology 1984; 86:174–193.
3. Goldin BR, Lichtenstein AH, Gorbach SL. Nutritional and metabolic roles of intestinal bacteria. In: Shils ME, Olson JA, Shike M, eds. Modern Nutrition in Health and Disease. Philadelphia: Lea & Febiger, 1994, pp 569–580.
4. Zajicek G. Antibiotic resistance and the intestinal flora. *Cancer J* 1996; 9:214–215.
5. Midtvedt T. Microbial functional activities. In: Hanson LA, Yolken RH, eds. Probiotics, Other Nutritional Factors and Intestinal Microflora. Nestlé Nutrition Workshop Series. New York: Lippincott-Raven, 1999, pp 79–96.
6. Ballongue J, Shumann C, Quignon P. Effects of lactulose and lactitol on colonic microflora and enzymatic activity. Scand J Gastroenterol Suppl 1997; 222:41–44.
7. Gibson GR, Collins MD. Concept of balanced colonic microbiotica, prebiotics, and synbiotics. In: Hanson LA, Yolken RH, eds. Probiotics, Other Nutritional Factors and Intestinal Microflora. Nestlé Nutrition Workshop Series. New York: Lippincott-Raven, 1999, pp 139–159.
8. Elmer GW, Surawicz CM, McFarland LV. Biotherapeutic agents: A neglected modality for the treatment and prevention of selected intestinal and vaginal infections. JAMA 1996; 275:870–876.
9. Alm L, Petterson L. Survival rate of lactobacilli during digestion: An in vitro study. Am J Clin Nutr 1980; 33:2543.
10. Marteau P, Rambaud JC. Potential of using lactic acid bacteria for therapy and immunomodulation in man. FEMS Microbiol Rev 1993; 12:207–220.
11. Marteau P, Pochert P, Bouhnik Y, Zidi S, Goderel I, Rambaud JC. Survie dans l'intestin grêle de *Lactobacillus acidophilus* et *Bificobacterium* sp, ingérés dans un lait fermenté. Gastroenterol Clin Biol 1992; 16:25–28.
12. Hamilton-Miller JMT, Shah S, Smith GT. ''Probiotic'' remedies are not what they seem. BMJ 1996; 312:55–56.
13. Canganella F, Paganini S, Ovidi M, Vettraino AM, Bevliacque L, Mass S, Trovatelli LD. A microbiological investigation on probiotic pharmaceutical products used for human health. Microbiol Res 1997; 152:171–179.
14. Coconnier MH, Liévin V, Bernet-Camard MF, Hudault S, Servin AL. Antibacterial effect of adhering human *Lactobacillus acidophilus* strain LB. Antimicrob Agents Chemother 1997; 41:1046–1052.
15. Hudault S, Liévin V, Bernet-Camard MF, Servin AL. Antagonistic activity exerted in vitro and in vivo by *Lactobacillus casei* (strain GG) against *Salmonella typhimurium C5* infection. Appl Environ Microbiol 1997; 63:513–518.
16. Borgia M, Sepe N, Brancaro V, Borgia R. A controlled clinical study on *Streptococcus faecium* preparation for the prevention of side reactions during long-term antibiotic treatments. Curr Ther Res 1982; 31:265–271.
17. Borgia M, Sepe N, Brancaro V, Simone P, Borgia R. Effect of *Streptococcus* lactic-acid producing bacteria (SF68 strain) on body weight in man: a double-blinded controlled clinical study. Curr Ther Res 1983; 33:214–218.

18. McDonough FE, Wong NP, Hitchins A, Bodwell CE. Alleviation of lactose malabsorption from sweet acidophilus milk. Am J Clin Nutr 1985; 42:345–346.

19. Hove H, Nordgaard-Andersen I, Mortensen PB. Effect of lactic acid bacteria on the intestinal production of lactate and short-chain fatty acids, and the absorption of lactose. Am J Clin Nutr 1994; 59:74–79.

20. Kaila M, Isolauri E, Saxelin M, Arvilommi H, Vesikari T. Viable versus inactivated *Lactobacillus* strain GG in acute rotavirus diarrhoea. Arch Dis Child 1995; 72:51–53.

21. Malin M, Suomalainen H, Saxelin M, Isolauri E. Promotion of IgA immune response in patients with Crohn's disease by oral bacteriotherapy with *Lactobacillus* GG. Ann Nutr Metab 1996; 40:137–145.

22. Malin M, Verronen P, Mykkanen H, Salminen S, Isolauri E. Increased bacterial urease activity in faeces in juvenile chronic arthritis: evidence of altered intestinal microflora? Br J Rheumatol 1996; 35:689–694.

23. Majamaa H, Isolauri E. Probiotics: A novel approach in the management of food allergy. J Allergy Clin Immunol 1997; 99:179–185.

24. Sutas Y, Soppi E, Korhonen H, Syvaoja EL, Saxelin M, Rokka T, Isolauri E. Suppression of lymphocyte proliferation in vitro by bovine caseins hydrolyzed with *Lactobacillus casei* GG derived enzymes. J Allergy Clin Immunol 1996; 98:216–224.

25. Braback L. Do infections protect against atopic diseases? Acta Paediatr 1999; 88:705–708.

26. Pekkanen J, Remes S, Kajosaari M, Husman T, Soininen L. Infections in early childhood and risk of atopic disease. Acta Paediatr 1999; 88:710–714.

27. Chauvière G, Coconnier MH, Kernies S, Darfeuille-Michaud A, Joly B, Servin AL. Competitive exclusion of diarrheagenic *Escherichia coli* ETEC from human enterocyte-like Caco-2 cells by heat-killed *Lactobacillus*. FEMS Microbiol Lett 1992; 91:213–218.

28. Vandenplas Y. Bacteria and yeast in the treatment of acute and chronic infectious diarrhoea: I. Bacteria. Clin Microbiol Infect 1993; 5:299–307.

29. Clements ML, Levine MM, Black RE, Robins-Browne LA, Cisneros RM, Drusano GL, Lanata CF, Saah AJ. *Lactobacillus* prophylaxis for diarrhea due to enterotoxigenic *Escherichia coli*. Antimicrob Agents Chemother 1981; 20:104–108.

30. Pozo-Olano JD, Warram JH, Gomez RG, Cavazos MG. Effect of a *Lactobacilli* preparation on traveller's diarrhea: a randomized double-blind clinical trial. Gastroenterology 1978; 74:829–830.

31. Tankanow RM, Ross MB, Ertel IJ, Dickinson DG, McCormick LS, Garfinkel JF. A double-blind, placebo-controlled study on the efficacy of Lactinex in the prophylaxis of amoxillin-induced diarrhea. DICP Ann Pharmacother 1990; 24:382–384.

32. Gotz V, Romankiewicz JA, Moss J, Murray HW. Prophylaxis against ampicillin-associated diarrhea with *Lactobacillus* preparations. Am J Hosp Pharm 1979; 36:754–757.

33. Heimburger DC, Sockwell DG, Geels WJ. Diarrhea with enteral feeding: prospective reappraisal of putative causes. Nutrition 1994; 10:392–396.

34. Kollaritsch HH, Kemsner P, Wiedermann G, Scheiner O. Prevention of traveller's diarrhoea: comparison of different non-antibiotic preparations. Travel Med Int 1989; 9–17.
35. Katelaris PH, Salam I, Farthing MJG. *Lactobacilli* to prevent traveler's diarrhea? N Engl J Med 1995; 333:1360–1361.
36. Boulloche J, Mouterde O, Mallet E. Traitement des diarrhées aiguës chez le nourisson et le jeune enfant. Ann Pédiatr 1994; 41:457–463.
37. Colombel JF, Cortot A, Neut C, Romond C. Yoghurt with bifidobacterium longum reduces erythromycin-induced gastrointestinal effects. Lancet 1987; 2:43.
38. Kruis W, Schütz E, Fric P, Fixa B, Judmaiers G, Stolte M. Double-blind comparison of an oral *Escherichia coli* preparation and mesalazine in maintaining remission of ulcerative colitis. Aliment Pharmacol Ther 1997; 11:853–858.
39. Rembacken BJ, Snelling AM, Hawkey PM, Axon ATR. A double-blind trial of non-pathogenic *E. coli* vs. mesalazine for the treatment of ulcerative colitis. Gut 1997; 41:A70.
40. Tanaka R, Shimosaka K. Investigation of the stool frequency in elderly who are bed ridden and its improvements by ingestion of bifidus yogurt. Nippon Ronen Igakkai Zasshi 1982; 19:557–582.
41. Hentschel C, Bauer J, Dill N. Complementary medicine in non-ulcer dyspepsia: Is alternative medicine a real alternative? A randomised placebo-controlled double blind clinical trial with two probiotic agents (HYLAC N and HYLAC N forte). Gastroenterology 1997; 112:A146.
42. Oksanen PJ, Salminen S, Saxelin M, Hämäläinen P, Ihantola-Vormisto A, Muurasiemi-Isoviita L, Nikkari S, Oksanen T, Pörsti I, Salminen E, Siitonen S, Stuckey H, Toppila A, Vapaatalo H. Prevention of traveller's diarrhoea by Lactobacillus GG. Ann Med 1990; 22:53–56.
43. Isolauri E, Juntunen M, Rautanen T, Sillanaukee P, Koivula T. A human *Lactobacillus* strain (*Lactobacillus casei* sp strain GG) promotes recovery from acute diarrhea in children. Pediatrics 1991; 88:90–97.
44. Millar MR, Bacon C, Smith SL, Walker V, Hall MA. Enteral feeding of premature infants with *Lactobacillus* GG. Arch Dis Child 1993; 69:483–487.
45. O'Sullivan M, Morain C. Probiotics in the treatment of irritable bowel syndrome (IBS)—A randomised double blind placebo controlled crossover study. Gastroenterology 1996; 110:A385.
46. The ESPGHAN working group on acute diarrhoea. *Lactobacillus* GG administered in oral rehydration solution to children with acute diarrhea: a multicenter European trial. J Pediatr Gastroenterol Nutr 1998; 26:547(A).
47. Raza S, Graham SM, Allen SJ, Sultana S, Cuevas L, Hart CA. *Lactobacillus* GG promotes recovery from acute nonbloody diarrhea in Pakistan. Pediatr Infect Dis 1995; 14:107–112.
48. Siitonen S, Vapaatalo H, Salminen S, Gordin A, Saxelin M, Wikberg R, Kirkkola AL. Effect of *Lactobacillus* GG yoghurt in prevention of antibiotic associated diarrhoea. Ann Med 1990; 22:57–59.
49. Gorbach SL, Chang TW, Goldin B. Successful treatment of relapsing *Clostridium difficile* colitis with Lactobacillus GG. Lancet 1987; 2:1519.

50. Shornikova AV, Isolauri E, Burkanova L, Lukonikova S, Vesikari T. A trial in the Karelian Republic of oral rehydration and *Lactobacillus* GG for treatment of acute diarrhea. Acta Paediatr 1997; 86:460–465.

51. Stotzer PO, Blomberg L, Conway PL, Henriksson A, Abrahamsson H. Probiotic treatment of small intestinal bacterial overgrowth by *Lactobacillus fermentum* KLD. Scand J Infect Dis 1996; 28:615–619.

52. Wunderlich PF, Braun L, Fumagalli I, D'Apuzzo V, Heim F, Karly M, Lodi R, Politta G, Vonbank FR, Zeltner L. Double blind report on the efficacy of lactic acid-producing *Enterococcus* SF68 in the prevention of antibiotic-associated diarrhoea and in the treatment of acute diarrhoea. J Int Med Res 1989; 17:333–338.

53. Mitra AK, Rabbani GH. A double-blind, controlled trial of Bioflorin (*Streptococcus faecium* SF68) in adults with acute diarrhea due to vibrio cholerae and enterotoxigenic *Escherichia coli*. Gastroenterology 1990; 99:1149–1152.

54. Buydens P, Debeuckelaere S. Efficacy of SF 68 in the treatment of acute diarrhea. Scand J Gastroenterol 1996; 31:887–891.

55. Shornikova AV, Casas IA, Isolauri E, Mykkanen H, Vesikari T. *Lactobacillus reuteri* as a therapeutic agent in acute diarrhea in young children. J Pediatr Gastroenterol Nutr 1997; 24:399–404.

56. Shornikova AV, Casas AI, Mykkänen H, Salo A, Vesikari T. Bacteriotherapy with *Lactobacillus reuteri* in rotavirus gastroenteritis. Pediatr Infec Dis J 1997; 16:1103–1107.

57. Chicoine L, Joncas JH. Emploi des ferments lactiques dans la gastro-entérite non bactérienne. Union Med Can 1973; 102:1114–1115.

58. Pearce JL, Hamilton JR. Controlled trial of orally administered *Lactobacilli* in acute infantile diarrhea. J Pediatr 1974; 84:261–262.

59. Black FT, Anderson PL, Orskov J, Gaarslev K, Laulund S. Prophylactic efficacy of *lactobacilli* on traveler's diarrhea. Travel Med 1989; 7:333–335.

60. Saavedra JM, Bauman NA, Oung I, Perman JA, Yolken RH. Feeding of *Bifidobacterium bifidum* and *Streptococcus thermophilus* to infants in hospital for prevention of diarrhea and shedding of rotavirus. Lancet 1994; 344:1046–1049.

61. Chouraqui JP, Van Egroo LD, Fichot MC. Prevention of diarrhea by feeding infants with an acidified milk formula containing *Bifidobacterium bifidum*. J Pediatr Gastroenterol Nutr 1998; 26:539(A).

62. Ribeiro H, Vanderhoof JA. Reduction of diarrheal illness following administration of *Lactobacillus plantarium* 299V in a daycare facility. J Pediatr Gastroenterol Nutr 1998; 26:561(A).

63. Kotz CM, Peterson LR, Moody JA, Savaiano DA, Levitt MD. Effect of yoghurt on clindamycin-induced *Clostridium difficile* colitis in hamsters. Dig Dis Sci 1992; 37:129–132.

64. Coconnier MH, Liévin V, Bernet-Camard MF, Hudault S, Servin AL. Antibacterial effect of adhering human *Lactobacillus acidophilus* strain LB. Antimicrob Agents Chemother 1997; 41:1046–1052.

65. Kabier G, Aiba Y, Takagi A, Kamiya S, Miwa T, Koga Y. Prevention of *Helicobacter pylori* infection by lactobacilli in a gnotobiotic murine model. Gut 1997; 41:49–55.

66. Coronado BE, Opal SM, Yoburn DC. Antibiotic-induced D-lactic acidosis. Ann Intern Med 1995; 122:839–842.
67. Perlmutter DH, Boyle JT, Campos JM, Egler JM, Watkins JB. D-Lactic acidosis in children: an unusual metabolic complication of small bowel resection. J Pediatr 1983; 102:234–238.
68. Stolberg L, Rolfe R, Giltin N, Merrit J, Mann L, Linder J, Finegold S. D-Lactic acidosis due to abnormal gut flora. N Engl J Med 1982; 306:1344–1348.
69. Oh MS, Phelps KR, Traube M, Barbarosa-Saldivar JL, Boxhill C, Carroll HJ. D-Lactic acidosis in a man with short-bowel syndrome. N Engl J Med 1979; 301: 249–252.
70. Traube M, Bock JL, Boyer JL. D-Lactic acidosis after jejunoileal bypass: identification of organic anions by nuclear magnetic resonance spectroscopy. Ann Intern Med 1983; 98:171–173.
71. Majamaa H. Lactic acid bacteria in the treatment of acute rotavirus gastroenteritis. J Pediatr Gastroenterol Nutr 1995; 20:333–338.
72. Sussman JI, Baron EJ, Goldberg SM, Kaplan MH, Pizzarello RA. Clinical manifestations and therapy of *Lactobacillus endocarditis*: report of a case and review of the literature. Rev Infect Dis 1986; 8:771–776.
73. Rahman M. Chest infection caused by *Lactobacillus casei* ss rhamnosus. Br Med J 1982; 284:471–472.
74. Saxellin M, Chuang N, Chassy B, Rautelin H, Mäkelä PH, Salminen S, Gorbach SL. *Lactobacilli* and bacteremia in Southern Finland, 1989–1992. Clin Infect Dis 1996; 22:564–566.
75. Saxelin M, Rautelin H, Salminen S, Makela PH. Safety of commercial products with viable *Lactobacillus* strains. Infect Dis Clin Proc 1996; 5:331–335.
76. Rogasi PG, Vigano S, Pecile P, Leoncini F. *Lactobacillus casei* pneumonia and sepsis in a patient with AIDS: Case report and review of the literature. Ann Ital Med Int 1998; 13:180–182.
77. Schoon Y, Schuurman B, Buiting AG, Kranendonk SE, Graafsma SJ. Aortic graft infection by *Lactobacillus casei*: a case report. Neth J Med 1998; 52:71–74.
78. Dobson SRM, Baker CJ. Enterococcal sepsis in neonates: features, by age at onset and occurrence of focal infection. Pediatrics 1990; 85:165–171.
79. Edmond MB, Ober JF, Weibaum DL, Pfaleer MA, Hwang T, Sanford MD, Wenzel RP. Vancomycin-resistant *Enterococcus faecium* bacteremia: risk factors for infection. Clin Infect Dis 1995; 20:1126–1131.
80. Boyce JM, Opal SM, Chow JW, Zervos MJ, Pottor GP, Sherman CB, Romulo RLC, Fortna S, Medeiros AA. Outbreak of multidrug-resistant *Enterococcus faecium* with transferable B class vancomycin resistance. J Clin Microbiol 1994; 32: 1148–1153.
81. Richard V, Van der Auwera P, Snoeck R, Daneau D, Meunier F. Nosocomial bacteremia caused by *Bacillus* species. Eur J Microbiol Infect Dis 1988; 7:783–785.
82. Lanco S, Guillot M, Eckart P, Paris C, Amiour M, Al-Jazayri Z, Gaudelus J, Jokic M, Lecacheux C. Infections systémiques sévères à bacille cereus: aspects actuels de la pathogénicité des bactéries du genre *Bacillus*. Arch Pédiatr 1997; 4:1144–1155.

83. Gasser F. Safety of lactic acid bacteria and their occurrence in human clinical infection. Bull Inst Pasteur 1994; 92:45–67.

84. Jacobsen BL, Brockmann E, Hertel C, Ludwig W, Schleifer KH. In: Hashimoto K et al., eds. Germfree and Its Ramifications. Proceedings XII. Shizawa, Japan: ISG Publishing Committee, 1996, pp 51–54.

85. Vanderhoof JA, Young RJ. Use of probiotics in childhood gastrointestinal disorders. J Pediatr Gastroenterol Nutr 1998; 27:323–332.

86. Léonard F, Andremont A, Leclerq B, Labia R, Tancrède C. Use of β-lactamase-producing anaerobes to prevent ceftriaxone from degrading intestinal resistance to colonization. J Infect Dis 1989; 160:274–280.

87. Murray BE. Editorial response: what can we do about vancomycin-resistant enterococci? Clin Infect Dis 1995; 20:1134–1136.

88. Mills JA. Do bacteria cause chronic polyarthritis? N Engl J Med 1989; 320:245–256.

89. Kohashi O, Kohashi Y, Takashi T, Ozawa A, Shigematsu N. Reverse effect of gram-positive bacteria vs gram-negative bacteria on adjuvant-induced arthritis in germfree rats. Microbiol Immunol 1985; 29:487–497.

90. Hagiage M. La flore intestinale. In: Hagiage M, ed. De l'equilibre au déséquilibre. Paris, France: Vigot, 1994, 99.

91. Granfors K, Jalkanen S, Lindberg AA, Mäki-Ikola O, Von Essen R, Lahesmaa-Rantala R, Isomäki H, Saario R, Arnold WJ, Toivanen A. Salmonella lipopolysaccharide in synovial cells from patients with reactive arthritis. Lancet 1990; 335:685–688.

92. McFarland LV, Bernasconi P. *Saccharomyces boulardii*: a review of an innovative biotherapeutic agent. Microb Ecol Health Disease 1993; 6:157–171.

93. Klein SM, Elmer GW, McFarland LV, Surawicz CM, Levy RH. Recovery and elimination of the biotherapeutic agent, *Saccharomyces boulardii* in healthy human volunteers. Pharm Res 1993; 10:1615–1619.

94. Boddy AV, Elmer GW, McFarland LV, Levy RH. Influence of antibiotics on the recovery of *Saccharomyces boulardii* in rats. Pharm Res 1991; 8:796–800.

95. Elmer G, Moyer K, Vega R, Surawicz C, Collier A, Hooton M, McFarland L. Pharmacokinetic studies of *Saccharomyces boulardii* in patients with HIV-related chronic diarrhea in healthy volunteers. XIX International Congress on Microbial Ecology and Disease. Rome, September 18–21, 1994.

96. Vandenplas Y. Bacteria and yeast in the treatment of acute and chronic infectious diarrhoea. II. Yeast. Clin Microbiol Infect 1999; 5:389–395.

97. Brugier S, Patte F. Antagonisme in vitro entre Perenterol et différents germes bactériens. Méd Paris 1975; 45:3–8.

98. Bergogne-Bérézin E, Bornet M. In vitro antagonistic effect of *Saccharomyces boulardii* against bacteria involved in diarrhea in intensive-care-unit patient. Sci Aliments 1986; 6:63–73.

99. Rigothier MC, Maccario J, Gayral P. Inhibitory activity of *Sacharomyces* yeasts on the adhesion of Entamoeba histolytica trophozoites to human erythrocytes in vitro. Parasitol Res 1994; 80:10–15.

100. Czerucka D, Roux I, Rampal P. *Saccharomyces boulardii* inhibits secretagogue-mediated adenosine 3′,5′-cyclic monophosphate induction in intestinal cells. Gastroenterology 1994; 106:65–72.

101. Brandao RL, Castro IM, Bambirra EA, Amaral SC, Fietto LG, Tropia MJ, Neves MJ, Dos-Santos RG, Gomes NC, Nicoli JR. Intracellular signal triggered by cholera toxin in *Saccharomyces boulardii* and *Saccharomyces cerevisiae*. Appl Environ Microbiol 1998; 64:564–568.

102. Castagliuolo I, Lamont JT, Nikulasson ST, Pothoulakis C. *Saccharomyces boulardii* protease inhibits *Clostridium difficile* toxin A effects in the rat ileum. Infect Immun 1996; 64:5225–5232.

103. Castex F, Corthier G, Jouvert S, Elmer GW, Lucas F, Bastide M. Prevention of *Clostridium difficile*–induced experimental pseudomembraneous colitis by *Saccharomyces boulardii*: A scanning electron microscopic and microbiological study. J Gen Microbiol 1990; 136:1085–1089.

104. Capano G, Bloch KJ, Carter EA, Dascoli JA, Schoenfeld D, Harmatz PR. Polyamines in human and rat milk influence intestinal cell growth in vitro. J Pediatr Gastroenterol Nutr 1998; 27:281–286.

105. Tutton PJ, Barkla DH. Biogenic amines as regulaters of the proliferative activity of normal and neoplastic intestinal epithelial cells. Anticancer Res 1987; 7:1–12.

106. Buts JP, De Keyser N, Kolanowski J, Sokal E, Van Hoof F. Maturation of villus and crypt cell functions in rat small intestine role of dietary polyamines. Dig Dis Sci 1993; 38:1091–1098.

107. Jahn HU, Ullrich R, Schneider T, Liehr RM, Schieferdecker HL, Holst H, Zeitz M. Immunological and trophical effects of *Saccharomyces boulardii* on the small intestine in healthy human volunteers. Digestion 1996; 57:95–104.

108. Johnson LR, Brockway PD, Madsen K, Hardin JA, Grant Gall D. Polyamines alter intestinal glucose transport. Am J Physiol 1995; 31:G416–G423.

109. Buts JP, De Keyser N, De Raedemaeker L. *Saccharomyces boulardii* enhances rat intestinal enzyme expression by endoluminal release of polyamines. Pediatr Res 1994; 36:552–557.

110. Vanderhoof JA, Kollman K, Goulet O. *Saccharomyces boulardii* does not stimulate mucosal hyperplasia following intestinal resection in the rat. J Pediatr Gastroenterol Nutr 1998; 26:567(A).

111. Zaouche A, Loukil C, Peuchmaur M, Macry J, D Lagausie P, Fitoussi F, Bléhaut H, Bernasconi P, Bingen E, Cézard JP. Effects of oral *Saccharomyces boulardii* on bacterial overgrowth, translocation and intestinal adaptation after small bowel resection in growing rats. J Pediatr Gastroenterol Nutr 1998; 26:570(A).

112. Buts JP, De Keyser N, Marandi S, Hermans D, Sokal EM, Chae YHE, Lambotte L, Chanteux H, Tulkens PM. *Saccharomyces boulardii* upgrades cellular adaptation after proximal enterectomy in rats. Gut 1999; 45:89–96.

113. Adam P. Essais cliniques controlés en double insu de l'ultra-levure lyophilisée (étude multicentrique par 25 médecins de 388 cas). Méd Chir Dig 1976; 5:401–406.

114. Surawicz CM, Elmer GW, Speelman P, McFarland LV, Chinn J, Van Belle G. Prevention of antibiotic-associated diarrhea by *Saccharomyces boulardii*: A prospective study. Gastroenterology 1989; 96:981–988.

115. McFarland LV, Surawicz CM, Greenberg RN, Elmer GW, Moyer KA, Melcher SA, Bowen KE, Cox JL. Prevention of beta-lactam-associated diarrhea by Saccharomyces boulardii compared with placebo. Am J Gastroenterol 1995; 90:439–448.

116. Lewis SJ, Potts LF, Barry RE. The lack of therapeutic effect of *Saccharomyces*

boulardii in the prevention of antibiotic-related diarrhoea in elderly patients. J Infect 1998; 36:171–174.

117. Templé JD, Steidel AL, Bléhaut H, Hasselman M, Lutun Ph, Maurier F. Prévention par *Saccharomyces boulardii* des diarrhées de l'alimentation entérale à débit continu. La Semaine des Hôpitaux de Paris 1983; 59:1409–1412.

118. Schlotterer M, Bernasconi P, Lebreton F, Wasserman D. Intére//t de *Saccharomyces boulardii* dans la tolérance digestive de la nutrition entérale à débit continu chez le brûlé. Nutr Clin Metabol 1987; 1:31–34.

119. Bleichner G, Bléhaut H, Mentec H, Moyse D. *Saccharomyces boulardii* prevents diarrhea in critically ill tube-fed patients. Intensive Care Med 1997; 23:517–523.

120. Kollaritsch H, Holst H, Grobara P, Wiederman G. Prophylaxe der reisdiarrhöe mit *Saccharomyces boulardii*. Fortschr Med 1993; 111:152–156.

121. McFarland LV, Surawicz CM, Greenberg RN, Feketey R, Elmer GW, Moyer KA, Melcher SA, Bowen KE, Cox JL, Noorani Z, Harrington G, Rubin M, Greenwald D. A randomized placebo-controlled trial of *Saccharomyces boulardii* in combination with standard antibiotics for *Clostridium difficile* disease. JAMA 1994; 271:1913–1918.

122. Höchter W, Chase D, Hagenhoff G. *Saccharomyces boulardii* in acute adult diarrhoea. Münch Med Wochenschr 1990; 132:188–192.

123. Cetina-Sauri G, Sierra Basto G. Evaluation Thérapeutique de *Saccharomyces boulardii* chez des enfants souffrant de diarrhée aiguë. Ann Pédiatr 1994; 41:397–400.

124. Chapoy P. Traitement des diarrhées aiguës infantiles: essais contrôlé de *Saccharomyces boulardii*. Ann Pédiatr Paris 1985; 32:561–563.

125. Castanada C. Effects of *Saccharomyces boulardii* in children with chronic diarrhea, especially due to giardiasis. Rev Mex Puericult Pediatr 1995;2.

126. Saint-Marc T, Bléhaut H, Musial Ch, Touraine JL. Diarrhöea im Zusammenhang mit AIDS (Doppelblindstudie mit *Saccharomyces boulardii*). Semin Hôp Paris 1995; 71:735–741.

127. Plein H, Hotz J. Therapeutic effects of *Saccharomyces boulardii* on mild residual symptoms in a stable phase of Crohn's disease with special respect to chronic diarrhea—A pilot study. Z Gastroenterol 1993; 31:129–134.

128. Attar A, Bouhnik Y, Flourié B. Efficacy of two antibiotics and a probiotic in the treatment of small intestinal bacterial overgrowth. Gut 1996; 39:A173.

129. Berg R, Bernasconi P, Fowler D, Gautreux M. Inhibition of Candida albicans translocation from the gastrointestinal tract of mice by oral administration of *Saccharomyces boulardii*. J Infect Dis 1993; 168:1314–1318.

130. Cartwright-Shamoon J, Dickson GR, Dodge J, Carr KE. Uptake of yeast (*Saccharomyces boulardii*) in normal and rotavirus treated intestine. Gut 1996; 39:204–209.

131. Saint-Marc T, Rossello-Prats L, Touraine JL. Efficacité de *Saccharomyces boulardii* dans le traitement des diarrhées du SIDA. Ann Méd Interne Paris 1991; 142:64–65.

132. Grillot R, Lebeau B, Gouillier-Fleuret A, Chouraqui JP, Andrini P. De deux maux il faut choisir le moindre ou du caractere opportuniste de *Saccharomyces boulardii*. Société Française de Mycologie Médicale 1986: Résumé des Rapports.

133. Zunic P, Lacotte J, Pegoix M, Buteux G, Leroy G, Mosquet B, Moulin M. Fongémie a *Saccharomyces boulardii*. Therapie 1991; 45:497–501.

134. Forge G, Aznar C, Marguet F, Polomeni P, Bouchet R, Manicacci M. *Saccharomyces fungemia* in AIDS patients after treatment for chronic diarrhea. The Fifth European Conference on Clinical Aspects and Treatment of HIV Infection, Copenhagen, Denmark, September 26–29, 1995.

135. Pletincx M, Legein J, Vandenplas Y. Fungemia with *Saccharomyces boulardii* in a 1-year-old girl with protracted diarrhea. J Pediatr Gastroenterol Nutr 1995; 21: 113–115.

136. Viggiano M, Badetti C, Bernini V, Garabedian M, Manelli JC. Fongémie à *Saccharomyces boulardii* chez un brûlé grave. Ann Fr Anesth Réanim 1995; 14:356–358.

137. Boucaud C, Berrada K, Bouletreau P. Septicémie à *Saccharomyces boulardii* après administration orale d'ultra-levure. Réan Urg 1996; 5:665.

138. Piarroux R, Millon L, Bardonnet K, Vagner O, Koenig H. Are live *Saccharomyces* yeasts harmful to patients? Lancet 1999; 353:1851–1852.

139. Niault M, Thomas F, Prost J, Hojjat Ansari F, Kalfon P. Fungemia due to *Saccharomyces* species in a patient treated with enteral *Saccharomyces boulardii*. CID 1999; 28:930.

140. Kirjavainen PV, Ouwehand AC, Isolauri E, Salminen SJ. The ability of probiotic bacteria to bind to human intestinal mucus. FEMS Microbiol Lett 1998; 167:185–189.

141. Pessi T, Stas Y, Marttinen A, Isolauri E. Probiotics reinforce mucosal degradation of antigens in rats: implications for therapeutic use of probiotics. J Nutr 1998; 128: 2313–2318.

6

Breastfeeding: Current Recommendations and Management Issues

Richard J. Schanler
Baylor College of Medicine, Houston, Texas

1 INTRODUCTION

The Committees on Nutrition of the American Academy of Pediatrics and the Canadian Paediatric Society have strongly recommended breastfeeding for full-term infants (1,2). Human milk is recommended as the exclusive nutrient source for feeding full-term infants during the first 6 months after birth and should be continued, with the addition of solid foods, at least through the first 12 months (1). The recommendation for human milk feeding arises because of its acknowledged benefits with respect to infant nutrition, gastrointestinal function, host defense, and psychological well-being. It is important to note that favorable outcomes of breastfeeding are reported both for infants and mothers. The unique species-specificity of human milk should be considered in any discussion of the merits of breastfeeding. The incidence of breastfeeding in the United States increased during the 1970s and peaked in the mid-1980s. Nationwide figures for 1983 indicated that 62% of women chose to breastfeed their newborns (3). Recent data suggest that rates of initiation and maintenance of breastfeeding are increasing (4). To meet the challenge imposed by this increased awareness, pediatricians must expand their knowledge base to understand the reasons for breastfeeding as well as the potential difficulties that may be encountered, and the solutions to those difficulties (5). This chapter describes the reasons behind the recommendations for the exclusive use of human milk and current management issues in the breastfed infant.

2 MILK COMPOSITION

2.1 Nutritional Aspects

Many of the components in human milk have dual roles, one as a nutrient source or to facilitate nutrient absorption and the other as an enhancer of host defense or gastrointestinal function. The composition of human milk is also remarkable for its variability, as the content of certain nutrients changes during lactation or throughout the day or differs among women (6). This variability in component composition probably adapts the nutrient composition to specifically meet the needs of the infant, while the lack of homogeneity possibly allows better acceptance of new flavors and foods (7). A comparison of the composition of human milk and bovine milk is depicted in Table 1.

2.1.1 Protein (Nitrogen)

In the first few weeks after birth, the total nitrogen content of milk from mothers who deliver premature infants (*preterm milk*) is greater than of milk obtained from women delivering full-term infants (*term milk*) (8–11). Usually, beyond the first few weeks of lactation, the total nitrogen content in both milks declines similarly to approach what we call *mature milk* (10,11). Despite the decline in nitrogen content, the protein status of breastfed infants is normal at 1 year of age (12). Approximately 20% of the total nitrogen is in the form of nonprotein nitrogen-containing compounds, such as free amino acids and urea, in contrast to bovine milk, which has 5% nonprotein nitrogen (13,14). There is debate as to how much these nonprotein nitrogen-containing compounds contribute to nitrogen utilization (15,16). The rate of absorption of nonprotein nitrogen, determined by stable isotope methods, has been estimated at 13 to 43% (15,16).

    The protein quality (proportion of whey and casein proteins) of human milk (30% casein, 70% whey) differs from that in bovine milk (82% casein, 18% whey) (14). The caseins are a group of proteins with low solubility in acid media. Whey proteins remain in solution after acid precipitation. Generally, the soluble proteins in the whey fraction are more easily digested and tend to facilitate more rapid gastric emptying (17). The whey protein fraction provides lower concentrations of phenylalanine, tyrosine, and methionine and higher concentrations of taurine than the casein fraction of milk (18–21). The pattern of amino acids in the plasma of breastfed infants is used as a reference in infant nutrition (22).

TABLE 1 Composition of Mature Human Milk
and Bovine Milk

Component, unit/L	Human milk	Bovine milk
Energy, kcal	680	680
Protein, g	10	33
% Whey/casein	72/28	18/82
Fat, g	39	38
% MCT/LCT	2/98	8/92
Carbohydrate, g	72	47
% Lactose	100	100
Calcium, mg	280	1200
Phosphorus, mg	140	920
Magnesium, mg	35	120
Sodium, mg	180	480
Potassium, mg	525	1570
Chloride, mg	420	1020
Zinc, μg	1200	3500
Copper, μg	250	100
Iron, μg	300	460
Vitamin A, IU	2230	1000
Vitamin D, IU	22	24
Vitamin E, IU	2.3	0.9
Vitamin K, μg	2.1	4.9
Thiamin (vitamin B_1), μg	210	300
Riboflavin (vitamin B_2), μg	350	1750
Pyridoxine (vitamin B_6), μg	93	470
Niacin, mg	1.5	0.8
Biotin, μg	4	35
Pantothenic acid, mg	1.8	3.5
Folic acid, μg	85	50
Vitamin B_{12}, μg	1	4
Ascorbic acid, mg	40	17

Sources: Refs. 47, 59, 125–128.

As such, potentially toxic imbalances in the levels of various amino acids are avoided.

The types of proteins contained in the whey fraction differ between human and bovine milks. The major human whey protein is α-lactalbumin, a protein involved in the mammary gland synthesis of lactose and a nutritional protein for the infant. Lactoferrin, lysozyme, and secretory immunoglobulin A (sIgA) are specific human whey proteins involved in host defense (23–25). Because these host-defense proteins resist proteolytic digestion, they are capable of a first line of defense by lining the gastrointestinal tract. The three host-defense proteins are essentially absent in bovine milk. The major whey protein in bovine milk is β-lactoglobulin (14).

2.1.2 Lipid

The lipid system in human milk, responsible for providing approximately 50% of the calories in the milk, is structured to facilitate superior fat digestion and absorption (26). The lipid system comprises an organized milk fat globule, a pattern of fatty acids (high in palmitic 16:0, oleic 18:1, and the essential fatty acids, linoleic 18:2ω6 and linolenic 18:3ω3) characteristically distributed on the triglyceride molecule (the major fatty acid, 16:0, esterified at the 2 position of the molecule), and bile salt–stimulated lipase (27,28). As the lipase is heat-labile, it is important to recognize that the superior fat absorption from human milk is reported only when unprocessed milk is fed (29). Most manufacturers of infant formulas have attempted to modify their fat blends to mimic the fat absorption in human milk. Thus, the mixture of fatty acids in commercial formulas differs from that in human milk. Generally, to meet the fat absorption from human milk, commercial formulas have a greater quantity of medium-chain fatty acids than human milk.

Of the macronutrients in human milk, fat is the most variable in content (30). The fat content rises slightly throughout lactation, changes over the course of the day, increases within-feed, and varies from mother to mother (6). Some investigators comment that the variability in fat content is related to the degree of breast emptying (31). The interindividual variation tracks through lactation, and although it is not affected by diet, it may be affected by maternal body composition (32,33).

The pattern of fatty acids in human milk is also unique in its composition of very long chain fatty acids. Arachidonic acid (20:4ω6) and docosahexaenoic acid (22:6ω3), derivatives of linoleic and linolenic acids, respectively, are found in human but not bovine milk. Arachidonic and docosahexaenoic acids functionally have been associated with cognition, growth, and vision (34–36).

2.1.3 Carbohydrate

The carbohydrate composition of human milk is important as a nutritional source of lactose, the major carbohydrate in milk, and for the presence of oligosaccharides. Although studies in full-term infants demonstrate a small proportion of unabsorbed lactose in the feces, the presence of lactose is assumed to be a normal physiological effect of feeding human milk (37,38). A softer stool consistency, more nonpathogenic bacterial fecal flora, and improved absorption of minerals have been attributed to the presence of small quantities of unabsorbed lactose from human milk feeding (39). Oligosaccharides are carbohydrate polymers and glycoprotein that are important in the host defense of the infant because their structure mimics specific bacterial antigen receptors (40). By preventing bacterial attachment to the host mucosa, oligosaccharides serve a protective role in the infant (41) (see Chap. 4).

2.1.4 Mineral and Trace Elements

The concentration of calcium and phosphorus in human milk is significantly lower than in bovine milk and infant formula. The content of these macrominerals is relatively constant throughout lactation. The macrominerals in human milk are more bioavailable than those in infant formula because of the manner in which they are packaged. In human milk, the minerals are bound to digestible proteins and also present in complexed and ionized states, which are readily bioavailable (42). Thus, despite differences in mineral intake, bone mineral content of breastfed infants is similar to that of infants fed formula (43).

The concentrations of iron, zinc, and copper decline throughout lactation (44,45). The concentrations of copper and zinc, despite their decline, appear adequate to meet the infant's nutritional needs. The concentration of iron, however, may not meet the infant's needs beyond 6 months of breastfeeding (46). At that time, most authorities agree that an iron supplement is indicated to prevent subsequent iron-deficiency anemia.

2.1.5 Vitamins

Maternal vitamin status may affect the content of vitamins in the milk. Generally, maternal deficiency may result in low concentrations in milk that increase in response to dietary supplementation. This is more common for water-soluble than fat-soluble vitamins. Vitamin K deficiency may be a concern in the breastfed infant. Bacterial flora are responsible for providing adequate vitamin K. The intestinal flora of the breastfed infant make less menaquinone, and the content of vitamin K in human milk is low. Therefore, to meet vitamin K needs, a single dose of vitamin K is given at birth (47).

2.2 Nonnutritional Factors

2.2.1 Nucleotides

Although they can be synthesized endogenously, it appears that exogenous nucleotides may have a role in a variety of metabolic functions (48). Nucleotides, consisting of either a purine (uracil, cytosine, thymine) or pyrimidine (adenine, guanine, hypoxanthine, xanthine) base and a pentose sugar (ribose or deoxyribose), joined by mono-, di-, or triphosphate esters, serve as immediate precursors in the synthesis of RNA and DNA. Nucleotides represent 2 to 5% of the nonprotein nitrogen in human milk (49). Numerous functions have been attributed to dietary nucleotide, including effects on lymphoid, intestinal, and hepatic tissues and on lipid metabolism (48,49). In addition, the growth of bifidobacteria in stool flora is enhanced by exogenous nucleotides (49).

2.2.2 Oligosaccharides

Human milk is unique in its content of complex carbohydrates. Free oligosaccharides and glycoproteins function as inhibitors of bacterial adhesion to epithelial surfaces (40) (see Chap. 5).

2.3 Components Affecting Gastrointestinal Function

Many hormones (cortisol, somatomedin-C, insulin-like growth factors, insulin, thyroid hormone) and growth factors (epidermal growth factor, nerve growth factor) and gastrointestinal mediators (neurotensin, motilin) are present in human milk that may affect gastrointestinal function. Epidermal growth factor (EGF) is a polypeptide that stimulates DNA synthesis, protein synthesis, and cellular proliferation in intestinal cells (50). EGF resists proteolytic digestion and is found in the intestinal lumen in suckling animals. Nerve growth factor may play a role in the innervation of the intestinal tract. The hormonal components in milk may affect intestinal growth and mucosal function. Free amino acids may exert dual roles in infants. Taurine may be trophic for intestinal growth and glutamine may be a fuel for the small intestine (50) (see Chap. 3).

2.4 Components Affecting Host Defense

A variety of heterogeneous agents that possess antimicrobial activity are found in human milk (23,25,41,51). Many of these agents persist throughout lactation and are resistant to the digestive enzymes in the infant's gastrointestinal tract. The antimicrobial activities are generally found at mucosal surfaces, such as the gastrointestinal, respiratory, and urinary tracts.

Specific factors such as lactoferrin, lysozyme, and sIgA comprise the whey fraction of human milk protein, generally resist proteolytic degradation, and line mucosal surfaces preventing microbial attachment and inhibiting microbial activity (23–25,52). Lactoferrin has antimicrobial activity when not conjugated to iron (apolactoferrin). It may function with other host-defense proteins to effect microbial killing. Lysozyme is active against bacteria by cleaving cell walls. SIgA is synthesized by plasma cells against specific antigens. The enteromammary and bronchomammary immune systems summarize the important part of the protective nature of human milk (53,54). In these systems the mother produces sIgA antibody when exposed via either her respiratory or gastrointestinal tract to foreign antigens. The plasma cells traverse the lymphatic system and are secreted at mucosal surfaces, including the mammary gland. Ingestion of milk, therefore, provides the infant with passive sIgA antibody against the offending antigen. The systems are active in infants against a variety of antigens (23,53,54).

The products of lipid hydrolysis, free fatty acids, and monoglycerides may exhibit antimicrobial activity against a variety of pathogens (55). These lipid end products may prevent attachment and infection with viruses and protozoa, such as *Giardia*. The activity of human milk bile salt–stimulated lipase also may affect host defense.

The class of carbohydrates including the oligosaccharides and glucoproteins affects intestinal bacterial flora to facilitate the growth of *Lactobacillus* species. These agents also mimic bacterial epithelial receptors in the respiratory tract and, in doing so, prevent attachment of pathogenic agents to epithelial lining of mucosal surfaces. There are a variety of oligosaccharides and glycoproteins that act as receptor analogues for multiple antimicrobial agents (41,56).

There are specific enzymes in human milk, such as platelet activating factor (PAF)-acetylhydrolase. This enzyme degrades PAF, a potent mediator in the intestinal injury induced during necrotizing enterocolitis (57). The cytokine interleukin-10 also functions as an anti-inflammatory mediator and may have a role in protecting the infant from necrotizing enterocolitis (58).

There are white cells (90% of which are neutrophils and macrophages) in human milk that contribute to the antimicrobial activity through phagocytosis and intracellular killing (24). The lymphocytes in human milk may contribute to cytokine production (T cells) or IgA production (B cells) (24,51).

2.5 Effect of Maternal Nutrition on Milk Composition

Evidence from diverse populations indicates that the capacity to produce milk of sufficient quantity and quality to support the growth of infants is satisfactory even when the mother's dietary supply of nutrients is limited (59). The additional nutritional needs imposed by lactation do not require drastic alterations in diet. Around the world, vastly diverse diets support adequate milk production. On the other hand, a chronically deficient diet resulting in depletion of maternal nutrient stores may adversely affect milk composition. With the exception of extreme dietary deprivation, maternal energy intake seems to have only a weak effect on milk volume (33). Short-term diet restriction to 1500 kcal per day for 1 week did not compromise milk production rates; however, there was some suggestion that diets with less than 1500 kcal per day compromised subsequent milk production (60).

The types of fatty acids in human milk are influenced primarily by the type and proportion of fat in the mother's diet (61). The fraction of milk lipids derived from endogenous fat synthesis within the mammary gland is increased on low-fat diets. A shift in dietary fat from 40 to 10% of total calories caused an increase in the milk content of short-chain saturated fatty acids (62).

In general, the fat-soluble vitamins are susceptible to the vitamin status of the mother and the water-soluble vitamins in milk are more responsive to maternal diet. Maternal vitamin A deficiency is associated with decreased levels of vitamin A in milk (63). Milk vitamin D is directly affected by maternal vitamin D status (64). The vitamin K concentration in human milk is also responsive to supplementation (65). The vegan mother who eats no meat products is at risk of vitamin B_{12} deficiency. Her infant may be at risk for vitamin B_{12} deficiency and may show signs of deficiency before the mother (66).

3   BENEFITS OF BREASTFEEDING FOR THE INFANT

3.1   Body Composition

Although lower concentrations of calcium and phosphorus are observed in human milk compared with formula, measures of bone mineralization are similar between human milk– or formula-fed full-term infants during the first year of life (43,67). Children who were breastfed had nearly one-half the prevalence of obesity as children fed formula, and the prevalence of obesity was inversely related to the dose of human milk received by the infant (68).

3.2   Gastrointestinal Function

Gastric emptying is faster following the feeding of human milk than with commercial bovine formula (17,69). The clinical impression is that large gastric residual volumes are reported less frequently in premature infants fed human milk. Many factors in human milk may stimulate gastrointestinal growth and motility and enhance maturity of the gastrointestinal tract.

3.3   Morbidity

Numerous studies conducted in developing countries delineate the protective effects of breastfeeding. In developing areas, the incidence of gastroenteritis and respiratory disease and overall morbidity and mortality are lower in breastfed infants than infants fed milk substitutes (70,71). In developed countries such as in the United States, breastfed infants have lower rates of diarrhea as well as lower respiratory tract illness, acute and recurrent otitis media, and urinary tract infection (72–74). Not only is the attack rate lower, but the duration and severity of illness appear to be shortened in the breastfed infant (75).

In developed countries, even in higher socioeconomic groups, a reduction is found in the incidence of gastroenteritis (70,76). The incidence of diarrheal disease in infants breastfed for 12 months was half that of formula-fed infants (75). After adjusting for potential confounding variables such as sibling number and day-care attendance, the same differences were observed. Infants who were breastfed for at least 13 weeks were found to have a significantly lower incidence of gastroenteritis (vomiting or diarrhea as a discrete illness lasting 48 hr or more) to 1 year of age than infants who were fed formula from birth (77). These observations were significant even when controlled for confounding variables such as social class, maternal age, and smoking.

Respiratory illnesses are reduced in frequency and/or in duration in breast-fed infants (76–79). The incidence of wheezing is less and, overall, lower respiratory tract infection is decreased (76,79). The incidence of otitis media and recurrent otitis media was reduced in infants breastfed for 4 or more months (80,81). This protective effect was observed even when the data were controlled for confounding variables, such as family history of allergy, family size, use of day care, and smoking. Not only was the incidence of otitis media reduced in infants breastfed for 1 year but the duration of each episode was reduced significantly compared with that in formula-fed infants (75).

A case-controlled study reported that the incidence of urinary tract infection was reduced in breastfed infants when compared with formula-fed infants matched for hospitalization, age, gender, social class, birth order, and smoking status of the mother (82). A mechanism for this protection has been suggested. Oligosaccharide excretion in the urine has been shown to prevent bacterial adhesion to urinary epithelial cells (83). Alternate mechanisms may be suggested because the host-defense proteins, lactoferrin and sIgA, also are excreted in the urine of human milk–fed premature infants (84).

The incidence of sepsis and a variety of neonatal infections is reduced in premature infants receiving human milk (85–88). Premature infants fed human milk have a lower incidence of necrotizing enterocolitis (NEC) if they receive human milk as opposed to commercial formula (86,88,89). The lower incidence of NEC is observed even if the supply of mother's milk is low and formula is used as a supplement. Thus, partial and exclusive use of mother's milk appears to protect the premature infant from this condition. Although the mechanism for the protection from NEC is unclear, the feeding of IgA-IgG preparations appears to reduce its incidence (90). Additional studies suggest that human milk containing PAF-acetylhydrolase as well as interleukin-10 might also reduce the severity of NEC or prevent it (57,58). These data suggest that by lining the gastrointestinal tract with host defense factors, the infant may be protected.

3.4 Chronic Disease in Pediatrics

Perhaps the most intriguing data are those suggesting that specific chronic pediatric disorders have a lower incidence in children who were breastfed as infants. There may be protective effects of breastfeeding against Crohn's disease, lymphoma, specific genotypes of type I juvenile diabetes mellitus, and certain allergic conditions (91–93). There are conflicting data regarding the protection against allergy afforded by breastfeeding (94). In some reports, maternal diet may not have excluded the potentially offending antigens. Breastfeeding appears to be protective against food allergies (25,41). Atopic dermatitis may be lessened in infants whose mothers follow a restricted diet. A lower incidence of atopic conditions is reported in breastfed infants with a family history of atopy (95).

There appears to be a relationship between breastfeeding and the development of type I insulin-dependent diabetes mellitus (IDDM) (93). IDDM was more likely when breastfeeding lasted for less than 3 months and bovine milk proteins were introduced before 4 months (93). Elevated concentrations of specific IgG antibody to bovine serum albumin that cross reacts with β cell–specific surface protein have been identified in children with insulin-dependent diabetes mellitus (96). It is estimated that up to 30% of type I IDDM could be prevented by removing bovine milk from the diet for the first 3 months (93).

3.5 Neurobehavioral Aspects

Maternal-infant bonding is enhanced during breastfeeding. In addition, improved long-term cognitive and motor abilities in full-term infants have been directly correlated with the duration of breastfeeding. Even when adjusted for socioeconomic status and parent education, there were significant increments in a limited set of cognitive test scores at 3, 4, and 5 years that paralleled the duration of breastfeeding (97). Improved long-term cognitive development in premature infants has also been correlated with the receipt of human milk during their hospitalization (98,99). A series of studies have indicated that human milk–fed full-term and premature infants have improved visual function compared with infants not receiving these fatty acids in their diet (34,35,100,101).

4 BENEFITS OF BREASTFEEDING TO THE MOTHER

Recovery from childbirth is accelerated by the action of oxytocin on uterine involution (102). Although breastfeeding should not be considered an entirely reliable means of contraception, it prolongs the period of postpartum anovulation (103). The frequency, intensity, and timing of feeds affect the endocrinological responses modulating ovulatory status (104).

Prolonged breastfeeding may confer some advantage in terms of weight loss (105). Bone demineralization occurs during lactation, with a compensatory remineralization after weaning (106,107). Lactation has been shown to confer a protective effect against osteoporosis and bone fracture in later life (108), but this has not been confirmed in all studies (109).

A protective effect of breastfeeding against breast cancer has been found in a number of studies (110–112). The effects were even greater in premenopausal women who had a cumulative total of 24 months of breastfeeding or who were 20 years of age or younger when they first lactated.

5 MANAGEMENT ISSUES

5.1 Prenatal Considerations

The successful management of lactation begins during pregnancy. The pediatrician should discuss feeding plans along with issues of infant care during a prenatal office visit. This is an ideal time to inquire about choice of infant feeding and to provide information, so that families can make informed choices about the benefits of breastfeeding. Although some studies have shown that infant feeding decisions are made before the third trimester, choices may have been influenced by certain misconceptions or fears held by the expectant mother or father, such as fear of inadequate milk supply because of small breast size, possible loss of sexual breast activity during lactation, cosmetic breast changes as a result of lactation, being a failure at breastfeeding, beliefs that breast milk is ''not rich enough,'' difficulties in learning how to breastfeed, as well as disapproval of the spouse, poor public acceptance, and possible loss of freedom or spontaneity (3). Unfortunately, recent data suggest that only 11% of pediatricians see parents for a prenatal visit (5). Thus, the early obstetric visit must take advantage of the opportunity to discuss and promote breastfeeding.

At the prenatal visit, a medical history describing any breast surgery should be sought and the breasts should be examined to identify potential problems with the nipple, areola, or the breasts themselves. For example, if the nipples are very inverted, the mother may benefit from using a breast shield in the last months of pregnancy to facilitate eversion. Physicians should become familiar with local community breastfeeding resources, including lactation specialists and support groups, and they should encourage parental participation.

5.2 The Early Lactation Experience

The early days of lactation are critical to the establishment of a good milk supply and effective let-down reflex. The Baby Friendly Hospital Initiative outlines 10 steps to ensure breastfeeding success (Table 2). Mother and infant should not be separated unless medically indicated. The mother should be offered the opportunity to nurse her infant as soon after delivery as possible. She should be offered as much assistance as necessary in positioning herself comfortably and facilitating the infant's proper grasp of the breast. Enough of the areola should be in the infant's mouth to permit the tongue to compress the areola overlying the collecting ducts against the hard palate. This will provide a good seal and proper emptying or milking of these ampullae. After suckling at the first breast, the infant is then repositioned on the second breast. The time for suckling should be unrestricted. Infants should be nursed approximately 8 to 12 times every 24 hr until satiety, usually 10 to 15 min at each breast (1). Breastfeeding should continue

TABLE 2   Ten Steps to Successful Breastfeeding

1. Written breastfeeding policy should be available.
2. Health care staff should be trained to implement the policy.
3. Educate pregnant women in prenatal classes and visits.
4. Initiate breastfeeding within 1 hr of birth.
5. Demonstrate how to breastfeed and maintain lactation.
6. Use only breast milk unless medically not indicated.
7. Practice rooming-in 24 hr/day.
8. Encourage breastfeeding on demand.
9. Give no artificial nipples or pacifiers.
10. Facilitate the development of breastfeeding support groups.

Sources: Refs. 129 and 130.

when the infant is wakeful and at least every 2 to 3 hr to stimulate milk production and facilitate bilirubin excretion. A normal infant will be alert and attentive and should root, grasp, and suckle well. It is important to recognize, however, that occasional infants may not demand feed in the first few days and that parents should be instructed to wake them for feedings.

In the first weeks, infants should go no longer than 4 hr between feeding (1). Each feeding should include nursing on both sides to enhance the stimulation of milk production. It is appropriate to alternate the side that is used to initiate the feeding and to equalize the time spent at each breast in a day's feedings. Most mothers who have delivered by cesarean section find that nursing in a semirecumbent position in bed is most comfortable. With a standard pillow on the mother's abdomen and the infant lying on the pillow, the full weight of the infant is not on the mother's incision. After vaginal delivery, many mothers prefer positioning on the side or sitting up.

Families should have access to knowledgeable information on breastfeeding well before the first follow-up visit. They should be encouraged to keep in touch with their physicians if questions arise. In the case of early hospital discharge, signs of hydration and the adequacy of feeding should be monitored by a health care provider knowledgeable in breastfeeding soon after discharge.

The infants should not be given supplements of water, glucose water, or formula unless medically indicated. If the appetite or the sucking response is partially satiated by water or formula, the infant will take less from the breast, causing diminished milk production, which may lead to lactation failure. Water and glucose water supplements may exacerbate hyperbilirubinemia because they prevent adequate milk (calorie) intake and gastrocolic stimulation (113). It must be realized that unconjugated (indirect) bilirubin is not water-soluble, must be eliminated in the feces, and is not excreted in the urine (47). The use of a pacifier in the early weeks should also be avoided, as any need for sucking should be satisfied with breastfeeding.

5.3 Is My Baby Receiving Enough Milk?

Many mothers discontinue breastfeeding from fear that their infants are not receiving enough milk. Newspaper headlines have identified isolated tragedies of breastfeeding due to catastrophic cases of dehydration. Most importantly, the mother as well as the health care provider can be taught simple methods to monitor the hydration status and milk intake of the breastfed infant.

In the first few weeks after birth, an infant is adequately nourished if at least 8 to 12 feedings are received every 24 hr and the infant sleeps contentedly between feedings. The adequacy of milk intake can be assessed daily by counting the number of wet diapers, the number and quantity of stools, and weight gain (avoiding body weight loss $> 7\%$) (114). In the first day, the infant should go no longer than 24 hr without a wet diaper and 24 hr without a stool. On day 3, breastfed infants usually have three or four wet diapers and one or two stools that no longer look like meconium but are beginning to appear yellow. Later in the first week after birth, there should be six pale yellow diapers per day and a yellow stool with each feeding. Later in the month, the stool frequency may diminish to three per day. Maternal fatigue and/or anxiety are important contributors to problems with breastfeeding and should be avoided. Family support is especially helpful in reducing fatigue and anxiety. A simple chart can be used by families or health care providers to assess adequacy of milk intake, but this should not take the place of the physical examination if there are any concerns (Table 3).

TABLE 3 Is My Baby Getting Enough Milk? Record for Breastfed Infants in Their First Week

Day	Hour	Number of feedings	Number of wet diapers	Number of stools	Stool color
1	0–24	8–12	1	1	Meconium
2	24–48	8–12	2	2	Brown
3	48–72	8–12	3	2	Green
4	72–96	8–12	4	3	Yellow
5	96–120	8–12	6	3	Yellow
6	120–144	8–12	6	3–4	Yellow
7	144–168	8–12	6–8	4	Yellow

Source: Adapted from Lisbeth Gabrielski, R.N., B.S.N., I.B.C.L.C. 1994. Revised 4/95. Lactation Support Service, The Children's Hospital, 1056 E. 19th Ave., B535, Denver, CO 80218; telephone: (303) 861-6548.

Early hospital discharge programs (<48 hr after delivery) pose a concern for monitoring the breastfed infant. A knowledgeable health care provider should see the infant between 2 and 4 days of age (1). This first visit should assess the adequacy of hydration, milk intake, and body weight, the presence of jaundice, and the state of the mother (anxiety, concerns). One breastfeeding episode should be observed during this first visit. Telephone contact should be encouraged if questions arise. Families should be made aware of the availability of community, office, and/or hospital lactation resources.

It also is important to recognize "appetite spurts" in the infant. These are characterized by periods of crying and apparent insatiability on the part of the infant, usually occurring at 8 to 12 days, 3 to 4 weeks, 3 months of age, and variable times thereafter. Frequent nursing will increase milk production to meet these changing needs of the infant.

5.4 Breast Changes and Care

Lactogenesis, or the onset of milk secretion, usually occurs on the second to fourth postpartum day and is associated with engorgement or swelling of the breasts. Engorgement can cause the nipple/areola junction to be tense and convex, hence difficult for the infant to grasp correctly. Manual or mechanical (breast pump) expression of milk prior to nursing will soften the areola area and facilitate the infant's latch-on.

Breast engorgement is an uncomfortable and sometimes painful swelling. It is due to increased blood and lymph flow to the breast at the onset of lactogenesis. Poor or infrequent emptying of the breast exacerbates this condition. Fortunately, the condition is easily managed by frequent emptying of the breast through feeding or milk expression by manual or mechanical methods.

The infant's initial grasp and suck of the nipple may cause pain during the first few days of lactation. This sensation is the result of negative pressure on the empty ductules. Sore nipples can be exacerbated by incorrect latch-on or impaired milk let-down. Usually this condition begins during the first few days of feeding and is greatest at the onset of feeding. Once lactation is well established, the tenderness diminishes.

Cracked or fissured nipples are usually the result of improper latch-on, improper disengagement, or the use of abrasive soaps or alcohol on the breast. Treatment of this condition involves keeping the nipples dry and avoidance of soaps and alcohol. Because the glands of Montgomery provide the best of lubrication for the areola and nipple throughout pregnancy, no additional lubricants are needed. Occasional application of milk, which is allowed to dry on the nipple, may assist the healing process. Alternatively, the application of dry heat may improve the healing of cracked or fissured nipples.

Chronically sore nipples, or a burning pain throughout the breast, may be caused by candidal infection. There is often concomitant thrush or fungal diaper rash in the infant. Treatment of both maternal and infant sources of infection with topical antifungal agents, coupled with air-drying of the nipples, is needed.

Localized areas of breast discomfort may be due to plugged ducts. These are focal areas of breast engorgement caused by milk stasis. The condition results from irregular nursing, skipped feedings, and inadequate breast emptying. This condition of localized tenderness and mass in an area of the breast should be differentiated from mastitis. The plugged duct may be a precursor of mastitis. Treatment of a plugged duct involves starting consecutive feedings on the affected side and changing nursing position to facilitate the emptying of different lobes of the breast. Additional relief is provided by gently massaging the affected area during nursing or pumping while applying moist heat. Frequent nursing is recommended.

Mastitis is a cellulitis of the interlobar connective tissue of the breast. Affected women experience pain, swelling, erythema, and fever. Sometimes mothers report that they feel as if they are getting the flu. The infection is usually due to *Staphylococcus aureus* and occasionally to *Streptococcus* species. Predisposing factors to mastitis include cracked nipples, incomplete breast emptying, plugged ducts, and breast trauma.

The treatment for mastitis is antibiotic therapy, which should be instituted promptly and offer coverage against staphylococcal bacteria. The duration of treatment is usually 10 days. Bed rest and analgesics may be necessary. Breastfeeding, however, should not be stopped during therapy, especially because breast emptying may facilitate the healing process. The mother may find it more comfortable to initiate nursing on the unaffected side and then move to the affected breast once let-down has been triggered. Occasionally, let-down becomes difficult. An electric breast pump may help to facilitate milk expression, especially from the affected breast.

5.5 Jaundice in Breastfed Infants

Jaundice due to unconjugated hyperbilirubinemia may be associated with breastfeeding in two circumstances: during the first week and beyond the first week of age (115). In the first week after birth, the entity "jaundice in a breastfed infant," may be related to inadequate milk intake and poor lactation performance. The treatment is aimed at decreasing the enterohepatic recirculation of bilirubin by increasing milk intake through an increase in the frequency of breastfeeding. By increasing the frequency of breastfeeding, the milk supply will increase and jaundice will decline (116). If hyperbilirubinemia is advanced and milk production is low, formula may be given to the infant after each breastfeeding while a manual or mechanical method for milk expression is used by the mother to stimulate milk production. Alternatively, supplemental formula can be fed by other means (e.g., through a tube or cup) during the breastfeeding or soon after. This entity may be avoided by appropriate lactation counseling early after delivery and appropriate follow-up of infants after hospital discharge.

The classic entity "breast milk jaundice" usually begins insidiously and peaks after the first week of age. Despite adequate maternal lactation performance and infant milk intake and growth, the infant remains jaundiced. This entity is thought to be related to one or more factors in human milk or to a combination of specific milk factors and a susceptible recipient infant (117). It is believed that the presence of these factors stimulates the enterohepatic recirculation of bilirubin. In extreme circumstances, usually when the serum bilirubin concentration exceeds 20 mg/dL, the hyperbilirubinemia can be reduced by interrupting breastfeeding for 2 to 4 days. If this course is chosen, the mother must be encouraged to maintain her milk supply with a manual or mechanical method while the infant receives commercial formula. When breastfeeding resumes, the serum bilirubin may rise slightly; but once the cycle is interrupted, the recurrence of jaundice is unlikely. This entity is unrelated to maternal lactation performance. The infants appear healthy and well-nourished.

5.6   Xenobiotics

A number of drugs may be secreted into human milk, but only a few are thought to be contraindications to breastfeeding (118). These include chemotherapeutic agents, radioactive isotopes, drugs of abuse, lithium, ergotamine, and drugs that suppress lactation. In addition, anticonvulsants, antihistamines, sulfa drugs, and salicylates may have effects on some breastfeeding infants. Potential exposures from environmental agents should also be considered. Caffeine may enter milk, but maternal consumption of one or two caffeine-containing beverages per day may not be associated with significant manifestations in the infant. The use of alcohol is controversial. Some studies have indicated that alcohol may affect the infant's behavior adversely. Some changes on developmental tests at 1 year have also been attributed to the maternal ingestion of alcohol. Cigarette smoking may affect milk volume.

Secretion of medications into milk is affected by dose schedule and duration, the feeding pattern of the infant, and the infant's total diet and age. The timing of breastfeeding should avoid peak blood concentrations of selected medications. For some medications, the stage of lactation (age of the infant) will determine the safety of the agent. Sulfa drugs would not be indicated in the first month of lactation but may pose no concern to the infant who is several months of age. The mother should be encouraged to discuss any medication with her physician.

The American Academy of Pediatrics periodically reports on drugs and their compatibility with breastfeeding (118).

5.7 Dietary Supplements for Breastfed Infants

Under usual circumstances, the healthy breastfed full-term infant requires little in the way of vitamin and mineral supplements. The breastfed infant, however, must rely on a vitamin K supplement to normalize the prolonged prothrombin time observed at birth (47). All infants receive sufficient vitamin K at birth. The vitamin D concentration in human milk may be insufficient to prevent rickets, especially in dark-skinned infants receiving little sun exposure (119). These infants may need a vitamin D supplement even if exposed to minimum amounts of sunlight (120). Iron absorption from human milk is excellent, but because the concentration of iron declines during lactation, the breastfed infant requires an iron supplement after 6 months of age (45).

6 CONTRAINDICATIONS TO BREASTFEEDING

There are cases in which breastfeeding is not in the best interests of the infant (1). These include infants with galactosemia, infants of mothers using illicit drugs, infants of mothers with active miliary tuberculosis, and, in the United States, infants born to mothers positive for human immunodeficiency virus.

It is appropriate to recommend breastfeeding to the mother who has mastitis and is undergoing treatment for the condition. Maternal herpes infections localized to the perineal area or the oral mucosa do not pose a risk to the breastfed infant (121). Maternal herpetic lesions localized to the areola, however, do pose a risk, and the infant should not be breastfed while these lesions remain. Cytomegalovirus excretion is common in human milk, the mothers being seropositive for cytomegalovirus (122). In the full-term infant, this is not a concern with respect to breastfeeding. Maternal rubella or maternal rubella immunization does not increase the risk of disease in the breastfed infant (121,123). To date, most authorities recommend breastfeeding for mothers exposed to and infected with the hepatitis viruses. Although mothers with active miliary tuberculosis should not breastfeed, those who are seroconverters or are receiving antituberculosis therapy may breastfeed their infants.

The data for human immunodeficiency virus are a concern (121). Although transplacental transmission may occur in 30% of cases when the mother is seropositive, the data for lactation are less clear. The virus has been isolated from human milk and there are suggestions of transmission of HIV from breastfeeding. There are also reports, however, that human milk protects the recipient infant from HIV. Until more data are accumulated, the guidelines from the Centers for Disease Control and Prevention in Atlanta suggest that mothers who are seropositive for HIV should not breastfeed. The World Health Organization advises that because the transmission of HIV in milk is uncertain, breastfeeding should be encouraged, especially in developing countries. In that recommendation, the risk/benefit ratio of not breastfeeding was greater in developing countries than the risk of transmission of HIV.

Most medications are compatible with breastfeeding. In specific situations where the data indicate an increased risk by taking the medication while breastfeeding, alternative medications should be sought. However, certain medications, such as radioactive isotopes, antimetabolites, and other cancer chemotherapeutic agents, necessitate interruption of breastfeeding for variable periods of time.

7 HOSPITAL LACTATION PROGRAMS

Successful initiation and continuation of breastfeeding results from hospital routines that facilitate this process. The 10 steps of the Baby Friendly Hospital Initiative will ensure successful early lactation in the postpartum unit. In order to accomplish successful breastfeeding, postpartum units must maintain a written policy on breastfeeding that is communicated to the entire staff. All health care staff must be trained in the implementation of this policy. Pregnant women should be informed of the benefits of breastfeeding. Breastfeeding should commence within 1 hr of birth unless medically not indicated. Health care staff must be able to demonstrate appropriate breastfeeding skills to mothers. Infants should be given nothing but breast milk unless medically indicated. There is no reason to supply glucose water or formula to the exclusively breastfed infant who is otherwise healthy. Rooming-in for 24 hr per day should be practiced to allow unrestricted breastfeeding. No pacifiers should be given to the infants, as any need for sucking should be met with breastfeeding. Each hospital should establish breastfeeding support groups or work with organized community support groups so that families have a resource upon leaving the hospital. These 10 steps represent a model program to promote a philosophy of maternal and infant care that advocates breastfeeding in a normal physiologic manner (124).

ACKNOWLEDGMENTS

This study was supported by the National Institute of Child Health and Human Development, Grant No. RO-1-HD-28140, and the General Clinical Research Center, Baylor College of Medicine/Texas Children's Hospital Clinical Research Center, Grant No. MO-1-RR-00188, National Institutes of Health. Partial funding also has been provided from the USDA/ARS under Cooperative Agreement No. 58-6250-6-001. This work is a publication of the USDA/ARS Children's Nutrition Research Center, Department of Pediatrics, Baylor College of Medicine and Texas Children's Hospital, Houston, Texas. The contents of this publication do not necessarily reflect the views or policies of the USDA, nor does mention of trade names, commercial products, or organizations imply endorsement by the U.S. government.

REFERENCES

1. American Academy of Pediatrics, Work Group on Breastfeeding. Breastfeeding and the use of human milk. Pediatrics 1997; 100:1035–1039.
2. Nutrition Committee of the Canadian Paediatric Society, Committee on Nutrition of the American Academy of Pediatrics. Breast-Feeding. Pediatrics 1978; 62:591– 601.
3. Freed GL, Landers S, Schanler RJ. A practical guide to successful breastfeeding management. Am J Dis Child 1991; 145:917–921.
4. Ryan AS. The resurgence of breastfeeding in the United States. Pediatrics 1997; 99:www.pediatrics.org/cgi/content/full/99/4/el2
5. Schanler RJ, O'Connor KG, Lawrence RA. Pediatricans' practices and attitudes regarding breastfeeding promotion. Pediatrics 1999; 103:http://www.pediatrics. org/cgi/content/full/103/3/e35
6. Neville MC, Keller RP, Seacat J, Casey CE, Allen JC, Archer P. Studies on human lactation: I. Within-feed and between-breast variation in selected components of human milk. Am J Clin Nutr 1984; 40:635–646.
7. Mennella JA. Mother's milk: A medium for early flavor experiences. J Hum Lact 1995; 11:39–43.
8. Atkinson SA, Bryan MH, Anderson GH. Human milk: Difference in nitrogen concentration in milk from mothers of term and premature infants. J Pediatr 1978; 93: 67–69.
9. Butte NF, Garza C, Johnson CA, Smith EO, Nichols BL. Longitudinal changes in milk composition of mothers delivering preterm and term infants. Early Hum Dev 1984; 9:153–162.
10. Schanler RJ, Oh W. Composition of breast milk obtained from mothers of premature infants as compared to breast milk obtained from donors. J Pediatr 1980; 96: 679–681.
11. Gross SJ, David RJ, Bauman L, Tomarelli RM. Nutritional composition of milk produced by mothers delivering preterm. J Pediatr 1980; 96:641–644.
12. Dewey KG, Cohen RJ, Rivera LL, Canahuati J, Brown KH. Do exclusively breastfed infants require extra protein? Pediatr Res 1996; 39:303–307.
13. Carlson SE. Human milk nonprotein nitrogen: occurrence and possible functions. In: Barness LA, ed. Advances in Pediatrics. Chicago: Year Book, 1985, pp 43– 70.
14. Hambraeus L. Proprietary milk versus human breast milk in infant feeding: A critical appraisal from the nutritional point of view. Pediatr Clin North Am 1977; 24: 17–35.
15. Heine W, Tiess M, Wutzke KD. 15N tracer investigations of the physiological availability of urea nitrogen in mother's milk. Acta Paediatr Scand 1986; 75:439– 443.

16. Fomon SJ, Bier DM, Matthews DE, Rogers RR, Edwards BB, Ziegler EE, Nelson SE. Bioavailability of dietary urea nitrogen in the breastfed infant. J Pediatr 1988; 113:515–517.

17. Billeaud C, Guillet J, Sandler B. Gastric emptying in infants with or without gastro-oesophageal reflux according to the type of milk. Eur J Clin Nutr 1990; 44:577–583.

18. Rassin DK, Gaull GE, Raiha NCR, Heinonen K. Milk protein quantity and quality in low-birth-weight infants: IV. Effects on tyrosine and phenylalanine in plasma and urine. J Pediatr 1977; 90:356–360.

19. Gaull GE, Rassin DK, Raiha NCR, Heinonen K. Milk protein quantity and quality in low-birthweight infants: III. Effects on sulfur amino acids in plasma and urine. J Pediatr 1977; 90:348–355.

20. Jarvenpaa AL, Raiha NC, Rassin DK. Feeding the low-birth-weight infant: I. Taurine and cholesterol supplementation of formula does not affect growth and metabolism. Pediatrics 1983; 71:171–178.

21. Jarvenpaa AL, Rassin DK, Raiha NCR, Gaull GE. Milk protein quantity and quality in the term infant: II. Effects on acidic and neutral amino acids. Pediatrics 1982; 70:221–230.

22. Picone TA, Benson JD, Moro G, Minoli I, Fulconis F, Rassin DK, Raiha NCR. Growth, serum biochemistries, and amino acids of term infants fed formulas with amino acid and protein concentrations similar to human milk. J Pediatr Gastroenterol Nutr 1989; 9:351–360.

23. Goldman AS, Chheda S, Keeney SE, Schmalsteig FC, Schanler RJ. Immunologic protection of the premature newborn by human milk. Semin Perinatol 1994; 18: 495–501.

24. Lonnerdal B. Biochemistry and physiological function of human milk proteins. Am J Clin Nutr 1985; 42:1299–1317.

25. Hanson LA, Ahlstedt S, Andersson B, Carlsson B, Fallstrom SP, Mallander L, Porras O, Soderstrom T, Svanborg C. Protective factors in milk and the development of the immune system. Pediatrics 1985; 75(suppl):172–176.

26. Jensen RG. The lipids in human milk. Prog Lipid Res 1996; 35:53–92.

27. Hernell O, Blackberg L. Human milk bile salt-stimulated lipase: Functional and molecular aspects. J Pediatr 1994; 125:S56–S61.

28. Jensen RG, Jensen GL. Specialty lipids for infant nutrition: I. Milks and formulas. J Pediatr Gastroenterol Nutr 1992; 15:232–245.

29. Jensen RG, Hagerty MM, McMahon KE. Lipids of human milk and infant formulas: A review. Am J Clin Nutr 1978; 31:990–1016.

30. Butte NF, Garza C, Smith EO. Variability of macronutrient concentrations in human milk. Eur J Clin Nutr 1988; 42:345–349.

31. Daly SE, Di Rosso A, Owens RA, Hartmann PE. Degree of breast emptying explains changes in the fat content, but not fatty acid composition, of human milk. Exp Physiol 1993; 78:741–755.

32. Nommsen LA, Lovelady CA, Heinig MJ, Lonnerdal B, Dewey KG. Determinants of energy, protein, lipid, and lactose concentrations in human milk during the first 12 months of lactation: the DARLING study. Am J Clin Nutr 1991; 53:457–465.

33. Butte NF, Garza C, Stuff JE, Smith EO, Nichols BL. Effect of maternal diet and body composition on lactational performance. Am J Clin Nutr 1984; 39:296–306.

34. Uauy R, Hoffman DR. Essential fatty acid requirements for normal eye and brain development. Semin Perinatol 1991; 15:449–455.

35. Carlson SE, Werkman SH, Rhodes PG, Tolley EA. Visual-acuity development in healthy preterm infants: Effect of marine-oil supplementation. Am J Clin Nutr 1993; 58:35–42.

36. Morley R, Lucas A. Nutrition and cognitive development. Br Med Bull 1997; 53: 123–134.

37. Whyte RK, Homer R, Pennock CA. Faecal excretion of oligosaccharides and other carbohydrates in normal neonates. Arch Dis Child 1978; 53:913–915.

38. MacLean WC, Fink BB. Lactose malabsorption by premature infants: magnitude and clinical significance. J Pediatr 1980; 97:383–388.

39. Ziegler EE, Fomon SJ. Lactose enhances mineral absorption in infancy. J Pediatr Gastroenterol Nutr 1983; 2:288–294.

40. Kunz C, Rudloff S. Bilogical functions of oligosaccharides in human milk. Acta Paediatr 1993; 82:903–912.

41. Hanson LA, Adlerberth I, Carlsson B, Castrignano SB, Dahlgren U, Jalil F, Khan SR, Mellander L, Eden CS, Svennerholm A-M, Wold A. Host defense of the neonate and the intestinal flora. Acta Paediatr Scand Suppl 1989; 351:122–125.

42. Neville MC, Watters CD. Secretion of calcium into milk: A review. J Dairy Sci 1983; 66:371–380.

43. Venkataraman PS, Luhar H, Neylan MJ. Bone mineral metabolism in full-term infants fed human milk, cow milk–based, and soy-based formulas. Am J Dis Child 1992; 146:1302–1305.

44. Casey CE, Hambidge KM, Neville MC. Studies in human lactation: Zinc, copper, manganese, and chromium in human milk in the first month of lactation. Am J Clin Nutr 1985; 41:1193–1200.

45. Dallman PR, Siimes MA, Stekel A. Iron deficiency in infancy and childhood. Am J Clin Nutr 1980; 33:86–118.

46. Lonnerdal B, Hernell O. Iron, zinc, copper and selenium status of breastfed infants and infants fed trace element–fortified milk-based infant formula. Acta Paediatr 1994; 83:367–373.

47. Greer FR, Suttie JW. Vitamin K and the newborn. In: Tsang RC, Nichols BL, eds. Nutrition During Infancy. Philadelphia: Hanley & Belfus, 1988, pp 289–297.

48. Carver JD, Walker WA. The role of nucleotides in human nutrition. Nutr Biochem 1995; 6:58–72.

49. Uauy R, Quan R, Gil A. Role of nucleotides in intestinal development and repair: Implications for infant nutrition. J Nutr 1994; 124:1436S–1441S.

50. Sheard NF, Walker WA. The role of breast milk in the development of the gastrointestinal tract. Nutr Rev 1988; 46:1–8.

51. Goldman AS, Sharpe LW, Goldblum RM. Anti-inflammatory properties of human milk. Acta Paediatr Scand 1986; 75:689–695.

52. Goldman AS, Smith CW. Host resistance factors in human milk. J Pediatr 1973; 82:1082–1090.

53. Kleinman RE, Walker WA. The enteromammary immune system. Dig Dis Sci 1979; 24:876–882.

54. Fishaut M, Murphy D, Neifert M, McIntosh K, Ogra PL. Bronchomammary axis in the immune response to respiratory syncytial virus. J Pediatr 1981; 99:186–191.

55. Isaacs CE, Kashyap S, Heird WC, Thormar H. Antiviral and antibacterial lipids in human milk and infant formula feeds. Arch Dis Child 1990; 65:861–864.

56. Brand-Miller JC, McVeagh P, McNeil Y, Messer M. Digestion of human milk oligosaccharides by healthy infants evaluated by the lactulose hydrogen breath test. J Pediatr 1998; 133:95–98.

57. Caplan MS, Lickerman M, Adler L, Dietsch GN, Yu A. The role of recombinant platelet-activating factor acetylhydrolase in a neonatal rat model of necrotizing enterocolitis. Pediatr Res 1997; 42:779–783.

58. Garofalo R, Chheda S, Mei F, Palkowetz KH, Rudloff HE, Schmalsteig FC, Rassin DK, Goldman AS. Interleukin-10 in human milk. Pediatr Res 1995; 37:444–449.

59. Institute of Medicine, Subcommittee on Nutrition During Lactation. Nutrition During Lactation. Washington, D.C.: National Academy Press, 1991.

60. Strode MA, Dewey KG, Lonnerdal B. Effects of short-term caloric restriction on lactational performance of well-nourished women. Acta Paediatr Scand 1986; 75: 222–229.

61. Jensen RG. The Lipids of Human Milk. Boca Raton, FL: CRC Press, 1989.

62. Hachey DL, Silber GH, Wong WW, Garza C. Human lactation II: Endogenous fatty acid synthesis by the mammary gland. Pediatrics 1989; 25:63–68.

63. Butte NF, Calloway DH. Evaluation of lactational performance of Navajo women. Am J Clin Nutr 1981; 34:2210–2215.

64. Hollis BW, Lambert PW, Horst RL. Factors affecting the antirachitic sterol content of native milk. In: Holick MF, Gray TK, Anast CS, eds. Perinatal Calcium and Phosphorous Metabolism. Amsterdam: Elsevier, 1983, pp 157–182.

65. von Kries R, Shearer M, McCarthy PT, Haug M, Harzer G, Gobel U. Vitamin K_1 content of maternal milk: Influence of the stage of lactation, lipid composition, and vitamin K_1 supplements given to the mother. Pediatr Res 1987; 22:513–517.

66. Higginbottom MC, Sweetman L, Nyhan WL. A syndrome of methylmalonic aciduria, homocystinuria, megaloblastic anemia and neurologic abnormalities in a vitamin B_{12}–deficient breastfed infant of a strict vegetarian. N Engl J Med 1978; 299: 317–323.

67. Greer FR, Searcy JE, Levin RS, Steichen JJ, Steichen-Asche PS, Tsang RC. Bone mineral content and serum 25-OH D concentrations in breastfed infants with and without supplemental vitamin D: One year follow-up. J Pediatr 1982; 100:919–922.

68. von Kries R, Koletzko B, Sauerwald T, von Mutius E, Barnert D, Grunert V, von Voss H. Breast feeding and obesity: Cross sectional study. BMJ 1999; 319:147–150.

69. Van Den Driessche M, Peeters K, Marien P, Ghoos Y, Devlieger H, Veereman-Wauters G. Gastric emptying in formula-fed and breastfed infants measured with the ^{13}C-octanoic acid breath test. J Pediatr Gastroenterol Nutr 1999; 29:46–51.

70. Popkin BM, Adair L, Akin JS, Black R, Briscoe J, Flieger W. Breast-feeding and diarrheal morbidity. Pediatrics 1990; 86:874–882.

71. Glass RI, Stoll BJ. The protective effect of human milk against diarrhea. Acta Paediatr Scand 1989; 351:131–136.

72. Cunningham AS. Morbidity in breastfed and artificially fed infants. J Pediatr 1977; 90:726–729.

73. Cunningham AS. Morbidity in breastfed and artificially fed infants. II. J Pediatr 1979; 95:685–689.
74. Cunningham AS, Jelliffe DB, Jelliffe EFP. Breast-feeding and health in the 1980s: A global epidemiologic review. J Pediatr 1991; 118:659–666.
75. Dewey KG, Heinig MJ, Nommsen-Rivers LA. Differences in morbidity between breastfed and formula-fed infants. J Pediatr 1995; 126:696–702.
76. Kovar MG, Serdula MD, Marks JS, Fraser DW. Review of the epidemiologic evidence for an association between infant feeding and infant health. Pediatrics 1984; 74:S615–S638.
77. Howie PW, Forsyth JS, Ogston SA, Clark A, Florey CV. Protective effect of breastfeeding against infection. BMJ 1990; 300:11–16.
78. Frank AL, Taber LH, Glezen WP, Kasel GL, Wells CR, Paredes A. Breast-feeding and respiratory virus infection. Pediatrics 1982; 70:239–245.
79. Wright AL, Holberg CJ, Martinez FD, Morgan WJ, Taussig LM, Group Health Medical Associates. Breast feeding and lower respiratory tract illness in the first year of life. BMJ 1989; 299:945–948.
80. Rubin DH, Leventhal JM, Krasilnikoff PA, Kuo HS, Jekel JF, Weile B, Levee A, Kurzon M, Berget A. Relationship between infant feeding and infectious illness: A prospective study of infants during the first year of life. Pediatrics 1990; 85: 464–471.
81. Duncan B, Ey J, Holberg CJ, Wright AL, Martinez FD, Taussing LM. Exclusive breastfeeding for at least 4 months protects against otitis media. Pediatrics 1993; 91:867–872.
82. Pisacane A, Graziano L, Mazzarella G, Scarpellino B, Zona G. Breast-feeding and urinary tract infection. J Pediatr 1992; 120:87–89.
83. Coppa GV, Gabrielli O, Giorgi P, Catassi C, Montanari MP, Varaldo PE, Nichols BL. Preliminary study of breastfeeding and bacterial adhesion to uroepithelial cells. Lancet 1990; 335:569–571.
84. Goldblum RM, Schanler RJ, Garza C, Goldman AS. Human milk feeding enhances the urinary excretion of immunologic factors in low birth weight infants. Pediatr Res 1989; 25:184–188.
85. Narayanan I, Prakash K, Gujral VV. The value of human milk in the prevention of infection in the high-risk low-birth-weight infant. J Pediatr 1981; 99:496–498.
86. Schanler RJ, Shulman RJ, Lau C. Feeding strategies for premature infants: Beneficial outcomes of feeding fortified human milk vs preterm formula. Pediatrics 1999; 103:1150–1157.
87. Hylander MA, Strobino DM, Dhanireddy R. Human milk feedings and infection among very low birth weight infants. Pediatrics 1998; http://www.pediatrics.org/cgi/content/full/102/3/e38
88. Contreras-Lemus J, Flores-Huerta S, Cisneros-Silva I, Orozco-Vigueras H, Hernandez-Gutierrez J, Fernandez-Morales J, Chavez-Hernandez F. Disminucion de la morbilidad en neonatos pretermino alimentados con leche de su propia madre. Biol Med Hosp Infant Mex 1992; 49:671–677.
89. Lucas A, Cole TJ. Breast milk and neonatal necrotizing enterocolitis. Lancet 1990; 336:1519–1523.
90. Eibl MM, Wolf HM, Fürnkranz H, Rosenkranz A. Prevention of necrotizing entero-

colitis in low-birth-weight infants by IgA-IgG feeding. N Engl J Med 1988; 319: 1–7.

91. Davis MK, Savitz DA, Graubard BI. Infant feeding and childhood cancer. Lancet 1988; 1:365–368.

92. Koletzko S, Sherman P, Corey M, Griffiths A, Smith C. Role of infant feeding practices in development of Crohn's disease in childhood. BMJ 1989; 298:1617–1618.

93. Gerstein HC. Cow's milk exposure and type I diabetes mellitus. Diabetes Care 1994; 17:13–19.

94. Kramer MS. Does breast feeding help protect against atopic disease? Biology, methodology, and a golden jubilee of controversy. J Pediatr 1988; 112:181–190.

95. Saarinen UM, Backman A, Kajosaari M, Siimes MA. Prolonged breastfeeding as prophylaxis for atopic disease. Lancet 1979; 2:163–166.

96. Karjalainen J, Martin JM, Knip M, Ilonen J, Robinson BH, Savilahti E, Akerblom HK, Dosch HM. A bovine albumin peptide as a possible trigger of insulin-dependent diabetes mellitus. N Engl J Med 1992; 327:302–307.

97. Rogan WJ, Gladen BC. Breast-feeding and cognitive development. Early Hum Dev 1993; 31:181–193.

98. Lucas A, Morley R, Cole TJ, Gore SM. A randomised multicenter study of human milk versus formula and later development in preterm infants. Arch Dis Child 1994; 70:F141–F146.

99. Lucas A, Morley R, Cole TJ, Lister G, Leeson-Payne C. Breast milk and subsequent intelligence quotient in children born preterm. Lancet 1992; 339:261–264.

100. Crawford MA. The role of essential fatty acids in neural development: Implications for perinatal nutrition. Am J Clin Nutr 1993; 57:703S–710S.

101. Anderson GJ, Connor WE, Corliss JD. Docosahexaenoic acid is the preferred dietary n-3 fatty acid for the development of the brain and retina. Pediatr Res 1990; 27:89–97.

102. Riordan J. Anatomy and psychophysiology of lactation. In: Riordan J, Auerbach KG, eds. Breastfeeding and Human Lactation. Boston: Jones and Bartlett, 1993: 81–104.

103. Wang IY, Fraser IS. Reproductive function and contraception in the postpartum period. Obstet Gynecol Surv 1994; 49:56–63.

104. Campbell OM, Gray RH. Characteristics and determinants of postpartum ovarian function in women in the United States. Am J Obstet Gynecol 1993; 169:55–60.

105. Dewey KG, Heinig MJ, Nommsen LA. Maternal weight-loss patterns during prolonged lactation. Am J Clin Nutr 1993; 58:162–166.

106. Specker BL, Tsang RC, Ho ML. Changes in calcium homeostasis over the first year postpartum: Effect of lactation and weaning. Obstet Gynecol 1991; 78:56–62.

107. Sowers MF, Corton G, Shapiro B, Jannausch ML, Crutchfield M, Smith ML, Randolph JF, Hollis B. Changes in bone density with lactation. JAMA 1993; 269:3130–3135.

108. Cumming RG, Klineberg RJ. Breastfeeding and other reproductive factors and the risk of hip fracture in elderly women. Int J Epidemiol 1993; 2:684–691.

109. Bauer DC, Browner WS, Cauley JA, Orwoll ES, Scott JC, Black DM, Tao JL,

Cummings SR. Factors associated with appendicular bone mass in older women. Ann Intern Med 1993; 118:657–665.

110. Yoo K, Tajima K, Kuroishi T, Hirose K, Yoshida M, Miura S, Murai H. Independent protective effect of lactation against breast cancer: A case control study in Japan. Am J Epidemiol 1992; 135:726–733.

111. Newcomb PA, Storer BE, Longnecker MP, Mittendorf R, Greenberg ER, Clapp RW, Burke KP, Willett WC, MacMahon B. Lactation and a reduced risk of premenopausal breast cancer. N Engl J Med 1994; 330:81–87.

112. Furberg H, Newman B, Moorman P, Millikan R. Lactation and breast cancer risk. Int J Epidemiol 1999; 28:396–402.

113. DeCarvalho M, Hall M, Harvey D. Effects of water supplementation on physiological jaundice in breastfed babies. Arch Dis Child 1981; 56:568–569.

114. Neifert MR. Clinical aspects of lactation: promoting breastfeeding success. Clin Perinatol 1999; 26:281–306.

115. Gartner LM, Lee K. Jaundice in the breastfed infant. Clin Perinatol 1999; 26:431–445.

116. DeCarvalho M, Klaus MH, Merkatz RB. Frequency of breastfeeding and serum bilirubin concentration. Am J Dis Child 1982; 136:737–738.

117. Gartner LM, Arias IM. Studies of prolonged neonatal jaundice in the breastfed infant. J Pediatr 1966; 68:54–66.

118. American Academy of Pediatrics, Committee on Drugs. The transfer of drugs and other chemicals into human milk. Pediatrics 1994; 93:137–150.

119. Bachrach S, Fisher J, Parks JS. An outbreak of vitamin D deficiency rickets in a susceptible population. Pediatrics 1979; 64:871–877.

120. Greer FR, Searcy JE, Levin RS, Steichen-Asche JJ, Tsang RC. Bone mineral content and serum 25-hydroxyvitamin D concentration in breastfed infants with and without supplemental vitamin D. J Pediatr 1981; 98:696–701.

121. Ruff AJ. Breastmilk, breastfeeding, and transmission of viruses to the neonate. Semin Perinatol 1994; 18:510–516.

122. Dworsky M, Yow M, Stagno S, Pass RF, Alford C. Cytomegalovirus infection of breast milk and transmission in infancy. Pediatrics 1983; 72:295–299.

123. Krogh V, Duffy C, Wong D, Rosenband M, Riddlesberger KR, Ogra PL. Postpartum immunization with rubella virus vaccine and antibody response in breastfeeding infants. J Lab Clin Med 1989; 113:695–699.

124. Powers NG, Naylor AJ, Wester RA. Hospital policies: Crucial to breastfeeding success. Semin Perinatol 1994; 18:517–524.

125. American Academy of Pediatrics, Committee on Nutrition. Zinc. Pediatrics 1978; 62:408–412.

126. Blanc B. Biochemical aspects of human milk—Comparison with bovine milk. World Rev Nutr Diet 1981; 36:1–89.

127. Dallman PR. Nutritional anemia in infancy: iron, folic acid, and vitamin B_{12}. In: Tsang RC, Nichols BL, eds. Nutrition During Infancy. Philadelphia: Hanley & Belfus, 1988, pp 216–235.

128. Schanler RJ. Water soluble vitamins: C, B_1,B_2,B_6, niacin, biotin, and pantothenic acid. In: Tsang RC, Nichols BL, eds. Nutrition During Infancy. Philadelphia: Hanley & Belfus, 1988, pp 236–252.

129. World Health Organization, UNICEF. Protecting, Promoting, and Supporting Breastfeeding: The Special Role of Maternity Services. Geneva, Switzerland: World Health Organization, 1989.
130. UNICEF. Take the Baby-Friendly Hospital Initiative! A Global Effort with Hospitals, Health Services, and Parents to Breastfeed Babies for the Best Start in Life. New York: UNICEF, 1991.

7

Calcium Intake Requirements of Infants, Children, and Adolescents

Steven A. Abrams
Baylor College of Medicine and USDA/ARS Children's Nutrition
Research Center, Houston, Texas

1 OVERVIEW

Dietary calcium requirements are established for children in order to prevent childhood calcium-deficient disorders (e.g., fractures and rickets) and to help reduce the risk of adult mineral deficiency conditions (e.g., osteoporosis) (1). The goal is to establish intake guidelines that will maximize the bone mass of each child based on his or her genetic potential. In this chapter, the physiological basis for current dietary recommendations (2,3) for calcium are reviewed, including data suggesting that calcium intakes currently achieved by most children are suboptimal.

It is important to note that bone mineralization is significantly affected by factors besides calcium intake. These factors include other dietary constituents, such as sodium; genetic factors, such as ethnicity and gender; exercise; smoking; medication usage; disease processes; and hormonal status. Conversely, calcium may be important for purposes other than bone mineralization, such as preventing hypertension and decreasing the risk of colon cancer (4). The interactions of all these factors make it impossible to identify a single number as the calcium "requirement" of all children. Nonetheless, data are available to establish general guidelines, based on the known physiology of calcium metabolism and recent research regarding the consequences of various calcium intakes on mineral metabolism and health.

2 INTRODUCTION: REGULATION OF CALCIUM ABSORPTION AND METABOLISM

Virtually all (>98%) the calcium in the body is found in the skeleton. Calcium in the serum exists in three fractions: ionized (approximately 50%), protein-bound (approximately 40%), and a small amount that is complexed, primarily to citrate and phosphate ions. Calcium absorption occurs either via a passive, vitamin D–independent route or an active, vitamin D–dependent route (5).

Active transport indicates that the transcellular movement of calcium requires metabolic energy. This process occurs primarily in the upper duodenum. Three steps occur in calcium movement into the circulation. First, calcium enters across the brush border into the intestinal cell down an electrochemical gradient. Subsequently, intracellular diffusion of the calcium ion occurs. This step is rate-limiting and occurs via the vitamin D–dependent cytosolic calcium-binding protein calbindin. In the absence of vitamin D, self-diffusion of calcium within the cell occurs at only a very small fraction of this rate. Finally, calcium is extruded from the intestinal cell against an electrochemical gradient (6).

In contrast, passive, vitamin D–independent absorption of calcium takes place via a paracellular pathway and occurs throughout the length of the small intestine. Although human data are not available, evidence suggests that some absorption via this pathway may also occur in the colon.

The relative proportion of calcium absorbed by these two pathways in the presence of adequate vitamin D is largely dependent on the dietary calcium intake. At low intakes, the active pathway predominates, whereas at high intakes, this pathway is downregulated and most calcium absorption is passive. The exact distribution of calcium absorbed by each of these pathways in children of different ages is unknown. However, in premature infants and possibly during the neonatal period in full-term infants, transcellular absorption is not yet activated and, regardless of intake, calcium absorption occurs predominantly via the passive route (7).

3 CALCIUM EXCRETION

There are three primary methods by which absorbed calcium can be lost from the body: first, secretion into the GI tract and subsequent excretion (referred to as *endogenous fecal excretion*); second, urinary excretion; and third, glandular, especially sweat, losses. Although minimal data regarding regulation of calcium excretion specific to children are available, some information may be extrapolated from animal data or adult human studies.

Endogenous fecal calcium excretion increases at higher calcium intakes in older children and adults. It is markedly higher in premature infants than in older children and adults. It is not, however, a primary site of calcium metabolic regulation (8).

In children, urinary calcium excretion is significantly related to calcium intake, but this correlation is not as close as in adults. This is because of the rapid utilization of absorbed calcium for bone mineralization. There is a close relationship between dietary calcium and urinary sodium and calcium excretion in children, similar to that found in adults (9,10). Urinary calcium excretion in children usually totals between 1 and 4 mg/kg/day, although higher levels are commonly seen, especially in premature infants (8).

There are virtually no data on sweat losses of calcium in children. These may be substantial in adults and of comparable magnitude to urinary or endogenous fecal losses during periods of exercise (3).

4 IDENTIFICATION OF MINERAL REQUIREMENTS DURING CHILDHOOD

Identifying an endpoint goal is the first step in establishing a nutrient intake requirement. In adults, fracture risk is frequently identified as the ultimate endpoint for calcium intake, with closely related surrogates, such as regional (e.g., spinal) bone mass or density being assessed. In children, comparable endpoints are less readily identified. For example, based on current knowledge, it is impossible to reliably predict the risk of postmenopausal osteoporosis based on information obtained during childhood. Instead, most research efforts have been based on identifying those factors that lead to a maximum peak bone mass in children. Available evidence has linked peak bone mass to the ultimate adult risk of osteoporosis, although further supporting research is needed (1). The nature of this hypothesized relationship is shown in Figure 1.

Although a direct relationship between low calcium intake and clinical symptoms is not usually identified in healthy children, it is recognized that a very low calcium intake can contribute to the development of rickets in infants and children. This is usually seen in children receiving very restrictive diets (e.g., a macrobiotic diet) (11). This risk may be present even if vitamin D status is adequate, as there is a maximum ability to adapt absorption to extremely low intakes. There are no reliable data on the lowest calcium intake needed to prevent rickets or on the relationships between ethnicity, vitamin D status, physical activity, and diet in the causation of rickets in children fed low-calcium diets. It is likely that

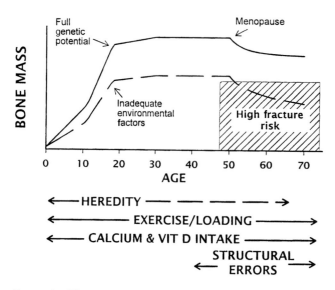

FIGURE 1   Diagrammatic representation of the bone mass lifeline in individuals who achieve their full genetic potential for skeletal mass and in those who do not (the magnitude of the difference between the curves is not intended to be to scale). Along the bottom of the graph are arrayed several of the factors known to be of particular importance. (Copyright Robert P. Heaney, 1999.)

intakes below 200 to 300 mg/day, especially if combined with a low or marginal vitamin D intake or limited sunshine exposure, may place toddlers and preschool children at risk for rickets.

In addition, a low bone mass may be a contributing factor to some fractures in otherwise healthy children. Lower bone mass at multiple sites was reported in a group of girls with distal forearm fractures compared with a healthy age-matched group (12). However, further data on the relationship between calcium intake and fractures are needed before it is possible to assess the magnitude of increased fracture risk at different calcium intake levels. In children with chronic illnesses, fractures may occur during childhood secondary to mineral deficiency associated with either the disease process or the effects of therapeutic interventions (i.e., corticosteroids) on calcium metabolism.

4.1   Methodologies to Assess Calcium Status

Multiple approaches are utilized to assess the calcium status of children (Table 1). Measuring calcium balance is the approach most commonly used to estimate

TABLE 1 Methods for Assessing Calcium and Bone Mineral
Status in Individuals

Method	Comment
Serum calcium	Not a reliable marker of whole-body calcium status
Serum alkaline phosphatase activity	May be increased during normal growth and by other conditions
Serum 25-hydroxyvitamin D	Lower in African-American and Hispanic children
Bone mineral content	Clinical standards not always available in children
	Still primarily a research tool, especially in small children
Metabolic balance studies	Research technique, difficult to perform in children
Stable isotope studies	Research technique, useful to establish dietary interrelationships
Bone biopsy	Definitive technique for establishing rickets; not appropriate for pediatric use
Skeletal x-rays	Used to establish rickets; not reliable for less severe bone loss

the requirement for the mineral. Its utility is based on the rationale that virtually all retained calcium must be utilized, especially by children, to enhance bone growth and mineralization. Therefore, the dietary calcium intake leading to the greatest calcium retention will lead to the greatest long-term benefit (13,14).

Unfortunately, significant limitations affect the collection and interpretation of calcium-balance data. These include substantial technical problems measuring calcium excretion and the difficulty of controlling the dietary intake of children. Both of these are necessary for adequate balance studies. These problems have been partly overcome in recent years by the development of stable-isotope methods to assess calcium absorption and excretion (15). Nonetheless, more data are needed to establish both the ''optimal'' level of calcium retention at different ages and the effects of development on calcium balance (3).

A significant advance in the field over the last 25 years has been the development and improvement of methods to measure both total-body and regional bone mineral content using various bone-density techniques. The technique currently utilized in many studies of children is dual-energy x-ray absorptiometry (DXA). This technique can rapidly measure the bone mineral content and bone mineral density of the entire skeleton or of regional sites with a virtually negligible level of radiation exposure. Furthermore, recent enhancements in the precision of the technique have made it particularly suitable for assessing the effects of calcium supplementation on bone mass in children of all ages (16).

Numerous studies have directly assessed the effects of calcium supplementation on bone mass using DXA or similar techniques (17,18). These studies, however, also have limitations. First, most supplementation studies done in children have involved a relatively short-term supplementation period, such as 12 months. This time period may be inadequate to fully assess the long-term benefits of calcium supplements on bone mineral density. The second limitation is that these studies generally have been done using only one level of supplementation, which frequently has been given in pill form. This limited-dosing approach makes it difficult to identify an optimal intake level or determine the relative benefits of dietary calcium versus supplements as a method of increasing calcium intake in children.

Several investigators have performed population-based epidemiological studies relating childhood or adult bone mass or fracture risk to calcium intake in childhood. Although many of these studies are limited by their retrospective design, they have generally shown a positive association between calcium intake in childhood and childhood and adult bone mass. Not all studies have shown a benefit, however, and further data regarding this relationship are needed (3,19).

5   RECOMMENDATIONS BY AGE GROUP

5.1   Overview

In 1997, the Food and Nutrition Board of the Institute of Medicine of the National Academy of Sciences released new dietary guidelines for calcium intake for healthy infants, children, and adults (3). A summary of these recommendations is shown in Table 2. Descriptions of these recommendations are provided below, based on age groups.

5.2   Full-Term Infants

It is possible to provide enough calcium in infant formulas that the calcium absorbed by the formula-fed infant exceeds the amount of calcium absorbed by the infants fed human milk; however, there is no evidence that this is beneficial. Long-term studies to determine the effects of different infant calcium intakes on peak bone mass have not been performed. These are very unlikely to be conducted in the near future owing to the long follow-up time needed for such studies.

The bioavailability of calcium from human milk is greater than that from infant formulas or cow's milk, although this comparison generally has not been made at intake concentrations similar to those of human milk (20). Nonetheless,

TABLE 2 Dietary Calcium Intake
(mg/day) Recommendations in the
United States[a,b]

0 to 6 months[b]	210
6 months–1 year[b]	270
1 through 3 years	500
4 through 8 years	800
9 through 18 years	1300

[a] The Food and Nutrition Board of the
National Academy of Sciences (NAS)
released new mineral recommended
dietary allowances (RDAs) in 1997. For
calcium, the board chose to use the term
adequate intake for its calcium intake recommendations but indicated that these
values were to be used as RDAs. NAS's
dietary recommendations are set to meet
the needs of 95% of the identified population of healthy subjects.
[b] For infant values, previous RDAs indicated values for formula-fed infants,
whereas the 1997 NAS report uses the human milk–fed infant as the standard by
which recommendations are made. It is
recognized that greater calcium intakes
should be provided to formula-fed infants
based on the possibility of lower bioavailability of calcium from formula relative to
that of human milk.
Sources: Refs. 2, 3, and 41.

it has been deemed prudent to increase the concentration of calcium in all infant
formulas relative to human milk to assure comparable levels of calcium retention.

Relatively greater calcium concentrations are found in specialized formulas
such as soy formulas and casein hydrolysates to account for the potentially lower
bioavailability of the calcium in these formulas relative to that of cow's milk–
based formula. Specific concentration requirements cannot readily be set, but
optimally, all formulas marketed should ensure a total dietary calcium absorption
that has been shown to be comparable to that of human milk.

Lactose may enhance the absorption of calcium in both infants and older
children. Data are sparse regarding lactose-free infant formulas, which utilize
cow's milk protein. It would be reasonable to increase the calcium intake in

lactose-free formulas relative to that of lactose-containing formulas, but the percentage increase needed is unknown.

5.3 Premature Infants

Osteopenia of prematurity is a condition in which the bone mineralization of a premature infant is significantly decreased relative to the expected level of mineralization of a fetus or infant of comparable size or gestational age. It may occur in as many as half of all infants weighing less than 1000 g at birth who are fed either unfortified human milk or formulas designed for full-term rather than preterm infants. The term *osteopenia of prematurity* is used in place of the older term, *rickets of prematurity*, to identify infants who have evidence of decreased bone mineralization without the presence of the classic radiological signs of rickets (21).

To prevent osteopenia of prematurity, infants of less than approximately 1800 g birth weight are usually fed either human milk fortified with additional calcium and phosphorus or formulas specially designed for premature infants that have very high mineral levels (22). The use of these approaches has markedly reduced the frequency with which rickets is identified in premature infants. However, special cases occur, especially in premature infants requiring prolonged parenteral nutrition (Fig. 2).

A major unresolved question at present is whether it is beneficial to continue supplemental calcium and phosphorus after the preterm infant is discharged. If energy and/or mineral intakes higher than those provided by routine formula are desired postdischarge, several means are available: first, concentrating a "routine" formula (i.e., by adding less water to the powdered formula); second, using a preterm formula; or third, using a formula that is specially designed for postdischarge use by preterm infants. Such formulas usually provide nutrients about the mean of those in routine (full-term) and preterm formulas. No data are available that directly compare the benefits and potential risks of these options. Mineral bioavailability studies as well as long-term growth and development studies may be required before these issues can be resolved. At present, the routine use of special formulas after hospital discharge cannot be recommended for all preterm infants.

A special disclosure situation to consider is the very low birth weight (VLBW) infant (especially less than 1200 g birth weight) whose mother intends to breast-feed exclusively. Although most VLBW infants will do very well under this circumstance, it is reasonable to assess these infants for evidence of mineral deficiency at some point, perhaps 4 to 8 weeks after discharge. This assessment might include a physical examination and measurement of serum phosphorus and alkaline phosphatase activity. If evidence of significant abnormality exists, an x-ray of the wrist may be obtained; depending on the findings of these evalua-

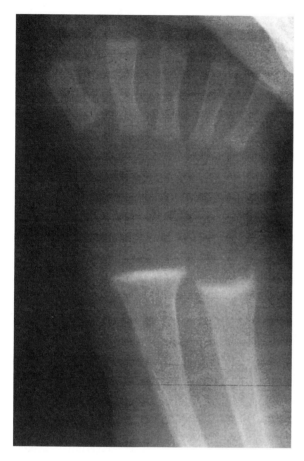

FIGURE 2   Rickets in a premature infant weighing less than 1000 g at birth who required prolonged parenteral nutrition due to bowel surgery.

tions, the provision of supplemental minerals may be considered. Supplemental minerals can be given by adding a small number of daily feedings of a high-mineral formula using a bottle or specialized infant feeding device. If the mother is giving the infant breast milk via a bottle, powdered formula can be added to the milk prior to feeding, although use of this approach postdischarge has not been evaluated in a controlled trial. In circumstances where supplemental formula is not feasible or desired (i.e., severe allergy to cow's milk protein), direct mineral supplementation of both calcium and phosphorus (and possibly zinc) may be advisable, with careful follow-up of growth and bone mineralization.

5.4 Toddlers and Small Children

Few data are available regarding the calcium requirements of children prior to puberty. Calcium retention is relatively low in toddlers and slowly increases as puberty approaches. Most available data indicate that calcium intake levels of about 500 mg/day in small children (ages 1 to 3 years) and 800 mg/day for older children (ages 4 to 8 years) are associated with adequate bone mineral accumulation at prepubescence. The benefits of greater levels of intake in this age group are unknown, although a recent study has suggested that intakes as low as 500 mg/day may not lead to maximal levels of calcium absorption by preschool children (23).

One study found a benefit to calcium supplements to children as young as 6 years of age (18). However, further supporting data are needed for this finding. Perhaps of most importance in this age group is the development of eating patterns that will be associated with adequate calcium intake later in life.

High levels of calcium intake may negatively affect other minerals, especially iron. As these minerals are important for growth and development, and may be marginal in toddlers and preschool children, more data regarding the risks and benefits of high calcium intake are needed.

5.5 Preadolescents and Adolescents

There is a rapid escalation in the rate of bone calcification and growth during adolescence (Fig. 3) (24). The efficiency of calcium absorption increases during puberty, and the majority of bone formation occurs during this time period. Data from balance studies suggest that, for most healthy children in this age range, the maximal net calcium balance (plateau) is achieved with intakes between 1200 and 1500 mg/day (3,14,15). That is, at intake levels above this, nearly all of the additional calcium is excreted and not utilized. It should be noted that virtually all the data used to establish this intake level are from Caucasian children. There are few comparable data for other ethnic groups.

Several controlled trials have found an increase in bone mineral content in adolescents who have received calcium supplementation (17,18). However, available data suggest that if calcium is supplemented for only relatively short time periods (1 to 2 years), there may not be long-term benefits to establishing and maintaining a maximum peak bone mass (25). This emphasizes the importance of diet in achieving adequate calcium intake, and in establishing dietary patterns consistent with a calcium intake near recommended levels throughout childhood and adolescence. Unfortunately, long-term studies evaluating the consequences of maintaining currently recommended calcium intakes beginning in childhood or early adolescence are not presently available. Most available epidemiological data support the view that maintaining such a diet will increase peak bone mass and lower fracture incidence (2,3).

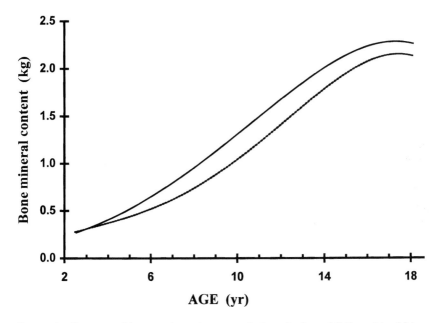

FIGURE 3   Pattern of bone mineral accumulation during childhood in African Americans (top curve) and non-Hispanic Caucasians (lower curve).

5.6   Pregnancy and Lactation

At birth, the fetus contains approximately 30 g of calcium. This represents approximately 2.5% of typical maternal body calcium stores (20). In a pregnant young adolescent, who has not achieved peak bone mass, this percentage may be somewhat higher. In a pregnant adult female, much of this 30 g comes from increases in dietary calcium absorption during pregnancy (26). Specific studies have not been performed to identify the ability of adolescents to increase calcium absorption during pregnancy. A period of 6 months of exclusive breast-feeding would lead to the secretion of an additional 45 g of calcium by the mother. Although some of this is accounted for by decreased urinary calcium excretion, there is extensive evidence demonstrating a loss of maternal bone calcium during lactation. In adults, however, bone remineralization occurs after weaning, and neither pregnancy nor lactation is associated with persistent bone gain or loss. Calcium supplementation during lactation does not significantly alter lactation-associated bone loss or enhance post-weaning bone mass recovery (27). Therefore the revised dietary recommendations do not increase the suggested calcium intake for healthy adult women who are pregnant or lactating above the 1000 mg/day, the amount recommended for nonlactating adult women. Similarly, the recommendations do not suggest increased intake of calcium for pregnant or lactating adolescents above the age-appropriate maximum for adolescents (1300 mg/day) (3). However, it should be noted that these recommended intake levels are substantially above those typical of the diet of most adolescents.

It is not clear whether the continuation of bone formation, especially in younger adolescents (i.e., less than 16 years of age), will lead to a competition between mother and baby and a loss of maternal peak bone mass. As rates of bone formation greatly diminish within 2 to 3 years of menarche, it seems less likely that excessive or unrecoverable bone loss occurs in lactating adolescents. The available evidence supports the position that the benefits of breast-feeding greatly outweigh any demonstrated risk to adolescents in terms of achieving either optimal growth or peak bone mass. Further studies are necessary to consider the impact of pregnancy and lactation on maternal bone mass in adolescent mothers.

Women who are nursing more than one child or women with closely spaced pregnancies may be at increased risk for bone loss during lactation. With regard to women nursing multiple infants, it is noteworthy that some lactating women can have very high levels of milk output that completely support the milk needs of twins or triplets. Daily human milk volumes of 1 to 2 liters or more are possible. It is likely that the secretion into milk of, for example, 400 to 600 mg/day of calcium would lead to greater loss of maternal bone mass than the 200 to 250 mg/day associated with nursing one child. However, there are no trials of calcium supplementation in women who are providing milk for more than one infant.

6 METHODS FOR INCREASING CALCIUM INTAKE IN CHILDREN

6.1 Dietary Interventions

There is a large gap between recommended calcium intakes and typical intakes of children, especially those 9 to 18 years of age. The vast majority of adolescents, especially females, have calcium intakes below the recommended levels. Mean calcium intakes in older children and adolescents are approximately 700 to 1000 mg/day, with values at the higher end of this range occurring in males (3). Preoccupation with being thin is common in this age group, especially among females, as is the misconception that all dairy foods are fattening. Many children and adolescents are unaware that low-fat milk has at least as much calcium as whole milk.

Knowledge of dietary calcium sources is a first step toward increasing intake of calcium-rich foods. Although milk and other dairy products are the primary sources of calcium in the American diet, additional sources of calcium are important in achieving adequate calcium intakes. Most vegetables contain calcium, although at low density; therefore, relatively large servings are needed to equal the total intake achieved with typical servings of dairy products. The bioavailability of calcium from vegetables is generally high. An exception is spinach, which is high in oxalate, making the calcium virtually nonbioavailable (28).

Recently, several calcium-fortified products have been introduced. These products, most notably orange juice and similar beverages, are fortified to achieve a calcium concentration similar to that of milk. It is likely that more such products will soon become available. Breakfast foods also are frequently fortified with calcium. However, this practice is not consistent, and families must read the food label to determine if the food is calcium-fortified. Calcium intakes on food labels are indicated as a percentage of the ''daily value'' in each serving. This daily value is currently set as 1000 mg/day.

6.2 Lactose Intolerance and Calcium Intake

Many children with lactose intolerance can drink small amounts of milk without discomfort (see Chaps. 14 and 22). Alternatives include the use of other dairy products, such as solid cheeses and yogurt, which may be better tolerated than milk. Lactose-free and low-lactose milks are available, as are tablets to facilitate lactose digestion. Increasing intake of nondairy products such as vegetables may be helpful, as well as the calcium-supplemented foods.

These measures alone, however, are not likely to achieve the recommended calcium intake of 1300 g/day in 9- to 18-year-old children. Other strategies will have to be used. Besides asking questions about the use of fortified foods discussed above, many families will inquire about providing mineral supplements for lactose-intolerant children. No absolute answer can be given, but a few principles should be considered.

First, when a calcium supplement is given, it provides only one nutrient. Optimal calcium utilization requires an adequate supply of other minerals, including phosphorus and magnesium, and vitamin D. Furthermore, calcium tablets do not provide the other nutrients contained in food and needed for optimal growth. Finally, supplements vary in their bioavailability, and the tolerance of each child to the supplements also varies. Ultimately, although supplements are useful when other sources of calcium are inadequate, decisions regarding their use must be made on an individual basis, keeping in mind the usual dietary habits of the subject, individual risk factors for osteoporosis, and the likelihood that supplementation usage will be maintained.

6.3 Children with Chronic Illnesses

Many chronic illnesses in children have been associated with decreased bone mineralization and fractures. The relationship between delayed growth and pubertal maturation frequently associated with chronic illnesses and slower bone growth has not always been clarified. It remains uncertain, for example, what the appropriate "normal" total-body bone calcium content is in a 10-year-old child with cerebral palsy whose growth is severely delayed. Ultimately, however, it is likely that many children with chronic disorders will survive to old age, and the possibility that their lives will be affected by inadequate bone mineralization during childhood is of concern. To appreciate the complex interactions among genetics, an individual medical disorder and its therapy, and growth failure, it is of value to examine a specific example. In this case, a brief review is presented below of the evidence related to calcium requirements in children with juvenile rheumatoid arthritis (JRA) as an example of a chronic disorder possibly associated with decreased bone mineralization.

6.4 Bone Loss in Children with Juvenile Rheumatoid Arthritis

There are multiple etiologies of bone loss in children with JRA. These include the effects of the medications used for its treatment; the systemic inflammation associated with the disease; the immobility due to decreased physical activity associated with the disease process; and the poor dietary mineral intake (29). The situation is further complicated by the fact that medications such as corticosteroids may decrease the inflammation but also subject the child to bone loss. Nonetheless, there is a general consensus that maximal peak bone mass, especially at cortical sites, is impaired in children with JRA, and that this impairment is positively correlated to disease severity.

A frequent question regarding the treatment of children with JRA and those with similar disorders is whether increasing calcium intake will ameliorate the bone loss. In children with JRA, bone mineral content is positively correlated to both physical activity and calcium intake. There is a trend toward decreased calcium absorption in children with JRA; however, it is unlikely that high-dose calcium can have a large impact (30). On the other hand, it is also likely that the combination of suboptimal calcium intake with an inflammatory disease is particularly harmful. It is rational to maintain calcium and vitamin D intake in children with JRA and other chronic disorders at least at the level of the dietary guidelines. This approach has been successful in small trials of children with rheumatic disorders. There is no evidence, however, of any beneficial effect of very high levels of calcium intake.

7 CONCLUSIONS

Recent studies and dietary recommendations have emphasized the importance of adequate calcium nutriture in children, especially those who are undergoing the rapid growth and bone mineralization associated with pubertal development. Current dietary intake of calcium by children and adolescents is well below recommended optimal levels. Available data support recent recommendations for calcium intakes of 1300 mg/day, beginning in the preteen years and continuing throughout adolescence, as recommended by the National Academy of Sciences. At the present time, there is inadequate evidence to alter dietary recommendations for children with chronic illnesses or those taking medications such as steroids, which alter bone metabolism. However, an effort should be made to achieve at least the recommended intake levels in these children.

REFERENCES

1. Matkovic V, Ilich J. Calcium requirements for growth: Are current recommendations adequate? Nutr Rev 1993; 51:171–180.
2. National Institute of Health Consensus Conference. Optimal calcium intake. JAMA 1994; 272:1942–1948.
3. Institute of Medicine, Food and Nutrition Board. Dietary Reference Intakes for Calcium, Phosphorus, Magnesium, Vitamin D, and Fluoride. Washington, DC: National Academy Press, 1997.
4. Gillman MW, Ellison RC. Childhood prevention of essential hypertension. Pediatr Clin North Am 1993; 40:179–194.
5. Wasserman RH, Fullmer CS. Vitamin D and intestinal calcium transport: Facts, speculations and hypothesis. J Nutr 1995; 125:1971S–1979S.
6. Bronner F, Pansu D. Nutritional aspects of calcium absorption. J Nutr 1999; 129: 9–12.
7. Bronner F, Salle BL, Putet G, Rigo J, Senterrre J. Net calcium absorption in premature infants: Results of 103 metabolic balance studies. Am J Clin Nutr 1992; 56: 1037–1044.
8. Abrams SA, Schanler RJ, Yergey AL, Vieira NE, Bronner F. Compartmental analysis of calcium metabolism in very low birth weight infants. Pediatr Res 1994; 36: 424–428.
9. Bronner F, Abrams SA. Development and regulation of calcium metabolism in healthy girls. J Nutr 1998; 128:1474–1480.
10. O'Brien KO, Abrams SA, Stuff JE, Liang LK, Welch TR. Predictors of urinary calcium excretion in children. J Pediatr Gastroenterol Nutr 1996; 23:8–12.
11. Dagnelie PC, Vergote F, Staveren WA, van den Berg H, Dingjan P, Hautvast J. High prevalence of rickets in infants on macro-biotic diets. Am J Clin Nutr 1990; 51:202–208.
12. Goulding A, Cannan R, Williams SM, Gold EJ, Taylor RW, Lewis-Barned NJ. Bone mineral density in girls with forearm fractures. J Bone Min Res 1998; 13:143–148.
13. Jackman LA, Millane SS, Martin BR, Wood OB, McCabe GP, Peacock M, Weaver CM. Calcium retention in relation to calcium intake and postmenarcheal age in adolescent females. Am J Clin Nutr 1997; 66:327–333.
14. Matkovic V, Heaney, RP. Calcium balance during human growth: evidence for threshold behavior. Am J Clin Nutr 1992; 55:992–996.
15. Abrams SA, Stuff JE. Calcium metabolism in girls: current dietary intakes lead to

low rates of calcium absorption and retention during puberty. Am J Clin Nutr 1994; 60:739–743.

16. Ellis KJ, Abrams SA, Wong WW. Body composition in a young multiethnic female population. Am J Clin Nutr 1997; 65:724–731.

17. Lloyd T, Andon MB, Rollings N, Martel JK, Landis JR, Demers LM, Eggli DF, Kieselhorst K, Kulin HE. Calcium supplementation and bone mineral density in adolescent girls. JAMA 1993; 270:841–844.

18. Johnston CC, Miller JZ, Slemenda CW, Reister TK, Hui S, Christian JC, Peacock M. Calcium supplementation and increases in bone mineral density in children. N Engl J Med 1992; 327:82–87.

19. Matkovic V, Kostial K, Simonovic I, Buzina R, Brodarec A, Nordin BEC. Bone status and fracture rates in two regions of Yugoslavia. Am J Clin Nutr 1979; 32: 540–549.

20. Fomon SJ, Nelson SE. Calcium, phosphorus, magnesium, and sulfur. In: Fomon SJ, ed. Nutrition of normal infants. St. Louis: Mosby–Year Book, 1993, pp 192–218.

21. Steichen J, Gratton T, Tsang R. Osteopenia of prematurity: The cause and possible treatment. J Pediatr 1980; 96:528–534.

22. Schanler RJ, Abrams SA. Can we meet intrauterine macromineral accretion rate postnatally in low birth weight infants fed fortified human milk? J Pediatr 1995; 126:441–447.

23. Ames SK, Gorham BM, Abrams SA. Effects of high vs low calcium intake on calcium absorption and red blood cell iron incorporation by small children Am J Clin Nutr 1999; 70:44–48.

24. Ellis KJ, Abrams SA, Wong WW. Body composition in a young multiethnic female population. Am J Clin Nutr 1997; 65:724–731.

25. Lee WTK, Leung SSF, Leung DMY, Cheng JCY. A follow-up study on the effects of calcium-supplement withdrawal and puberty on bone acquisition of children. Am J Clin Nutr 1996; 64:71–77.

26. Heaney RP, Skillman TG, Calcium metabolism in normal human pregnancy. J Clin Endocrinol Metab 1971; 33:661–670.

27. Abrams SA. Bone turnover during lactation—Can calcium supplementation make a difference? J Clin Endocrinol Metab 1998; 43:1056–1058.

28. Weaver CM. Calcium bioavailability and its relation to osteoporosis. Proc Soc Exp Biol Med 1992; 200:157–160.

29. Cassidy JT, Hillman LS. Abnormalities in skeletal growth in children with juvenile rheumatoid arthritis. Pediatr Rheum 1997; 23:499–522.

30. Abrams SA, Lipnick RN, Vieira NE, Stuff J, Yergey AL. Calcium absorption in children with juvenile rheumatoid arthritis assessed using stable isotopes. J Rheumatol 1993; 20:1196–1200.

8

Feeding Strategies of the Premature/Sick Infant

Josef Neu
University of Florida College of Medicine, Gainesville, Florida

1 INTRODUCTION

Advances in mechanical ventilation, the use of pulmonary surfactants, improved pharmacological management of expectant mothers and preterm infants, and greater confidence in our overall intensive care techniques have resulted in a marked increase in the number of very immature infants who survive. The same ethical controversies surrounding whether or not to resuscitate 26- to 28-week gestation prematures 20 years ago are now focused on 22- to 24-week preemies. Those involved with the care of these survivors are faced with a constellation of problems that include prevention of morbidity and fulfillment of genetic potential. Nutrition is becoming a key factor not only for the growth of these infants during their stay in the neonatal intensive care unit (NICU) but also for their lifelong well-being. Much of what we know about nutrition of low–birth weight infants stems from studies done on growth during fetal development and in large preterm (>1250 g) infants who are not critically ill. We also have derived information from studies in various animals. Thus, our knowledge of human growth and body composition changes during fetal life may not directly translate to an understanding of nutritional needs and gastrointestinal and metabolic capabilities of this new generation of very low birth weight (VLBW: < 1250 g) infants while they are undergoing high-level NICU care.

A major goal of this chapter is to provide the reader with an overview of recent research and clinical experience that can be applied in the daily care of these infants. A few emerging concepts that may become important in the future care of these infants are also presented.

2 NUTRITIONAL NEEDS OF THE VLBW PRETERM INFANT

2.1 Energy Requirements

The fetus gains approximately 5 g/day at 16 weeks of gestation, 10 g/day at 21 weeks, and 20 g/day at 29 weeks (1). Between 24 and 40 weeks' gestation, water content declines from approximately 87 to 71%, protein rises from 8.8 to 12%, and fat from 1 to 13%. The American Academy of Pediatrics has recommended that the caloric average intake of the growing preterm infant be approximately 120 to 130 kcal/kg/day (2). However, this is based on the assumption that postnatal growth should approximate the growth in utero of a normal fetus of the same postconceptional age. This does not take into account the increased caloric needs of a sick premature infant. Currently, we do not have clear data to make valid recommendations with regard to the optimal energy requirements for extremely low–birth weight or critically ill infants except that their caloric requirements are most likely higher than those of stable, growing low–birth weight infants.

2.2 Carbohydrates

Both hyper- and hypoglycemia are common problems in VLBW infants. Glucose utilization and production rates in VLBW average from 6 to 10 mg/kg/min (3). Infusion rates greater than these may lead to hyperglycemia, fat deposition, and increased CO_2 production, which may increase the ventilatory requirements of these infants. Sick VLBW infants requiring mechanical ventilation appear to have a particularly high glucose production rate secondary to enhanced gluconeogenesis (4). Early infusion of amino acids in the first several days of life may decrease glucose production, increase insulin secretion, and enhance insulin action, thus decreasing the need for insulin infusions (5). What constitutes ''hypoglycemia'' in the preterm infants is somewhat controversial. Fetal plasma glucose levels over the second half of gestation are usually greater than 50 to 55 mg/dL (6). These levels are barely greater than those below which repeated measurements of low glucose concentrations are associated with increased risk of mental and motor developmental delay (7). Thus, a 50 to 55-mg/dL range of plasma glucose concentration should be the lower limit for VLBW preterm infants.

The capability of the VLBW infant to digest and absorb carbohydrates, proteins, and lipids increases with maturation and enteral exposure. The developmental aspects are described in detail elsewhere (8). Figure 1 provides a chart of the development of several digestive-absorptive secretions and enzymes. A brief summary of these processes is provided here.

Amylase, secreted from the salivary glands and the pancreas, cleaves internal α-1-4 glucose bonds to maltose, maltotriose, limit dextrin, and glucose. It is the major enzyme that hydrolyzes starches. Pancreatic secretion is poorly developed in the first several months of life; therefore at least this mode of starch hydrolysis could serve as a limiting factor and leave a lot of undigested starch in the intestine (8). There is some information suggesting that glucose polymers (18 to 29 glucose units) can be hydrolyzed by salivary amylases, but this digestion still falls substantially short of that accomplished by usual concentrations of pancreatic amylase (9). Many infant formulas including those formulated for preterm infants contain corn syrup solids or tapioca, which are partially hydrolyzed starches. The more extensively hydrolyzed the starch, the less reliance is placed on an immature digestive capability but the greater the osmolality. High osmolality can cause feeding intolerance—i.e., vomiting and/or diarrhea. Whether there is any advantage of these hydrolyzed starch formulas over those containing disaccharides or lactose has not been established.

The major carbohydrate in human milk and most infant formulas is lactose. Studies of fetal lactase activity and intestinal H_2 formation secondary to bacterial salvage of hydrolyzed disaccharides (via distal intestinal and colonic bacterial fermentation) suggest that lactose digestion is inefficient in the preterm and possibly even the term infant, whereas clinical observations and assessments of weight gain suggest efficient lactose assimilation (10). Colonic fermentation of lactose is a process known to occur in premature neonates and serves to (1) conserve a fraction of dietary carbohydrate that is not absorbed, (2) prevent osmotic diarrhea, and (3) produce short-chain fatty acids that stimulate sodium and water absorption. Short-chain fatty acids also serve as fuel for colonocytes and stimulate cell replication in colon and small intestine (10).

The presence of a high lactose concentration in human milk should not be a contraindication for its use in the VLBW infant. Feedings for VLBW infants are rarely initiated at levels intended to meet the infant's entire nutritional requirements and are usually advanced slowly in the first 1 to 2 weeks (see Figure 2). The rationale for using a lactose-free formula instead of human milk or lactose-containing formula is weak and may theoretically be harmful (11). Slow initiation of enteral feedings is unlikely to exceed the lactose hydrolytic and salvage capability of the small and large intestine, especially when less than 50% of the caloric requirement is provided via the gastrointestinal tract (unless the infant has a bowel that has been radically shortened by surgery) (see Chap. 29). Feeding lactose may also promote the growth of nonpathogenic *Lactobacillus*, which provides a

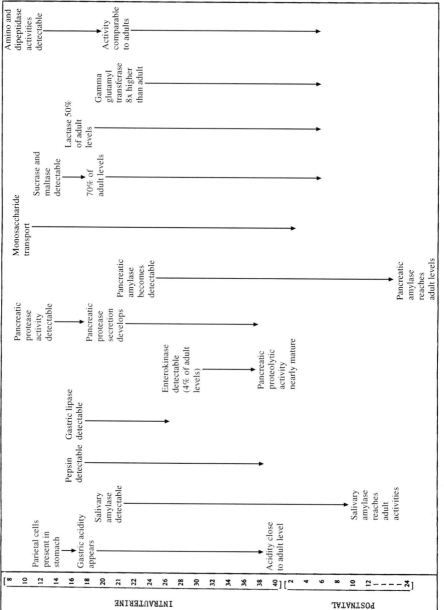

FIGURE 1 Appearance and development of digestive and absorptive capabilities in the human fetus.

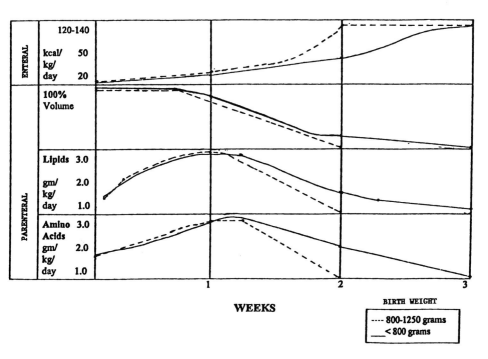

FIGURE 2 A proposed strategy for macronutrient intake in very low birth weight infants.

tamer intestinal microenvironment that is not as conducive to translocation by more pathogenic species such as *Klebsiella*, *Escherichia coli*, or *Enterobacter*. Human milk also contains several lactose-derived oligosaccharides and other gly-coconjugates that may play an important role in the infant's host defense (12) (see Chaps. 5 and 6).

2.3 Amino Acids and Protein

Growth cannot be attained without protein or amino acids. The growth rate of lean body mass of the normally growing human fetus is about 3.6 to 4.8 g/kg/day (13,14). This is greater than the amount of amino acid or protein intake that these infants are usually fed (14). With current human milk or formula feeding regimes, it is practically impossible to achieve and maintain the desired rates of protein intake (14). This becomes especially critical in sick VLBW infants. If they receive glucose alone, they lose in excess of 1.2 g/kg/day of endogenous protein (15). Provision of amino acids, even if total energy intake is low, spares endogenous protein stores by enhancing the rate of protein synthesis. Providing

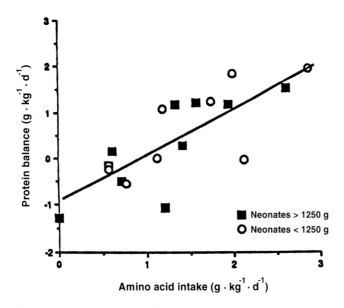

FIGURE 3   Relationship of intravenous amino acid intake to protein balance. (From Ref. 17.)

30 kcal/kg/day with 1.1 to 1.5 g of intravenous amino acid changes the balance of protein from substantially negative to zero or slightly positive (16). Increased amino acid intake in the first week of life correlates with increased protein balance (Fig. 3). Unfortunately, many VLBW infants do not receive even such modest intravenous amino acid intakes during their first several days of life, nor do they receive enough enteral feedings to meet these requirements, thus assuring the development of a catabolic state. Exacerbation of this catabolic state occurs when these infants are given glucocorticoids (dexamethasone) to facilitate weaning from mechanical ventilation.

Even when high quantities of amino acid or protein are provided, an inadequate intake of certain "conditionally essential" amino acids may exist (18). Examples of these include glutamine, glycine, histidine, taurine, and tyrosine. If these are not provided, essential amino acids are diverted away from protein synthesis. One such amino acid that has recently received increasing attention is glutamine (see Chaps. 1 and 18). Glutamine supplementation in adults has resulted in improved survival (19), decreased hospital-acquired sepsis in bone marrow transplant (20) and trauma (21) patients, along with improved nitrogen balance and decreased costs of hospitalization. One study of parenteral glutamine supplementation has shown a decreased requirement for mechanical ventilation in neonates with a birth weight of less than 800 g (22). Another study of enteral glutamine supplementation has demonstrated decreased hospital-acquired sepsis, decreased catabolism and/or improved amino acid utilization, improved tolerance to enteral feedings, and decreased cost of hospitalization; such supplementation appeared safe at the doses used (23–25).

The rationale for supplementing glutamine is based on its versatile metabolic role in energy metabolism (especially in the intestine and lymphocytes), nucleotide synthesis, glucosamine synthesis, and as an antioxidant precursor (26). Studies in animals have demonstrated both intravenous and enteral glutamine to be protective against various forms of experimentally induced enterocolitis, and it has been found to be a "conditionally essential" amino acid during times of stress (27). Although VLBW infants are catabolic and highly stressed during their first weeks of hospitalization, glutamine is not added to their total parenteral nutrition (TPN) and they do not receive glutamine unless they are enterally fed (they frequently are not).

Another amino acid that some consider as either essential or conditionally essential in the neonate is arginine. This amino acid plays a critical role in immune function, as a stimulant to the production of growth hormone, and as a precursor to energy carriers such as creatine. In a study of amino acid concentrations in low–birth weight infants (28), it was found that patients who subsequently developed necrotizing enterocolitis (NEC) had a lower plasma concentration of arginine. Further studies of glutamine, arginine, and other conditionally essential nutrients for VLBW infants are warranted.

As with carbohydrates, there are some limitations of protein digestion and absorption in the VLBW infant. Digestion begins in the acid environment of the stomach, where pepsin is also secreted and starts the proteolytic process. Even very preterm neonates are able to secrete hydrogen ion from the parietal cells of their stomachs, making the stomach pH chlorhydric with a pH <4.0 (29,30). The gastric acid output is related to gestational age and increases in the first couple weeks of life. It can also be stimulated by pentagastrin (Fig. 4). Pepsin secretion is lower in preterm infants than in full-term infants (31). Pepsin output in preterm infants (29 weeks gestation) has been compared with that of healthy adults. Mean postprandial pepsin output in infants fed mother's milk was 639 ± 142 U/kg body weight compared with 3352 ± 753 U/kg body weight in adults. Gastric contents of gavage-fed premature infants maintain a pH greater than 5.0 for the entire postprandial period. This pH is above that which is optimal for pepsin activity. How much the stomach contributes to overall protein digestion in the preterm infants is thus questionable.

Pancreatic proteases are secreted as inactive zymogens. These are activated by the action of enterokinase, an enzyme originating from the intestinal mucosa. Enterokinase activity cannot be detected before the 26th week of gestation (32). Between the 26th and 40th weeks of gestation, enterokinase activity increases

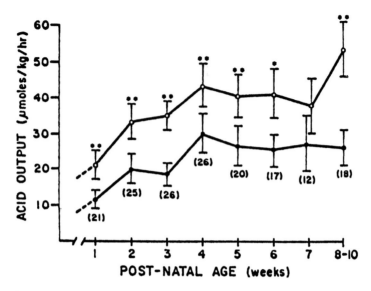

FIGURE 4   Basal acid output (solid circles) and pentagastrin-stimulated gastric acid output (open circles) in preterm infants. Number of subjects is given in parentheses. *$p < 0.05$. **$p < 0.01$. (From Ref. 29.)

and approximates 25% of that found in babies younger than 1 year of age. This may also limit luminal protein digestion.

The limitations in acid output and enterokinase activity are also theoretically important to a greater passage of microorganisms to the small intestine. It has been speculated that gastric acid production may protect the infant from bacteria in the milk (33). The results of one study also suggest a decrease in necrotizing enterocolitis with acidification of formula (34). The common practice of giving premature infants H_2-blocking agents in order to decrease acid output has not been demonstrated to have any clinical efficacy in VLBW infants and may be detrimental because it allows more microorganisms from the NICU environment to pass into the intestine. The relative risk of sepsis has been found to be 4.2 in prematures treated with H_2 blockers over controls (35).

The peptides produced by pancreatic enzyme digestion are hydrolyzed by intestinal brush border and intracellular peptidases. There are different transport systems involving the different categories of amino acids. Some amino acids are absorbed from the intestinal lumen more rapidly in the form of peptides than when they are presented as an equimolar mixture of free amino acids (36).

There is an apparent trend toward greater use of partially hydrolyzed proteins in formulas for preterm infants. Whether these formulas decrease the inci-

dence of atopy and are better tolerated than the nonhydrolyzed products is not
yet clear.

2.4 Lipids

Lipid requirements are limited to the essential fatty acids (linoleic or linolenic
acid). Although lipid makes up about 50% of the nonprotein energy content of
human milk and formulas, both of which contain these fatty acids, the frequent
practice of limiting enteral intake precludes the supply of these essential fatty
acids unless they are provided intravenously. Parenteral lipid emulsions provide
these essential fatty acids, but their use is often delayed or limited by concerns
of adverse effects. These putative effects include impaired oxygenation, impaired
lung function, impaired immune function, decreased platelets, and increased free
bilirubin levels. Despite in vitro studies suggesting deleterious effects of lipid
emulsion on immune function (37,38), there is no conclusive evidence for in vivo
effects. In vitro studies have shown that unesterified fatty acids can displace
bound bilirubin from albumin, thus increasing free bilirubin. However, clinical
studies have shown that infusion of lipid at rates up to 3 g/kg/day do not increase
plasma concentrations of free fatty acids or free bilirubin (39). Provision of lipid
infusions at rates less than 0.2 g/kg/hr does not result in deterioration of oxygenation or lung function (40). Although thrombocytopenia is frequently listed as
a side effect of intravenous lipids, provision of up to 3.3 g/kg/day has been
shown to have no effect on platelet concentrations even if given for up to 4 weeks
(41). There remains controversy about whether intravenous lipids are associated
with an increased incidence of sepsis (42,43). At this time there is no convincing evidence that lipids should be withheld because of an increased risk of
sepsis.

Failure to provide essential fatty acids in the VLBW infant results in biochemical signs of deficiency within 72 hr (44). This can be prevented by the
administration of as little as 0.5 g/kg/d of lipid emulsions. Although these emulsions contain high concentrations of linoleic and linolenic acid, they do not contain the long-chain polyunsaturated fatty acids (LC-PUFAs) arachidonic or docosahexaenoic acid. These are thought to be critical nutrients for the developing
central nervous system. The qualitative composition of lipids in these intravenous
emulsions is quite different from that in normal tissue, plasma lipids, and human
milk. The high content of linoleic and linolenic acid but low content of saturated
and monounsaturated fatty acids along with the absence of LC-PUFAs raises
questions about the propriety of the present solutions for the VLBW infant.

As with carbohydrates and proteins, there are some limitations of lipid digestion and absorption in the gastrointestinal tract of VLBW infants. The digestion and absorption of lipid can be split into several phases. These are discussed in
detail elsewhere (45) but are briefly summarized here. The luminal phase involves

deesterification of triglycerides to 3-monoglycerides and free fatty acids and bile acid–mediated micellar solubilization. This latter process is limited in VLBW infants because the duodenal concentration of bile acids is low due to lower synthesis and ileal reabsorption. Lower micellar solubilization leads to inefficient cell-mucosal interaction and subsequently lower absorption of the molecules of the mucosal–cell surface interface. Long-chain fatty acids but not medium-chain fatty acids depend on bile acids for solubilization and thus are the most susceptible to inefficient absorption.

The permeation of fatty acids and 2-monoglycerides from the lumen into the cell, intracellular reesterification, chylomicron formation, and transport of the chylomicrons from the cell into the circulation are the primary absorptive events. After luminal digestion, fatty acids and monoglycerides must approximate the absorptive surface, where the assembly of these substances into a form that can enter the intracellular milieu occurs. The medium-chain triglycerides undergo a relatively simple process of digestion and absorption compared to the long-chain triglycerides, but the long-chain triglycerides must still be supplied to prevent deficiencies of essential fatty acids and optimize central nervous system development.

2.5 Vitamins, Minerals, and Trace Elements

Recent data suggests that vitamin A is deficient in premature infants who develop chronic lung disease, and a multicenter trial is currently under way to determine the efficacy of supplementation (46). Several lines of evidence suggest that VLBW infants require more zinc than term infants. Higher intake of dietary zinc has been shown to improve growth and motor development as well as development and function of the immune system, especially in VLBW infants with intrauterine growth retardation (47). The optimal range of zinc intake is not known. Optimal iron intake is also not known. Iron intake in high doses can cause oxidative membrane damage to red blood cells and other cell types. Present recommendations are daily intakes of between 2 and 4 mg/kg/day of elemental iron for prematures (48), depending on their birth weight. The optimal intake of iron with concomitant erythropoietin therapy is not known. In addition, the ideal balance between iron therapy, antioxidants such as vitamin E, and selenium and polyunsaturated fatty acids remains poorly defined.

3 CONSIDERATIONS FOR ENTERAL FEEDING OF THE SICK PREMATURE INFANT

3.1 Gastrointestinal Development

One of the major excuses neonatologists give for not using the gastrointestinal (GI) tract of the premature infant for long periods of time after birth is that the

GI tract of these infants is poorly developed. What are these immaturities? They can be divided into mechanical ones, which include suck-swallow coordination and motility, and immaturities of luminal digestion and mucosal absorption. Immaturities of luminal digestion and mucosal absorption have already been discussed. An argument can be made in support of using the GI tract whenever possible in VLBW infants.

3.1.1 Suck-Swallow Coordination

It is a common belief that the very premature infant prior to about 32 weeks of gestation has a suck-swallow pattern that differs from that of the infant closer to term in that the very preterm infant will not be able to continue sucking activities during the swallowing process. This results in an inefficient and potentially dangerous pattern if these infants are fed by mouth rather than by a tube. Thus most VLBW infants are tube-fed.

Feeding performance of preterm infants has been studied in order to determine whether milk flow could affect their feeding performance (49). The investigators compared ''restricted'' flow, during which the nipple hole is not large enough for milk to flow freely, to unrestricted flow; they observed that the use of a restricted pattern of milk flow facilitates oral feeding, especially for those born at 30 weeks' gestation or earlier. With this type of flow, milk will not continue to drip into the oral cavity, as it would with the unrestricted flow, giving the infant time to rest without choking or to catch up with breathing bursts. From these studies it appeared that the term sucking pattern was not always necessary for successful oral feeding, especially when restricted nipple flow was used.

3.1.2 Immature Motility

Ganglia are present in the esophagus at 5 weeks' gestation and complete their migration to the rectum by 24 weeks' gestation. Despite this, the esophagus of the premature demonstrates slower propagation velocities and a contraction duration that is more prolonged than in the older child. At about 28 weeks' gestation, the lower esophageal sphincter resting pressure is only 4 mmHg, but it increases to adult values (18 mmHg) by term (50,51). The relationship of this factor to the putative high incidence of gastroesophageal reflux (GER) in premature infants is reviewed elsewhere (52), but it is likely that increases in intra-abdominal pressure may be a contributory factor. Dramatic increases in GER have been seen after diaper changes, an intervention that results in increased intra-abdominal pressure (53). Delayed gastric emptying is also a factor related to GER, because gastric emptying is slower in prematures than in term infants (54). In the adult, the rate of gastric emptying is controlled by feedback from the small and large intestines. Stimulation of duodenal receptors by acid, fat, carbohydrate, tryptophan, or increasing osmolality decreases rates of gastric emptying. Studies of the effects of various formula components on gastric emptying have yielded conflicting results. Siegel, et al. (55), studying infants between 32 and 39 weeks' gestation, demonstrated that progressive increments of caloric density from 0.2 cal/mL to 0.66 cal/mL decreased the rate of gastric emptying, but they found no differences in formula between 0.6 to 0.8 cal/mL. However, despite the reduction in emptying rate at higher caloric density, the quantity of calories delivered into the duodenum from the stomach increased with concentrated formula. Changes in osmolality from 279 to 448 mOsm/kg do not significantly alter the rates of gastric emptying of isocaloric formulas. No information on the ability of duodenal feedback to control the rate of gastric emptying in the VLBW infant between 25 and 32 weeks' gestation is available. Inadequate control of emptying could overwhelm the intestinal tract, leading to malabsorption and feeding intolerance. Therapeutic agents that increase gastric emptying rates in children and adults are also effective in premature infants. Metoclopramide increases the gastric emptying rate in preterm and term infants (56). Cisapride (57) increases gastric emptying rates in preterm infants. However, the efficiency and safety of these agents must be studied in larger randomized trials and cisapride is no longer available in the U.S. market. Nasojejunal feeding may provide only limited improvement in feeding tolerance, because intestinal motility is also immature (58).

The motility patterns of the small bowel are poorly developed before 28 weeks' gestation. In studies by Berseth et al. (59), the small intestine showed disorganized motility patterns between 27 and 30 weeks' gestation, progressing to a more mature pattern, so that migrating myoelectric complexes are present at 33 to 34 weeks' gestation. Gastroanal transit ranges from 8 to 96 hr in preterm infants as compared with 4 to 12 hr in adults. In preterm infants, the motilin receptor is not present until 32 weeks gestation, and the cyclic release of motilin is not present. This suggests that the use of erythromycin would not be effective prior to 32 weeks gestation.

When we decide on feeding strategies for premature infants, it is important to remember that infants given early minimal enteral nutrition show faster maturation of motor patterns and release of gastrointestinal hormones than infants given no enteral feedings (59). Early-fed infants have less feeding intolerance, establish oral feedings sooner, and do not differ in their incidence of NEC (60). Motor responses appear to be less intense on the more diluted formulas (59). The amount of volume does not appear to have a benefit in maturing motor function. Motor responses are equally intense whether feedings are instilled intragastrically or transpylorically. They are similar whether feedings are given chilled, at room temperature, or warmed to body temperature (61). When infants are fed a slow infusion over 120 min, they display an intense fed response that is accompanied by brisk gastric emptying. However, when the same volume is fed over 15 min, duodenal motor responses are far less intense and are accompanied by delayed gastric emptying (62). Because two-thirds of all preterm infants display an immature duodenal fed pattern that is accompanied by delayed gastric emptying, many preterm infants may not be as physiologically prepared to process bolus feedings as well as slow infusion feedings from the viewpoint of motor activity. Nevertheless, whether accomplished by bolus or continuous administration, enteral feeding is a major stimulus to motility and other maturational factors in the GI tract.

4 WHAT CAN GO WRONG?

Table 1 lists some of the problems associated with feeding practices for VLBW infants and some of the potential results of these problems. These include undernutrition, prolonged use of TPN, and overly rapid advancement of enteral feeding. The consequences of undernutrition have already been discussed. Several situations commonly seen in preterm infants have been used as contraindications to institute or advance enteral feedings leading to prolonged use of exclusive TPN. These include hypoxic/ischemic insults at birth (low Apgar scores), the presence of apnea and/or bradycardia, sepsis, the presence of an umbilical catheter, the use of indomethacin, the use of inotropic agents such as dopamine, and the presence of heme-positive stools. These practices are largely based on anecdotal associations between these practices and the common finding of intolerance to enteral feedings as determined by large gastric residuals, abdominal distention, and the occurrence of NEC. Withholding of enteral feedings is occasionally taken to the extreme; infants may have all enteral feedings withheld for several weeks after birth and/or several days after a mild episode of intolerance or the presence of heme-positive stools. This can lead to undernutrition and its consequences.

The ability to nourish VLBW infants by the parenteral route has provided an alternative that is believed by most neonatal caregivers to be completely acceptable. However, the use of TPN is not free of complications. It is widely

TABLE 1 Problems Associated with Feeding Practices

What can go wrong?	Potential effects
Undernutrition	Catabolism leading to poor muscle function, difficulty weaning from mechanical ventilation, prolonged hospitalization, increased costs, subsequent neurodevelopmental delays
Prolonged use of exclusive total parenteral nutrition	Sepsis, intestinal atrophy, subsequent feeding intolerances, liver damage, thrombosis, metabolic imbalances, requirement for frequent monitoring of electrolytes
Overly rapid advancement of feedings	Necrotizing enterocolitis, feeding intolerance, vomiting and aspiration, reflux

thought that the use of TPN catheters contributes to the high incidence of sepsis seen in LBW infants. The mechanism of this is widely thought to be via introduction of micro-organisms through the catheters. Alternative hypotheses, which are not as popular but tenable, are based on the fact that the use of TPN without trophic nutrition to the intestine is associated with gut atrophy, which could, in turn, lead to a greater propensity for translocation of micro-organisms across the intestinal mucosal barrier (63). Liver damage (cholestesis and fibrosis), catheter thrombosis, and metabolic imbalances and the need for more frequent blood draws for monitoring of electrolytes are other effects of prolonged TPN. These can also markedly increase the costs of caring for VLBW infants.

It is common practice in many NICUs to withhold enteral feedings when premature infants are having apneic spells, which are very common in VLBW infants. Mandich et al. (64) studied this systematically and found that infants who experienced apnea had a significantly longer transition time to the initiation of oral feeding (10.3 to 11.3 days) than infants who did not experience apnea (5.4 to 6.6 days). One reason commonly given for not feeding an infant with apnea is that the apnea causes transient ischemia to the intestine, and this may lead to NEC. However, epidemiological investigations have not found an increased risk (65).

The use of umbilical arterial catheters has also been implicated as a risk factor in the development of NEC. Many neonatologists do not feed enterally if an umbilical artery catheter is in place. This can lead to undernutrition and its consequences. The basis of this practice stems from the observation that many if not most umbilical catheters have thrombi at the ends and these may dislodge and embolize to the intestine. In addition, frequent blood draws and flushes may cause hemodynamic compromise to the intestine. Although, these theoretical possibilities exist, neither a true cause-and-effect relationship nor a strong association between the use of umbilical arterial catheters and NEC has been demonstrated (65).

Indomethacin is one of the most commonly used drugs in the NICU. The major indications are to close a patent ductus arteriosus and for the prophylaxis of intraventricular hemorrhage. Many neonatologists withhold enteral feedings entirely during the time that indomethacin is administered. The theoretical basis for withholding feedings during indomethacin administration is that there may be a reduction of splanchnic blood flow, and this compromised flow may cause hypoxic-ischemic injury to the intestine. Although there is a suggestion that the use of indomethacin may be a risk factor for the development of NEC or spontaneous perforation (66), others do not support this notion (67). There are now approximately 10 comparisons of early minimal enteral nutrition to late enteral nutrition. In the infants receiving minimal enteral nutrition, the presence of apneic spells, the use of umbilical catheters, or indomethacin did not appear to predispose for NEC or feeding intolerance (60). However, this does not preclude caution in the advancement of enteral feedings while infants are receiving these supportive measures.

5 FEEDING ADVANCEMENT (TPN AND ENTERAL)

How then should we proceed to nourish the VLBW infant in the NICU? The above information suggests that, ideally, we should not interrupt the flow of nutrition that the fetus has been obtaining from its mother and not hesitate to provide nutrition to the infant immediately after birth. Because of gastrointestinal immaturities, it is neither possible nor prudent to attempt full nutrition by the enteral route immediately after birth. However, there are very few if any convincing reasons to withhold intravenous glucose, amino acids, lipids, vitamins, and trace elements beyond the immediate stabilization period after birth. There is a tendency to begin parenteral amino acid intake at only 0.5 g/kg/day or less, gradually achieving an intake of 2.5 to 3.0 g/kg/day over a period of 7 to 10 days to avoid protein "intolerance and toxicity." This practice should become obsolete, since studies have demonstrated that intakes up to 2.6 g/kg/day revealed little evidence of protein toxicity as measured by hyperammonemia, azotemia, or metabolic acidosis (15,68). There are also no convincing reasons—other than a known gastrointestinal anomaly such as volvulus, atresia, tracheoesophageal (T-E) fistula, etc.—that should preclude placing small amounts of milk or formula into the gastrointestinal tract shortly after birth.

How quickly should we advance enteral feedings? Because of the individual characteristics of each patient, one feeding advancement schedule or guideline cannot be used for all infants. An example is given in Figure 2. Clinical judgment based on available scientific data and experience presently appears to be the best criterion on which we should base our feeding practices. From the available studies, minimal enteral feedings should be instituted within the first days of life. There is no clear evidence that the concomitant use of umbilical catheters, continuous positive airway pressure, mechanical ventilation, indomethacin, or the presence of apneic and bradycardic episodes preclude the use of minimal enteral nutrition because of an increased risk of NEC.

Clear evidence for advantages of diluted versus undiluted milk during minimal enteral feeding is not yet available. At least one study suggests an advantage of bolus over continuous feedings (69). Placement of food into the stomach rather than administering it transpylorically utilizes the capability of the stomach to partially hydrolyze proteins and lipids. Minimal enteral feedings of less than 20 kcal/kg/day for several days are safe and may improve subsequent tolerance to the advancement of enteral feedings. Enteral increments of less than 20 kcal/kg/day appear advisable in most VLBW infants (70), although some can clearly tolerate more.

TABLE 2   Recommendations for Enteral Feeding

Indications to continue enteral feeds with caution or to temporarily withhold enteral feedings	1. An increase in abdominal girth of 2 cm or more over the previous measurement. Abdominal girth is measured prior to every enteral feeding. 2. A single gastric residual fluid volume of >3 mL/kg body weight. 3. Emesis. 4. Sudden onset of guaiac-positive stools. These are very common in tube-fed infants and are most significant if concomitant with one of the other factors listed here.
Indications to withhold feeding until more extensive workup indicates it is safe to continue enteral feedings	1. Grossly bloody stools. 2. Ileus. 3. Radiological evidence of necrotizing enterocolitis (pneumatosis intestinalis or free intraperitoneal air). 4. Slightly greenish or dark yellow gastric residuals. These are common in very low birth weight infants. Feedings can be carefully continued if there is no abdominal distention, x-rays are normal, and infant is otherwise stable.

How can we monitor "tolerance" to enteral feedings? There are several criteria that can be used to determine "intolerance." We have used the guidelines shown in Table 2 to temporarily withhold and proceed with caution or definitively withhold enteral feedings until the problem is resolved and/or until further, more extensive workup or treatment indicates it is safe to continue enteral feeding. Close monitoring of tolerance and adjusting of intake according to individual tolerance during advancement is *always* indicated.

REFERENCES

1. Sparks JW. Human intrauterine growth and nutrient accretion. Semin Perinatol 1984; 8(2):74–93.
2. Committee on Nutrition, American Academy of Pediatrics. Nutritional needs for low birthweight infants. Pediatrics 1985; 75:976.
3. Sunehag A, Ewald U, Larsson A, Gustafsson J. Glucose production rate in extremely immature neonates (<28 weeks) studied by use of deuterated glucose. Pediatr Res 1993; 33:97–100.
4. Keshen T, Miller R, Jahoor F, Jaksic T, Reeds PJ. Glucose production and gluconeogenesis are negatively related to body weight in mechanically ventilated, very low birth weight neonates. Pediatr Res 1997; 41(1):132–138.
5. Michael JL, Schutz Y, Jequier E. Protein metabolism of the newborn. In: Polin RA, Fox WW, eds. Fetal and Neonatal Physiology. Philadelphia, Saunders, 1992, pp 462–471.
6. Srinivasan G, Pildes RS, Cattamanchi G, Voora S, Lilien LD. Plasma glucose values in normal neonates: A new look. J Pediatr 1986; 109:114–117.
7. Lucas A, Morley R, Cole TJ. Adverse neurodevelopmental outcome of moderate neonatal hypoglycemia. BMJ 1988; 297:1304–1308.
8. Koldovsky O. Small and large intestine. In: Polin RA, Fox WW, eds. Fetal and Neonatal Physiology. Vol 2. Philadelphia, Saunders, 1992, p 1059.
9. Murray RD, Kerzner B, Sloan HR, McClung HJ, Gilbert M, Ailabouni A. The contribution of salivary amylase to glucose polymer hydrolysis in premature infants. Pediatr Res 1986; 20(2):186–191.
10. Kien CL. Digestion, absorption, and fermentation of carbohydrates in the newborn. Clin Perinatol 1996; 23(2):211–228.
11. Neu J, Koldovsky O. Nutrient absorption in the preterm neonate. Clin Perinatol 1996; 23(2):229–243.
12. Kunz C, Rudloff S. Biological functions of oligosaccharides in human milk. Acta Paediatr 1993; 82:903–912.
13. Widdowson EM. Changes in body proportions and composition during growth. In: Davis JA, Dobbing J, eds. Scientific Foundations of Pediatrics. Philadelphia: Saunders, 1974, pp 153–163.
14. Ziegler EE. Protein in premature feeding. Nutrition 1994; 10:69–71.
15. Mitton SG, Calder AG, Garlick PJ. Protein turnover in sick, premature neonates during the first few days of life. Pediatr Res 1991; 30:418–422.
16. Rivera A Jr, Bell EF, Bier DM. Effect of intravenous amino acids on protein metabolism of preterm infants during the first three days of life. Pediatr Res 1993; 33:106–111.
17. Thureen PJ, Anderson AH, Baron KA, Melara DC, Hay WW, Fennessey PV. Protein balance in the first week of life in ventilated neonates receiving parenteral nutrition. Am J Clin Nutr 1998; 68:1228–1235.
18. Rassin DK. Essential and non-essential amino acids in neonatal nutrition. In: Raiha NCR, ed. Protein Metabolism During Infancy. New York: Raven Press, 1994; pp 183–195.

19. Griffiths RD. Six-month outcome of critically ill patients given glutamine-supplemented parenteral nutrition. Nutrition 1997; 13:295–302.
20. Ziegler TR, Young LS, Benfell K, et al. Clinical and metabolic efficacy of glutamine-supplemental parenteral nutrition after bone marrow transplantation. Ann Intern Med 1992; 1126:821–828.
21. Houdijk AP, Rijnsburger ER, Jansen J, Wesdorp RI, Weiss JK, McCamish MA, Teerlink T, Meuwissen SG, Haarman HJ, Thijs LG, van Leeuwen PA. Randomized trial of glutamine-enriched enteral nutrition on infectious morbidity in patients with multiple trauma. Lancet 1998; 352(9130):772–776.
22. Lacey JM, Crouch JB, Benfell K, Ringer SA, Wilmore CK, Maguire D, Wilmore DW. The effects of glutamine-supplemented parenteral nutrition in premature infants. J Parenter Enter Nutr 1996; 20(1):74–80.
23. Neu J, Roig JC, Meetze WH, Veerman M, Carter C, Millsaps M, Bowling D, Dallas MJ, Sleasman J, Knight T, Auestad N. Enteral glutamine supplementation in very low-birthweight infants decreases morbidity. J Pediatr 1997; 131(5):691–699.
24. Roig JC, Meetze WH, Auestad N, Jasionowski T, Veerman M, McMurray CA, Neu J. Enteral glutamine supplementation for the very low birthweight infant: Plasma amino acid concentrations. J Nutr (Suppl) 1996; 126:1155–1120S.
25. Dallas MJ, Bowling D, Roig JC, Auestad N, Neu J. Enteral glutamine supplementation for very-low-birthweight infants decreases hospital costs. J Parenter Enter Nutr 1998; 22(6):352–356.
26. Neu J, Shenoy V, Chakrabarti R. Glutamine nutrition and metabolism: Where do we go from here? FASEB J 1996; 10:829–837.
27. Lacey JM, Wilmore DW. Is glutamine a conditionally essential amino acid? Nutr Rev 1990; 48:297–309.
28. Zamora SA, Amin HJ, McMillan DD, Kubes P, Fick GH, Butzner JD, Parsons HG, Scott RB. Plasma L-arginine concentrations in premature infants with necrotizing enterocolitis. J Pediatr 1997; 131(2):226–232.
29. Hyman PE, Clarke DD, Everett SL, Sonne B, Stewart D, Harada T, Walsh JH, Taylor IL. Gastric acid secretory function in preterm infants. J Pediatr 1985; 106(3):467–471.
30. Kelly EJ, Newell SJ, Brownlee KG, Promrose JN, Dear PR. Gastric acid secretion in preterm infants. Early Hum Dev 1993; 35(3):215–220.
31. Armand M, Hamosh M, Mehta NR, Angelus PA, Philpott JR, Henderson TR, Dwyer NK, Lairon D, Hamosh P. Effect of human milk or formula on gastric function and fat digestion in the premature infant. Pediatr Res 1996; 40(3):429–437.
32. Antonowicz I, Lebenthal E. Developmental pattern of small intestinal enterokinase and disaccharidase activities in the human fetus. Gastroenterology 1977; 72(6):1299–1303.
33. Usowicz AG, Dab SB, Emery JR, McCann EM, Brady JP. Does gastric acid protect the preterm infant from bacteria in unheated human milk? Early Hum Dev 1988; 16(1):27–33.
34. Carrion V, Egan EA. Prevention of neonatal necrotizing enterocolitis J Pediatr Gastrentrol Nutr 1990; 11(3):317–323.
35. Beck-Sague CM, Azimi P, Fonseca SN, Baltimore RS, Powell DA, Bland LA, Arduino MJ, McAllister SK, Huberman RS, Sinkowitz RL, et al. Bloodstream infections in neonatal intensive care unit patients: Results of a multicenter study. Pediatr Infect Dis J 1994; 13(12):1110–1116.

36. Matthews DM. Intestinal absorption of peptides. Physiol Rev 1976; 55:337.
37. Sirota L, Straussberg R, Notti I, Bessler H. Effect of lipid emulsion on IL-2 production by mononuclear cells of newborn infants and adults. Acta Paediatr 1997; 86(4): 410–413.
38. Salo M. Inhibition of immunoglobulin synthesis in vitro by intravenous lipid emulsion (Intralipid). J Parenter Enter Nutr 1990; 14(5):459–462.
39. Rubin M, Naor N, Sirota L, Moser A, Pakula R, Harell D, Sulkes J, Davidson S, Lichtenberg D. Are bilirubin and plasma lipid profiles of premature infants dependent on the lipid emulsion infused? J Pediatr Gastroenterol Nutr 1995; 21(1): 25–30.
40. Brans YW, Ritter DA, Kenny JD, Andrew DS, Dutton EB, Carrillo DW. Influence of intravenous fat emulsion on serum bilirubin in very low birthweight neonates. Arch Dis Child 1987; 62(2):156–160.
41. Spear ML, Spear M, Cohen AR, Pereira GR. Effect of fat infusions on platelet concentration in premature infants. J Parenter Enter Nutr 1990; 14(2):165–168.
42. Avila-Figueroa C, Goldmann DA, Richardson DK, Gray JE, Ferrari A, Freeman J. Intravenous lipid emulsions are the major determinant of coagulase-negative staphylococcal bacteremia in very low birth weight newborns. Pediatr Infect Dis J 1998; 17(1):10–17.
43. Druml W, Fisher M, Ratheiser K. Use of intravenous lipids in critically ill patients with sepsis without and with hepatic failure. J Parenter Enter Nutr 1998; 22(4):217–223.
44. Foote KD, MacKinnon MJ, Innis SM. Effect of early introduction of formula vs fat-free parenteral nutrition on essential fatty acid status of preterm infants. Am J Clin Nutr 1991; 54(1):93–97.
45. Hamosh M. Digestion in the newborn. Clin Perinatol 1996; 23(2):191–209.
46. Kennedy KA, Stoll BJ, Ehrenkranz RA, Oh W, Wright LL, Stevenson DK, Lemons JA, Sowell A, Mele L, Tyson JE, Verter J. Vitamin A to prevent bronchopulmonary dysplasia in very-low-birth-weight infants: has the dose been too low? The NICHD Neonatal Research Network. Early Hum Dev 1997; 24;49(1):19–31.
47. Friel JK, Andrews WL. Zinc requirement of premature infants. Nutrition 1994 Jan–Feb; 10(1):63–65.
48. Siimes MA. Iron requirement in low birthweight infants. Acta Paediatr Scand Suppl 1982; 296:101–103.
49. Lau C, Schanler RJ. Oral motor function in the neonate. Clin Perinatol 1996; 23(2): 161–178.
50. Boix-Ochoa J, Canals J: Maturation of the lower esophagus. J Pediatr Surg 1976; 11:749.
51. Newell SJ, Sarkar PK, Durbin G: Maturation of the lower oesophageal sphincter function in the preterm baby. Gut 1988; 29:1677.
52. Novak DA. Gastroesophageal reflux in the preterm infant. Clin Perinatol 1996; 23(2):305–320.
53. Newell SJ, Booth IW, Morgan MEI, Durbin GM, McNeish AS. Gastro-oesophageal reflux in preterm infants. Arch Dis Child 1989; 64(6):780–786.
54. Cavell B. Reservoir and emptying function of the stomach of the premature infant. Acta Paediatr Scand 1982; 296:60.

55. Siegel M. Gastric emptying time in premature and compromised infants. J Pediatr Gastroenterol Nutr 1983; 2(suppl 1):S136.
56. Hyman PE, Abrams C, Dubors A. Effect of metaclopramide and bethanechol on gastric emptying in infants. Pediatr Res 1985; 19:1029.
57. Janssens G, Melis K, Vaerenberg M. Long-term use of cisapride (Propulsid) in premature neonates of <34 weeks gestational age. J Pediatr Gastroenterol Nutr 1990; 11:420.
58. Leung AK, Liay PC. Use of metoclopramide in the treatment of gastroesophageal reflux in infants and children. Curr Ther Res 1984; 36:911.
59. Berseth CL. Gastrointestinal Motility in the neonate. Clin Perinatol 1996; 23(2): 179–190.
60. La Gamma EF, Browne LE. Feeding practices for infants weighing less than 1500 g at birth and the pathogenesis of necrotizing enterocolitis. Clin Perinatol 1994; 21(2):271–306.
61. Anderson CA, Berseth CL. Milk temperature affects gastric emptying in the preterm infant. Pediatr Res 1994; 35:307A.
62. DeVille KT, Shulman RJ, Berseth CL. Slow infusion feeding enhances gastric emptying in preterm infants compared to bolus feeding. Clin Res 1993; 41:787A.
63. Pierro A, van Saene HK, Donnell SC, Hughes J, Ewan C, Nonn AJ, Lloyd DA. Microbial translocation in neonates and infants receiving long-term parenteral nutrition. Arch Surg 1996; 131(2):176–179.
64. Mandich MB, Ritchie SK, Mullett M. Transition times to oral feeding in premature infants with and without apnea. J Obstet Gynecol Neonatal Nurs 1996; 25(9):771–776.
65. Covert RF, Neu J, Elliott MJ, Rea JL, Gimotty PA. Factors associated with age of onset of necrotizing enterocolitis. Am J Perinatol 1989; 6(4):455–460.
66. Grosfeld JL, Chaet M, Molinari F, Engle W, Engum SA, West KW, Rescorla FJ, Scherer LR III. Increased risk of necrotizing enterocolitis in premature infants with patent ductus arteriosus treated with indomethacin. Ann Surg 1996; 224(3):350–355.
67. Kumar RK, Yu VY. Prolonged low-dose indomethacin therapy for patent ductus arteriosus in very low birthweight infants. J Pediatr Child Health 1997; 33(1): 38–41.
68. Van Goudoever JB, Colen T, Wattimena JL, Huijmans JG, Carnielli VP, Sauer PJ. Immediate commencement of amino acid supplementation in preterm infants: Effect on serum amino acid concentrations and protein kinetics on the first day of life. J Pediatr 1995; 127(3):458–465.
69. Schanler RJ, Schulman RJ, Lau C, Smith EO, Heitkemper MM. Feeding strategies for premature infants: Randomized trial of gastrointestinal priming and tube feeding method. Pediatrics 1999; 103(2):434–439.

9

Anorexia Nervosa and Bulimia Nervosa

Carmen Mikhail
Baylor College of Medicine, Houston, Texas

The Duchess of Windsor is reputed to have said that ''no woman can be too rich or too thin.'' The ''too thin'' aspect of this adage is emphasized in the eating disorders anorexia nervosa and bulimia nervosa, which occur primarily in females. Anorexia nervosa is characterized by a relentless pursuit of thinness, dread of weight gain, food restriction, and overactivity. Bulimia nervosa, which originally appeared in the literature as a symptom of anorexia nervosa, involves episodic binge eating of substantial quantities of food followed by purging. As both disorders are complex and multiply determined, their comprehensive assessment is often difficult.

1 DEFINITION OF THE DISORDERS

1.1 Diagnostic Criteria and Guidelines

Patients with anorexia nervosa and bulimia nervosa differ in kind and severity of their symptomatology, generating some debate over which characteristics are unique to these disorders. The most widely used criteria for a diagnosis of anorexia nervosa are those of the *Diagnostic and Statistical Manual of Mental Disorders*, fourth edition (DSM-IV) (1), presented in Table 1. DSM-IV suggests but

TABLE 1   DSM-IV Criteria for Anorexia Nervosa

A. Refusal to maintain body weight at or above a minimally normal weight for age and height (e.g., weight loss leading to a maintenance of body weight less than 85% of that expected or failure to make expected weight gain during periods of growth, leading to body weight less than 85% of that expected).
B. Intense fear of gaining weight or becoming fat, even though underweight.
C. Disturbance in the way in which one's body weight or shape is experienced, undue influence of body weight or shape on self-evaluation, or denial of the seriousness of the current low body weight.
D. In postmenarcheal females, amenorrhea, i.e., the absence of at least three consecutive menstrual cycles. [A woman is considered to have amenorrhea if her periods occur only following hormone (e.g., estrogen) administration.]
Specify type:
Restricting type: During the current episode of anorexia nervosa, the person has not regularly engaged in binge eating or purging behavior (i.e., self-induced vomiting or the misuse of laxatives, diuretics, or enemas).
Binge eating/purging type: During the current episode of anorexia nervosa, the person has regularly engaged in binge eating or purging behavior (i.e., self-induced vomiting or the misuse of laxatives, diuretics, or enemas).

Source: Ref. 1.

does not require a minimum body weight for a diagnosis. Although DSM-IV criteria stipulate fear of weight gain and body-image disturbance, we are not provided with specific standards for their measurement. DSM-IV adds two further requirements: (1) the centrality of weight and shape to the subject's self-evaluation and (2) denial of the seriousness of the low weight. The DSM-IV criteria also specify amenorrhea as a requirement. Some researchers debate the necessity of including this criterion, as amenorrhea sometimes occurs only as a result of starvation.

DSM-IV delineates two subtypes of anorexia nervosa. Descriptions of anorexics who strictly limit food intake, as opposed to those who binge and purge, indicate that the groups differ in terms of premorbid adjustment, development of the disorder, and family characteristics, highlighting the need to distinguish between the two subgroups. Moreover, anorexia nervosa is classified as a disorder of adolescence in DSM-IV, and there are special considerations in using the criteria for younger children. Prepubescent girls have a smaller percentage of body

TABLE 2 ICD-10 Diagnostic Guidelines for Anorexia Nervosa

1. Body weight is maintained at least 15% below that expected, or body mass index (BMI) is 17.5 or less. Prepubertal patients may fail to make expected weight gains.
2. The weight loss is self-induced by avoidance of "fattening foods" and by the use of self-induced vomiting, self-induced purging, excessive exercise, appetite suppressants, and/or diuretics.
3. There is a body image distortion whereby a dread of fatness persists as an intrusive, overvalued idea and patients impose a low weight threshold on themselves.
4. An endocrine disorder involving the hypothalamic-pituitary-gonadal axis is present, manifest in the female as amenorrhea and in the male as loss of sexual interest and potency.
5. If onset is prepubertal, the sequence of pubertal events is delayed or even arrested. In girls, breasts do not develop and there is amenorrhea; in boys, the genitals remain juvenile.

Source: Ref. 2.

fat than do their postpubescent counterparts. This could affect their fulfilling the weight criterion, although it must be remembered that the weight criterion is only a suggested guideline. In DSM-IV the amenorrheal requirements are limited to postmenarcheal females, allowing younger girls to meet the criteria for anorexia nervosa.

Another classification system, which is in close agreement with that of DSM-IV, is the 10th revision of the *International Classification of Diseases* (ICD-10) (2). Five disturbances, presented in abbreviated form in Table 2, are necessary for a diagnosis of anorexia nervosa. As in DSM-IV, the ICD-10 includes patients with bulimic episodes in the diagnosis of anorexia nervosa. The ICD-10 also requires a fear of fatness. Unlike the DSM-IV, the ICD-10 requires the presence of an endocrine disorder. This requirement may result in more false negatives, as not all anorexics suffer from an endocrine disorder. Furthermore, it is not clear whether the endocrinological changes are due to primary hypothalamic disease or are secondary to weight loss alone (3).

The DSM-IV criteria for bulimia nervosa are presented in Table 3. The amount of food characterizing a "binge" is specified as being larger than most people would eat given the same period of time and circumstances. Additionally, the binge eating and inappropriate compensatory behavior must occur at least twice a week and last for 3 months. The DSM-IV criteria also add the stipulation that these individuals place an excessive emphasis on body shape and weight in their self-evaluation. Other additions are the clarification that the diagnosis not be given when the disturbance occurs only in anorexia nervosa, and the inclusion

Table 3 DSM-IV Criteria for Bulimia Nervosa

A. Recurrent episodes of binge eating. An episode of binge eating is characterized by both of the following: (1) Eating, in a discrete period of time (e.g., within any 2-hr period) an amount of food that is definitely larger than most people would eat during a similar period of time and under similar circumstances. (2) A sense of lack of control over eating during the episode (e.g., a feeling that one cannot stop eating or control what or how much one is eating).

B. Recurrent inappropriate compensatory behavior in order to prevent weight gain, such as self-induced vomiting; misuse of laxatives, diuretics, enemas, or other medications; fasting; or excessive exercise.

C. The binge eating and inappropriate compensatory behaviors both occur, on average, at least twice a week for 3 months.

D. Self-evaluation is unduly influenced by body shape and weight.

E. The disturbance does not occur exclusively during episodes of anorexia nervosa.

Specify type:

Purging type: during the current episode of bulimia nervosa, the person has regularly engaged in self-induced vomiting or the misuse of laxatives, diuretics, or enemas.

Nonpurging type: during the current episode of bulimia nervosa, the person has used other inappropriate compensatory behaviors, such as fasting or excessive exercise, but has not regularly engaged in self-induced vomiting or the misuse of laxatives, diuretics, or enemas.

Source: Ref. 1.

of purging and nonpurging subtypes. Diagnosis of bulimia nervosa, which is also described as a disorder of adolescence, will be valid only if subjects acknowledge bingeing and purging behaviors. As these are usually secretive and adolescents may fear censure from parents, the behaviors may be difficult to detect. Furthermore, care must be taken to ensure that younger adolescents understand the terms *bingeing* and *purging* during the diagnostic interview.

The ICD-10 guidelines (2) for bulimia nervosa are presented in Table 4. These guidelines also include the DSM-IV requirements of bingeing and purging. The ICD-10 includes a dread of fatness, whereas DSM-IV lists an overemphasis on body size. In this respect, ICD-10 has satisfied earlier criticisms of diagnosis placing inadequate emphasis on the patient's fear of fatness. The third guideline of ICD-10 acknowledges this disorder as being related to anorexia nervosa and encourages the confirmation of an earlier anorexic episode. The ICD-10 also provides separate diagnostic guidelines for normal-weight bulimia and other eating disorders.

TABLE 4   ICD-10 Diagnostic Guidelines for Bulimia Nervosa

1. Patients exhibit a preoccupation with eating and engage in episodes of overeating (large amounts in a short period of time).
2. Patients attempt to counteract fattening effects of food by one or more of the following:
   Self-induced vomiting
   Purging
   Starvation
   Use of drugs (appetite suppressants, thyroid pills, diuretics)
   Neglect of insulin treatment (diabetics)
3. There is a morbid dread of fatness; patients set themselves a stringent weight threshold. A history of a previous episode of anorexia nervosa is often but not always present.

Source: Ref. 2.

The usefulness of a diagnostic category or label is based in part upon its ability to specify homogeneous and distinct disorders. In this respect, anorexia nervosa and bulimia nervosa are less than desirable diagnostic labels. There is some debate as to whether bulimia nervosa is a separate syndrome or merely a manifestation of anorexia nervosa. About half of female anorexic patients develop bulimia nervosa at a later stage. Also interesting is the finding of Garner et al. (4) that bulimics who had never met the weight loss criteria for anorexia nervosa were more similar to bingeing anorexics than either group was to restricting anorexics on demographic, clinical, and psychometric variables. If normal-weight bulimics and bingeing anorexics are similar, it might make sense to group these two populations together.

1.2   Differential Diagnosis with Psychiatric Disorders

1.2.1   Anorexia Nervosa Versus Bulimia Nervosa

Differential diagnosis between anorexia nervosa and bulimia nervosa is difficult, as the disorders share some common features, including body image distortion, overemphasis on body weight in self-evaluation, and anxiety after eating. Anorexics are 15% or more below normal weight, whereas bulimics are within 10% of normal weight. Anorexics engage in binge eating only occasionally, but bulimics do so frequently. Furthermore, anorexics typically fast and avoid forbidden food, whereas bulimics binge on forbidden food and purge to control weight.

1.2.2   Depression

The psychiatric disorder most readily confused with an eating disorder is depression. Patients with both depression and eating disorders may present with depressed mood, low self-esteem, and neurovegetative symptoms including decreased or increased appetite, sleep disturbance, and decreased sexual interest. Symptoms distinguishing those with an eating disorder include body image distortion, preference for thinness, overemphasis on body weight as determining self-worth, fear of weight gain, and use of inappropriate means to control weight. Weight loss may bring about sincere concern in those with depression but secretive satisfaction in those with an eating disorder. Since starvation itself may produce cognitive changes resembling depression, a diagnosis of depression in a patient with recent weight loss should be delayed until the weight is at least partially restored.

1.2.3   Obsessive-Compulsive Disorder

Obsessional and phobic anxiety symptoms are sometimes prominent in anorexia nervosa, leading to a possible misdiagnosis with obsessive-compulsive disorder. The basis of both disorders involves an irrational fear, paired with a behavioral habit designed to reduce anxiety surrounding the fear. Differential diagnosis is based on the content of the fears and corresponding behaviors. If the content is related solely to food or eating, an additional diagnosis of obsessive-compulsive disorder is not warranted. Moreover, obsessional and compulsive symptoms in anorexia nervosa may be exacerbated by dieting and consequent starvation and may abate with weight restoration.

1.2.4   Schizophrenia

Patients with schizophrenia may present with self-imposed starvation, avoidance of specific foods, and vomiting. However, starvation is due to delusions about the food—e.g., concerns about poisoning; therefore food avoidance and vomiting are designed to prevent undesirable effects on the body. Those with schizophrenia do not display an intense drive for thinness, body-image disturbance, or abuse of laxatives or diet pills.

1.3   Differential Diagnosis with Medical Disorders

It is important to rule out medical conditions that may mimic anorexia nervosa and bulimia nervosa and to recognize the interaction of medical illness with eating disorders. Misdiagnosis may lead to inappropriate interventions, which may exacerbate symptoms and delay appropriate treatment. The most common medical conditions to be considered in the differential diagnosis include gastrointestinal diseases, endocrine diseases, central nervous system disorders, and chronic infections.

1.3.1   Gastrointestinal Diseases

Common gastrointestinal causes of weight loss in adolescents include Crohn's disease and ulcerative colitis, both chronic inflammatory bowel diseases (see Chap. 27). Symptoms include weight loss, anorexia, fever, fatigue, diarrhea, nausea, and vomiting. As these symptoms overlap with those of eating disorders, patients with inflammatory bowel disease have been mistakenly diagnosed as having anorexia nervosa (e.g., Ref. 5). Distinction is made on the basis of laboratory evidence of inflammation, i.e., elevated erythrocyte sedimentation rate (ESR) and malabsorption. Additionally, iron stores are usually not depleted and cholesterol level is usually high rather than low in anorexia nervosa. Weight loss of patients with inflammatory bowel disease is not deliberate. Their decreased food intake may be due to abdominal pain, nausea, and genuine appetite loss; increased caloric requirements may be due to fever and inflammation; malabsorption may be due to the disease, bowel resection, or lactose intolerance secondary to lactase deficiency. There have been several reports of coexistence of Crohn's disease with an eating disorder. In one report (6), two lactose-intolerant patients used milk ingestion as a purgative and two patients did not take required corticosteroids or sulfasalazine, resulting in diarrhea and weight loss. In another report (7), weight gain on steroids triggered excessive dieting in one case and misuse of laxatives in another.

Eating disorder patients with vomiting and parotid gland hypertrophy may be mistakenly diagnosed as having pancreatitis due to elevated serum amylase. However, in eating disorders, hyperamylasemia is salivary rarely pancreatic in origin, and seldom exceeds twice the normal values. In pancreatitis, food intake may be restricted to avoid abdominal pain, and resolution of pancreatitis should reverse this restriction. Bulimia nervosa was found on follow-up in 5 of 21 patients with hyperlipidemic pancreatitis (8). The development of the eating disorder was attributed to the restrictive nature of the prescribed diet together with emotional stressors associated with the illness.

Malabsorption syndrome may result in weight loss, diarrhea, and abdominal complaints. While patients with this disorder suffer abnormal fecal fat loss, those with anorexia nervosa exhibit negligible fecal fat loss due to restrictive fat intake. Loss of protein resulting in hypoalbuminemia is found in patients with malabsorption but not in those with eating disorders.

Superior mesenteric artery syndrome may mimic or exacerbate anorexia nervosa. This syndrome involves compression of the third portion of the duodenum by the superior mesenteric neurovascular bundle. Patients present with vomiting, abdominal pain, and eventual weight loss. In this case patients avoid food to control postprandial vomiting and distress rather than to pursue thinness.

1.3.2 Endocrine Diseases

Because the endocrine system plays a role in weight regulation, appetite, and metabolism, differential diagnosis with endocrine disease must be addressed. Hyperthyroidism, diabetes mellitus, and Addison's disease all present with weight loss. In hyperthyroidism, elevated pulse rate, respiration rate, blood pressure, and sweaty extremities signal a hypermetabolic rate. However, patients with anorexia nervosa rarely have a primary thyroid abnormality. They often display a *euthyroid sick pattern*, with thyroid indices in the low or normal range secondary to starvation. This pattern should not be treated with thyroid hormone therapy, as such therapy is abused by patients with eating disorders in order to facilitate weight loss or counter binge eating.

Patients with diabetes mellitus present with polydipsia and polyuria. While those with eating disorders may also drink large quantities of water, the motive is to reduce hunger, facilitate vomiting, or increase weight monitored at a physician's office. In this case, polydipsia is not due to increased thirst, nor is it accompanied by polyuria. As patients with diabetes mellitus are required to follow a low-carbohydrate, low-fat diet, dietary restraint may precipitate an eating disorder in vulnerable individuals. Comorbidity of insulin-dependent diabetes mellitus and eating disorders increases diabetic complications (9). Diabetic control is poor due to insulin misuse and binge eating. Patients are likely to omit or reduce insulin levels to induce glycosuria (loss of glucose in the urine) and weight loss. Additionally, the erratic caloric intake of bulimics or severe restriction and overexercising of anorexics can make determination of required insulin levels difficult.

Symptoms of Addison's disease include weight loss, reduced food intake, vomiting, hypoglycemia, and hypotension. However, while patients with Addison's disease report extreme weakness and fatigue, those in early stages of anorexia nervosa display hyperactivity and rarely complain of fatigue. Tests of adrenocortical function assist in the differential diagnosis.

1.3.3   Central Nervous System Disorders

Central nervous system lesions can impair the regulation of eating. Hypothalamic lesions may result in hypo-or hyperphagia. Differential diagnosis is based on the existence of symptoms suggestive of an intracranial lesion, such as headache, increased or decreased thirst, spontaneous vomiting, diplopia, and coarse or diminished hair rather than lanugo. Traumatic brain injuries, especially of the frontal or bilateral temporal lobes, may produce transient hyperphagia. With temporal lobe damage, the hyperphagia often appears as part of Kluver-Bucy syndrome, including placidity, hypersexuality, visual agnosias, hyperorality, and exploration of the environment via touch. Hyperphagia has also been known to occur with central nervous system (CNS) infections, seizure disorders, and Prader-Willi syndrome, a congenital disorder.

Brain imaging studies have shown enlarged ventricles and external cerebrospinal fluid spaces in many patients with anorexia nervosa and some patients with bulimia nervosa (10). This *pseudoatrophy* reflects a compromised nutritional state and usually resolves with weight gain.

1.3.4   Chronic Infections

Chronic infections, especially tuberculosis and AIDS, may cause weight loss secondary to anorexia and acceleration of metabolic requirements. Differential diagnosis is based on signs of inflammation, including fever and increased ESR.

1.4   Age of Onset

Epidemiological investigations support the belief that anorexia nervosa develops in adolescence. Martin (11) described 25 anorexic patients (2 males and 23 females) who averaged 14.9 years of age, with the time between onset of illness and referral being approximately 8 months. In another study (12) 20 anorexic patients' age of onset was 16.2 ± 3.4 years. While these ages can be targeted, there is evidence suggesting that anorexic symptoms develop over time and have a relatively predictable sequence. Beumont et al. (13) have collected data suggesting that there is a temporal sequence to the development of anorexic symptoms. Concern about body weight and engagement in relatively reasonable weight-control efforts precede preoccupation with weight and food and bizarre methods of weight control, with the last of these increasing over time.

A number of reports have described anorexia nervosa in young children. Fosson et al. (14) described 48 children 14 years of age and younger who met modified diagnostic criteria for anorexia nervosa. Russell (15) and Jacobs and Isaacs (16) each followed their own groups of 20 female patients with anorexia nervosa that had developed before menarche. In a summary of eating disturbance seen in children 8 to 14 years old, the authors described anorexia nervosa, food avoidance emotional disorder, food refusal, pervasive refusal, selective eating, bulimia nervosa, and appetite loss secondary to depression (17). Gowers et al. (18) utilized a database of 650 female anorexics to identify 30 girls who developed the disorder before menarche. In a retrospective and longitudinal study of a child psychiatry service, 27 out of 8051 children met the criteria for anorexia nervosa; it was found that early-onset anorexia nervosa showed a nature, course, and outcome similar to those of the adult disease (19).

A survey of 499 bulimic women recruited through a popular women's magazine placed the mean age of onset of bulimia nervosa at 18.4 years (20). In Agras and Kirkley's (21) sample of 76 bulimic women, the mean age of onset was 19.3 years. Separating the onset of binge eating and of vomiting, Mitchell et al. (22) found that their sample of 275 bulimic women began bingeing at a mean age of 17.7 years and vomiting at a mean age of 18.8 years. While results are not altogether unambiguous, the accumulating evidence seems to suggest that anorexia nervosa is a problem of early adolescence and bulimia nervosa is a disorder of late adolescence.

1.5   Epidemiology

A survey of nine girls' schools in England found 1 case of severe anorexia nervosa in every 250 girls; in private schools, 1 in 200 girls under the age of 16 and 1 in 100 girls between 16 and 18 years of age had the disorder (23). Moss et al. (24) found that 18 of 151 tenth-grade girls scored in a range indicating the presence of anorexic symptoms. In a screening study of 1010 girls 14 to 16 years old, a prevalence rate of 0.99% was detected for clinical eating disorder and 1.78% for the partial syndrome of eating disorder (25).

In a review of 11 studies of bulimia in high school students (26), the prevalence rates for bulimia nervosa ranged from 1.2 to 16% in girls. A nationwide study of U.S. high school students with a large sample size of 5596 students and a 91% completion rate yielded a prevalence rate for bulimia nervosa of 1.2% for girls and 0.4% for boys (27). Johnson et al. (28) found that 4.9% of a sample of 1268 female high school students were engaging in clinically significant levels of bulimic behavior. Differences in these rates may be due to variation in the populations, discrepancies in self-report, or differences in criteria for inclusion.

Approximately 5 to 10% of patients with an eating disorder are male. The clinical features and outcome of Anorexia Nervosa and Bulimia Nervosa in males are relatively similar to those in females (29) with the obvious exception of amenorrhea. (Because the ratio of male to female patients with these disorders is so low, feminine nouns and pronouns are used in the remainder of this chapter to refer to patients.)

2 ASSESSMENT OF THE EATING-DISORDERED INDIVIDUAL

The clinician should be prepared for eating-disordered patients to be very difficult to assess. Anorexics deny their disorder and their need for treatment. Since they are usually referred by concerned family members, they can be resistant to evaluation. While the family may be motivated for assessment and symptom relief, the patient may not. The clinician must be careful not to be perceived as siding with the family against the patient. It is crucial to establish rapport and a positive relationship with the anorexic patient prior to information collection.

Bulimics may present a slightly different set of difficulties. They tend to be embarrassed and secretive about their unusual eating and purging behaviors, and since the clinician may be the first person they have told about their problems, they may be rebellious or oppositional. Their noncompliance may extend to the assessment procedures. In such cases, the clinician must be skilled in eliciting information.

Patients with anorexia nervosa and bulimia nervosa frequently elicit strong negative feelings in the first interview. When attempts are made to collect information and work with these patients, they can be defensive, secretive, disagreeable, and attacking. Their behavior may seem so unreasonable and provocative that it is difficult for the interviewer not to become angry. To counteract such negative feelings, it is sometimes helpful for the interviewer to view the symptoms as a reaction to a very disordered environment. The style of interacting may have been very adaptive and self-preserving within the context in which it developed. The interviewer may be seen as trying to dismantle the scheme these

TABLE 5   Warning Signs of Anorexia Nervosa

Low body weight and weight loss
Agitation/hyperactivity
Constipation
Abdominal bloating/pain
Bradycardia
Hypotension
Dry skin
Brittle hair/nails
Hypothermia, cold intolerance
Lanugo
Amenorrhea
Peripheral edema
Recent switch to vegetarianism
Obsession with exercise
Perfectionism, compulsivity, rigidity, feelings of ineffectiveness
Social and/or sexual disinterest

patients have developed to preserve themselves, their sense of independence, or their feelings of self-control. Care should be taken to not label the individual with the eating disorder as *being* "the problem" when the eating disorder might more appropriately be attributed to the social or family situation or to cultural factors.

Assessment should cover a wide range of behaviors and problem areas. The manner and sequence in which one approaches a patient should be designed to match the patient's view of the problem, insofar as this is possible. The patient's view of the problem can be solicited upon initial inquiry. This can be adopted, with adjustments, as the rationale or justification for the collection of information that might otherwise be objectionable or provoke noncompliance. Given the possibility of obtaining skewed information from patients, interview material should be supplemented with information collected from family members, teachers, coaches, counselors, or other individuals in close contact with the patient. Additionally, Tables 5 and 6 provide warning signs to alert the clinician to the presence of anorexia nervosa or bulimia nervosa, respectively. If the patient is in an end stage or physically compromised stage of anorexia nervosa, medical considerations must come first and foremost.

2.1 Assessment of Medical Symptoms

Anorexia nervosa and bulimia nervosa are medically assessed in terms of endocrinological/metabolic, cardiovascular, renal, gastrointestinal, hematologi-

TABLE 6 Warning Signs of Bulimia Nervosa

Bruises on dorsum of hands
Parotid gland swelling
Dental enamel erosion
Peripheral edema
Fatigue
Heartburn
Constipation
Abdominal bloating
Irregular menses
Electrolyte abnormalities
Cardiovascular problems, including hypotension and arrhythmias
Patient consumes large amounts of food in a short period of time
Patient disappears after meals
Impulsivity, irritability, depression
Experimentation with alcohol, drugs, sex

cal, and pulmonary dysfunction (for excellent reviews, see Refs. 30 and 31). Physical examination, standard laboratory tests, multiple-channel chemistry analysis, complete blood count, and urinalysis should be routine. Recommended laboratory tests are presented in Table 7. It is well known that anorexia is a potentially life-threatening disorder. Approximately 10 to 15% of untreated cases end in death (32). Medical complications of bulimia have also proven fatal. While these are reviewed below in detail, it is also important to note that the leading cause of death in bingeing anorexics is suicide (33).

The most dangerous complication of vomiting and purgative (laxative and diuretic) abuse is the depletion of the electrolytes potassium, chloride, and sodium

TABLE 7 Recommended Laboratory Tests

Complete blood count
Electrolytes (potassium, chloride, sodium, CO_2)
Chemistry panel
Albumin, transferrin
Liver function tests
Calcium
Thyroid function tests
Urinalysis
Electrocardiogram

(30). The clinician should be alert to complaints of weakness, tiredness, constipation, and depression, which can be produced by electrolyte abnormalities (34). Electrolyte abnormalities may result in cardiac arrhythmias and sudden death or in kidney disturbances (31). Mitchell et al. (35) found electrolyte disturbances in almost 49% of their nonanorexic bulimic patients. Neurological disturbances have also been documented; some are associated with electrolyte disturbances (36), while others have included muscular spasms and tingling sensations in the extremities (37) and swollen salivary glands accompanied by facial swelling (38).

Gastrointestinal disturbances associated with bulimia include abdominal pain, spontaneous regurgitation of food, extreme dilation of the stomach (leading to rupture and death in some cases), permanent loss of bowel reactivity, and serious tearing of mouth and throat tissue. Gastric acid from self-induced vomiting leads to dental erosion, and loss of enamel causes color changes, caries, and periodontal disease (39). Edema is common after vomiting and laxative abuse have ceased; many patients notice swelling or "puffiness" caused by excessive water retention. Menstrual irregularities are common among bulimics, even those of normal weight (40). Johnson et al. (41) found that 20% of a sample of 50 bulimics had experienced amenorrhea following the onset of eating disorders and that 50% were experiencing menstrual irregularities at the time of the survey.

2.2 Assessment of Behavior

2.2.1 Weight Regulation

One of the most striking symptoms in anorexia nervosa and bulimia nervosa is the preoccupation with weight and thinness. Weight history as well as preoccupation with weight should be thoroughly assessed, including the following: current weight and height; ideal weight; highest and lowest weight since early adolescence; fluctuations and their relationship to major life events and changes; actual or perceived consequences of weight loss and gain (including occupational and interpersonal); family and peer attitudes toward thinness, dieting, and appearance; and history of weight loss (speed and method). Weight should be taken with the subject dressed in a gown. If anxiety regarding weight is too high, the subject can turn away from the reading on the scale.

More general eating habits are also significant. Food intake, regularity-irregularity of eating habits, nutritional adequacy of intake, purging, and exercise behavior are likely to play some role in the maintenance or development of the disorder. Patients might be asked to explain what calories are, how food is digested, the function of fat, and how most fad diets work in order that the clinician may assess superstitious and magical thinking associated with food. A prolonged period of restrictive eating is the most commonly cited precipitant of binge eating.

Loss or separation from a significant other, interpersonal conflict, and difficulty handling sexuality and emotions such as anger, loneliness, and depression are also cited.

Important questions regarding dieting include how long the patient has been involved in dieting behavior; when, why, and with whose encouragement the dieting first began; and what the role of dieting and weight problems was in the patient's family of origin. The extent and function of weighing and exercise behaviors are also of interest, since they can often become ritualistic and self-defeating.

2.2.2   Binge Behavior

Assessment of the binge behavior includes information about when, where, and with whom it occurs and about its frequency and length. What is consumed (type and quantity), antecedents and consequences of the binge behavior, onset, initial precipitants, associated feelings, and length and circumstances surrounding the longest asymptomatic period are also assessed. A binge-purge diary can be helpful in obtaining some of this information. It has been found that patients with eating disorders who monitor their behavior progress better than those who do not. Self-report methods have been criticized for being too removed from the behavior of interest; an alternate is the direct measurement of eating during a test meal.

Most bulimics begin to binge approximately 1 1/2 years after beginning to diet (42) and to purge (usually in the form of self-induced vomiting) approximately 1 year after the onset of binge eating (43). A group of 40 bulimic patients studied by Mitchell et al. (44) reported a mean of 11.7 binge episodes per week (range of 1 to 46), averaging 1.18 hr in length (15 min to 8 hr), with an average consumption of 3415 calories (1200 to 11,500). It is common to find that a patient binges on certain foods and that these foods have acquired a forbidden status, such that the patient perceives that his or her consumption alone has the power to trigger a binge.

Psychological as well as physical deprivation may trigger binge eating or specific food cravings. Dissatisfaction with body image and poor self-esteem have been shown to be significant predictors of the severity of binge eating (45). Binge eating occurs most often in the afternoon and evening; when patients are at home alone; on foods of which they normally deprive themselves (carbohydrates and sweets); and typically after not eating during the day. Binge eaters tend to have the most difficulty with unstructured time and with making transitions between settings (e.g., going from school to home).

2.2.3   Purge Behavior

Purge behavior can take many different forms, including laxative abuse, self-induced vomiting, diuretic abuse, amphetamine abuse, fasting or strict dieting, and excessive exercise. Purging serves to protect patients against the dreaded weight gain and may also be a way to express anger, to punish themselves, or to regain a sense of control. Initial research (46) suggests that the act of purging may be more tension-regulating than the binge eating, and that while patients may begin to purge so that they can eat, they later binge eat in order to be able to purge.

3 MODELS OF ANOREXIA NERVOSA AND BULIMIA

Relevant dimensions or variables for assessment and treatment are chosen on the basis of a theoretical model about the nature of the disorder, the nature of individuals, and the nature of change. Virtually all current models of anorexia nervosa and bulimia nervosa begin with an explanation of the most salient features of the disorders. With anorexia nervosa, these include the time of onset, male-female ratio, weight loss, the disturbed body image, desire to be thin, and the refusal to maintain adequate or moderate/regular dietary intake. The most salient characteristics of bulimia nervosa are the binge eating and the purging behaviors. Related features vary greatly among different orientations. The following discussion reviews major theoretical orientations.

3.1 Biological Models

There are essentially three types of biological models of the eating disorders. One emphasizes the hormonal changes that occur at puberty; another emphasizes statistical relationships between depression and eating disorders, such as incidence of mood disorders in first-degree relatives of eating-disordered patients; and a third emphasizes brain functioning.

The first model suggests that there are abnormalities in hormone output and regulation mechanisms, such that the changes occurring at puberty in these processes make these abnormalities evident and interfere with normal eating behavior and weight control. However the endocrine abnormalities that have been found in anorexics seem to be secondary to the starvation process itself, since they can be found in nonanorexic persons who have reached starvation weights (47).

The second and most prominent biological model of anorexia nervosa and bulimia nervosa assumes the existence of a genetic predisposition toward the development of such disorders and links them to affective disorders, including depression (48). Abnormally high incidences of major affective disorder in first-degree relatives and bulimics' response to imipramine treatment are cited as supporting evidence.

Representing the third type of biological model, Wurtman and Wurtman (49) have proposed that there may be a disturbance in the feedback mechanism in bulimia, whereby carbohydrate intake registers in the brain in an abnormal fashion. They suggest that the concentration of the neurotransmitter serotonin is abnormal and that an abnormal craving for carbohydrates is thereby produced. Finally, Rau and Green (50) have asserted that a small number of bulimics have an epileptic-like, neurologically based disorder of impulse control. They argue that the psychologically based disorder is different and distinguishable from the neurologically based disorder. They claim that in the neurologically based disorder the patients may experience an aura; the patients see binge-purge behavior as inconsistent with their self-image; there is no psychological pattern to the binge eating; postictal phenomena may be present (extended period of sleeping unconsciousness, confusion, memory loss or disruption, headaches, or loss of bladder control); and/or the patients may exhibit various neurological "soft signs."

3.2 Psychodynamic Models

According to psychodynamic theory, the eating disorders, like any other syndrome or symptom complex, are the expression of unconscious internal conflicts that stem from early development. In anorexia nervosa and bulimia nervosa, these conflicts are thought to involve sexuality, autonomy, and identity. The severe food restriction seen in anorexia nervosa patients is considered symbolic of severe sexual conflicts, since the pattern of dieting and self-starvation often begins at the prepubertal period and delays or reverses the development of secondary sexual characteristics. The amenorrhea associated with anorexia nervosa is seen as both a denial of sexuality and a defense against pregnancy.

Bruch (51) believes that anorexia nervosa stems from core developmental conflicts and deficits relating to autonomy and initiative. She has observed that anorexia nervosa patients are typically model children with outstanding performance records who can be considered overly compliant. They subsequently experience themselves as acting only in response to demands coming from others and not in accordance with their own needs and wants. The illness is an attempt to break away from this dependence on others, a desperate fight against feeling enslaved, and a declaration of ownership and control over their own bodies.

Bulimia nervosa as a distinct syndrome has not been given wide attention from psychodynamically oriented theorists. Coffman (52) presents a clinical model of the "binge-purge" syndrome that draws heavily upon Bruch's (51) discussions of issues of personal authority, effectiveness, and power over a person in authority, such as a parent. In fact, Coffman cautions against focusing exclusively or too heavily on the binge-purge behaviors, as this might be perceived as a demand and thus as a threat to these clients' weak sense of personal control, which might provoke them to maintain or increase the binge eating and purging.

Bruch doubts the existence of bulimia nervosa as a separate clinical entity. She views it as a treatment complication of anorexia nervosa (not as the manifestation of a separate disorder), although an increasingly common one. In keeping with this conceptualization, Bruch has identified deficits in self-knowledge and self-definition in bulimics.

From a psychodynamic perspective, then, assessment and treatment of anorexia nervosa and bulimia nervosa is directed at fundamental ambivalences and conflicts centering around issues of control, personal autonomy, initiative, effectiveness, power, and sexuality.

3.3 Cognitive-Behavioral Models

The cognitive-behavioral approach emphasizes the analysis of functional relationships among antecedents, consequences, and individual behaviors as the proper units for studying, eventually understanding, and changing the behaviors of anorexia nervosa and bulimia nervosa patients. The literature on these disorders has focused on describing the parameters of the maladaptive behaviors and the development of behavioral and cognitive-behavioral treatment programs rather than specifying the types of pathogenic social learning experiences. Leon (53), in contrast, has proposed that extremely negative thoughts and feelings about weight and weight gain become associated with the consumption of food over time, such that it becomes reinforcing to refuse food in order to avoid these negative thoughts and feelings. Crisp (54) conceptualizes anorexic patients' symptomatic behavior as an avoidance response whereby psychosexual maturity is avoided or reversed. These patients' behavior not only helps them to avoid negative thoughts, feelings, and fears but also provides opportunities for much cognitive self-reinforcement through the sense of mastery, virtue, and self-control that it provides. Thus, contingencies of both positive and negative reinforcement are used to explain the development and the maintenance of anorexia nervosa.

Several approaches have been generated within the cognitive-behavioral orientation regarding bulimia nervosa. Orleans and Barnett (55) argue that ''bulimarexia'' (a term used to describe a pattern of behavior that includes binge eating and purging and occurs in normal-weight individuals) is initially acquired as a weight-control tactic. They hypothesize that bulimarexia ''develops as a faulty weight control practice in an environment where problematic self-control patterns are modeled'' (p. 148). Theorists also emphasize the positive, non-eating-related outcomes associated with bingeing and purging. Binge eating provides comfort and distraction from anxiety and depression over interpersonal rejection or academic stress. The binge eater defines her problem as being uncontrolled eating, which is something she can master, if only theoretically. She avoids the more difficult and emotionally challenging interpersonal and academic problems. The binge also provides an opportunity for renewed self-determination, which the binge eater does by making what theorists call the ''purification promise'': ''If only I could lose 20 pounds,'' or ''if only I would never eat any more sweets, then all my problems would be solved.'' Time-consuming rituals also drive persons who binge and purge into social isolation, which offers similar protection from possible rejection and negative evaluation by others.

In summary, the cognitive-behavioral approach directs its assessment efforts at the individual by delineating the antecedents and consequences (cognitive, behavior, affective, and interpersonal) of the maladaptive behaviors and the associated skills deficits; this delineation is aimed primarily at treatment planning. These approaches have identified areas of difficulties that involve basic knowledge about diet and nutrition, cognitions and emotions (particularly self-evaluative), and interpersonal difficulties.

4 TREATMENT CONSIDERATIONS

4.1 Outpatient Treatment

Outpatient treatment is best managed by a multidisciplinary eating disorders team capable of addressing medical, psychological, and nutritional aspects of care. Psychotherapy is central to the treatment of eating disorders. The duration and frequency of individual therapy sessions is dictated by the severity of symptomatology and rapidity of weight loss; they are usually conducted one to three times per week. As patients obtain only minimal benefit from psychotherapy when their weight is low, weight restoration is a primary goal in recovery. Family therapy is indicated with younger patients still living at home and with older patients who appear overinvolved with their families. Family therapists address dysfunctional roles, conflicts, alliances, and patterns which the eating disorder is precipitating or maintaining and provide family members with assistance in dealing with the eating disorder. Group therapy is an effective and economical adjunct to individual and family therapy, providing psychoeducation and social support to members.

4.2 Inpatient Treatment

Hospitalization provides the opportunity to treat a patient more intensively than permitted during outpatient treatment. Indications for hospitalization are summarized in Table 8. The decision to hospitalize should be made by the entire treatment team in conjunction with the patient and family members. Inpatient treatment is best administered in a psychiatric residential facility specializing in eating disorders. Serious medical complications may warrant brief admission to a medical hospital prior to transfer to a residential facility.

Family members and patients react to the decision to hospitalize with a myriad of emotions, including guilt, shame, fear, anger, confusion, and feelings

TABLE 8 Indications for Hospitalization

Rapid weight loss (e.g., > 7 kg in 4 weeks)
Weight below 70–75% ideal body weight
Hypokalemia from vomiting, laxative/diuretic abuse
Severe bradycardia
Other cardiac arrhythmias
Major gastrointestinal bleeding
Severe depression/suicidal ideation
Resistance to outpatient treatment
Nonfunctioning family
Lack of local outpatient treatment facility

---

of failure. It is important for the patient to be informed of possible benefits to her, such as increased self-esteem or lessened depression. Care should be taken to present inpatient treatment as an opportunity for more comprehensive assistance and support rather than as a punitive act for slow recovery. A preadmission tour of the facility dispels fears and clarifies expectations prior to admission while also reducing the chance of leaving against medical advice.

The initial phase of treatment involves nutritional rehabilitation. Given current insurance limitations, most inpatient programs aim for a weight gain to approximately 85 to 90% of ideal body weight. Once patients' concentration and judgment are improved, intensive individual and group psychotherapy are added. A good program should make provisions for resolution of family dysfunction, preferably in the form of a family therapy week. While most patients have at least a partial improvement following treatment, the relapse rate after discharge is approximately 30%. Indications for good prognosis include younger age at admission, shorter duration of illness, fewer prior hospitalizations, greater body weight on admission and at follow-up, slower weight increase during treatment, absence of purging, stable family relationships, and good premorbid social functioning (56,57).

4.3 Weight Management

Weight restoration avoids serious medical complications and restores cognitive functioning for maximum benefit from psychotherapy. This may be accomplished through oral, nasogastric, or intravenous feeds. Choice of intervention depends on current medical and nutritional status, severity of weight loss, and psychological symptomatology. Team members should initially enforce the least intrusive methods, resorting to nasogastric or intravenous feeds only when other strategies have failed. The goal should be slow, steady weight gain of approximately 1 kg per week. Caution should be exercised in pushing for rapid weight gain, which is likely to result in excessive anxiety or depression in the patient and may precipitate bulimia.

On an outpatient basis, weight management is accomplished with behavioral contracting between the patient and therapist or other team member. Contracts must be negotiated with the patient to increase her feelings of control and responsibility over her recovery. Realistic weight goals are set for the next session, with subsequent rewards for attainment or consequences for nonattainment. Recommended rewards include special privileges or outings, while consequences include lessened exercise or consumption of a feared food. If weight loss continues to be a problem, contracts can stipulate weights at which nasogastric feeding or hospitalization will occur. Consistency in reinforcing rewards and consequences is central to the success of behavioral contracting.

On an inpatient unit, contracting for daily food intake can be a useful tool for increasing patient food consumption, the units for negotiation being calories or food exchanges. Levels of daily caloric intake may begin at approximately 1200 kcal per day, gradually increasing by approximately 100 kcal per day. Patients should be closely supervised by nursing staff during and for 1 to 1 1/2 hours following food consumption. If the patient is unable to consume the required intake by the end of the day, she could be required to take the remainder in the form of a nutritional supplement.

When all attempts at voluntary food intake have failed and the patient is medically compromised, nasogastric feeds can be implemented. On an outpatient basis the tube feeds may be administered at night so as not to interfere with daily activities, possibly being monitored by a home care assistant. The patient should receive approximately 1500 kcal per night and be encouraged to eat regular meals during the day. It is preferable to use a supplement that is high in phosphate and potassium. Once a weight gain of approximately 2 kg is established, further efforts should be made toward voluntary food intake. The patient should be informed a priori of the weight at which the tube is to be removed. If the patient is being monitored in an inpatient unit, the amount of food voluntarily consumed could be deducted from calories administered via nasogastric feeding. Because nasogastric feeding may produce dependency on tube feeds, is invasive, and often exacerbates issues of control in the patient, it is recommended only as a time-limited intervention.

If the patient cannot tolerate nasogastric feeding, she may be fed intravenously using total parenteral nutrition via an indwelling needle or catheter. Since concentrated solutions are difficult to tolerate, the patient may have to be fed continuously, thereby restricting her daily activities. The same considerations addressed earlier for nasogastric feeding apply. Enteral and parenteral nutrition are discussed more comprehensively in Chapter 17.

4.4 Pharmacotherapy

Prompted by obsessive-compulsive, depressive, or what may appear to be delusional symptomatology in patients, a wide variety of pharmacological treatments have been investigated for eating disorders. The mechanism of action of pharmacological treatment in highly complex disorders such as anorexia nervosa and bulimia nervosa is not well understood, and there is a lack information to enable the physician to predict patient response to pharmacological agents. Pharmacotherapy should never be the sole treatment for an eating disorder but rather an adjunct to psychotherapy, weight restoration, and nutritional rehabilitation. A comprehensive review of the existing literature on pharmacological treatment for eating disorders is found in Crow and Mitchell (58).

While medications have been used since 1960 in treatment of anorexia nervosa, there is little empirical evidence for their efficacy. Early reports exploring the utility of antipsychotic medications found no beneficial effect over placebo and a variety of unwanted side effects. Later studies investigated tricyclic antidepressants and fluoxetine, an antidepressant belonging to the group known as selective serotonin reuptake inhibitors (SSRIs). While there has been little empirical evidence in general for the efficacy of antidepressants in treating anorexia nervosa, fluoxetine has been found to be helpful in relapse prevention when administered to nutritionally rehabilitated patients. However, there is the possibility of abuse, given the drug's known potential to promote weight loss. Appetite-enhancing agents have been found to provide little benefit, most likely due to the lack of true appetite in this disorder coupled with patients' fears of losing control and consequent hypervigilance over food consumption. Prokinetic agents may be useful in facilitating food intake when there is evidence of delayed gastric emptying. The use of anxiolytic agents has been suggested as an adjunct to psychotherapeutic measures to reduce anxiety around mealtimes, but lack of controlled studies precludes any definitive statements.

Investigations of the application of pharmacotherapy in bulimia nervosa have been more promising than for anorexia nervosa. Antidepressants—including tricyclic antidepressants, monoamine oxidase inhibitors, and SSRIs—have all been shown to provide some benefit in controlled trials. However, dropout rates have been high due to side effects and patient attitudes. Additionally, few long-term studies exist, although bulimia nervosa often requires extended treatment. SSRIs have recently been the drugs of choice in treatment of bulimia nervosa, given their minimal side effects and lower risk of suicidal overdose. The proven effective daily dose of fluoxetine is 60 mg.; the drug may be started at a daily dose of 20 mg and gradually increased to 60 mg. The physician must be aware that accurate dosing may be problematic in patients who purge very frequently. Responders should be maintained on the drug for at least 4 to 6 months, although patients have been known to relapse while on the medication. Research studies indicate that cognitive-behavioral therapy is superior to antidepressant medication alone in reducing bulimic symptoms, and antidepressant medication provides only modest additional benefit to cognitive-behavioral therapy. The additional gains must always be balanced against the side effects in each case. Since psychotherapy alone has been shown to provide substantial benefit in bulimia nervosa, the decision to administer pharmacotherapy should be made only after poor response to competent psychotherapy or in the case of comorbidity with depression or anxiety.

4.5 What Can Go Wrong

Eating disorders are complex and multifaceted and as such pose several difficulties for the practitioner. Due to denial of illness, patients with eating disorders often refuse or sabotage treatment efforts by health care providers. Decisions regarding imposing treatment must be made with consideration for ethical ramifications. It is tempting for the clinician to utilize scare tactics or engage in battles with these patients. However, power struggles with these patients only escalate the eating disorder symptomatology, given that control issues are often central to the development of eating disorders. Power struggles can be kept in check by forming an alliance with the patient, viewing the patient as part of the treatment team, and negotiating treatment options when possible. Least intrusive interventions should be attempted first and be given adequate time to work before resorting to more intrusive interventions. It is important to clarify for patients the point at which they will be tube-fed or hospitalized so that they may make informed decisions about their courses of action. All team members should be in agreement with the treatment philosophy and protocol in so that the patient will not be likely to "split" the members. Treating patients with respect ensures preservation of their self-esteem, a necessary factor for successful recovery.

REFERENCES

1. American Psychiatric Association. Diagnostic and Statistical Manual of Mental Disorders (4th ed). Washington, DC: Author, 1994.
2. World Health Organization. Mental and behavioral disorders. In: International Classification of Diseases, rev 10. Geneva: author, 1992, chap 5.
3. Bhanji S, Mattingly D. Medical Aspects of Anorexia Nervosa. London: Wright, 1988.
4. Garner DM, Garfinkel PE, O'Shaughnessy M. The validity of the distinction between bulimia with and without anorexia nervosa. Am J Psychiatry 1985; 142:581–587.
5. Rickards H, Prendergast M, Booth IW. Psychiatric presentation of Crohn's disease. Br J Psychiatry 1994; 164:256–261.

6. Gryboski JD. Eating disorders in inflammatory bowel disease. Am J Gastroenterol 1993; 88:293–296.
7. Meadows G, Treasure J. Bulimia nervosa and Crohn's disease: Two case reports. Acta Psychiatr Scand 1989; 79:413–414.
8. Gavish D, Eisenberg S, Berry EM, Kleinman Y, Witztum E, Norman J, Leitersdorf E. Bulimia. An underlying behavioral disorder in hyperlipidemic pancreatitis: A prospective multi-disciplinary approach. Arch Intern Med 1987; 147:705–708.
9. Cantwell R, Steel M. Screening for eating disorders in diabetes mellitus. J Psychosom Res 1996; 40:15–20.
10. Krieg JC. Eating disorders as assessed by cranial computerized tomography. In: Vranic M, ed. Fuel Homeostasis and the Nervous System. New York: Plenum Press, 1991, pp 223–229.
11. Martin F. Subgroups in anorexia nervosa: A family systems study. In: Darby PL, Garfinkel PE, Garner DM, Coscina DV, eds. Anorexia Nervosa: Recent Developments in Research. New York: Liss, 1983, pp 57–63.
12. Garfinkel PE, Kaplan AS, Garner DM, Darby PL. The differentiation of vomiting/weight loss as a conversion disorder from anorexia nervosa. Am J Psychiatry 1983; 140:1019–1022.
13. Beumont PJV, Booth AL, Abraham SF, Griffiths DA, Turner TR. A temporal sequence of symptoms in patients with anorexia nervosa: A preliminary report. In: Darby PL, Garfinkel PE, Garner DM, Coscina DV, eds. Anorexia Nervosa: Recent Developments in Research. New York: Liss, 1983, pp 129–136.
14. Fosson A, Knibbs J, Bryant-Waugh R, Lask B. Early onset anorexia nervosa. Arch Dis Child 1987; 62:114–118.
15. Russell GFM. The changing nature of anorexia nervosa: an introduction to the conference. J Psychiatr Res 1985; 19:101–109.
16. Jacobs BW, Isaacs S. Pre-pubertal anorexia nervosa: A retrospective controlled study. J Psychol Psychiatry 1986; 27:237–250.
17. Bryant-Waugh R, Kaminski Z. Eating disorders in children: An overview. In: Lask B, Bryant-Waugh R, eds. Childhood Onset Anorexia Nervosa and Related Eating Disorders. Hillsdale, NJ: Erlbaum, 1993, pp 17–30.
18. Gowers S, Crisp A, Joughin N, Bhat A. Premenarcheal anorexia nervosa. J Child Psychol Psychiatry 1991; 32:515–524.
19. Higgs J, Goodyer I, Birch J. Anorexia nervosa and food avoidance emotional disorder. Arch Dis Child 1989; 64:346–351.
20. Fairburn CG, Cooper PJ. Self-induced vomiting and bulimia nervosa: An undetected problem. BMJ 1982; 184:1153–1155.
21. Agras WS, Kirkley BG. Bulimia: theories of etiology. In: Brownell KD, Foreyt JP, eds. Handbook of Eating Disorders: Physiology, Psychology, and Treatment of Obesity, Anorexia, and Bulimia. New York: Basic Books, 1986, pp 367–378.
22. Mitchell JE, Hatsukami D, Eckert ED, Pyle RL. Characteristics of 275 patients with bulimia. Am J Psychiatry 1985; 142:482–485.
23. Crisp AH, Palmer RL, Kalucy RS. How common is anorexia nervosa? A prevalence study. Br J Psychiatry 1976; 128:549–554.
24. Moss RA, Jennings G, McFarland JH, Carter P. Binge eating, vomiting, and weight fear in a female high school population. J Fam Pract 1984; 18:313–320.

25. Johnson-Sabine E, Wood K, Patton G, Mann A, Wakeling A. Abnormal eating attitudes in London schoolgirls—A prospective epidemiological study. Factors associated with abnormal response on screening questionnaires. Psychol Med 1988; 18: 615–622.

26. Crowther JH, Tennenbaum DL, Hobfoll SE, Stephens MAP. The Etiology of Bulimia Nervosa: the Individual and Familial Context. Philadelphia: Hemisphere, 1990.

27. Whitaker A, Johnson J, Shaffer D, Rapoport JL, Kalikow K, Walsh BT, Davies M, Braiman S, Dolinsky A. Uncommon troubles in young people: Prevalence estimates of selected psychiatric disorders in a non-referred psychiatric population. Arch of Gen Psychiatry 1990; 47:487–496.

28. Johnson CL, Lewis C, Love S, Lewis L, Stuckey M. Incidence and correlates of bulimic behavior in a female high school population. J Youth Adolesc 1984; 13: 15–26.

29. Anderson, AE. Males with Eating Disorders. New York: Brunner/Mazel, 1990.

30. Garner DM, Rockert W, Olmsted MP, Johnson C, Coscina, DV. Psychoeducational principles in the treatment of bulimia and anorexia nervosa. In: Garner DM, Garfinkel PE, eds. Handbook of Psychotherapy for Anorexia Nervosa and Bulimia. New York: Guilford Press, 1985, pp 513–572.

31. Mitchell JE, Pomeroy C, Adson DE. Managing medical complications. In: Garner DM, Garfinkel PE, eds. Handbook of Treatment of Eating Disorders. New York: Guilford Press, 1997, pp 383–393.

32. Schwartz DM, Thompson MG. Do anorectics get well? Current research and future needs. Am J Psychiatry 1981; 138:319–323.

33. Crisp AH. Anorexia nervosa with normal body weight: The abnormal normal weight control syndrome. Int J Psychiatry Med 1982; 11:203–233.

34. Webb WL, Gehi M. Electrolyte and fluid imbalance: Neuropsychiatric manifestations. Psychosomatics 1983; 22:199–203.

35. Mitchell JE, Pyle RL, Eckert ED, Hatsukami D, Lentz R. Electrolyte and other physiological abnormalities in patients with bulimia. Psychol Med 1983; 13:273–278.

36. Mitchell JE, Pyle RL. The bulimic syndrome in normal weight individuals: A review. Int J Eating Disord 1982; 1(2):61–73.

37. Fairbum C. Binge-eating and bulimia nervosa. Smith, Kline and French Laboratory Research 1982; 1:1–20.

38. Levin PA, Falko JM, Dixon K, Gallup EM, Saunders W. Benign parotid enlargement in bulimia. Ann Intern Med 1980; 93:827–829.

39. Stege P, Visco-Dangler L, Rye L. Anorexia nervosa: Review including oral and dental manifestations. J Am Dent Assoc 1982; 104:648–652.

40. Pirke KM. Menstrual cycle and neuroendocrine disturbances of the gonadal axis in bulimia nervosa. In: Fichter MM, ed. Bulimia Nervosa: Basic Research, Diagnosis, and Therapy. New York: Wiley, 1990, pp 223–234.

41. Johnson CL, Stuckey MK, Lewis LD, Schwartz D. A descriptive survey of 509 cases of self-reported bulimia. In: Darby PL, Garfinkel PE, Garner DM, Coscina DV, eds. Anorexia Nervosa: Recent Development in Research. New York: Liss, 1983, pp 159–171.

42. Garfinkel PE, Moldofsky H, Garner DM. The heterogeneity of anorexia nervosa. Arch Gen Psychiatry 1980; 37:1036–1040.

43. Johnson CL, Stuckey MK, Lewis LD, Schwartz D. Bulimia: A descriptive survey of 316 cases. Int J Eating Disord 1982; 2(1):3–16.

44. Mitchell JE, Pyle RL, Eckert ED. Frequency and duration of binge-eating episodes in patients with bulimia. Am J Psychiatry 1981; 138:835–836.

45. Wolf EM, Crowther JH. Personality and eating habit variables as predictors of severity of binge eating and weight. Addict Behav 1983; 8:335–344.

46. Rosen JC, Leitenberg H. Bulimia nervosa: Treatment with exposure and response prevention. Behav Ther 1982; 13:117–124.

47. Barbosa-Salvidar JL, Van Itallie TB. Semi-starvation: An overview of an old problem. Bull NY Acad Med 1979; 55:774–797.

48. Hudson JI, Pope HG, Jonas JM, Yurgelun-Todd D. Family history study of anorexia nervosa and bulimia. Br J Psychiatry 1983; 142:133–138.

49. Wurtman RJ, Wurtman JJ. Nutrients, neurotransmitter synthesis, and the control of food intake. In: Stunkard AJ, Stellar E, eds. Eating and Its Disorders. New York: Raven Press, 1984, pp 77–86.

50. Rau JH, Green RS. Neurological factors affecting binge eating: Body over mind. In: Hawkins RC, Fremouw WJ, Clement PF, eds. The Binge-Purge Syndrome: Diagnosis, Treatment and Research, New York: Springer, 1984, pp 123–143.

51. Bruch H. Eating Disorders: Obesity, Anorexia Nervosa and the Person Within. New York: Basic Books, 1973.

52. Coffman DA. A clinically derived treatment model for the binge-purge syndrome. In: Hawkins RC, Fremouw WJ, Clement PF, eds. The Binge-Purge Syndrome: Diagnosis, Treatment, and Research. New York: Springer, 1984, pp 211–226.

53. Leon GR. Cognitive-behavior therapy for eating disturbances. In Kendall PC, Hollon SD, eds, Cognitive-Behavioral Interventions: Theory, Research, and Procedures New York: Academic Press, 1979, pp 357–388.

54. Crisp AH. Anorexia Nervosa: Let Me Be. London: Academic Press, 1980.

55. Orleans CT, Barnett LR. Bulimarexia: Guidelines for behavioral assessment and treatment. In: Hawkins RC, Fremouw WJ, Clement PF, eds. The Binge-Purge Syndrome: Diagnosis, Treatment, and Research. New York: Springer, 1984, pp 144–182.

56. Bryant-Waugh R, Knibbs J, Fosson A, Kaminski J, Lask J. Long-term follow-up of patients with early onset anorexia nervosa. Arch Dis Child 1988; 63:5–9.

57. Hsu LKG. Outcome of anorexia nervosa: A review of the literature (1954–1978). Arch Gen Psychiatry 1980; 37:1041–1046.

58. Crow SL, Mitchell, JE. Pharmacologic treatments for eating disorders. In: Thompson JK, ed. Body Image, Eating Disorders, and Obesity. Washington, DC: American Psychological Association, 1996, pp 345–360.

10

Obesity

Andrew M. Tershakovec, and
Virginia A. Stallings
University of Pennsylvania School of Medicine and The Children's
Hospital of Philadelphia, Philadelphia, Pennsylvania

Andrea S. Hiralall
The Children's Hospital of Philadelphia, Philadelphia, Pennsylvania

1 EPIDEMIOLOGY

The prevalence of obesity in children has increased dramatically over the last 20
to 30 years. Between 1988 and 1991, the overall prevalence of all children with
a body-mass index (BMI) greater than the 95th percentile was 11%, while 22%
were above the 85th percentile (1). Data from the National Health and Nutrition
Examination Surveys (NHANES), completed intermittently from 1963 to 1991,
demonstrated a 39 to 43% increase in the prevalence of 6- to 17-year-old white
children above the 85th percentile for BMI, while the prevalence of white children with BMI above the 95th percentile increased 68 to 167% over the same
period (Table 1).

Even more disturbing is the fact that the prevalence of overweight and
obesity increased even more dramatically in other ethnic groups, such as African-
American children. Though in most cases African-American children had a lower
prevalence of overweight and obesity than white children in the 1963–1970 time
period, that has changed in the most recent survey. Over the 1963–1991 time
period, the prevalence of 6- to 17-year-old African-American children with a

249

TABLE 1 Prevalence of Overweight (>85th percentile BMI) and Obesity (>95th percentile BMI) in Children and Adolescents (%)

Age, years	>85th percentile		>95th percentile	
	White	Black	White	Black
Boys 6–11				
1963–70	16.0	10.3	5.6	2.0
1971–74	19.5	12.3	6.7	5.6
1976–80	20.8	15.1	7.9	7.9
1988–97	22.3	27.2	10.4	13.4
Girls 6–11				
1963–70	15.7	12.1	5.1	5.3
1971–74	13.4	16.8	4.5	3.5
1976–80	15.4	18.4	6.4	11.3
1988–97	22.0	30.7	10.2	16.2
Boys 12–17				
1963–70	15.8	10.4	5.4	3.7
1971–74	15.3	12.3	5.5	4.3
1976–80	16.6	14.5	5.4	6.3
1988–97	22.6	23.3	14.4	9.4
Girls 12–17				
1963–70	15.0	16.6	5.0	6.6
1971–74	19.7	20.8	6.6	12.2
1976–80	15.6	18.2	5.3	10.4
1988–97	20.3	29.9	8.4	14.4

Source: Ref. 1.

BMI greater than the 85th percentile increased 81 to 164%, while the prevalence of BMI greater than the 95th percentile increased 118 to 570% over this period. Thus, the greatest increases in the prevalence of obesity were in minority groups and in the proportion of children who were more severely overweight.

A comparison of NHANES I (completed 1971–1974) and NHANES III (completed 1988–1994) demonstrated that the prevalence of overweight 4- to 5-year-old children increased significantly over this time period; however, no such increase was observed in the 1- to 3-year-old children. Though the prevalence of overweight children increased among Mexican-American, non-Hispanic black, and non-Hispanic white children, the highest prevalence was observed among the Mexican-American children. These results suggest that efforts to prevent the onset of obesity must begin in very young children.

Obese children are at risk for becoming obese adults. The risk of remaining obese increases with age and the degree of obesity. For example, 11-year-old children who are overweight are more than twice as likely to remain overweight at the age of 15 than are 7-year-old overweight children. Even during infancy, a high weight (>90th percentile during the first 6 months of life) is associated with a twofold increase in the rate of obesity in adults 20 to 30 years later.

The risk of becoming obese as a child and remaining obese as an adult is also influenced by family history. Forty percent of children with one overweight parent have been noted to be overweight, while 80% of children with two overweight parents become overweight. Only 10% of children with no overweight parents become overweight. The interaction between age and the degree of obesity, mentioned above, and the family history are well demonstrated (see Table 2). A survey of medical records of a Washington State health maintenance organization demonstrated that older children, more obese children, and children with an obese mother or father were much more likely to be obese as young adults (21 to 29 years of age) (2). Family history of cardiovascular disease has been utilized to identify children at risk for premature heart disease. Given the clustering of obesity within families, it would seem appropriate to utilize a similar strategy with obesity and to institute anticipatory health promotion efforts for children of obese or overweight parents.

Other factors in the family and environment of a child have been associated with obesity, including single parents, only children, nonworking parents, parents

TABLE 2 Risk of Young Adult Obesity According to Child's Age and Parents' Relative Weight

Child's age, years	Parent's weight status	Odds ratio
3–5	Mother not obese	1.0
	Mother obese	3.6
	Father not obese	1.0
	Father obese	2.9
10–14	Mother not obese	1.0
	Mother obese	3.1
	Father not obese	1.0
	Father obese	2.4
3–5	Child not obese	1.0
	Child obese/very obese	4.1
	Child very obese	7.9
10–14	Child not obese	1.0
	Child obese/very obese	28.3
	Child very obese	44.3

Source: Ref. 2.

with lower educational levels, and the quality of the home environment. However, when other potentially important covariates are included in the analyses, some of these factors are not independently associated with childhood obesity. For example, if obesity occurs at a higher rate among adults with low educational levels, a higher rate of obesity in the children of these adults could be associated with their parents' higher relative weight and/or lower educational level. In addition, much of the data relating to sociodemographic factors and obesity are conflicting or rather complex. For example, obesity has been positively associated with lower socioeconomic status in women but not in men (3). Differences in reported results may be due to differences between the groups studied.

In addition, the causative agents linking obesity with other factors are not always well explained. For example, as described in Section 3.4, obese children have been noted to suffer from a variety of psychosocial problems. Whether these problems predispose the children to the development of obesity or obesity predisposes to the development of psychosocial problems is not known. Despite these unknowns and inconsistencies, it seems clear that children from altered or stressed psychosocial environments are at greater risk to develop obesity. This also suggests that an evaluation and therapeutic plan for the obese child must include these factors in order to maximize the opportunity for success.

2   ETIOLOGY OF OBESITY

In simple terms, obesity is caused by an energy imbalance in which the individual expends less energy than he or she takes in. A chronic, small energy imbalance can have a profound effect on weight gain. For example, a positive energy balance of 100 kcal/day would induce a weight gain of approximately 4.5 kg. per year, or 45 kg. over 10 years. [Note that 100 kcal represents the caloric content of less than an average can of a carbonated beverage or a chocolate bar, or the energy expended walking approximately 30 min at a moderate pace (3 mi/hr; 4–6 km/hr) for the average man or woman.] The fact that such a small difference in energy balance over an expended period of time can have such a dramatic effect makes investigations into the causes of obesity and therapeutic attempts at treating obesity frustratingly difficult. Despite these challenges, the search for the causes for obesity has focused on four general areas: genetics, environment, energy expenditure, and dietary factors.

2.1   Genetics

Certain genetic syndromes, most prominently Prader-Willi syndrome, are associated with an increased rate of obesity. However, it must be noted that identifiable syndromes associated with obesity are very rare. For example, the genetic and other syndromes associated with childhood obesity listed in Table 3 represent less than 1% of the cases of obesity in children.

TABLE 3 Differential Diagnosis: Syndromes Associated
with Obesity in Childhood

Alström-Hallgren syndrome
Carpenter syndrome
Cohen syndrome
Cushing syndrome
Growth hormone deficiency
Hyperinsulinemia
Hypothalamic dysfunction
Hypothyroidism
Laurence-Moon-Biedl (Bardet-Biedl) syndrome
Polycystic ovary (Stein-Leventhal) syndrome
Prader-Willi syndrome
Pseudohypoparathyroidism (type I)
Turner syndrome

Source: Ref. 34.

The clustering of obesity within families also suggests a potential genetic and/or shared-environment input. As described in Section 1, children of obese parents are at significantly increased risk for the development of obesity. Useful information attempting to define the genetics versus environmental influence on the development of obesity is gained from studies comparing twins reared together and twins reared apart as well as from studies of adopted children. A strong relationship exists between the relative weight of adults who were adopted as children and the relative weight of their biological parents, while no relationship exists between the relative weight of the adults who were adopted as children and their adoptive parents (4). Similarly, the correlation between the BMI of twins reared apart was only slightly lower than that for twins reared together (5). Further, of the potential environmental factors assessed, only those specific to the individual but not shared family characteristics were significantly associated with BMI. The authors of these two papers concluded that the family and childhood environment have little or no influence on adult relative weight.

Much current research is focused on specific genetic factors potentially related to the development of obesity. Much of the work involves the identification of genetic factors in animal models of obesity and attempts to identify these genetic factors in humans. One well-described example of this is the *ob* mouse and leptin (6). The *ob* strain of mice, which develops severe obesity, was found to be missing the *ob* gene, which codes for the production of leptin. In normal mice, leptin was found to be positively associated with relative weight (e.g., heavier mice have higher leptin levels). *Ob* mice were found to have very low leptin levels. When given leptin, an *ob* mouse decreases its caloric intake and loses weight. Therefore it was proposed that leptin acts in a feedback loop to report relative body size to centers of the body that control dietary intake. Hypothetically, for example, as the mouse gained weight, the leptin level rose, presumably inducing eating control centers to decrease dietary intake, which caused the mouse to lose weight. It was therefore postulated that obese humans were leptin-deficient. However, of the many obese humans who have been screened, only a handful have been identified as being leptin-deficient. In most cases, leptin levels have been shown to correlate with relative weight in humans as in genetically normal mice. This example and subsequent experience suggest that the control of weight and eating is a very complex process, and single genetic factors that individually act to promote the development of obesity in large numbers of individuals may not exist.

The rapid rise in the prevalence of obesity also argues against a purely genetic cause. Our genetic makeup cannot have changed so dramatically over the last 30 years as to explain the rapid increase in the prevalence of obesity over this time. Most experts believe that certain people have a genetic makeup that predisposes them to the development of obesity, given the appropriate environment. Thus, it is suggested that the gene-environment interaction, along with a changing environment, have supported the rapid increase in obesity.

2.2 Environment

In contrast to the findings relating to adopted children and twins described in the discussion of genetics (Sec. 2.1), several environmental factors have been associated with a greater risk of obesity in children. These include socioeconomic factors, parental education, and family size. Other environmental factors have also been described. A large national survey of 6- to 11-year-old children showed that rates of obesity were higher in the fall and winter, in metropolitan areas, and in the U.S. Northeast and Midwest. It has been suggested that the common thread in these observations is that the regions and seasons that allow and support more outdoor activities are also associated with less obesity. Children playing outdoors are more active than children playing indoors.

One of the more important environmental factors relating to the increasing prevalence of obesity in children seems to be the introduction of television, computers, and video games into children's environments. Television watching is associated with less physical activity, even in children as young as 3 to 4 years old. Though television watching has not been associated with increased relative weight in children younger than 8 years of age, a relationship between television watching and obesity has been clearly described in older children, including a clear dose response (7,8). For example, 10- to 15-year-old children were 5.5 times as likely to be overweight if they watched more than 5 hr of television per day as compared to those who watched less than 2 hr per day. Overweight remission over the next 4 years was also 8.3 times less likely in the children who watched more than 5 hr of television per day as compared to those watching less than 2 hr per day (7,8). Although excessive use of computer and video games has not been extensively studied, a similar effect is likely.

Though much of the effect of television seems to be related to decreased physical activity, other factors seem to play a role also. Children who watch more television ask their parents more frequently to buy food. In addition, the mothers of children who watch more television subsequently buy their children the requested foods more frequently. This suggests that the food-oriented advertising aimed at children encourages them to ask their parents for the advertised foods. In turn, the more the children ask for these foods, the more the parents go and buy the foods. Thus, television watching seems to alter the child's and the parent's behavior.

2.3 Energy Expenditure

Three main aspects of energy expenditure have been evaluated in considering energy expenditure and energy imbalances as potential causes of excessive weight gain—resting energy expenditure or resting metabolic rate, energy of physical activity, and total energy expenditure.

It is a commonly held belief among families of overweight children that their children must have a "low metabolism," supporting their excess weight gain. However, the data supporting this are mixed. Studies of infants and children who had at least one overweight parent suggested that those children who gained excess weight did have lower resting or total energy expenditure (9). The risk of gaining over 7.5 kg over a 4-year period was increased fourfold for southwestern adult Native Americans who were found to have a low total energy expenditure. Similarly, those who gained more than 10 kg over the 4-year period were noted to have an adjusted resting metabolic rate that was 70 kcal/day lower than the rate of those who gained less than 10 kg over this time period (10).

However, more recent data relating to energy expenditure and weight gain are more conflicting. In these studies, energy expenditure was not found to be predictive of excess weight gain or increased fat mass in infants or children (11,12). In our clinical experience despite the family's belief, it is rare to document a truly low resting energy expenditure adjusted for body composition in an obese child.

Given the high and rapidly rising prevalence of obesity in African Americans, especially African-American women, ethnic differences in resting energy expenditure have also been reviewed. Though most of the data support the existence of lower resting energy expenditure among African-American females (especially among premenarcheal girls) when compared to white females, these data are also somewhat conflicting.

It has also been suggested that obese individuals are less physically active. The decreased energy for physical activity could induce a positive energy balance, inducing excessive weight gain. Though some studies have suggested that obese children may be less physically active than nonobese children, it seems that obese individuals expend so much extra energy to carry their excess body mass through these activities that they expend as much energy or more completing these activities as nonobese children. However, increasing physical activity in children as young as 3 to 5 years of age has been associated with decreasing relative weight over the next 2 years. This observation, the previously cited association between television watching and prevalence of obesity, and the improved outcome with weight management that includes formal exercise support the influence of sedentary activity and physical activity on the development and treatment of obesity. However, the negative findings described above also suggest that alterations in the energy expended during physical activity are only a portion of the puzzle relating to the development of obesity.

It is also somewhat frightening to see how sedentary some children are. Parents have reported that 5-year-old children spent an average of 10.3 to 16.0 hr playing and an average of 24.5 to 28.7 hr watching television per week (13). Clearly, preventive health efforts and therapeutic programs for obese children must work to encourage them to be more active.

2.4 Dietary Intake

Data relating to dietary intake and obesity suggest that obese children tend to consume diets higher in fat. High-fat foods tend to have higher caloric density owing to such factors as lower fiber and water content and the higher caloric density of fat (9 kcal/g for fat versus 4 kcal/g for carbohydrates and protein). The body also expends less energy metabolizing and storing fat. Thus eating an equivalent volume or weight of high-fat foods will support the ingestion of more calories.

Recent information also suggests that humans have a preference for foods of high caloric density (14). In an environment where food is relatively scarce (as is thought to have been the case on earth for thousands of years), a preference for such foods created a survival advantage. In our current environment, where most people have easy access to an abundance of such foods, this preference may be supporting the increasing prevalence of obesity.

One of the main public health messages relating to diet over the last 20 years has been to lower the fat content of the American diet so as to help lower cholesterol levels and the rate of cardiovascular disease. Nutrition surveys document significant decreases in the proportion of calories ingested as fat over this time. Despite the success of this campaign, it has had one fairly negative impact: many people have adopted the attitude that since high-fat foods are "bad" for you, low-fat foods must be good for you. This attitude may be appropriate for foods of high nutrient density, such as low-fat milk and meats, but not for foods of low nutrient density, such as cookies and cakes. Thus, following such a broad-based low-fat diet, including high-calorie, low-fat products, may actually increase caloric intake.

Despite this, following a low-fat, low-caloric-density diet does seem to have utility in weight management. A survey of obese adults who have been successful at maintaining 13.6 kg of weight loss for at least 1 year demonstrates that these persons almost universally follow a low-fat diet (15).

There has been recent interest in and promotion of low-carbohydrate diets. It is proposed that eating a diet high in high-glycemic-index foods induces a high insulin response, which sets off a cascade of negative health consequences and promotes excessive food intake and, potentially, excessive weight gain. The data supporting this theory are very limited, especially relating to children (16). Clearly, this approach must be studied before it is implemented in children, especially given the described long-term success with weight loss and maintenance described above with a low-fat and low-caloric-density diet.

It is difficult to assess the caloric intake and the caloric needs of children and adolescents, and the impact of caloric intake on excessive weight gain. Most people tend to underreport caloric intake; obese adolescents underreport caloric intake more than nonobese adolescents. Surveys suggest that obese adolescents may underreport caloric intake by 40 to 60%. Thus, diet recalls or other methods to assess the caloric of obese individuals must be "taken with a grain of salt." Furthermore, standardized equations designed to calculate the resting energy requirements of children have been shown to overestimate the true caloric needs of obese children and adolescents.

There is increasing evidence that parenting style can also influence dietary behavior. It has been postulated that children have an inherent ability to regulate their own caloric intake appropriately. However, it has been shown that overweight preschool children are less able to control their caloric intake appropriately. Furthermore, the best predictor of the child's ability to regulate his or her own caloric intake is parental control during meals [e.g., children whose mothers imposed more control on them during meals (e.g., "clean off your plate, "just take another bite") were less able to control their caloric intake appropriately] (17). It has been suggested that when external control is imposed on children during meals, they lose the natural ability to control their own intake. These children are then at risk for eating inappropriately in response to external cues, having lost their natural internal control mechanisms.

3 HEALTH CONSEQUENCES OF OBESITY

In adults, obesity is associated with an increased risk for mortality, coronary heart disease, hypertension, lipid disorders, non-insulin-dependent diabetes mellitus (NIDDM), orthopedic problems, stroke, gall bladder disease, sleep apnea and some cancers (18–20). Similar medical problems can develop or begin to develop in obese children. Though acute medical problems that require immediate intervention are rare in obese children, the practitioner should screen all obese children for these acute issues and consider implementing interventions that have potential for long-term prevention.

3.1 Cardiovascular Disease Related Comorbidity

Obesity, abdominal fat, and visceral fat have been shown to be associated with cardiovascular disease (CVD) risk factors in children and adults (21). For example, an association between a central fat distribution and less favorable lipoprotein levels and increased blood pressure has been described in 9- to 17-year-old children. Similarly, a central fat distribution and higher visceral abdominal fat have been shown to be associated with higher insulin levels in Japanese as well as in both black and white Americans (21).

Most commonly, obesity is associated with elevations in triglyceride level and decreases in the level of high-density-lipoprotein cholesterol (HDL-C) (see Chap. 11). However, even relatively small reductions in weight in adults (10% of body weight) have been associated with improvement in CVD risk (22). Though the data are more limited in children, it appears that relatively small changes in overweight status have similar effects on CVD risk.

Recent information expands the list of CVD risk factors associated with obesity to include such things as low antioxidant intake or status, small LDL-C particle size, altered hemostatic/fibrinolytic factors, and altered sympathetic nervous system tone. These factors also interact with the previously noted factors. For example, higher levels of nonesterified fatty acids, abdominal fat, obesity, and insulin resistance are associated with thrombosis and thrombotic potential (22) and small LDL-C size has been associated with a poor lipoprotein profile, increased glucose and insulin levels, and insulin resistance. Similarly, weight loss has been associated with short-term improvement in many of these factors, including blood pressure, lipoprotein profile, hemostatic activity, norepinephrine level, total body fat, and visceral abdominal fat) (23). However, the degree of weight loss needed to induce a significant change in these factors has not been defined.

3.2 Non-Insulin-Dependent Diabetes Mellitus

Though non-insulin-dependent diabetes mellitus (NIDDM) was once a relatively rare problem in children, it is now becoming more common. For example, the incidence of NIDDM in adolescents was estimated to increase tenfold from 1982 to 1994 in the greater Cincinnati area (24). The mean age of the newly presenting patients with NIDDM was 13.8 years, while the mean BMI was 37.7. The high relative weight of these children, along with the known association between obesity and NIDDM, suggests that this rapid rise in NIDDM among adolescents is related to the rapid rise in obesity. In addition, data from the Pathobiological Determinants of Atherosclerosis in Youth Study describe the association between elevated glycohemoglobin, increased adiposity, and atherosclerosis in young adults (24). This suggests that we will soon see an epidemic of adults with obesity and diabetes-related comorbidities. In addition, experience with adults suggests that weight management and/or weight maintenance after weight loss may be more difficult in persons with NIDDM. This clearly supports the need for preventive and therapeutic efforts for obesity and NIDDM that begin in childhood.

3.3 Other Medical Factors

Other factors that may be primarily or secondarily related to obesity are listed in Table 4. Recent experience has added nonalcoholic steatohepatitis to this list (25). In children, nonalcoholic steatohepatitis usually presents when an obese child is unexpectedly found to have mildly elevated liver function tests without an obvious cause and a liver biopsy shows steatosis. As the liver function abnormalities have been shown to resolve with weight loss and no other etiology for the steatosis has been identified, this entity seems to be related to obesity. Adults with obesity-related steatohepatitis have developed cirrhosis, and in some instances have gone on to liver failure and liver transplant. Given the epidemic of childhood obesity, one would expect to see an epidemic of such cases, though for unknown reasons this does not seem to be the case.

3.4 Psychological Factors

Pediatric obesity is often associated with negative psychosocial complications for children and adolescents. For example, obese children and adolescents tend to suffer from low self-esteem, poor body image, depression, and learning problems more than their nonobese peers do. Some experts in weight management believe that the psychological complications of obesity are more pervasive and damaging to the growing child than the physiological problems these children endure (26). It is not known whether these psychosocial problems develop as a consequence of the child's obesity or are factors that increase the child's vulnerability to becoming obese. What is known is that obese children and adolescents are frequently the target of early discrimination and stigmatization. As the obese child ages, the effects of discrimination and stigmatization become more salient and may spread to several aspects of his or her life including social, economic, and educational areas (3,26).

For many obese children, the stigma of being obese carries with it potentially harmful psychosocial problems. Peer rejection accompanied by social isola-

TABLE 4 Assessment of Medical Conditions Related to Obesity and Its Diagnosis: What Can Go Wrong—Warning Signs

Findings	Potential conditions
History	
Developmental delay	Genetic
Poor linear growth	Hypothyroidism, Cushing syndrome, Prader-Willi syndrome
Headaches	Pseudotumor cerebri
Nighttime breathing difficulty	Sleep apnea, obesity hypoventilation syndrome
Daytime somnolence	Sleep apnea, obesity hypoventilation syndrome
Abdominal pain	Gallbladder disease
Hip or knee pain	Slipped capital femoral epiphysis
Oligomenorrhea or amenorrhea	Polycystic ovary syndrome
Family history	
Obesity	
NIDDM	
Cardiovascular disease	
Hypertension	
Dyslipidemia	
Gallbladder disease	
Social/psychological history	
Tobacco use	
Depression	
Eating disorder	
Social isolation, depression	Lowered self-esteem (if program unsuccessful)
Increased family conflicts	
Refusal of insurance to cover obesity management	
Physical examination	
Height, weight, and BMI	
Excessive and rapid weight loss, arrhythmia, muscle spasm	Inadequate nutrition, provision of unbalanced diet
Triceps skinfold thickness	
Blood pressure	Risk of cardiovascular disease; Cushing syndrome
Truncal obesity	
Dysmorphic features	Genetic disorders, including Prader-Willi syndrome
Acanthosis nigricans	NIDDM, insulin resistance
Hirsutism	Polycystic ovary syndrome; Cushing syndrome
Violaceous striae	Cushing syndrome
Optic disks	Pseudomotor cerebri
Tonsils	Sleep apnea
Abdominal pain, vomiting	Gallbladder disease
Undescended testicles	Prader-Willi syndrome
Limited hip range of motion	Slipped capital femoral epiphysis
Lower leg bowing	Blount's disease

Key: NIDDM, non-insulin-dependent diabetes mellitus; BMI, body-mass index.
Source: Ref. 29.

tion is one such problem. A number of studies have shown that children as young as age 6 have already incorporated preferences for "thinness." Results from preference tests—including sociometric ratings and other checklists that assess social acceptance—suggest that children would prefer to have as friends other children with a wide variety of handicaps rather than children who are overweight. In fact, overweight children are ranked lowest as preferred playmates. Furthermore, even young children already associate several negative characteristics to peers that are overweight, such as "sloppy," "lazy," and "slow" (3). Obese peers are viewed as unable to play and run like other peers, which makes them less attractive to other children.

More recent studies of social acceptance among obese children indicate that these children are less likely to be rejected by peers when there is a medical explanation for the child's obese condition. In this case, the obese child is not "blamed" for being obese and fewer negative characteristics are assigned to the child. On the other hand, peers are more likely to tease and reject an obese child, who is seen as being at fault for his or her obesity. Such a child is thought to "eat too much" and "does not care about being overweight." The most unfortunate outcome of such early discrimination is that it puts the obese child at risk for increased negative social experiences that can persist into adolescence and adulthood (26). For example, an obese child who is discriminated against at an early age may shy away from future social interaction in order to avoid further humiliation and rejection by peers. Continued social isolation is associated with the development of depression, emotional disturbance, and other behavioral problems. A metanalysis of research studies on the treatment of pediatric obesity estimated that approximately 25% of obese children entering treatment meet or exceed clinical levels for psychological problems on standardized measures of behavior, with the most prevalent abnormalities in the areas of depression and social problems.

Although obese children are at high risk for poor peer relation and depression, obese adolescents appear to suffer more from low self-esteem than their prepubescent counterparts. Unlike younger children, obese adolescents tend to derive their self-esteem from cultural messages and peer evaluations. Thus, social rejection may have more serious implications for self-esteem and emotional development during adolescence.

In general, the results of research on the self-esteem of obese children and adolescents has been inconsistent. Some studies have found that obese children exhibit lower levels of self-esteem than their nonobese peers, while other studies have shown no difference between the two groups. More recent examinations of self-esteem among obese children and adolescents have demonstrated that what obese children believe to be the cause of their weight problem is associated with the way they feel about themselves. Children who make internal attributions (i.e., blame themselves) about their obesity are more likely to have low self-esteem and experience depression than those children who believe that external forces play a greater role in their weight problem (i.e., genetic predisposition, or a medical problem). The external attribution seems to function as a form of self-protection for these children. Because children's interpretation of the negative feedback they receive from others in reference to their weight may serve to modulate their self-esteem and affect, positive feedback and support from parents can act as a "buffer."

Low self-esteem is often a precursor to the negative body image found among adolescent girls. Caucasian female adolescents who have a negative body image are at greater risk for eating disorders, including bulimia, binge eating disorder, and anorexia nervosa. In a cross-sectional study of obese children 7 to 13 years of age, it was found that over 50% reported being very concerned about their weight, and over one-third of these had tried to lose weight by dieting. Not surprisingly, older females made up the largest percentage of children who displayed dieting behaviors and concerns with weight. A relatively large proportion of morbidly obese adolescent girls have also been described as having characteristics of binge eating disorder. African-American females exhibit a substantially lower rate of eating disorders, which is partially attributed to the greater acceptance of overweight in this culture.

Poor family functioning is yet another psychosocial factor associated with obesity. Severely obese children tend to come from families in which the parents have difficulty in placing appropriate limits on the child's eating as well as other aspects of behavior. One study of family functioning found that mothers of obese children had significantly less control over their child's environment and provided less structure to their children than mothers of nonobese children. Furthermore, other studies have shown that increased parental distress and psychopathology are associated with childhood obesity as well.

Other work examining the relationship between family functioning and children's eating behavior suggests that children's food choices are also heavily shaped by the food selections and eating habits observed in their parents. This may have important implications for families in which obesity, dieting, and weight control are issues. For example, children's eating patterns may be altered by the parents' degree of dietary restraint, levels of hunger, and disinhibition. Parents who report dietary disinhibition and problems in controlling their eating are more likely to have daughters with similar problems and difficulties with weight control (27).

Unfortunately, obesity in children and adolescents may have long-term psychosocial implications. The National Longitudinal Survey of Youth, which surveyed 10,000 individuals 16 to 24 years of age, demonstrated that obese females were less likely to marry, had lower incomes, and achieved lower levels of education than nonobese females. In contrast, obese males did not differ from nonobese males on any of these variables (3).

4 EVALUATION AND TREATMENT

4.1 Anthropometric Assessment

Strictly speaking, *obesity* refers to excess body fat. Unfortunately, real body composition assessment using accurate body composition assessment methods, such as underwater weighing or dual-energy absorptiometry, are not easily accessible for practicing physicians. Therefore, other methods, which estimate or act as a proxy measure for adiposity are utilized.

Obtaining age- and gender-specific weight and height percentiles from the regular National Center for Health Statistics growth curves is the easiest way to qualitatively assess relative weight for children. A more quantitative assessment of relative weight can be gained from the weight-for-height percentile curves; however, these curves can only be used for younger children. Percent ideal body weight can also be estimated from the growth curves, though this cannot be completed for tall adolescents.

To calculate ideal body weight:

Plot the child's height on the growth curve.
Draw a horizontal line to the 50th percentile height curve.
At this point of intersection, draw a vertical line down to the 50th percentile weight curve. This point of intersection represents the child's ideal body weight.
About 90 to 110% of ideal body weight is considered the normal range.
More than 110% is considered overweight.
More than 120% is considered obese.

One of the most commonly used measures to assess relative weight is the body mass index [BMI = weight (kg)/height (m)^2]. In adults, a BMI above 25 defines overweight and above 30 defines obesity. In addition, the First Federal Obesity Clinical Guidelines also use the waist measurement along with the BMI to set priorities for clinical intervention in adults. Unfortunately, these guidelines cannot be applied to children.

BMI changes with age in children. Therefore we are not able to set a particular BMI cut point to define obesity in children. It is generally acknowledged that a BMI above the 95th percentile (age- and gender-specific) (28,29) usually identifies an obese child, while a BMI above the 85th percentile identifies an overweight child. The introduction of the new growth charts, which will include age versus BMI gender-specific curves, will make the use of BMI to assess relative weight in children more practical.

Measurements of skinfold thickness do specifically provide some indication of subcutaneous adiposity; however, these measurements are difficult to complete accurately, especially with very obese individuals. Few practicing physicians are trained to complete these measurements accurately, though some dietitians do use these measurements in their regular clinical practice. In general, a triceps skinfold >85th percentile is considered overweight and >95th percentile indicates obesity. Equations have been developed that estimate body composition based upon measurements of skinfold thickness. As previously mentioned, these are not very practical for use by primary care providers. However, if they are utilized, one must make sure that the specific equation has been validated for use with the age, gender, and ethnic group of interest.

4.2 Medical Assessment

The assessment of an obese child should include a routine history and physical. Though genetic or other syndromes associated with obesity are rare, the signs of such conditions should be reviewed. The practitioner should also be familiar with the secondary medical problems associated with obesity.

The specific signs and symptoms associated with obesity or the treatment of obesity are listed in Table 4. All of these should be reviewed in assessing an obese child. Further assessment should be dependent on specific physical findings (e.g., violaceous striae). In addition, screening for dyslipidemia and insulin resistance should be considered. Given the association between dyslipidemia and obesity, the clustering of CVD risk factors in obese individuals, and the relatively poor predictive value of family history to predict child hyperlipidemia, lipid profile screening (total cholesterol, triglycerides, HDL-C) should be considered as part of the initial evaluation of the obese child. Similarly, a fasting glucose and insulin level or formal glucose tolerance testing should be considered for those with acanthosis nigricans. Though families will commonly state that they feel their child's obesity is related to endocrinological causes, thyroid function testing or other screening without specific indications has a very low yield.

Measurement of resting metabolic rate should be considered for several reasons. The resting energy expenditure prediction equations are relatively inaccurate for obese children and adolescents. Actually completing the measurement and using this individualized information will allow more appropriate dietary counseling. This is especially important given inaccuracies in diet recall. In addition, many families feel that their child's obesity is linked to a low metabolic rate and that intervention is therefore futile. Concrete assessment of metabolic rate allows a factual discussion of the child's condition.

4.3 Psychological Assessment

Given that there is increased risk for psychosocial problems among obese children and their families, a psychological evaluation should be included as part of the overall assessment of the obese child. It is known that the presence of psychosocial problems can have detrimental effects on treatment outcomes in general.

Furthermore, research on treatment outcomes specific to the obese population indicates that obese adults with psychosocial difficulties are less likely to benefit from therapy for weight problems. Similarly, it is often difficult for obese children to make adequate progress if underlying issues of family dysfunction and psychological problems are not identified or addressed (26).

A psychological evaluation will help a practitioner determine if more intensive psychological treatment is needed for a given child or family. It can also help to pinpoint areas that may interfere with successful treatment. Although there are no standard test batteries available to assess the obese patient, it makes sense that a psychological evaluation should encompass those areas of psychosocial functioning known to be problematic within this population. In selecting tests and measures to include in a battery, the clinician should make an effort to include instruments that are standardized and have established reliability and validity; also, tests should be included that examine the behavioral and emotional status of the child, the parents, and the family as a whole.

To assess the child's psychosocial functioning, a battery should include a measure of overall behavior, a measure of depression, a self-esteem inventory, and an informal assessment of the child's and family's readiness to make dietary and exercise changes. Parental psychological functioning can be quickly examined using a brief self-report measure of psychological distress and/or psychopathology. Significant parental psychological dysfunction may interfere with the child's course of treatment. The parent's eating habits and the presence of eating disorders should also be assessed, given the important influence that parental eating behaviors can exert on children's eating behaviors.

Finally, an assessment of family functioning is useful to ascertain the family's strengths and weaknesses as they enter a weight management program. Successful treatment of obese children typically requires families to make a serious commitment to change lifestyle habits with regards to diet and physical activity. In examining family functioning, the clinician should obtain information about overall family interaction, including patterns of communication and how problems are handled. In addition, the assessment should provide insight into what types of rules and limits are set on the child's behavior and how these rules are enforced. Background information about the child's social environment should also be elicited, including information about who cares for the child and when, whether the child is ever left alone for prolonged periods (e.g., after school), and who prepares meals for the child and family.

After the completion of the psychological evaluation, the data should be combined with those obtained from the medical history and nutrition assessment in order to plan the most appropriate course of treatment for a given child. The psychological evaluation can help the clinician form the basis of recommendations for each child and family. For some children and families, the presence of mild psychological problems may be addressed within the context of a weight management program. Children and families with other, more significant psychosocial dysfunction may require further evaluation and intervention prior to starting weight management therapy.

4.4 Expert Panel Recommendations

There are few official or consensus guidelines relating to pediatric obesity. The Expert Panel on Clinical Guidelines for overweight in Adolescent Preventive Services was convened as an advisory group to two national health initiatives: (1) Bright Futures: National Guidelines for Health Supervision of Infants, Children, and Adolescents and (2) Guidelines for Adolescents Preventive Services. The Expert Panel guidelines were published in 1994 (28). A summary of the Expert Panel's recommendations are listed in Table 5.

The Expert Panel recommended the use of BMI to assess relative weight status. The new National Center for Health Statistics growth curves will include gender-specific curves showing BMI versus age, including percentile curves, thus supporting the easy application of this measurement to clinical practice.

TABLE 5 Expert Committee Goals of Therapy

Behavior
Develop awareness of current eating habits, activity, and parenting
  behavior
Identify problem behaviors
Modify current behavior
Continued awareness of behavior and recognition of changes that occur
  as child grows, gains independence, etc.
Medical
Improvement or resolution of secondary complications of obesity
Weight
Weight *maintenance* is the goal in the following situations:
2- to 7-year-old children
  BMI 85th–95th percentile
  BMI >95th percentile without complications of obesity
>7-year-old children
  BMI 85th–95th percentile without complications of obesity
Weight *loss* is the goal in the following situations:
2- to 7-year-old children
  BMI >95th percentile with complications of obesity
>7-year-old children
  BMI 85th–95th percentile with complications of obesity
  BMI >95th percentile

Source: Ref. 29.

In 1997, the Maternal and Child Health Bureau convened an Expert Committee on Obesity Evaluation and Treatment (29). This Expert Committee largely confirmed the previous recommendations listed in Table 5, with the following exceptions. The 1997 Expert Committee defined a rapid increase in BMI as an increase of 3 to 4 kg/m^2 in 1 year. In addition, this Expert Committee developed guidelines for medical, family and psychosocial screening and physical examinations (Table 6), including a listing of medical conditions associated with obesity (Table 4).

The 1997 Expert Committee also suggested the following indications for referral to a Pediatric Obesity Treatment Specialist: pseudotumor cerebri, sleep apnea, obesity-hypoventilation syndrome, orthopedic problems, massively overweight children or adolescents, and severely overweight children under 2 years of age. Though these conditions do define an urgent need to initiate weight management, the limited availability of pediatric obesity treatment centers and the

TABLE 6   Diagnostic Tests to Consider

Guidelines for preventive adolescent services
Utilize body-mass index (BMI) to define overweight
BMI ≥95th percentile or BMI >30 kg/m^2 defines overweight adolescents
  who should receive an in-depth medical assessment
Adolescents with a BMI between the 85th and 95th percentiles or equal to
  30 should be referred to second-level screening
Second level screening consists of the following:
• Review family history of cardiovascular disease or diabetes mellitus and
  parental hypercholesterolemia or obesity
• Blood pressure assessment
• Total cholesterol screening (elevated ≥200 mg/dL)
• Assess recent weight changes; rapid increase in weight (BMI increase in
  last year ≥2 kg/m^2)
• Assess adolescent's concern about current weight status or emotional or
  psychological manifestations thought to be related to overweight or
  perceptions of overweight
Adolescents with positive second-level screening should complete
an in-depth medical assessment
Suggestions for in-depth medical assessments:
• Physical examination, including assessment of sexual maturation
• Anthropometry to assess triceps and subscapular skinfolds
• Lipoprotein fractions (total cholesterol, HDL-C, triglyceride, and
  calculated LDL-C)

Key: HDL-C, high-density-lipoprotein cholesterol; LDL-C, low-density-lipoprotein cholesterol.
Source: Ref. 28.

need for a multidisciplinary approach to obesity evaluation and management may make it appropriate to assess all significantly obese children at an obesity specialty center.

The Expert Committee also recommends that the child and family's readiness to make changes be assessed. Families of young children may be able to institute changes in diet and physical activity by altering the child's environment without the direct cooperation of the child. However, trying to impose changes when the older child or adolescent is resistant or not interested, or the family is not willing or able to be supportive, will probably be futile and may induce family problems, discourage future attempts at weight control, and damage the child's self-esteem. Similarly, a psychosocial screen of the family is useful to identify issues that may impede initiation of a behavior modification program. Significant psychological problems, and eating disorders in particular, may need to be addressed initially and adequately before weight management is instituted. It is also our experience that many parents of obese children have difficulties with setting limits and with parenting skills. These issues should also be assessed prior to initiating therapy. In addition, the Expert Panel recommended assessment of diet and physical activity histories.

The 1997 Expert Committee also defined the goals of therapy (Table 5). In addition, the committee recommended the early initiation of therapy, educating the child and family about medical complications of obesity (including all caregivers in the program), and working to make small, gradual, but long-term changes. The chronicity of the risk of obesity needs to emphasized with all families, as promotion of a healthy lifestyle is a lifelong issue for the obese child.

4.5 Treatment of Obesity

4.5.1 Behavior Modification

Several treatment methods have been devised in an effort to help obese children attain a normal weight and improve health. These treatments include behavioral programs, dietary modification, exercise programs, and school-based programs. The majority of childhood weight-management programs have targeted younger age groups, such as children 7 to 12 years of age, rather than adolescents. A recent review of empirical investigations of pediatric obesity treatments concluded that the outcomes of most treatment programs are modest. Furthermore, most children in these programs do not maintain their weight loss. Treatment for pediatric obesity is more successful when a comprehensive behavioral program in conjunction with specific diet and exercise prescriptions is utilized (30).

Most comprehensive behavioral treatments for pediatric obesity contain five key components:

1. *Self-monitoring*: Children record dietary intake and physical activity on a regular basis.

2. *Stimulus control*: Families are taught how to modify aspects of the environment that may serve as cues for overeating, such as eating while watching television.

3. *Eating management*: Children learn strategies aimed at changing the way they actually eat, such as eating slowly.

4. *Contingency management*: Children are given the opportunity to earn rewards contingent upon reaching specific weight-related goals, including keeping records, engaging in physical activity, and eating certain foods.

5. *Cognitive-behavioral techniques*: Children and parents acquire coping skills and problem-solving techniques that can be used to facilitate weight stabilization and weight loss as well as prevent relapse. This could include practicing conflict-resolution skills and increasing communication between parent and child.

Another crucial component of pediatric weight management programs is adult caregiver participation. A number of studies have shown that obese children are more likely to lose weight and keep the weight off when their parents are involved in the treatment. Parental participation involves more than simply attending sessions with the child. To help the obese child succeed, the parent must learn to restructure the child's eating environment in ways that support changes in habits of eating and physical activity. For example, obese children whose parents had participated in a course in general behavior management had significantly better weight control than obese children in an intervention that focused only on weight reduction (30). Most parents seeking treatment for their child must not only be encouraged to exert a certain degree of control over their child's environment to promote healthy behaviors but also be taught how to do so. Thus, parent training in specific behavior modification methods should be integrated into pediatric weight management programs. Some examples of behavior modification methods include using positive reinforcement to increase healthy behaviors and implementing a token system for contingency contracting.

One of the best examples of a comprehensive behavioral treatment package is the program developed by Epstein and colleagues (30). This treatment program combines behavioral methods such as praise, goal setting, self-monitoring, and contingency contracting with nutrition education (i.e., ''the traffic light diet'').

In considering what treatment methods to use with a given child and family, it is important to consider the potential risk of developing an eating disorder. It has been suggested that caloric restriction that is a part of many behavioral treatments may trigger binge eating and eating disorders. Research with obese adults has found that although a low-calorie diet does not appear to exacerbate binge eating in those individuals already identified as binge eaters, there is evidence that suggests binge eating could develop in persons who have not binged before while following such a diet. Consequently, clinicians and parents must both carefully monitor children receiving treatment for signs and symptoms that could indicate an eating disorder. Finally, interventions for weight management must encourage healthy eating habits that promote gradual weight loss in the growing child, with treatment starting at as young an age as appropriate and practical (29).

4.5.2 Very Low Calorie Diets

Very low calorie diets have induced rapid weight loss in obese adults, children, and adolescents (31). In general, these diets provide 600 to 800 kcal/day and induce weight loss of approximately 2 to 4 lb per week. However, complications, including cardiac arrhythmias and sudden death, have occurred with such diets. It appears that the initial serious complications were related to poor-quality dietary protein, inadequate protein intake, or inadequate electrolyte intake. Electrolyte imbalances also occurred secondary to the osmotic diuresis due to the ketosis. (Note that some version of the very low calorie diet are very low in carbohydrate, and thus ketogenic.)

The very low calorie diet is sometimes provided with very small amounts of carbohydrate, inducing ketosis. It is commonly believed that ketogenic, very low calorie diets are associated with less hunger, though this belief is not supported by objective data. Furthermore, including significant amounts of carbohydrate in the diet has been associated with less protein loss. Diets made up of normal food products and special liquid diet formulations have been utilized. Though use of a liquid diet may provide practical advantages in ease of delivery, such diets are associated with more hunger.

Though some cases of longer-term success at maintaining loss of weight have been reported with very low calorie diets, the vast majority of individuals regain most or all of their weight after transitioning to a regular diet. Though this approach seems promising for initial weight loss, alternative methods for weight maintenance need to be developed before very low calorie diets can be widely utilized.

Due to their limited long-term success and the potential danger of a very low calorie diets, they should be utilized under strict supervision by practitioners with direct experience of using such diets with children or adolescents. It would also be prudent to limit the use of such diets to those children or adolescents suffering from significant obesity-related medical problems (such as sleep apnea or pseudotumor cerebri), which would be expected to remit or significantly improve with significant weight loss.

Whether using a commercial liquid product or regular food, adequate diet quality must be assured. Special attention must be paid to the provision of high-quality protein, an adequate protein intake, and adequate amounts of vitamins and minerals. Though there are no accepted guidelines relating to micronutrient supplementation during implementation of a very low calorie diet, most adolescents on very low calorie diets receive potassium, calcium, magnesium supplementation and other nutrients to protect against significant losses or inadequate supply in diet.

4.5.3 Medications

There are currently no weight-loss medications approved for use in children. Given the recent experience with the combination of the two medications phentermine and fenfluramine (associated with cardiac valve defects), practitioners need to carefully balance the potential risks and benefits of such therapy, especially if the drugs have not been studied in controlled trials with children. As new medications become available, there is a clear need to ensure the safety and efficacy of their use in children and adolescents. Even then, the use of medications for the treatment of obesity in children and adolescents may be appropriate only in extreme situations or with associated medical comorbidities.

4.5.4 Herbal and Other Nutrition-Related Products

Many herbal and other over-the-counter weight management products are available. As many of these are not marketed as medications, their safety and efficacy have generally not been demonstrated in adults or children. Therefore the use of such products is not recommended in children or adolescents.

4.5.5 Surgery

Surgical procedures that either make the stomach smaller or divert food around a certain portion of the gastrointestinal tract have been utilized in extreme cases. These procedures decrease food intake or absorption. Experience with the surgical treatment of severely obese adults describes a relatively high rate of morbidity and mortality. The limited experience in children and adolescents seems to confirm a similar rate of complications. Before considering surgical a procedure, all other treatment options should be considered and attempted and a careful risk/benefit analysis undertaken. Referral to a medical center with significant experience with such procedures should also be considered.

4.5.6 Outcome

Relatively few studies have been published that evaluate weight loss programs for children, though a comprehensive review of this topic is available (30). The data relating to weight management in children are even more limited by the short-term follow-up period of the studies. Epstein et al. (32) have described the 10-year follow-up of obese 6- to 12-year-old children who initially received a family-based intervention including diet, exercise, and behavior management lasting less than 1 year. At 10 years, the children who participated in the program together with their parents had decreased their relative weight by 7.5% while those in a control group increased their relative weight by 14.3%. Despite the relatively short-term nature of the intervention, the 22% difference in relative weight after 10 years supports the potential for positive long-term results with weight management for children. The data from this study indicate that the best predictor of outcome was change during the first 5 years following treatment. Other important predictors of outcome were the child's eating and exercise environment and support from family and friends. Further research by Epstein and colleagues has repeatedly demonstrated that behavioral methods are best administered in parent-child groups where the parents and children meet separately (30).

4.6 Insurance Coverage for Pediatric Weight Management Services

Many insurance companies will not cover pediatric weight management services (33). Even in instances where the child has an obesity-associated comorbidity, it is common for the treatment of the secondary problem but not the primary problem (obesity) to be covered. Though efforts to improve outcome with weight management need to continue, long-term moderate success in the treatment of childhood obesity has been demonstrated (32). Medical care providers should actively lobby insurance companies to cover these important prevention and therapeutic programs.

REFERENCES

1. Troiano RP, Flegal KM, Kuczmarski RJ, Campbell SM, Johnson CL. Overweight prevalence and trends for children and adolescents. Arch Pediatr Adolesc Med 1995; 149:1085–1091.
2. Bray GA. Obesity and the heart. Mod Concepts CVD 1987; 56(12):67–71.
3. Gortmaker SL, Must A, Perrin JM, Sobol AM, Dietz WH. Social and economic consequences of overweight in adolescence and young adulthood. N Engl J Med 1993; 329:1008–10012.
4. Stunkard AJ, Sorensen TIA, Hanis C, Teasdale TW, Chakraborty R, Schull WJ, Schulsinger F. An adoption study of human obesity. N Engl J Med 1986; 314:193–198.
5. Stunkard AJ, Harris JR, Pedersen, NL, McClearn GE. The body-mass index of twins who have been reared apart. N Engl J Med 1990; 322:1483–1487.
6. Mantzoros CM. The role of leptin in human obesity and disease: A review of current evidence. Ann Intern Med 1999; 130:671–680.
7. Gortmaker SL, Must A, Sobol AM, Peterson K, Colditz GA, Dietz WH. Television viewing as a cause of increasing obesity among children in the United States, 1986–1990. Arch Pediatr Adolesc Med 1996; 150:356–362.
8. Andersen RE, Crespo CJ, Bartlett SJ, Cheskin LJ, Pratt M. Relationship of physical activity and television watching with body weight and level of fatness among children. JAMA 1998; 279:938–942.
9. Roberts SB, Savage J, Coward WA, Chew B, Lucas A. Energy expenditure and

intake in infants born to lean and overweight mothers. N Engl J Med 1988; 318: 461–466.

10. Ravussin E, Lillioja S, Knowler WC, Christin L, Freymond D, Abbott WGH, Boyce V, Howard BV, Bogardus C. Reduced rate of energy expenditure as a risk factor for body-weight gain. N Engl J Med 1988; 318:467–472.

11. Goran MI, Shewchuk R, Gower BA, Nagy TR, Carpenter WH, Johnson RK. Longitudinal changes in fatness in white children: No effect of childhood energy expenditure. Am J Clin Nutr 1998; 67:309–316.

12. Stunkard AJ, Berkowitz RI, Stallings VA, Schoeller DA. Energy intake, not energy output is a determinant of body size in infants. Am J Clin Nutr 1999; 69:524–530.

13. Salbe AD, Fontvieille AM, Harper IT, Ravussin E. Low levels of physical activity in 5-year-old children. J Pediatr 1997; 131(3):423–429.

14. Rolls BJ, Bell EA, Castellanos VH, Pelkman CL, Thowart ML. Energy density but not fat content of foods affected energy intake in lean and obese women. Am J Clin Nutr 1999; 69(5):863–871.

15. Shick SM, Wing RR, Klem ML, McGuire T, Hill JO, Seagle H. Persons successful at long-term weight loss and maintenance continue to consume a low-energy, low-fat diet. J Am Diet Assoc 1998; 98(11):1273.

16. Ludwig DS, Majzoub JA, Al-Zahrani A, Dallal GE, Blanco I, Roberts SB. High glycemic index foods, overeating, and obesity. Pediatrics 1999; 103(3):1–6.

17. Johnson SL, Birch LL. Parents' and children's adiposity and eating style. Pediatrics 1994; 94(5):653–661.

18. National Heart, Lung and Blood Institute. Statement on First Federal Obesity Clinical Guidelines. NIH publication #984083. Bethesda, MD: NHLBI, 1998.

19. Lee IM, Manson JE, Hennekens CH, Paffenbarger RS. Body weight and mortality. A 27-year follow-up of middle-aged men. JAMA 1993; 270:2823–2828.

20. Manson JA, Willett WC, Stampfer MJ, Colditz GA, Hunter DJ, Hankinson SE, Hennekens CH, Speizer FE. Body weight and mortality among women. N Engl J Med 1995; 333:667–685.

21. Freedman DS, Srinivasan SR, Harsha DW, Webber LKS, Berenson GS. Relation of body fat patterning to lipid and lipoprotein concentrations in children and adolescents: The Bogalusa Heart Study. Am J Clin Nutr 1987; 46:403–410.

22. Van Gaal LF, Wauters MA, De Leeuw IH. The beneficial effects of modest weight loss on cardiovascular risk factors. Int J Obesity 1997; 21(suppl 1):S5–S9.

23. Rocchini AP, Katch V, Anderson J, Hinderliter J, Becque D, Martin M, Marks C. Blood pressure in obese adolescents effect on weight loss. Pediatrics 1988; 82(1): 16–23.

24. Pinhas-Hamiel O, Dolan LM, Daniels SR, Standiford D, Khoury PR, Zeitler P. Increased incidence of non-insulin-dependent diabetes mellitus among adolescents. J Pediatr 1996; 128:608–615.

25. McGill HC, McMahan A, Malcom GT, Oalmann MC, Strong JP, Pathobiological determinants of Atherosclerosis Research Group (PDAY). Relation of glycohemoglobin and adiposity to atherosclerosis in youth. Arterioscler Thromb Vasc Biol 1995; 15:431–440.

26. Dietz WH. Health consequences of obesity in youth: Childhood predictors of adult disease. Pediatrics 1998; (suppl): 101:518S–524S.

27. Birch LL, Fisher J. Development of eating behaviors among children and adolescents. Pediatrics 1998; (suppl): 101:539S–548S.

28. Himes JH, Dietz WH. Guidelines for overweight in adolescent preventive services: Recommendations from an expert committee. Am J Clin Nutr 1994; 59:307–316.

29. Barlow SE, Dietz WH. Obesity evaluation and treatment: Expert committee recommendations. Pediatrics 1998; 102:1–11.

30. Epstein LH, Myers MD, Raynor HA, Saelens BE. Treatment of pediatric obesity. Pediatrics 1998; 101:554–570.

31. Willi WM, Oexmann MJ, Wright NM, Collop NA, Key LL. The effects of a high-protein, low fat, ketogenic diet on adolescents with morbid obesity: Body composition, blood chemistries, and sleep abnormalities. Pediatrics 1998; 101:61–67.

32. Epstein LH, Valoski A, Wing RR, McCurley J. Ten-year follow-up of behavioral, family based treatment for obese children. JAMA 1990; 264(19):2550–2551.

33. Tershakovec AM, Watson MH, Wenner WJ, Marx AL. Insurance reimbursement for the treatment of obesity in children. J Pediatr 1999; 134:573–578.

34. Dietz WH, Robinson TN. Assessment and treatment of childhood obesity. Pediatr Rev 1993; 14(9):337–344.

11

Hyperlipidemias

Tracy Harpel Laird and J. Timothy Bricker
Baylor College of Medicine and Texas Children's Hospital,
Houston, Texas

1 OVERVIEW

The rationale for the detection and treatment of hyperlipidemia in children and young adults is to delay or prevent the onset of premature coronary artery disease. The validity of this goal depends on the establishment of the following principles. First, coronary artery disease is detrimental; second, coronary artery disease begins in childhood; third, coronary artery disease is related to blood cholesterol levels; and finally, lowering of cholesterol levels is effective in reducing coronary artery disease.

1.1 Coronary Artery Disease Is Detrimental

It is widely accepted that coronary artery disease is a cause of significant mortality, morbidity, and expense. American Heart Association statistics demonstrate that coronary artery disease is the leading cause of death in the United States, accounting for two of every five deaths, or more than 500,000 deaths annually (1). The AHA and the National Center for Health and Statistics estimate that more than 10 million people in the United States suffer from some form of cardiovascular disease at an annual cost of approximately $274 billion in medical expenses and lost productivity (2).

1.2 Coronary Artery Disease Begins in Childhood

Although the clinical sequelae of atherosclerosis do not occur until later in life, there is overwhelming evidence that the pathological changes begin years prior, during childhood. Atherosclerosis is a disease of medium- and large-sized arteries. It results from the progressive accumulation of smooth muscle cells and lipids within the intima of vessels. The advanced lesions of atherosclerosis are the final result of several complicated processes. First, there is proliferation of smooth muscle cells, T cells, and macrophages. This often occurs secondary to an exogenous injury. The smooth muscle cells then form a collagen matrix, and lipid accumulates in the macrophages to form large foam cells. The foam cells, together with the smooth muscle cells and T cells, form a fatty streak. As the lesion accumulates more cells, the fatty streak progresses to an intermediate fibrofatty lesion and ultimately to a fibrous plaque (3,4). With continued growth, the lesion encroaches on other layers of the arterial wall and narrows the arterial lumen.

The evidence that the atherosclerotic process begins in childhood is largely provided by autopsy studies. A study in 1955 found a 77% incidence of coronary artery disease among young U.S. soldiers killed in the Korean war (5). Similar evidence was provided by a 1971 investigation that found a 45% incidence of coronary artery disease in young soldiers killed in the Vietnam war (6). Multiple studies examining the coronary arteries of deceased subjects have found that coronary fatty streaks are rare in the first decade of life but common by age 20. Fibrous plaque formation is noted to occur in the second decade, with an increase in both extent and frequency during the third and fourth decades (7,8). The development and extent of atherosclerotic lesions in the aortas of young people has also been evaluated. A study of more than 500 subjects found fatty streaks in all individuals over 3 years of age (9). The extent of intimal surface involved progressed dramatically in the second decade of life. Fibrous plaques were seen by late adolescence; by 30 years of age, 90% of aortas contained fibrous plaques to some degree. Taken as a whole, these studies demonstrate that atherosclerosis is unquestionably a pediatric problem in that aortic fatty streaks develop extensively in childhood, coronary fatty streaks begin to form in adolescence, and fibrous plaques begin to develop in the teenage years.

1.3 Coronary Artery Disease Is Related to Blood Cholesterol Levels

The relationship of coronary artery disease and cholesterol levels has been established by a variety of animal, epidemiological, and autopsy studies. Studies in laboratory animals have shown that high blood cholesterol levels promote atherosclerosis. When fed high-cholesterol diets, many species develop atherosclerotic lesions that progress from fatty streaks to complicated fibrous plaques, similar to human atherosclerotic lesions (10,11). Epidemiological studies have demonstrated conclusively that an elevated blood cholesterol level (specifically LDL cholesterol) is one of several major risk factors for coronary artery disease. Comparisons of populations with low and high rates of coronary artery disease have shown that children from countries with a high incidence of coronary artery disease have higher total cholesterol levels than do children from countries with a low incidence (12,13). Several prospective observational studies have established that an elevated blood cholesterol level is a powerful and independent predictor of coronary artery disease (14–17). On the average, each 1% rise in cholesterol is associated with an approximate 2% increase in coronary artery disease risk. Autopsy studies have added even more supporting evidence that atherosclerosis is related to cholesterol levels. The Bogalusa Heart Study, a study of cardiovascular risk factors in children in the community of Bogalusa, Louisiana, routinely measured coronary risk factors of study participants. Children who had their cholesterol levels measured as participants and then who died accidentally were studied by autopsy. It was found that fatty streaks occurred in all subjects, and that the extent of fatty streaks was related to the total and LDL cholesterol levels. In addition, the frequency of fatty streaks was inversely related to HDL cholesterol levels (18).

1.4 Lowering Cholesterol Levels Is Effective in Reducing Coronary Artery Disease Risk

While there is undoubtedly a link between high blood cholesterol levels and atherosclerosis, evidence that lowering blood cholesterol levels is effective in reducing the risk of coronary artery disease also exists. Numerous clinical trials in adults have provided convincing evidence that decreasing cholesterol levels lessens the incidence of both fatal and nonfatal myocardial infarction (19–22). Several angiographic studies also support the assertion that lowering cholesterol levels is effective in reducing the risk of atherosclerosis. These studies have demonstrated that lowering elevated cholesterol levels results in the stabilization and even regression of atherosclerotic plaques (23–26).

1.5 Summary

The precursors to coronary artery disease begin at a young age. Elevated cholesterol levels have been shown to play an important role in the atherosclerotic process, and the beneficial effects of lowering cholesterol levels are clear. This provides the justification for efforts to detect, treat, and prevent hyperlipidemia beginning in childhood.

2   LIPOPROTEIN STRUCTURE AND METABOLISM

The primary lipids in plasma are cholesterol and triglycerides. Cholesterol forms part of the cell membrane structure and is necessary for cellular metabolism. Triglycerides are the storage form of fatty acids and are a major source of energy. Both are water-insoluble and are therefore carried in blood as components of lipid-protein macromolecules termed *lipoproteins* (Fig. 1) (27). These macromolecules contain a hydrophilic coat, comprised mainly of phospholipids, that surrounds the hydrophobic triglyceride and cholesterol core. Distributed throughout the phospholipid coat are free cholesterol and proteins, called apoproteins. The apoproteins serve as enzymatic cofactors and recognition elements in lipoprotein metabolism.

Four main classes of lipoproteins have been isolated and are separable on the basis of their densities and electrostatic charges: chylomicrons, very low-density lipoproteins (VLDL), low-density lipoproteins (LDL), and high-density lipoproteins (HDL). The properties of the lipoproteins are summarized in Table 1 (28). It is also useful to categorize the lipoproteins on the basis of their most abundant chemical component. Chylomicrons are 90% triglyceride, VLDLs are 55% triglyceride, HDLs are predominately protein, and LDLs are rich in cholesterol.

Each class of lipoprotein plays a different role in lipid metabolism (Fig. 2) (27). In the exogenous pathway of lipoprotein metabolism, chylomicrons are formed in the gastrointestinal tract from a combination of dietary fat (triglycer-

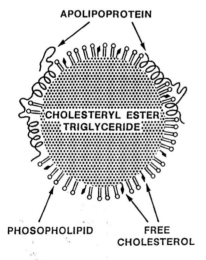

FIGURE 1   Lipoprotein structure. (From Ref. 27.)

TABLE 1 Properties of the Major Plasma Lipoproteins

	Chylomicron	VLDL	LDL	HDL
Chemical composition	Triglycerides, 90% Phospholipid, 6% Cholesterol, 3% Protein, 1%	Triglycerides, 55% Cholesterol, 22% Phospholipid, 15% Protein, 8%	Cholesterol, 50% Phospholipid, 25% Protein, 20% Triglycerides, 5%	Protein, 50% Phospholipid, 25% Cholesterol, 20% Triglycerides, 5%
Major apoproteins	ApoB-48 ApoC-I, II, III ApoA-I, II, IV ApoE	ApoB-100 ApoC-I, II, III ApoE	ApoB-100	ApoA-I, II ApoC-I, II, III ApoE
Origin	Intestine	Liver	Metabolic product of VLDL metabolism	Liver Intestine Catabolism of VLDL and chylomicrons
Function	Transports dietary triglycerides	Transports hepatic triglycerides and cholesterol to peripheral tissue	Provides cholesterol to peripheral tissues	Participates in reverse cholesterol transport
	Dietary fat	Endogenous triglyceride		

Key: VLDL, Very low-density lipoprotein; LDL, low-density lipoprotein; HDL, high-density lipoprotein.
Source: Ref. 28.

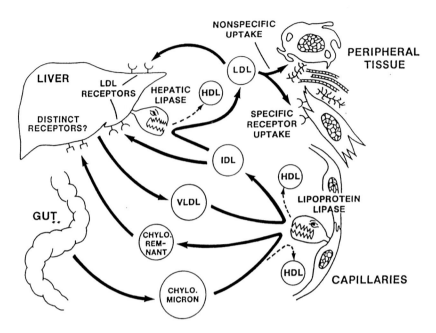

FIGURE 2   Lipoprotein metabolism pathways. (From Ref. 27.)

ides), esterified cholesterol, and apoproteins. Chylomicrons enter the circulation and are rapidly acted upon by the enzyme lipoprotein lipase (LPL). LPL cleaves the triglycerides from the chylomicrons, allowing the triglycerides to be stored in fat cells as fatty acids, thus leaving a cholesterol-rich chylomicron remnant that is rapidly taken up by hepatic cells. During the action of LPL, the surface components of chylomicrons, including apoproteins, are transferred to HDL particles. A deficiency of LPL activity results in an elevation of triglycerides in the form of chylomicrons.

In the endogenous pathway of lipoprotein metabolism, triglyceride-rich VLDLs are secreted by the liver and acted upon by LPL in much the same way as chylomicrons. The remnant produced is an intermediate density lipoprotein (IDL), which is either taken up by the liver or converted, by the enzyme hepatic lipase, to cholesterol-LDLs. LDL is the end product of VLDL metabolism and is the major carrier of cholesterol. It is LDL cholesterol that is associated with atherosclerosis. Uptake of plasma LDL by cells is regulated by LDL receptors located on cell membranes. Some genetic diseases result in a deficiency or malfunction of these receptors and cause elevated levels of plasma LDL cholesterol. HDLs are rich in protein and also important transporters of cholesterol. HDL carries cholesterol to the liver for secretion into bile, a process known as *reverse cholesterol metabolism*. Because HDL facilitates removal of cholesterol from the body, it is commonly referred to as "good" cholesterol and is protective against atherosclerosis.

Abnormalities in lipoprotein structure or metabolism can occur as a consequence of genetic, environmental, or acquired factors. Regardless of the cause, the outcome is an abnormal buildup of lipoproteins, with increases in cholesterol, triglycerides, or both depending on the composition of the lipoprotein accumulated.

3 CLASSIFICATION OF HYPERLIPIDEMIAS

3.1 Primary Versus Secondary

Hyperlipidemias can be categorized as either primary or secondary, depending on their cause. Primary hyperlipidemias are the result of a specific genetic defect or a combination of genetic and environmental factors. Secondary hyperlipidemias, on the other hand, may result from a multitude of metabolic diseases and exogenous causes.

The secondary causes of hyperlipidemia are listed in Table 2. In evaluating a patient with hyperlipidemia, a thorough history and physical examination are mandatory. Because hypothyroidism, diabetes mellitus, and nephrotic syndrome are among the most common metabolic causes of secondary hyperlipidemia, ap-

TABLE 2 Causes of Secondary Hyperlipidemia

Exogenous factors	Endocrine and metabolic
Drugs	Hypothyroidism
Corticosteroids	Diabetes mellitus
Anabolic steroids	Glycogen storage disease
Isotretinoin	Other storage diseases
Oral contraceptives	Lipodystrophy
Alcohol	Idiopathic hypercalcemia
Obesity	Pregnancy
Liver disease	Acute intermittent prophyria
Biliary atresia	Other
Biliary cirrhosis	Anorexia nervosa
Renal disease	Klinefelter's syndrome
Nephrotic syndrome	Systemic lupus erythematosus
Chronic renal failure	Progeria

Source: Ref. 28.

propriate testing of blood glucose as well as kidney and thyroid function may be indicated. During childhood and adolescence, exogenous factors are considered to be a major contributor to secondary hyperlipidemias. The most common of these include obesity, alcohol ingestion, oral contraceptive use, isotretinoin (Accutane) use, and steroid use. When a secondary cause of hyperlipidemia has been excluded, a diagnosis of primary hyperlipidemia can be made.

3.2 Fredrickson Classification

In their 1965 paper, Fredrickson and Lees were the first to devise a method to formally classify the lipoprotein abnormalities (29). The Fredrickson classification scheme is shown in Table 3. The hyperlipidemias are grouped into five major types according to the plasma lipoprotein patterns produced. The types define which lipoproteins (chylomicrons, VLDL, LDL, HDL) are elevated, and the resultant phenotype depends on the composition of the particular lipoproteins. There can be several different primary and/or secondary causes of the same Fredrickson phenotype.

TABLE 3 Fredrickson Classification of Dyslipidemias

Type	Lipoprotein abnormality	Resultant phenotype	Familial disorder
Type I	Chylomicrons	Very high triglycerides (TG)	Familial hyperchylomicronemia
Type IIa	LDL	High cholesterol	Familial hypercholesterolemia Familial defective apoB Familial combined hyperlipidemia
Type IIb	LDL and VLDL	High cholesterol and TG	Familial combined hyperlipidemia
Type III	Beta-VLDL	High cholesterol and TG	Familial dysbetalipoproteinemia
Type IV	VLDL	High TG	Familial hypertriglyceridemia Familial combined hyperlipidemia
Type V	Chylomicron and VLDL	Very high TG and slightly high cholesterol	Familial severe hypertriglyceridemia

3.3 Clinical Classification

Clinically, it is often more practical to separate the hyperlipidemias into categories of hypercholesterolemia, hypertriglyceridemia, and combined hyperlipidemia. This method of classification is less cumbersome and provides useful information for determining a cause, predicting clinical sequelae (such as the risk of atherosclerosis or pancreatitis), and planning treatment.

The ability to identify and quantify specific enzymes, apoproteins, and receptors has made it possible to determine many of the specific metabolic and genetic defects that result in hyperlipidemia. Testing techniques of this nature are currently available at some lipid research centers. However, such intricate description of lipoprotein abnormalities is usually not necessary or cost-effective. Currently available therapy is not specific; treatment plans are directed at the phenotypes of hypercholesterolemia and hypertriglyceridemia. In addition, hyperlipidemia in the majority of children results from a combination of genetic and environmental factors, not from an isolated defect in lipid metabolism.

4 HYPERCHOLESTEROLEMIA

4.1 Definition

The normal levels for total cholesterol, LDL cholesterol, HDL cholesterol, and triglycerides for children under 20 years of age are given in Table 4. Based on these values, the National Cholesterol Education Program (NCEP) Expert Panel on Blood Cholesterol Levels in Children and Adolescents (30) developed categories of acceptable (<75%), borderline (75 to 95%), and high (>95%) for total and LDL cholesterol levels (Table 5). Hypercholesterolemia in children is therefore defined as a total cholesterol of greater than 170 mg/dL or an LDL cholesterol of greater than 110 mg/dL.

The only Fredrickson phenotype that represents an elevation of cholesterol alone (without hypertriglyceridemia) is type IIa. There are both primary and secondary causes of this phenotype. The most common secondary causes include anorexia nervosa, hypothyroidism, Cushing's syndrome, glucocorticoid use, and the nephrotic syndrome. The most common primary cause is familial hypercholesterolemia. Familial combined hyperlipidemia, which causes a variety of phenotypes (including type IIa), is discussed in Section 6.1.

4.2 Familial Hypercholesterolemia

Familial hypercholesterolemia (FH) is the most commonly recognized form of familial hyperlipidemia in childhood. It is inherited in an autosomal dominant pattern, with the prevalence of heterozygotes approximately 1 in 500 and the

TABLE 4 Serum Levels of Lipids in U.S. Children and Adolescents (mg/dL)

Age (years)	Cholesterol					LDL-C				
	5%	25%	50%	75%	95%	5%	25%	50%	75%	95%
0–4										
Male	117	141	156	176	209	—	—	—	—	—
Female	115	143	161	177	206	—	—	—	—	—
5–9										
Male	125	147	164	180	209	65	82	93	106	133
Female	130	150	168	184	211	70	91	101	118	144
10–14										
Male	123	144	160	178	208	66	83	97	112	136
Female	128	148	163	179	207	70	83	97	113	140
15–19										
Male	116	136	150	170	203	64	82	96	112	134
Female	124	144	160	177	209	61	80	96	114	141

Age (years)	HDL-C					Triglycerides				
	5%	25%	50%	75%	95%	5%	25%	50%	75%	95%
0–4										
Male	—	—	—	—	—	30	41	53	69	102
Female	—	—	—	—	—	35	46	61	79	115
5–9										
Male	39	50	56	65	76	31	41	53	67	104
Female	37	48	54	63	75	33	45	57	73	108
10–14										
Male	38	47	57	63	76	33	46	61	80	129
Female	38	46	54	60	72	38	56	72	93	135
15–19										
Male	31	40	47	54	65	38	56	71	94	152
Female	36	44	53	63	76	40	55	70	90	136

Key: LDL-C, low-density-lipoprotein cholesterol; HDL-C, high-density-lipoprotein cholesterol.
Source: from the Lipid Research Clinic Data Book (1979).

TABLE 5   Categories of Cholesterol Levels (mg/dL)

Category	Total cholesterol	LDL-cholesterol
Acceptable	<170	<110
Borderline	170–199	110–129
High	≥200	≥130

Source: Ref. 30.

prevalence of the homozygous form 1 in 1 million. Increased LDL cholesterol levels result from abnormal interactions between LDL receptors on cell surfaces and the LDL lipoprotein (31,32). Most commonly, this altered interaction is the result of a mutation on the LDL receptor gene, located on the short arm of chromosome 19, which causes production of abnormal, nonfunctioning LDL receptors. Heterozygotes have about a 50% decrease in functioning LDL receptors and homozygotes have almost no receptor activity. A rare cause of FH is a defect of ApoB-100, the apoprotein on LDL particles (33). This abnormal apoprotein is unable to interact with LDL receptors and produces an outcome similar to that seen with LDL receptor abnormalities.

Children with heterozygous familial hypercholesterolemia usually have LDL cholesterol levels above the 95th percentile from birth. The levels remain elevated during childhood and adolescence, with an average total cholesterol in the range of 250 to 500 mg/dL and LDL cholesterol 200 to 300 mg/dL. Typically, these children are clinically asymptomatic. Tendon xanthomas are rarely found during the first 10 years of life; they develop during the second and third decades in only 10 to 15% of affected individuals. When they occur, these xanthomas are most common in the Achilles tendon and the extensor tendons of the hands. Some patients develop early corneal arcus. The most significant clinical manifestation, however, is premature coronary artery disease. Angina pectoris is rare in the teenage years but common after age 30. By 60 years of age, 50 to 75% of heterozygotic men will have a myocardial infaction (31).

The total cholesterol levels in patients with homozygous FH are generally 500 to 1000 mg/dL. Patients with this form of the disease classically present in early childhood (or even at birth) with planar and tendon xanthomas. Planar xanthomas are flat, yellow colored lesions that most commonly occur on the knees, elbows, hands, buttocks, and around the eyes. Other clinical findings include cholesterol deposits in the retinal fundus and corneal arcus. These patients develop coronary artery disease at a very young age, with angina and myocardial infarction during the teenage years not uncommon. Most patients have severe coronary artery disease before age 30. Lipid deposition also occurs on the aortic valve and along the ascending aorta, often resulting in aortic valve and supraval-vular stenosis.

5 HYPERTRIGLYCERIDEMIA

5.1 Definition

The normal levels of serum triglyceride levels in children and adolescents are shown in Table 4. Based on these values, hypertriglyceridemia is defined as a triglyceride level above 100 mg/dL in the first decade of life and greater than 130 mg/dL thereafter.

The relationship between hypertriglyceridemia and coronary artery disease risk is not as straightforward as that seen with hypercholesterolemia. Although several studies have shown a positive correlation between triglyceride levels and atherosclerosis, this association often disappears when factors such as LDL and HDL levels are controlled (34). However, it is firmly established that in-fants and children with severe elevations (>1000 mg/dL) of triglyceride levels are at risk for severe and recurrent pancreatitis.

There are several Fredrickson phenotypes that represent an isolated eleva-tion in triglyceride levels, including types I, IV, and V. Hypertriglyceridemia, like hypercholesterolemia, can be the result of environmental factors, secondary disease states, familial disorders, or any combination of these. Common environ-mental reasons for increased triglyceride levels include a high-fat diet, obesity, and lack of exercise. Other secondary causes include diabetes mellitus, alcohol ingestion, and oral contraceptive use. There are several primary genetic disorders that result in hypertriglyceridemia, including familial hyperchylomicronemia, fa-milial hypertriglyceridemia, and familial severe hypertriglyceridemia. Familial combined hyperlipidemia, which can cause isolated hypertriglyceridemia, is dis-cussed in Section 6.1.

5.2 Familial Hyperchylomicronemia

Familial hyperchylomicronemia is an elevation of triglycerides in the form of chylomicrons (Fredrickson phenotype I). The disorder is the result of deficient LPL activity. As mentioned earlier, LPL is the enzyme that promotes both the removal of triglycerides from lipoprotein particles and the uptake and storage of triglycerides by cells. A lack of active LPL results in a considerable increase in chylomicrons and marked hypertriglyceridemia, often in excess of 10,000 mg/dL. LPL deficiency is inherited in an autosomal recessive pattern, and the incidence of homozygous patients is approximately one in 100,000.

Patients with hyperchylomicronemia usually come to medical attention early in childhood with recurrent abdominal pain secondary to pancreatitis. Other clinical manifestations of the disorder include eruptive xanthomas, hepatospleno-megaly (secondary to uptake of chylomicrons by the reticuloendothelial system), and lipemia retinalis. The disease can often be diagnosed by observing the formation of a creamy layer of chylomicrons on top of plasma.

5.3 Familial Hypertriglyceridemia

Familial hypertriglyceridemia is characterized by increased triglycerides in the form of VLDLs (Fredrickson type IV). The disorder produces moderate increases in triglyceride levels, usually in the range of 200 to 500 mg/dL. The exact metabolic defect responsible for the disease is not known, but it is thought to be inherited in an autosomal dominant pattern. The disorder is frequently associated with obesity and diabetes and typically does not develop until adulthood.

5.4 Familial Severe Hypertriglyceridemia

Familial severe hypertriglyceridemia is the result of elevated triglyceride levels in the form of both chylomicrons and VLDL (Fredrickson phenotype V). Triglyceride levels in this disorder are usually greater than 1000 mg/dL. These patients do not usually present until adulthood, and symptoms include eruptive xanthomas, pancreatitis, and glucose intolerance. This condition is commonly associated with a variety of secondary disorders, such as diabetes, liver disease, and alcoholism.

6 COMBINED HYPERCHOLESTEROLEMIA AND HYPERTRIGLYCERIDEMIA

6.1 Familial Combined Hyperlipidemia

Familial combined hyperlipidemia (FCH) affects several members of the same family and may present clinically as hypercholesterolemia, hypertriglyceridemia, or both (31,32). Some family members have an elevation of LDL cholesterol alone (Fredrickson phenotype IIa), some have an elevation of triglycerides alone in the form of VLDL (type IV), and others have an elevation of LDL cholesterol and VLDL together (type IIb). The variable lipoprotein profiles seen within families can also be seen at different times within the same individual.

FCH is a common disorder, occurring in approximately 1 in 300 people. The disease is inherited in an autosomal dominant pattern, and diagnosis is based on finding multiple lipoprotein phenotypes within a family and a family history that supports this inheritance pattern (35,36). While most patients do not develop xanthomas or ocular abnormalities, there is a high incidence of premature atherosclerosis.

6.2 Familial Dysbetalipoproteinemia

Familial dysbetalipoproteinemia (Fredrickson type III), also known as *broad beta disease*, is defined by the presence of abnormal, cholesterol-rich VLDLs (called beta VLDLs) in the plasma. Accumulation of this abnormal lipoprotein results in increases of both cholesterol and triglycerides, usually to an equal degree. It is inherited in an autosomal recessive pattern and is rare, occurring in about 1 in 5000 people. Premature coronary artery disease, stroke, and peripheral vascular disease are common features in middle age (37). Xanthomas over the knees and elbows are common; nearly pathognomonic of the disease is xanthoma striata palmaris, or yellow deposits in the creases of the palms.

7 OTHER DYSLIPIDEMIAS

7.1 Hypoalphalipoproteinemia

High-density lipoproteins are responsible for reverse cholesterol metabolism and are thus protective against atherosclerosis. Conversely, low levels of HDL cholesterol are associated with an increased risk of coronary artery disease. Hypoalphalipoproteinemia is an HDL cholesterol level less than the 10th percentile for age. A familial form of hypoalphalipoproteinemia, inherited in an autosomal dominant pattern, is associated with premature atherosclerosis (38). In addition, there are several secondary causes of low HDL levels, including drugs and cigarette smoking, which are often modifiable.

8 CHOLESTEROL-LOWERING STRATEGIES

The National Cholesterol Education Program (NCEP) expert panel on blood cholesterol levels in children and adolescents has developed two strategies for lowering cholesterol levels: the population approach and the individual approach (30).

The population approach provides nutritional guidelines to the population at large with the intent of lowering the average cholesterol level of all children and adolescents and at the same time establishing a firm basis for healthy eating patterns that will be maintained throughout life. The foundation of the guidelines is a diet low in total fat, saturated fat, and cholesterol. Specifically, a diet that provides no more than 30% of total calories from fat and less than 10% of total calories from saturated fats; less than 300 mg/day of cholesterol is advised. Families are encouraged to select a variety of foods to guarantee adequate intake of other nutrients, including protein, carbohydrates, vitamins, and minerals. Because the rapid growth in children less than 2 years of age requires a higher percentage of calories from fat, the nutrient intake recommendations provided by the panel are not intended for children in this age group. Toddlers should instead make the transition to a lower-fat diet as they begin to eat with the family.

The goal of the individual approach is to identify and treat those children and adolescents who are at greatest risk for hypercholesterolemia and thus premature coronary artery disease. The NCEP recommends selective lipid screening of children and adolescents determined to be at high risk. Although the effectiveness of this selective screening approach remains somewhat controversial, neither the American Academy of Pediatrics nor the American Heart Association recommend routine cholesterol screening in all children (30,39–41). A detailed family history and assessment of other cardiovascular risk factors provide the groundwork for determining which children fall into a high-risk category and should be evaluated further.

9 RISK ASSESSMENT AND DETECTION OF HYPERLIPIDEMIA

9.1 Risk Factors

Based upon a comprehensive body of evidence demonstrating a familial clustering of coronary artery disease, high cholesterol levels, and other risk factors, it is generally accepted that the major risk factor for hypercholesterolemia in a child is a family history of premature coronary artery disease or high cholesterol. For this reason, the NCEP recommends cholesterol screening for any child or adolescent with a family history of premature coronary artery disease or parental high cholesterol. In this context, *family history* refers to a patient's parents or grandparents and *premature* is defined as occurring at age 55 or younger. Coronary artery disease extends to any evidence of atherosclerosis by diagnostic or therapeutic cardiac catheterization, documented myocardial infarction, angina pectoris, peripheral vascular disease, cerebrovascular disease, or sudden cardiac death. Parental high cholesterol is a total cholesterol level of 240 mg/dL, defined by the NCEP's Adult Treatment Panel as a high level (42). Cholesterol testing may also be appropriate in children whose family history is unknown or who are considered to be at higher risk for coronary artery disease independent of family history or parental hypercholesterolemia. For example, children and adolescents who are obese, have high blood pressure or diabetes, or who smoke may also deserve cholesterol screening. Table 6 outlines the recommended screening approach.

9.2 When and What to Measure

The NCEP recommends the screening of high-risk individuals at any time after 2 years of age. Cholesterol levels are relatively stable by this age and there are

TABLE 6   National Cholesterol Education Program
Screening Recommendations

Family history of premature coronary artery disease
Family history = parent or grandparent
Premature = age 55 or younger
Coronary artery disease = any evidence of atherosclerosis by:
diagnostic or therapeutic cardiac catheterization
documented myocardial infarction
angina pectoris
peripheral vascular disease
cerebrovascular disease
sudden cardiac death
Parental high cholesterol
Cholesterol level ≥ 240 mg/dL
Unavailable family history
Other significant coronary risk factors
Obesity
Hypertension
Smoking
Diabetes mellitus

Source: Ref. 30.

no treatment recommendations for children below age 2. If initial screening results are acceptable, they should be repeated in 5 years.

The initial screening test can be either a measurement of total cholesterol or
a complete lipoprotein analysis. A lipoprotein analysis measures total cholesterol,
HDL cholesterol, and triglycerides. LDL cholesterol is then calculated by a formula devised from the Lipid Research Clinics: LDL-C = total cholesterol −
(triglyceride level/5 + HDL-C). This formula is accurate if the triglyceride level
is less than 400 mg/dL. A lipoprotein analysis is more expensive than a measurement of total cholesterol and also requires a 12-hr fast.

As outlined in Figure 3, the recommended method of initial screening depends on the reason for testing. For those being tested because of a parent with
high cholesterol or because they have other concerning risk factors, a total cholesterol level should be obtained. If this level is in the acceptable range, education
should be given in regard to risk factors and nutrition and the testing of the
cholesterol level should be repeated in 5 years. If the level is high, a lipoprotein
analysis should be done. A borderline level should be retested and averaged; if
it is high, a lipoprotein analysis should be performed. For those being screened
secondary to a family history of premature coronary artery disease, a lipoprotein
analysis should be done from the start.

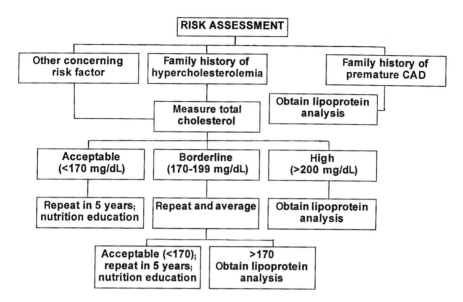

FIGURE 3 Risk-assessment algorithm. Lipoprotein analysis requires a 12-hr fast and measures the total cholesterol, HDL-C, and triglyceride levels. LDL-C is calculated: LDL-C = total cholesterol − (triglyceride level/5 + HDL-C). This formula is accurate only if the triglyceride level is <400 mg/dL. (From Ref. 30.)

10 TREATMENT OF HYPERCHOLESTEROLEMIA

Once a lipoprotein analysis is obtained, it should be repeated and the values averaged. Hypercholesterolemia is almost always secondary to an elevated LDL cholesterol, and it is the LDL cholesterol level that ultimately determines individual risk and treatment guidelines. Elevated HDL levels do not require treatment.

Figure 4 depicts the treatment algorithm recommended for elevated LDL cholesterol levels by the NCEP (30). Once determined, an average LDL level is classified as either acceptable, borderline, or high (see Table 5). If the value is acceptable, education should be given regarding nutrition and other coronary artery disease risk factors and a lipoprotein analysis should be repeated in 5 years. If the value is in the borderline range, risk-factor advice should be given and the Step One diet (see Section 10.1) initiated. A repeat lipoprotein analysis should be performed in 1 year. Values in the high category require intensive clinical intervention. An evaluation for secondary causes of hyperlipidemia (see Table 2) should be undertaken and all family members screened. Counseling on other

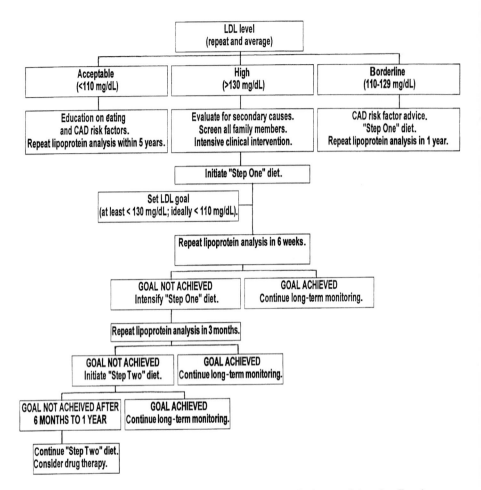

FIGURE 4 Treatment algorithm based on LDL cholesterol levels. For long-term monitoring, recheck lipoprotein analysis at least twice a year. (From Ref. 30.)

risk factors, nutrition, and exercise should be given. The Step One diet should be initiated after a goal LDL level is set. The minimum goal should be a LDL cholesterol level <130 mg/dL; less than 110 mg/dL is even better. A repeat lipoprotein analysis should be obtained in 6 weeks to evaluate progress. If the goal is not achieved, diet therapy should be intensified and lipoprotein analysis repeated in 3 months. If the goal is still not achieved, the Step Two diet should be initiated. If the goal is not achieved after 6 months to a year of diet therapy, drug therapy should be considered as a supplement to diet therapy.

10.1 Diet Therapy

Diet therapy is the primary approach to treating children and adolescents with elevated cholesterol levels. It is prescribed in two steps that progressively reduce saturated fatty acid and cholesterol intake (30). Table 7 summarizes the nutrient recommendations of these diets.

The Step One diet includes the same nutrient intake guidelines as recommended to the general population in the population approach to cholesterol reduction. That is, less than 30% of total calories from fat, less than 10% of total calories from saturated fatty acids, and less then 300 mg/day of cholesterol. The diet is considered therapeutic in this setting because it is prescribed and monitored by medical professionals.

The Step Two diet further reduces the amount of saturated fatty acids and cholesterol permitted. Specifically, saturated fatty acids are reduced to 7% of total calories and cholesterol intake to less than 200 mg per day. It is prescribed if, after strict adherence to the Step One diet for at least 3 months, the goals of therapy have not been achieved.

10.2 Drug Therapy

Drug therapy for hypercholesterolemia in children and adolescents is reserved for those cases that are both severe and refractory to diet therapy. The relative reluctance to use drug therapy in other cases is secondary to the potential side effects of the medications and the lack of definitive prospective data on the effect of such treatment in children. The NCEP recommends considering pharmacother-

TABLE 7 Summary of Step One and Step Two Diets

Nutrient	Step One Diet	Step Two Diet
Calories	To promote normal growth and development	Same
Total fat	No more than 30% of total calories	Same
Saturated fatty acids	<10% total calories	<7% total calories
Polyunsaurated fatty acids	Up to 10% total calories	Same
Monounsaturated fatty acids	Remaining fat calories	Same
Cholesterol	<300 mg/day	<200 mg/day
Carbohydrates	~55% of total calories	Same
Protein	~15–20% total calories	Same

Source: Ref. 30.

apy in children 10 years of age or older if 6 to 12 months of diet therapy and risk factor modification have not reduced LDL levels to less than 190 mg/dL, or less than 160 mg/dL if other risk factors coexist. Table 8 summarizes the specific indications of pharmacotherapy for hypercholesterolemia in children. If drug therapy is initiated, it must be used in conjunction with diet therapy. Follow-up should occur approximately 6 weeks after beginning the medication and every 3 months thereafter until the goal LDL level is met.

10.2.1 Bile Acid Sequestrants

The bile acid sequestrants cholestyramine and colestipol are the agents most commonly used to treat isolated hypercholesterolemia in children and adolescents (43). The sequestrants act as anion exchange resins by binding negatively charged bile acids in the intestinal lumen. The resin-bile complex is insoluble and excreted via the feces, thereby preventing enterohepatic circulation of the bile acids. Lowering of the bile acid concentration in hepatocytes results in an increase in the conversion of cholesterol to bile acids and causes a decrease in intracellular cholesterol. This stimulates an increased synthesis of LDL receptors, which, in turn, leads to enhanced uptake of LDL cholesterol. The final outcome is a decrease in plasma cholesterol.

Because they are not absorbed by the intestine, bile acid sequestrants generally lack systemic toxicity. The most common side effects are gastrointestinal and include constipation, nausea, bloating, and flatulence. Other potential side effects include malabsorption of folic acid, fat-soluble vitamins, and other drugs.

TABLE 8 Pharmacotherapy for Hyperlipoproteinemia in Children—When and Whom to Treat

Children 10 years of age or older
After failure of adequate trial of diet therapy (6 months to 1 year)
IF
1. LDL remains ≥ 190 mg/dL
2. LDL remains ≥ 160 mg/dL AND there is
   a. A positive family history of premature coronary artery disease
   OR
   b. Two or more of the following risk factors after attempts to control them
   Smoking
   Hypertension
   HDL < 35 mg/dL
   Severe obesity
   Diabetes mellitus
   Physical inactivity

Source: Ref. 30.

A daily multivitamin containing folic acid usually prevents vitamin deficiencies. Because resins can interfere with absorption of other drugs given at the same time, additional medications should be given 4 hr after or 1 hr before resins. Transient elevations in liver transaminases and alkaline phosphatase have occurred in some children but are not thought to represent hepatotoxicity. The bile acid sequestrants can sometimes increase plasma triglyceride levels. Lipid profiles must therefore be followed closely. Occasionally, the addition of niacin to the therapeutic regimen to treat the iatrogenic increase in triglycerides is necessary. Complete blood count, fat-soluble vitamin levels, folate, and liver function tests should be monitored yearly in children receiving bile acid sequestrants.

Cholestyramine and colestipol are both powders that must be mixed with water or juice before ingestion. Cholestyramine is also available as a flavored bar. They should be taken with meals, when bile acids are secreted. The choice of one over the other is usually a matter of individual taste and side effects. The dose depends on cholesterol levels, not body weight. In general, the lowest dose possible is started and increased one dose at a time until the goal cholesterol is achieved. An overview of treatment with bile acid resins is shown in Table 9.

10.2.2 Niacin

Niacin (nicotinic acid) has been used effectively in adults with hyperlipidemia for many years. Although it has been used in children as well (44), experience is still somewhat limited and the NCEP advises caution when using it in this age

TABLE 9 Treatment with Bile Acid Resins

"One dose" = 4-g packet or 1 scoop of cholestyramine
One bar of cholestryramine
5-g packet or 1 scoop of colestipol
Number of daily doses depends on cholesterol levels.

Daily doses	Total cholesterol	LDL cholesterol
1	<245	<195
2	245–300	195–235
3	301–345	236–280
4	>345	>280

Take immediately before, during, or after meals.
Supplement with daily multivitamin containing folic acid.
Administer other medications 4 hr after or 1 hr before resins.
Follow lipid profiles closely.
Monitor complete blood count, fat-soluble vitamin levels,
folate, and liver function tests annually.

group (30). In general, niacin should be used only if therapy with both diet and bile acid sequestrants fails to lower cholesterol to desirable levels or in cases of severe hypertriglyceridemia. Niacin is often used together with bile acid sequestrants and has been shown to be efficacious as part of combination therapy in patients with heterozygous and homozygous FH (45,46).

The usefulness of niacin is often limited by its relatively high frequency of side effects. These include liver disease, gastrointestinal discomfort, hyperuricemia, glucose intolerance, and an intense cutaneous flush. When used in children, niacin is usually started at a dose of 50 mg/day and increased very gradually. Aspirin can often attenuate the associated cutaneous flush. Liver function tests, glucose, and uric acid should be monitored regularly in children taking niacin.

10.2.3 HMG-CoA Reductase Inhibitors

The HMG-CoA reductase inhibitors, or "statins," are a group of drugs that inhibit the rate-limiting enzyme in cholesterol biosynthesis. They have long been used as effective cholesterol-lowering agents in adults. Some studies have shown statins to be effective and safe in children (45,47), and several other clinical trials are still ongoing. As more studies are completed, it is likely that the use of these agents in pediatric patients will increase. However, they are not as yet approved for use in the pediatric age group.

Side effects of statins in adults include hepatocellular toxicity and rhabdomyolysis, which can lead to renal failure. Close monitoring of liver enzymes and prompt evaluation of unexplained muscle pain during treatment is therefore essential.

10.2.4 Other Drugs

Although commonly used in adults, other pharmacotherapeutic agents—such as fibric acid derivatives (gemfibrozil and clofibrate), probucol, D-thyroxine, and para-aminosalicylic acid—are not recommended as routine agents for use in children and adolescents.

10.3 Other Forms of Therapy

Some patients with severe heterozygous or homozygous FH do not respond adequately to diet and drug management alone. These patients may require more aggressive therapies. Plasmapheresis, either by plasma exchange or LDL apheresis, has been successful at significantly reducing plasma LDL cholesterol levels in this population of patients (48–50). However, the reduction in LDL is transient, and apheresis must be repeated approximately every 2 to 3 weeks. Surgical treatments—in the form of partial ileal bypass, portacaval shunt, and liver transplantation—have had some degree of success but are rarely performed in children and are associated with significant morbidity and mortality (51–53).

11 TREATMENT OF HYPERTRIGLYCERIDEMIA

Dietary therapy and lifestyle modifications are the core of treatment for hypertriglyceridemia in children. The NCEP does not stress management and treatment of elevated serum triglycerides, likely because the risk of atherosclerosis associated with hypertriglyceridemia is not well defined (30). The most common cause of elevated triglyceride levels in childhood is a combination of poor diet, lack of exercise, and obesity. It is not surprising, then, that both familial and secondary elevations in serum triglycerides generally respond well to lifestyle modifications that include a low-fat diet, exercise, and weight reduction. The use of pharmacotherapy for hypertriglyceridemia in children is rarely necessary, and no pharmacological agents are approved for use in children. Niacin and fibric acid derivatives are common and effective treatments in adults.

Patients with familial chylomicronemia often require more specific and intensive therapy because the risk of pancreatitis increases markedly with triglyceride levels above 1000 mg/dL. Diet therapy in these patients should attempt to reduce fat intake to 10 to 15 g/day, although this diet can be difficult to maintain. Medium-chain triglycerides, which are absorbed directly through the portal vein rather than packaged into chylomicrons, can be substituted for fat in food preparation.

REFERENCES

1. American Heart Association. 1992 Heart and Stroke Facts Statistics. Dallas: American Heart Association, 1992.
2. American Heart Association. Epidemic of cardiovascular disease and stroke: The three main challenges. Circulation 1999; 99:1132–1137.
3. Ross R, Glomset JA. The pathogenesis of atherosclerosis. N Engl J Med 1976; 295: 369–377.
4. Ross R. Atherosclerosis: A defense mechanism gone awry. Am J Pathol 1993; 143: 987–1002.
5. Enos WF, Beyer JC, Holmes RH. Pathogenesis of coronary disease in American soldiers killed in Korea. JAMA 1955; 158:912–914.
6. McNamara JJ, Molot MA, Stremple JF, Cutting RT. Coronary artery disease in combat casualties in Vietnam. JAMA 1971; 216:1185–1187.
7. Strong JP, McGill HC Jr. The pediatric aspects of atherosclerosis. J Atheroscler Res 1969; 9:251–265.
8. Starry HS. Evolution and progression of atherosclerotic lesions in coronary arteries of children and young adults. Arteriosclerosis 1989; 9(suppl 1):I19–I39.

9. Holman RL, McGill HC Jr, Strong JP, Geer JC. The natural history of atherosclerosis: The early aortic lesions as seen in New Orleans in the middle of the 20th century. Am J Pathol 1968; 34:209–235.

10. LaRosa JC, Hunninghake D, Bush D, et al. The Cholesterol Facts. A summary of the evidence relating dietary fats, serum cholesterol, and coronary heart disease. Circulation 1990; 81:1721–1733.

11. Bullock BC, Lehner NDM, Clarkson TB, et al. Comparative primate atherosclerosis: I Tissue cholesterol concentration and pathologic anatomy. Exp Mol Pathol 1975; 22:151–175.

12. Conference on the Health Effects of Blood Lipids: Optimal Distributions for Populations. Workshop report: Epidemiologic Section III. The epidemiologic evidence from comparative childhood lipid distributions. Prev Med 1979; 8:644–652.

13. Hass J, Epstein FH, Lloyd J. Study of atherosclerosis precursors in children. Report of WHO Consultation, WHO CVD-74.4. Geneva: WHO, 1974.

14. Castelli WP, Garrison RJ, Wilson PWF, Abbott RD, Kalousdian S, Kannel WB. Incidence of coronary heart disease and lipoprotein cholesterol levels. The Framingham Study. JAMA 1986; 256:2835–2838.

15. Kannel WB, Neaton JD, Wentworth D, et al. Overall and coronary heart disease mortality rates in relation to major risk factors in 325,348 men screened for the multiple risk factor intervention trial (MRFIT). Am Heart J 1986; 112:825–836.

16. Stamler J, Wentworth D, Neaton JD. Is the relationship between serum cholesterol and risk of premature death from coronary heart disease continuous and graded? Findings in 356,222 primary screenees of the multiple risk factor intervention trial (MRFIT). JAMA 1986; 256:2823–2828.

17. Multiple Risk Factor Intervention Trial Research Group. Mortality rates after 10.5 years for participants in the MRFIT: Findings related to a priori hypotheses of the trial. JAMA 1990; 263:1795–1801.

18. Newman WPIII, Freedman DS, Voors AW, et al. Relation of serum lipoproteins and systolic blood pressure to early atherosclerosis: The Bogalusa Heart Study. N Engl J Med 1986; 314:138–144.

19. Lipid Research Clinics Program. The Lipid Research Clinic Coronary Primary Prevention Trial Results: II. The relationship of reduction in incidence of coronary heart disease to cholesterol lowering. JAMA 1984; 251:365–374.

20. Frick MH, Elo O, Haapa K, et al. Helsinki Heart Study: primary prevention trial with gemfibrozil in middle-aged men with dyslipidemia: Safety of treatment, changes in risk factors, and incidence of coronary heart disease. N Engl J Med 1987; 317:1237–1245.

21. Canner PL, Berge KG, Wenger NK, et al. Fifteen year mortality in Coronary Drug Project patients: Long-term benefit with niacin. J Am Coll Cardiol 1986; 8:1245–1255.

22. Yusif S, Wittes J, Friedman L. Overview of results of randomized clinical trials in heart disease: II. Unstable angina, heart failure, primary prevention with aspirin, and risk factor modification. JAMA 1988; 260:2259–2263.

23. Brensike JF, Levy RI, Kelsey SF, et al. Effects of therapy with cholestyramine on progression of coronary arteriosclerosis: Results of the NHLBI Type II Coronary Intervention Study. Circulation 1984; 69:313–324.

24. Blankenhorn DH, Nessim SA, Johnson FL, Sanmarco ME, Axen SP, Cahin-Hemphill L. Beneficial effects of combined colestipol-niacin therapy on coronary atherosclerosis and coronary venous bypass grafts. JAMA 1987; 257:3233–3240.

25. Brown G, Albers JJ, Fisher LD, et al. Regression of coronary artery disease as a result of intensive lipid-lowering therapy in men with high levels of apolipoprotein B. N Engl J Med 1990; 323:1289–1298.

26. Kane JP, Malloy MJ, Ports TA, Phillips NR, Diehl JC, Havel RJ. Regression of coronary atherosclerosis during treatment of familial hypercholesterolemia with combined drug regimens. JAMA 1990; 264:3007–3012.

27. Guyton JR. Lipoprotein metabolism and atherogenesis: genetics and pathophysiology. In: Garson AT, Bricker JT, Fisher DJ, Neish SR, eds. The Science and Practice of Pediatric Cardiology, 2nd ed. Baltimore: Williams & Wilkins, 1998, pp 491–509.

28. Kwiterovich P. Disorders of lipid metabolism. In: Rudolph AM, ed. Rudolph's Pediatrics, 20th ed. Stamford, Conn: Appleton & Lange 1996, pp 343–356.

29. Fredrickson DS, Lees RS. System for phenotyping hyperlipoproteinemia. Circulation 1965; 31:321–327.

30. National Cholesterol Education Program: Report of the Expert Panel on Blood Cholesterol Levels in Children and Adolescents. Pediatrics 1992; 89(suppl):525–584. (NIH Publication No. 91-2732, September 1991.)

31. Brown MS, Goldstein JL. The hyperlipoproteinemias and other disorders of lipid metabolism. In: Isselbacher KJ, Braunwald E, Wilson JD et al, eds. Harrison's Principles of Internal Medicine, 13th ed. New York: McGraw-Hill, 1994, pp 2062–2067.

32. Goldstein JL, Brown MS. Familial hypercholesterolemia. In: Scriver CR, Beaudet AC, Sly WS, Valle D, eds. The Metabolic Basis of Inherited Disease, 6th ed. New York: McGraw-Hill, 1989, pp 1215–1250.

33. Tybjaerg-Hansen A, Gallagher J, Vincent J, et al. Familial defective apolipoprotein B-100: Detection in the United Kingdom and Scandinavia, and clinical characteristics of ten cases. Atherosclerosis 1990; 80:235–242.

34. Austin MA. Plasma triglyceride and coronary heart disease. Arterioscler Thromb 1991; 11:2–4.

35. Goldstein JL, Hazzard WR, Shrott HG, et al. Hyperlipidemia in coronary heart disease: 1. Lipid levels in 500 survivors of myocardial infarction. J Clin Invest 1973; 52:1533–1543.

36. Goldstein JL, Hazzard WR, Shrott HG, et al. Hyperlipidemia in coronary heart disease: 2. Genetic analysis of lipid levels in 176 families and delineation of a new inherited disorder, familial combined hyperlipidemia. J Clin Invest 1973; 52:1544–1568.

37. Mahley RW, Rall SC. Type III hyperlipoproteinemia (dysbetalipoproteinemia): The role of apolipoprotein E in normal and abnormal lipoprotein metabolism. In: Scriver CR, Beaudet AC, Sly WS, Valle D, eds. The Metabolic Basis of Inherited Disease 6th ed. New York: McGraw-Hill, 1989, pp 1168–1214.

38. Genest JJ Jr, Bard JM, Fruchart JC, et al. Familial hypoalphalipoproteinemia in premature coronary artery disease. Arterioscler Thromb 1993; 13:1728–1737.

39. Stare TJ, Belamarich PF, Shea S, et al: Family history fails to identify many children with severe hypercholesterolemia. Am J Dis Child 1991; 145:61.

40. Committee on Nutrition: Indications for cholesterol testing in children. Pediatrics 1989; 83:141.
41. Committee on Atherosclerosis and Hypertension in Childhood of the Council on Cardiovascular Disease in the Young and the Nutrition Committee, American Heart Association: Diagnosis and treatment of primary hyperlipidemia in childhood. Circulation 1986; 74:1181A.
42. National Cholesterol Education Program. Report of the Expert Panel on Detection, Evaluation, and Treatment of High Blood Cholesterol in Adults. NIH Publication 89-2925. Bethesda, MD: U.S. Department of Health and Human Services, Public Health Service, National Institutes of Health, National Heart, Lung, and Blood Institute, January 1989.
43. Tonstad S, Knuatzan J: Efficacy and safety of cholestryramine therapy in peripubertal and prepubertal children with familial hypercholesterolemia. J Pediatr 1996; 129: 42.
44. Colletti RR, Neufled EJ, Roff NK, et al: Niacin treatment of hypercholesterolemia in children. Pediatrics 1993; 92:78.
45. Stein EA. Treatment of familial hypercholesterolemia with drugs in children. Arteriosclerosis 1989; 9:I145–I151.
46. Levy RI, Fredrickson DS, Shulman R, et al. Dietary and drug treatment of primary hyperlipoproteinemia. Ann Intern Med 1972; 77:267–294.
47. Dobocu J, Brasseur D, Chaudron JM, et al: Simvastatin use in children. Lancet 1992; 339:1488.
48. Thompson GR, Lowenthal R, Myant NB. Plasma exchange in the management of homozygous familial hypercholesterolemia. Lancet 1975; 1:1208–1211.
49. Yokoyama S, Hayashi R, Kikkawa T et al. Specific sorbent of apolipoprotein B– containing lipoproteins for plasmapheresis. Arteriosclerosis 1984; 4:276–282.
50. Gordon BR, Kelsey SF, Bilheimer DW, et al. Treatment of refractory hypercholesterolemia by low-density lipoprotein apheresis using an automated dextran sulfate cellulose adsorption system. Am J Cardiol 1992; 70:1010–1016.
51. Buchwald H, Varco RL, Matts JP, et al. Effect of partial ileal bypass surgery on mortality and morbidity from coronary heart disease in patients with hypercholesterolemia: Report of the Program on the Surgical Control of the Hyperlipidemias (POSCH). N Engl J Med 1990; 323:946–955.
52. Stein EA, Mieny C, Spitx L, et al. Portacaval shunt in four patients with homozygous hypercholesterolemia. Lancet 1975; 1:832–835.
53. Bilheimer DW, Grundy SM, Starzel TE, Brown MS. Liver transplantation to provide low density lipoprotein receptors and lower plasma cholesterol in a child with homozygous familial hypercholesterolemia. N Engl J Med 1984; 311:1658–1664.

12

Failure to Thrive

Jere Ziffer Lifshitz
Prime Health Consultants, Inc., Miami, Florida

Fima Lifshitz
State University of New York Health Science Center at Brooklyn,
New York, New York, and Miami Children's Hospital, Miami, Florida

1   DEFINITION

The term *failure to thrive* is used to describe infants and young children whose body weight and weight gain is substantially less than that of their peers. In children born at term with weight and length in the normal range, it is defined as growth deceleration to a point below the third percentile in weight; a child who has fallen across two or more percentiles; or a child whose weight is less than 80% of the ideal weight for age.

Failure to thrive (FTT) accounts for 1 to 5% of tertiary hospital admissions for patients less than 1 year of age (1). Many more children, perhaps 10% of a pediatric population, are managed as outpatients by physicians throughout the United States (2). Although the diagnosis of FTT is made frequently, both the term and its value as a diagnosis remain debatable. Despite its established status in medical terminology, the concept of FTT lacks a clarified definition and should be considered a sign or symptom, not a diagnosis or a disease (3).

The term *FTT* is used primarily to describe a failure to gain weight. The lack of weight gain may be due to a variety of medical and/or social conditions. Although many serious diseases can cause growth failure, *FTT* usually implies that the cause is not immediately apparent.

Children who are afflicted with FTT are typically diagnosed in the first few months of life, and their illness may persist for years. All FTT infants have physiological alterations due to malnutrition, but the causes can be categorized as organic or nonorganic (4). Organic FTT (OFTT) involves infants who have specific diagnosable disorders. It is only identified in 20 to 40% of children hospitalized with FTT and even less frequently in outpatient clinics.

Nonorganic failure to thrive (NOFTT) is a subtype of FTT that accounts for the majority of FTT infants, although the percentage varies from institution to institution. NOFTT does not imply a specific cause but merely suggests that the cause is primarily external to the infant (5). In addition, there may be an overlap between OFTT and NOFTT owing to the presence of minor infections, vomiting, and diarrhea together with behavioral problems and altered eating behavior. Therefore, several authors have questioned the adequacy of this dichotomous view, suggesting the need for a third category: ''mixed'' etiology (6). However most authors believe that this categorization or use of the mixed terminology fails to provide guidelines for diagnosis or treatment (7). FTT results from malnutrition that is manifest as poor growth, but in this chapter the term of FTT is used, as said previously, to denote a weight-related problem that would lead to growth failure. At times, however, the failure to gain adequate weight may not be associated with alterations in length. NOFTT is more than a growth problem. Children with NOFTT present a low rate of weight or length gain, delayed development, abnormal behavior, and distorted caretaker–infant interaction.

2 DIAGNOSTIC CRITERIA

The central issue in defining FTT is the choice of growth indices by which it is identified. Traditionally, growth parameters have been the major criteria for determining optimal health, nutritional status, and/or the presence of FTT in infants and children. Plotting body weight, length, and head circumference measurements on growth charts detects abnormalities in the growth pattern and can help to identify FTT. The advantage of this approach is its familiarity and simplicity; the disadvantage is its insensitivity (8). The most commonly used criteria are based on cross-sectional assessments of body weight and length that fail to ascertain growth progression longitudinally. Instead, growth velocity measurements plotted in charts are more accurate and should be used to establish adequacy or inadequacy of weight and length progression. Guo and colleagues (9) provided reference data on the expected incremental gains in weight and length for clinically relevant age intervals during the first 2 years of life.

The author has used the theoretical body weight of the patient as an index of malnutrition (10). *Theoretical body weight* is defined as the weight that the child should have at the time of the examination if the patient had continued to gain weight along the previously established percentile during the premorbid period. Using this method, nutritional growth problems may be detected even when there is no body-weight deficit for length and even when there is body-weight excess. However, longitudinal evaluation of growth is fraught with difficulties because often no length and weight data are available or the measurements are inaccurate (11).

A 1994 review (12) of the methods used to categorize undernutrition claimed that body weight and length may not inversely correlate with functional outcomes in longitudinal studies, thus the categorization of anthropometric deficits will remain arbitrary. Therefore, body weight and length should be used only to define a child as having a risk of possible adverse effects of FTT, not as being malnourished (13–15).

3 FAILURE TO THRIVE

FTT can be due to a variety of disorders that may have little in common except for poor body weight. Each one of them must be recognized and treated accordingly. However, the goals of nutritional rehabilitation are similar regardless of the cause. In this chapter, the presentation is limited to the syndrome of NOFTT; the reader is referred elsewhere for a review of OFTT (16–18). In the NOFTT syndrome, inadequate nutrition (i.e., nature) and distorted social stimulation (i.e., nurture) both contribute to poor weight gain, delayed development, and abnormal behavior.

3.1 Characteristics of the Child

The major clinical presentations in NOFTT infants include decreased rate of weight gain or, at times, weight loss. Lack of linear growth may also be observed over time, but body weight is more severely affected. Other characteristics of this type of FTT infants are shown in Table 1.

There has also been evidence that NOFTT infants may present a combination of biological vulnerability, environmental difficulties, and be the products of parents with poor marital relationships (19,20). Infants suffering from this type of FTT were more passive, more likely to sleep through meals or take longer to finish at each breast, and more likely to be diagnosed as hypotonic. There was also evidence that NOFTT infants received less appropriate developmental stimulation at home and have developmental delays.

Developmental delays have also been linked to oral-motor dysfunction (OMD), which is frequently found in FTT children (Table 2). In fact, when chil-

TABLE 1 Clinical Findings in Nonorganic Failure
to Thrive

Small for age
Thin for length
Wide-eyed expression or gaze aversion
Thin chest
Wasted buttocks
Prominent abdomen
Hanging skin folds under the arms
Expressionless face
Decreased vocalization, gross motor activity, and
    response to social stimuli
Lack of cuddling
Clenched fists

---

dren with FTT were compared with children of the same developmental age with
cerebral palsy, the oral-motor profiles were not remarkably different. Reilly and
colleagues (21) hypothesized that children with OMD might have subtle neurodevelopmental disorders. Their study was the first whole-population survey that
used direct assessment and observation showing that a substantial number of
children previously diagnosed with NOFTT in fact had significant OMD due
possibly to developmental delays (see chap. 13).

Wilensky and colleagues (19) measured FTT infants' mental and cognitive
development by administering the Bayley Scales of Mental Development. They
concluded that at 20 months of age, FTT infants were twice as likely to show
mental developmental quotients of less than 80. Behaviorally, the infants also
showed less sociability.

3.2 Assessment

Every child who fails to thrive has either not taken, has not been offered, or has
not retained adequate energy to meet his or her nutritional needs. Assessing in-

TABLE 2 Characteristics of Oral-Motor Dysfunction

Difficulties with sucking, chewing, and swallowing
Abnormally long feeding times
Poor appetite
Delayed texture tolerance
Difficult feeding behavior
Inappropriate hunger or satiety signal
Food refusal

---

fants with FTT demands a very careful history and physical examination. Questions should focus on diet, feedings, and family interaction (Table 3). Difficulties in breast-feeding that may lead to FTT include positioning during feeding (22), foremilk consumption associated with changing breasts before the infant can empty the breast (23,24), or insufficient milk produced by the mother due to a variety of factors (25,26). Dietary inadequacies may also result from exclusive breast-milk feedings for prolonged periods (27). However, FTT in breast-fed infants should not be confused with the normal growth-deceleration pattern of this type of infant observed after 4 to 6 months of age, as described below in Section 4.4. The physician should look for signs of neglect, abuse, or illness. It should be kept in mind that there are no specific laboratory data that will confirm the diagnosis. Confirmation of the diagnosis of NOFTT is always based on a positive growth and behavioral response to treatment.

3.2.1 Nutritional Evaluation

A careful nutritional evaluation must be performed, which should include collecting dietary intake data from a 24-hr recall or, more accurately, a food diary for 3 to 7 days. It should also address meal frequency, feeding patterns, and an assessment of all fluids given. It is also valuable to determine whether any particular food was restricted or promoted—i.e., increased fruit juice consumption (see below, Sec. 3.3). Often, the diet record suggests that the child is receiving adequate calories for weight and length but not for age. This level of intake allows the infant to maintain current weight but does not provide sufficient nutrients for

TABLE 3 Necessary Elements of History Taking

Feeding history	Family history	Psychosocial history
Method—breast or bottle	Heights	Family makeup
Timing—how often, how long	Weights	Employment status
Solids—when introduced, reaction	Illnesses	Financial status
Feeding advice compliance	Development problems	Stress
Caregiver—who feeds the child	Inherited diseases	Caretakers' history of neglect or abuse
Location—where the child is fed	Concerns with obesity, cholesterol, and/or junk food	Maternal depression
Elimination—stool or vomiting patterns	Allergies	

growth. Supplementation studies have demonstrated that improvements in nutrient intake result in improved growth, including bone mineralization and maturation (28–31). Sometimes the dietary intake is adequate in calories and protein but is deficient in specific nutrients—such as iron, zinc, and/or other micronutrients—resulting in growth faltering (32–34). Direct observation of mother-infant feeding interaction is a necessary part of the evaluation.

If decreased energy intake was the cause of inappropriate weight gain, the question becomes: Why are insufficient amounts of food consumed by infants with NOFTT? Are these children simply not offered enough? Do the infants fail to signal hunger or satiety? Do they have a poor appetite or refuse food?

Particular attention should be paid to nonspecific symptoms, such as intermittent vomiting, spitting up, diarrhea, and frequent upper respiratory tract infections that may be present in NOFTT and in other organic conditions. In most instances, as the child gains weight, regurgitation gradually ceases and the gastroesophageal reflux gradually improves. Changing to an antiregurgitation infant formula thickened with rice cereal and keeping the child upright after feedings may help in this transitional period (35). Recurrent respiratory infections, which are common in the malnourished child, may also alter the child's appetite. Dentition may make eating difficult or painful. Other conditions, such as mild brain injury (e.g., cerebral palsy), may lead to swallowing or sucking problems and OMD, as described above. The key pointers in evaluation of a patient with FTT are delineated in Table 4.

The dietary intake may or may not be adequate for the infants age and/or size; however, when the child presents a history of increased intake within the presence of FTT, an organic problem must be considered—i.e., malabsorption. Similarly, a history of weight loss should suggest the possibility of organic disease, as most infants with NOFTT cease gaining weight but do not show weight loss unless there is starvation. The presence of specific symptoms may also suggest a variety of disorders or possible pathogenic mechanisms and require specific assessment and/or treatment, such as gastroesophageal reflux and antiregurgitation formula (36).

3.3 Family Evaluation

FTT infants prove that nourishment involves much more than ingestion of food. In most instances, NOFTT results from a disruption in nurturing practices that ultimately affects the child's ability to obtain proper nourishment. These nurturing factors include the parents beliefs and their concepts of nutrition. Also the infant's behavior or adverse social or psychological environments may contribute to an inadequate nurturing environment leading to NOFTT. Therefore, direct observation of mother-infant feeding and social interaction is a necessary part of the evaluation. The clinician evaluating a child with FTT must also determine if

TABLE 4 Evaluating Failure to Thrive

Intake	Weight	Possible cause of symptom	Next steps

1. Adequate	Loss	1. Malabsorption
		   Organic disease
		   Biliary atresia or cirrhosis
		2. Diarrhea
		3. Liver disease
		4. Hirschsprung's disease
		5. Increased metabolism
		   Endocrine disorders
			Laboratory testing

2. Adequate or inadequate	Inappropriate	1. Lack of appetite
		   Anemia, iron deficiency
		   Psychosocial problems
		   Central nervous system disorder
		   Chronic infection
		2. Ingestion difficulties
		   Psychosocial problems
		   Central nervous system disorders
		   Impaired mental or motor development
		   Oral-motor dysfunction
		   Dyspnea
		   Muscle pathology
		   Genetic disorders
		3. Unavailability of food
		   Breast-feeding failure or error in feeding method
		   Incorrect feeding technique
		   Insufficient food
		   Inappropriate food
		   Bizarre diet or health belief
		4. Vomiting or regurgitation
		   CNS pathology
		   Reflux
		   Organic disease
			1. Nutrition assessment and counseling
			2. Education on feeding and nurturing
			3. If necessary, GI and neurological workup

any prenatal factor many play a role in the etiology of the problem. Small-for-date infants at birth need to be carefully investigated and their growth plotted in appropriate charts (see Sec. 4.3). The possibility of prenatal exposure to psychoactive substances must be ascertained, including exposure to alcohol, tobacco, and other drugs (37).

3.4 Parental Characteristics

Parents with misconceptions about nutrition require education to help manage an infant with FTT. Parents may limit their infant's nutrition by placing it on a diet because of certain health practices and beliefs recommended for adults by the medical community. Some parents cling to the belief that restricting excess food during childhood is a way to develop healthful nutritional patterns for their children later in life (38). For example, families concerned with cholesterol and atherosclerosis, obesity, or "junk food" may restrict and limit the nutritional intake of the infant (39). McCann et al (40) studied the eating habits and attitudes concerning body shape of mothers of children with NOFTT using the eating disorder examination. These mothers were found to have a higher level of dietary concern, and despite their child's weight deficits, 50% of them were restricting their child's intake of sweet foods and a further 30% were restricting food they considered "fattening" or "unhealthy."

Parents who want their children to ingest an appropriate diet and to avoid potentially harmful diets may offer low-cholesterol foods, avoid eggs, and provide low-fat milk to their infants. These nutritional practices may lead to nutritional growth retardation (41). Many parents may also offer "natural" juices instead of milk, sweets, and other snacks without realizing that excess of intake juice may be harmful, even though juice itself is not considered "junk food." Excess juice intake may result in an unbalanced diet and FTT (42). The author reported eight patients, aged 14 to 27 months, who were referred for FTT and whose deterioration of weight and linear growth progression coincided with excessive juice consumption. The children's diets were hypocaloric, providing 78 to 92% of recommended energy intake for age and weight. Dietary intake included considerable juice consumption (360 to 900 mL daily). Fruit juice, primarily apple juice, contributed to 25 to 60% of daily energy intakes. As a result, food consumption was reduced, lowering dietary protein, fat, and micronutrient intakes.

Fruit juices that contain higher concentrations of fructose than glucose, with or without sorbitol, are those that may be associated with malabsorption of these carbohydrates (43). Failure to absorb sugars from juice has been noted to be a factor in the development of chronic nonspecific diarrheal syndrome of children ingesting large quantities of fruit juice (44). Juices with equivalent fructose-glucose concentration and no sorbitol may be less likely to be associated with malabsorption and therefore may be a good substitute during the transition from juice dependence (45). Pediatricians investigating an infant with FTT should be aware of the dietary practices and beliefs of the parents and of the quantities and carbohydrate content of juice consumed, as not all juices are created equal.

Caregivers who are vegetarians may also feed an infant an inappropriate diet leading to FTT. This phenomenon has increased greatly during the past few years because of concerns about animal welfare, the environment, and "healthy eating." Growth failure has been reported in infants and toddlers fed inappropriate vegetarian diets (46,47). Other nutritional hazards of vegetarian diets have been identified, such as iron-deficiency anemia, vitamin B_{12} deficiency, and rickets; also, a bulky diet can restrict energy intakes, especially in the first few years of life, and then lead to impaired growth (48).

3.5 Infant Behaviors

"Feeding difficulties" may also be a cause of decreased nutrient intake in NOFTT infants (49). These infants exhibit unusual behaviors, such as wide-eyed staring, gaze avoidance, fist clenching, and apathy toward their caregivers (Table 1). Although apathy and decreased motor activity are recognized behaviors in malnourished infants, many of the abnormal behaviors of NOFTT patients are not attributable to malnutrition alone. The effects of malnutrition on behavioral development have been studied extensively, with data generated primarily from low-income populations (50–52).

Some nutritional alterations may influence the infant's behavior. Iron deficiency during infancy has been associated with anorexia, irritability, and lack of interest in the surroundings (53). Similarly, zinc deficiency may compound the course of FTT (54), and excess lead ingestion may complicate the clinical picture even before the blood lead levels reach a toxic concentration. NOFTT infants were shown to have blood lead levels in a range formerly thought to be safe (i.e., 15 to 20 mg/dL) (55). These elements should be monitored in all FTT patients and treatment should be given when alterations are demonstrated.

An infant behavior that typically leads to FTT is infantile anorexia nervosa, which is characterized by food refusal, extreme food selectivity, and undereating despite parental efforts to increase the infant's food intake. The onset of this disorder usually occurs between 6 months and 3 years of age, with a peak around 9 months of age (56). The feeding difficulties stem from the infant's thrust for autonomy; a striking observation of these infants being their willfulness. Mother and infant become embroiled in conflicts over autonomy and control, which become manifest primarily during the feeding time. This conflict leads to a battle of wills over the infant's food intake. Characteristically, parents mention that they have "tried everything" to get the infant to eat. Chatoor and colleagues (57) hypothesized that this separation-related conflict interferes with the infant development of somatopsychological differentiation. The process of distinguishing somatic sensations, such as hunger or satiety, from emotional feelings, such as affection, anger, or frustration, is clouded by noncontingent responses by the parents to cues coming form the infant. As a result of this confusion, the infant's eating becomes controlled by emotional experiences instead of physiological needs. The focus of the treatment is improving communications between the parents and the infant to facilitate the process of separation and individuality. In a cognitive-behavioral approach, the therapist explains the infant's behavior to the parents and suggests ways to structure mealtimes differently to modify it.

3.6   Adverse Social and Psychological Environment

Often, parental stress affects the way infants interact with their mothers (18). The quantity and quality of social and emotional stimulation between mother and child may be decreased even before clinical evidence of FTT. Many mothers of NOFTT infants are depressed, come from lower socioeconomic groups, lack a support group, and/or are under multiple stresses. Mothers from higher socioeconomic groups may also lack the emotional strength or motivation to interpret or respond to the needs of the infant. As more mothers become engaged in work outside of the home or involved in activities that are independent of their family responsibilities, their children may not be getting the appropriate attention to meet their needs for nurturing (58).

3.7   Physical Examination

Height, weight, and head circumference should be plotted on a standard growth chart. The results of these measurements will give a clue to the possible causes of FTT (Table 5). Physicians should examine the infant for signs of central nervous system, pulmonary, cardiac, or gastrointestinal disorders as well as for signs of abuse (i.e., poor hygiene, unexplained bruises or scars, or inappropriate behavior).

The assessment of the growth pattern is very helpful and may by itself

TABLE 5   Assessments of Growth in Infants

Measurements	Indication
Weight loss or lack of growth	Underlying organic disease
Measurements below third percentile, but showing same growth rate	Probably not FTT, but intrauterine growth retardation, familial-constitutional short stature
Median age for weight is less than median age for length	Child may be undernourished

distinguish infants with FTT of different types from those with other growth disorders and/or with factitious failure to thrive (see below, Sec. 4).

3.8 Laboratory Aids

Poor nutrition and psychosocial factors are by far the most frequent causes of FTT. Therefore, laboratory tests are of limited value in determining the etiology of growth deficiency and should be used only when the findings from the history and physical examination indicate something organic or the need to assess possible nutritional alterations. In some cases, the child's bone age should be determined radiologically to facilitate the process of ruling out systemic chronic diseases or a hormonal abnormality. This measurement may also be of help as a baseline for the future progression of growth and bone development.

Unless organic disease is suspected, detailed testing should be reserved for those patients for whom management of nutritional and psychosocial problems does not result in the expected improvement in the rate of growth. It has long been known that less than 1% of laboratory tests showed an abnormality that helped identify the etiology of FTT (59) (Table 6).

However, the laboratory evaluation of nutritional status should be comprehensive to assess for deficiencies that are not clinically apparent. A group of protein markers may be valuable in diagnosing suboptimal nutrition. Table 7 lists some of the proteins used and their relative pros and cons (60,61). Other nutritional measurements must be done in accordance with the dietary history—i.e., measurements of zinc or iron status. It should be kept in mind that iron deficiency without anemia may be present and be responsible for some of the clinical findings in the patient—i.e., anorexia—as well as some of the long-term consequences (53). Thus this deficiency needs to be appropriately diagnosed and promptly treated.

TABLE 6 Possible Laboratory Tests

Urinalysis with speciic gravity and urine culture
Serum bicarbonate with simultaneous urine pH
Sedimentation rate, c-reactive protein
Creatinine, electrolytes, glucose
Calcium and phosphorus
Bilirubin and liver enzymes
TSH and thyroxine
Lead and HIV serology
Stool pathogens, parasites, sugars, and pH
Tuberculin
Abdominal ultrasonography
Sweat test

TABLE 7   Protein Markers to Assess Nutritional Status

Protein	Pros	Cons
Albumin	Readily available	20-day half-life
Transferrin	Readily available	10-day half-life
Prealbumin	Half-life less than 2 days; rapid synthesis in the liver	Sensitive to infection and inflammatory response
Retinol binding protein (RBP)	Produced by the liver, half-life of 12 hr	Seems more affected by energy defi- ciency than by pro- tein deficits
Fibronectin		Further clinical studies needed to validate as a marker for malnu- trition

IGF-1 concentrations are also correlated with nutritional status; however, these measurements are of little value in infancy and there were no detectable differences in the IGF-1 concentrations in either patients with nutritional dwarfing compared with children with familial or constitutional short stature (62). In contrast, the author reported that children with nutritional dwarfing showed decreased activity of erythrocyte Na^+-K^+-ATPase (ENKA) compared with familial short-stature children (63). This enzyme is involved in the active transport of sugars and amino acids and with cellular thermogenesis. It usually accounts for approximately one-third of the basal energy requirements. A diminished energy intake lowers the basal metabolic rate and decreases ENKA activity. Furthermore, ENKA activity was positively correlated with mild degrees of suboptimal nutrition in an experimental model in rats (64,65). Therefore, ENKA activity may be a good marker of subtle malnutrition and prolonged energy deficits. To date, this assay has not been tested in NOFTT, nor has it been available for clinical purposes, and it can be applied only on a research basis.

If weight gain does not occur soon after advice is given to the parent(s) about feedings, the child must be evaluated more intensely. Usually these patients are admitted to the hospital to have any possible organic alterations ruled out and simultaneously to receive appropriate nutritional intake to induce weight gain (66).

4 MANAGEMENT

In the past, hospital care was routinely recommended as part of the initial management of FTT patients. The goals were to ensure an adequate dietary intake, observe the child's behavior, and watch the family-child interactions. Despite today's economic constraints, hospital care is justified when the patient has not responded to appropriate outpatient management; the severity of the malnutrition warrants it; or abuse, neglect, or both are suspected. Fryer, in a metanalysis with NOFTT, found that hospitalization significantly improved growth recovery and sustained catch-up growth (67). However, an aggressive outpatient management may also be appropriate. The use of a multidisciplinary team usually offers special advantages in the rapid correction of undernutrition in children with NOFTT. Bithoney and colleagues (68) showed that the multidisciplinary team treatment resulted in improved weight gain compared with children treated in a primary care setting. Growth outcomes over a 6-month follow-up evaluation were analyzed using growth quotient (GQ) analysis in 53 children with NOFTT compared with 107 children treated in the primary care clinic. The hospital-treated group grew better (i.e., GQ = 1.75 ± 0.39) than the group treated in primary care (i.e., GQ = 1.18 ± 0.42; $p < 0.001$).

4.1 Nutritional Management

Since children with FTT are unable to achieve an adequate caloric intake, nutritional management is the cornerstone of therapy. Nutritional therapy of FTT children has several goals: (1) achieving ideal weight for height; (2) correcting nutrient deficits; (3) allowing catch-up growth; (4) restoring optimal body composition; and (4) educating parents in the nutritional requirements and feeding of the child.

4.1.1 Achieving Ideal Height for Weight

Regardless of why a child fails to thrive, effective nutritional management consists primarily of providing enough calories to achieve a positive energy balance and growth. The World Health Organization Expert Consultation on Energy and Protein Requirements (1981) recommended that "whenever possible, energy requirements should be based on measurement of expenditure rather than intake" (69). One such way to measure the expenditure is to calculate resting energy expenditure (REE). REE is fairly stable in young, healthy children and is the largest single contributor to total energy requirements.

Since the standard equations to predict resting energy expenditure were all derived from data accumulated from healthy children, Sentongo and colleagues (70) set out to study the applicability of prediction equations in children with FTT. They measured REE in young children with FTT by indirect calorimetry and compared the results with predicted REE from the World Health Organization—Schofield weight-based, and Schofield weight height-based. The study of 45 children concluded that REE should be measured in young infants and children with moderate to severe FTT. The Schofield weight/height-based equation was least likely to underestimate REE and is therefore preferred when REE cannot be directly measured. Recently, REEs were measured most accurately by an enhanced metabolic testing activity chamber designed for infants; data obtained by this accurate method differ from those derived from the usual equations (71). Furthermore, the results obtained with this accurate method showed that the World Health Organization equations allowed for only about one-fourth of the true energy requirement.

Because nutritional intervention is usually the focus in treating children with FTT, high-calorie, adequate protein feeding has been advocated for many years. With this treatment the child recovers more rapidly, the stay in the hospital is shorter, and more children can be treated in a given period of time at less cost.

Nurses or trained therapists should feed the infant initially to allow identification of a feeding problem and ensure that intake will be adequate. Proper feeding of the FTT child can be achieved most often through the use of infant formula that is modified to meet the child's specific nutrient needs. Feeding formula alone allows for easy calculation of caloric intake and estimation of losses through vomiting. The number of calories per unit volume of formula can be increased in ready-to-feed formulas. Carbohydrate can be added in the form of glucose polymers—medium-chain triglycerides or corn oil will provide long-chain triglycerides and milk solids can improve the caloric density. Protein supplementation is usually not needed, but some products can be used when indicated.

Tube feedings are indicated only in cases of severe malnutrition or failure to induce weight gain in the hospital. They may be necessary if the child is severely debilitated, is metabolically unstable, or requires immediate restoration of fluid and electrolyte balance. Tube feedings may be useful for children with NOFTT as a temporary behavior modification modality or in patients who fail to respond to other methods of nutritional rehabilitation (72).

Many FTT children begin to gain weight with an intake of 630 kJ/kg (73). An almost linear relationship exists between the rates of weight gain and energy intake over the caloric intake of 420 to 1050 kJ/day. Foods that have minimal nutritional value should be discouraged and high-calorie meals and nutritious snacks should be recommended. Caution must be taken to preserve the ratio of calories derived from protein, fat, and carbohydrate as a percent of the total calories. Appropriate water intake in relation to the nutrients provided should also be maintained.

4.1.2 Correcting Nutrient Deficits

Many clinical trials have indicated that supplementation with micronutrients improves growth in growth-faltering patients. Single-nutrient deficiencies are cumbersome to document and micronutrient deficiencies commonly coexist. For example, iron deficiency may be present without iron-deficiency anemia, and zinc deficiency may be difficult to document by the lack of a good indicator. Yet clinical trials of iron supplementation have positive effects on weight gain, linear growth, and psychosocial behavior (74). Similar studies have revealed positive effects with zinc supplementation (75). Vitamin and mineral deficiencies sometimes become evident only after the infant starts growing and gaining weight. Therefore a multivitamin preparation that includes iron and zinc is recommended for all undernourished children.

4.1.3 Allowing Catch-Up Growth

Catch-up growth is defined as the acceleration in growth that occurs when a period of growth retardation ends and favorable conditions are restored. Catch-up growth in FTT depends on the provision of calories, protein, and other nutrients in excess of normal requirements. Whitehead and Biol (76) calculated that children need approximately 25 to 30% more energy and nearly double the amount of protein for catch-up growth.

For infants of about 6 months of age, a weight gain of 45 g/day (i.e., three times the usual weight gain in this age group) can be considered catch-up growth. Estimates of the energy cost for tissue anabolism range from 21 kJ/g to 42 to 53.8 kJ/g of weight gain. Increases in the caloric density of the diet are often necessary to ensure adequate caloric intake without increases in volume. One to two weeks of refeeding may be required to demonstrate initial weight gain. Efforts to promote catch-up growth should be sustained until the child reaches previous premorbid growth percentiles. Once the child has attained an appropriate weight-to-height ratio, velocity decelerates and nutrient intake should also be automatically reduced to recommended energy intakes for age.

4.1.4 Restoring Optimal Body Composition

The extent to which nutritional rehabilitation can restore normal body size and composition is a critical subject. Returning to one's previous growth curve does not indicate achievement of a normal body composition. For example, those with prior IUGR showed a propensity toward an increase in fat and a decrease in lean body mass after catch-up growth.

The effect of the diet fed to the recovering child and the rate of weight gain on the outcome have been investigated. Hospitalization for rehabilitation can be shortened if more rapid weight gain can be achieved without inducing undesirable changes in body composition especially fat accretion. Studies of malnourished children before and after recovery show that total body water and extracellular fluid decrease to values approximating the normal range. Individual values for total body water in malnourished children suggest that excessive adipose tissue was laid down during nutritional recovery (1,77). Studies based on nitrogen-creatinine turnover and biopsy material suggest that through both cellular hypertrophy and hyperplasia, muscle cell mass returns to values similar to those of children of normal height and weight (2). The enlargement of the adipocytes apparently leads to an increase in the fat content of adipose tissue.

The proportions of the weight gain accounted for by lean tissue and fat in recovering children have been estimated by studies of the energy cost of weight gain. The cost of laying down 1 g of fat is estimated to be approximately 33.6 to 42 kJ/g, whereas 1 g of muscle requires on 7.6 kJ/g. Intermediate values reflect the proportion of fat and lean tissue.

Fjeld (78) studied infants randomized to regimens that induced rates of weight gain of either 6 or 12 g/day until the weight-to-height ratio had been restored to the NCHS median (i.e., approximately 60 days and 30 days, respectively). Using a combination of measurements of nitrogen balance and energy turnover and body composition (D_2 ^{18}O), Fjeld concluded that more rapid recovery did not result in excessive fat deposition.

Kabir and coworkers (79) assessed body composition by bioelectrical impedance in malnourished children before and after dietary supplementation. They noted that a major determinant in restoring the reference body composition and accelerating the catch-up growth was the high protein content (15%) of the different diets. On the whole, the data suggest that, depending on the timing and severity of malnutrition, recovery of body mass to normal composition is a possible although not uniform occurrence.

4.1.5 Educating Parents

During the recovery period, parental nutrition education programs are extremely important. When a family's psychosocial maladaptations are determined to be major contributors to FTT, the physician must discuss them in a nonjudgmental way, so that guilt is not increased or compliance endangered. Parents should be reassured, and support should be provided for correction of the problems as much as possible.

To improve infants' eating habits, Chatoor (80) introduced an inpatient treatment program for food-refusing infants. Parents and infant were separated at mealtimes. The nurses fed the child with structured, time-limited meals. Parents were given individual therapy and were then reintroduced to the feeding situation. New and healthier guidelines for mealtimes were established. Once the infant no longer had a problem with feeding and adequate intake had been achieved, the mother was permitted to feed the infant under observation. Education of the parents concerning the infant's nutritional needs was an essential part of therapy.

Parents must be educated regarding the catch-up growth process and long-term growth goals. The baseline appearance of a cachectic child may bias the family's perception of recovery. The misperception that the recovering child is too plump may result in an abrupt diet change and abandonment of high-calorie feedings (Table 8).

TABLE 8 Behavioral Advice to Parents of Infants with Nonorganic Failure to Thrive

Relax.	Feedings and mealtimes should be pleasant. Avoid battles.
Use positive reinforcement.	Praise a child for eating well. Do not withhold food as a punishment.
Let child feed him/herself.	Allow self-feeding even if child makes a mess.
Provide good role models.	Eat as a family. Children will mimic other siblings and adults.
Establish food-free time.	There should be no food or drink (except water) for 1 hr before meals.
Limit consumption of juice.	Offer solid food before drinks at mealtime. Limit juice throughout the day.
Establish meal and snack times.	Set a time for meals and snacks. Avoid snacking after an unfinished meal.
Recognize feeding cues.	Learn your child's hunger and satiety cues.
Limit distractions.	Limit distractions, such as television or reading, during meals.

In all instances and at all stages of evaluation and treatment of FTT, a "working alliance" between key family members and professionals must be established (81). Developing such relationships can be a challenge, and it requires the availability and commitment of multidisciplinary teams to assist the family in the treatment of NOFTT.

5 FACTITIOUS FAILURE TO THRIVE

Pediatricians should always be aware of different patterns of growth in the first years of life that can be present as factitious failure to thrive, which does not require nutritional rehabilitation (58). These patterns include patients with familial short stature or constitutional growth delay, intrauterine growth retardation, and the breast-fed baby. Because the size of an infant at birth is more related to maternal size and intrauterine influences than to genetic factors, in some children an adjustment in growth velocity between birth and 2 years of age is to be expected. There may be a change in growth velocity of greater than 25% (across two percentile lines) as a recanalization of normal growth owing to a genetic adjustment. A significant decrease in growth rate may represent a physiological event in the first years of life and does not necessarily indicate FTT (82).

5.1 Familial Short Stature

Familial short stature (FSS) has been defined as genetic short stature. These patients are short throughout life. Their final height is consonant with parental height. However, they readjust their growth percentile according to their genetic potential before 3 years of age (83).

5.2 Constitutional Growth Delay

The growth pattern of patients with constitutional growth delay (CGD) is generally considered a normal variation of growth. CGD patients are typically "slow growers" and "late bloomers." They usually have a severe deceleration of growth within the first 2 years of life that may be confused with FTT. CGD patients have a subsequent definition of growth and weight gain and normal growth increments paralleling the normal curve until adolescence, when a growth spurt occurs.

However, significant differences have been found between patients with CGD and FSS in profiles of their weight-to-length and weight-to-height ratios from 4 months to 12 years of age (83). After 4 months of age, the weight-to-length ratio of the patients with CGD was significantly lower than that of the FSS population. Also, a significant weight deficit for length was noted by the sixth month of life in the CGD population. The difference became more evident by 18 months of age. In addition, nutritional parameters—such as mean creatinine-height index, retinol binding protein, serum iron, and transferrin saturation values—were lower among young CGD patients.

Because patients with CGD might have subtle nutritional deficiencies in early life, it is advisable to perform a workup to rule out any alteration, particularly during the deceleration phase of growth in infancy. Treatment is necessary only if deficits are detected. Otherwise, careful monitoring of growth suffices. In CGD patients, the suboptimal nutrition is usually mild, because growth progression proceeds with eventual recovery. In contrast, in patients with nutritional dwarfing, a more severe impairment of weight gain and abnormal growth pattern are present (10).

5.3 Intrauterine Growth Retardation

Intrauterine growth retardation (IUGR) should be considered when the patients fail to catch up in growth (84). The initial small size and the weight gain and growth progression of these patients may give the false impression of FTT, particularly when the growth pattern is not monitored on appropriate charts developed for small-for-date infants (85). However, if the patient doubles the birth weight by 4 months of age and triples it by 1 year of age, FTT must be excluded. Nevertheless, the absence of catch-up growth is of great concern to pediatricians and families, even when the child is growing at a normal rate. Under these circumstances, careful monitoring and reassurance are necessary and no nutritional therapy needs to be given.

IUGR refers to a heterogeneous group of patients who fail to grow in utero as a result of environmental, maternal, placental, or fetal factors. Due to the diversity of the etiologic factors and the variability in the period of time during pregnancy that the fetus was affected, different studies reached different conflicting results for the growth prognosis of IUGR infants (73,74). IUGR infants have been shown to catch up in growth during the first 6 months of life, although the growth patterns are diverse (86). In another large series (87), IUGR infants were reported to have an accelerated growth phase during the first 3 months after delivery; however, they persisted in being small compared with the control group through 1 year of age. In a long-term follow-up study (88) of IUGR infants, significant deficits in height and weight were found between 13 and 19 years of age, even after adjustment for differences in socioeconomic status and parental height. Early puberty in some of these patients may be a contributing factor for the unusually short adult height (89).

A recent review of intrauterine growth retardation and the long-term effects of this syndrome on size suggested that treatment with growth hormone may be of value (90). Trials with human growth hormone carried out by different investigators demonstrated that growth may be maximized in these patients. The final height potential appeared to be positively influenced by human growth hormone therapy for 2 to 4 years in dosages from 0.4 to 1.2 U/kg per week. Although these studies are promising, it is necessary to exercise caution when using such therapy, which at present can be considered only on an experimental basis.

5.4 The Breast-Fed Baby

Caution must be taken in labeling an infant who is exclusively breast-fed as having FTT. Because no growth charts for breast-fed infants are usually used, a normal growth pattern of a breast-fed baby may seem to be lower on the growth channel of the currently available growth charts, which are based on studies of infants who were mostly formula-fed (91). To date, no clear data would warrant discouraging breast-feeding of an infant whose growth seems to deviate across channels in such growth charts. Human milk is the ideal and most readily available nutrient and should therefore be continued and encouraged as much as possible. However, breast-feeding alone may not be adequate for a particular child who indeed may be failing to gain weight appropriately. Breast-feeding must be closely monitored to ensure that adequate lactation is present and that the infant thrives at an appropriate rate as plotted on growth charts for breast-fed infants.

The effect of prolonged breast-feeding on growth is controversial. One study (92) demonstrated that exclusively breast-fed infants had slower length velocity after 3 months of age compared with infants who were weaned early and given formula plus solids. This trend was more obvious at 9 months of age. In this study, relative weight had no deficit. More recently, the growth of breast-fed and formula-fed infants from 0 to 18 months of age was investigated in the "DARLING" study (93). The mean weight of breast-fed infants was shown to drop below the median of the formula-fed group between 6 and 18 months of age. In contrast, length and circumference values were similar between the two groups. The results of the study showed that breast-fed infants gain weight more slowly compared with formula-fed infants from similar socioeconomic and ethnic backgrounds during the first 9 months of life.

6 FOLLOW-UP EVALUATION AND LONG-TERM PROGNOSIS

Continued treatment after discharge from the hospital is necessary and the infant should be followed at regular intervals for a long time. Growth, development, and social behavior must be carefully and continually monitored. Temporary placement in a more favorable setting within the family or in a foster care environment may be necessary if the immediate family is judged as being incapable of following through on the recommended management.

There are few systematic long-term studies of growth and development in NOFTT infants. The longest follow-up study on growth, 14 years, has been reported by Oates (94), who found a difference between former FTT children and control children when the relationship between the height ages and weight ages of the children was compared with their chronological ages. Of the children with FTT, 6 out of 14 were 1 or more years below their chronological age for height and weight. In the comparison group it was 1 child out of 14 ($p < 0.04$).

Studies of catch-up growth show that NOFTT children continue to do poorly developmentally despite increased weight. A study by Singer (95) showed that even after extended hospitalization, NOFTT infants manifested persistent intellectual delays at a 3-year follow-up examination, despite maintenance of weight gains achieved during early hospitalization.

These children remained significantly behind in language development, reading age, and verbal intelligence compared to their control group (3). They also scored lower than the control group on a social maturity rating.

7 CONCLUSIONS

Children's eating patterns are very variable, with marked differences in intake from meal to meal—a frequent complaint by parents. However, energy intake is relatively constant on a daily basis, because children adjust their energy at successive meals (96). Parents who worry about the feeding behavior of their children should be reassured if body-weight and height progression is appropriate. In contrast, if FTT is present, regardless of the presence or absence of complaints by the family, a careful nutritional and nurturing assessment should be done with prompt treatment instituted.

Although FTT children may eventually reach normal size, they may fail to outgrow developmental deficits. Thus all interventions for the treatment of NOFTT must be instituted early, be comprehensive, and be long-term. Therapy must focus on improving nutrition, mother–infant interaction, and other social and environmental factors if this problem is to be correctly diagnosed and effectively treated. The physician faces specific additional problems when dealing with a NOFTT patient in the managed health care environment. The diagnostic coding of such children is fraught with "Catch-22" dilemmas (97). Medical, nutritional, development, and/or psychiatric diagnosis may be utilized, but no optimum classification and coding scheme exists for use in these patients. Additionally, the rapid growth of managed care has significant implications for access to care, quality of services, reimbursement, and payment for health care. The special needs of these patients amplify the issues and challenges in ensuring that managed care is an effective component of community resources that foster healthy growth and development (98). These patients are at risk for concurrent illness and adverse developmental outcomes. A healthier child ultimately requires fewer services and indirect benefits may also occur with fewer health care expenditures and lifelong productivity.

REFERENCES

1. Powell B, Skuse D. When does slow weight gain become failure to thrive? Arch Dis Child 1991; 66:905–906.
2. Mitchell WF, Gorell RW, Greenberg RA. Failure to thrive: A study in a primary care setting, epidemiology and follow-up. Pediatrics 1980; 65:971–977.
3. Wilcox WD, Nieburg P, Miller DS. Failure to thrive: A continuing problem of definition. Clin Pediatr 1989; 28:391–394.
4. Rosenn DW, Loeb LS, Jura MB. Differentiation of organic from nonorganic failure to thrive syndrome in infancy. Pediatrics 1980; 66:698–704.
5. Frank DA, Zeisel SH. Failure to thrive. Pediatr Clin North Am 1988; 35:1187–1206.
6. Casey PH. Failure to thrive: A reconceptualization. J Dev Behav Pediatr 1983; 4: 63–66.
7. Skuse D. Epidemiological and definitional issues in failure to thrive. Child Adolesc Psychiatr Clin North Am 1993; 2:37–59.
8. Formon SJ. Reference data for assessing growth of infants. J Pediatr 1991; 119: 415–416.
9. Guo S, Roche AF, Foman SJ, Nelson SE, Chumlea WC, Rogers RR, Baumgartner RN, Ziegler EE, Siervogel RM. Reference data on gains in weight and length during the first two years of life. J Pediatr 1991; 119:355–362.

10. Lifshitz F, Moses N. Nutritional growth retardation. In: Lifshitz F, ed. Pediatric
     Endocrinology. New York: Marcel-Dekker, 1990, pp 111–132.
11. Cooney K, Pathak U, Watson A. Infant growth charts. Arch Dis Child 1994; 71:
     159–160.
12. Wright JA, Ashenburg CA, Whitaker RC. Comparison of methods to categorize
     undernutrition in children. J Pediatr 1994; 124:944–946.
13. Edwards AG, Halse PC, Parkin JM, Waterson AJ. Recognising failure to thrive in
     early childhood. Arch Dis Child 1990; 65:1263–1265.
14. Leung AK, Lane W, Robson M. Failure to thrive—or physiologic adjustment to
     growth? J Pediatr 1992; 120:497–498.
15. Wright CM, Edwards AG, Halse PC, Waterson AJ. Weight and failure to thrive in
     infancy. Lancet 1991; 337:365–366.
16. Kirkland RT. Failure to thrive. In: Osky FA, et al, eds. Principles and Practice of
     Pediatrics, 2nd Philadelphia: JB Lippincott, 1994, pp 1048–1050.
17. Leung AK, Robson WM, Fagan JE. Assessment of the child with failure to thrive:
     Am Fam Physician 1993; 48:1432–1438.
18. Powell GF. Failure to thrive. In: Lifshitz F, ed. Pediatric Endocrinology 3rd ed. New
     York: Marcel Dekker, 1996, pp 121–130.
19. Wilensky DS, Ginsberg G, Altman M, Tullchinsky TH, Ben Yishay F, Auerbach
     J. A community based study of failure to thrive in Israel. Arch Dis Child 1996; 75:
     145–148.
20. Altemeier WA, O' Connor SM, Sherrod KB, Vietze PM. Prospective study of ante-
     cedents of nonorganic failure to thrive. J Pediatr 1985; 106:360–365.
21. Reilly SM, Skuse DH, Wolke D, Stevenson J. Oral-motor dysfunction in children who
     fail to thrive: Organic or nonorganic? Dev Med Child Neurol 1999; 41:115–122.
22. Morton JA. Ineffective suckling: A possible consequence of obstructive positioning.
     J Hum Lact 1992; 8:83–85.
23. Woolridge MW, Fisher C. Colic, ''overfeeding,'' and symptoms of lactose malab-
     sorption. Clin Pediatr 1998; 28:382–384.
24. Acs G, Lodolini G, Kaminsky S, Cisneros, GJ. Effect of nursing caries on body
     weight in a pediatric population. Pediatr Dent 1992; 14:302–305.
25. Hill PD. Insufficient milk supply syndrome. Clin Iss Perinat Womens Health Nurs
     1992; 3:605–612.
26. Motil KJ, Sheng H-P, Montando CM. Case report: Failure to thrive in a breast-fed
     infant is associated with maternal dietary protein and energy restriction. J Am Coll
     Nutr 1994; 13:203–208.
27. Weston JA, Stage AF, Hathaway P, Andrews DL, Stonington JA, McCabe EB. Pro-
     longed breast-feeding and nonorganic failure to thrive. Am J Dis Child 1987; 141:
     242–243.
28. Allen LH. Nutritional influences on linear growth: A general review. Eur J Clin Nutr
     1994; 48(suppl 1):S75–S89.
29. Martorell R. Results and implications of the INCAP follow-up study. J Nutr 1995;
     125:1127S–1138S.
30. Caulfield LE, Himes JH, Rivera JA. Nutritional supplementation during early child-
     hood and bone mineralization during adolescence. J Nutr 1995; 125:1104S–1110S.
31. Pickett KE, Haas JD, Murdoch S, Rivera JA, Martorell R. Early nutritional supple-

mentation and skeletal maturation in Guatemalan adolescents. J Nutr 1995; 125: 1097S–1103S.

32. Cook JD, Baynes RD, Skikne BS. The physiological significance of circulating transferrin receptors. Adv Exp Med Biol 1994; 352:119–126.
33. Cavan KR, Gibson RS, Grazioso CF, Isalgue AM, Ruz M, Solomons NW. Growth and body composition of periurban Guatemalan children in relation to zinc status: A cross-sectional study. Am J Clin Nutr 1993; 57:334–343.
34. Cavan KR, Gibson RS, Grazioso CF, Isalgue AM, Ruz M, Solomons NW. Growth and body composition of periurban Guatemalan children in relation to zinc status: A longitudinal zinc intervention trial. Am J Clin Nutr 1993; 57:344–352.
35. Hadi H, Stoltzfus R, Dibley MJ, Moulton LH, West KP Jr, Kejolhede CL, Sajimin T. Vitamin A supplementation selectively improves the linear growth of Indonesian children: Results from a randomized controlled trial. Am Soc Clin Nutr 2000; 71: 507–513.
36. Vandenplas Y, Lifshitz JZ, Orenstein S, Lifschitz CH, Shepherd RW, Casaubon PR, Muinos WI, Fagundes Neto U, Garcia Aranda JA, Gentles M, Santiago JD, Vanderhoof J, Yeung C-Y, Moran JR, Lifshitz F. Nutritional management of regurgitation in infants. J Am Coll Nutr 1998; 17:308–316.
37. Frank DA, Wong F. Effects of prenatal exposures to alcohol, tobacco and other drugs. Fail Thrive Pediat Undernutr 1999; 18:275–280.
38. Puglieese MT, Weyman-Daum M, Moses N, Lifshitz F. Parental health beliefs as a cause of nonorganic failure to thrive. Pediatrics 1987; 80:175–182.
39. Lifshitz F, Moses N. Growth failure: A complication of dietary treatment of hypercholesterolemia. Am J Dis Child 1989; 143:537–542.
40. McCann JB, Stein A, Fairburn CG, Dunger DB. Eating habits and attitudes of mothers of children with non-organic failure to thrive. Arch Dis Child 1994; 70:234–236.
41. Lifshitz F, Tarim O. Nutritional dwarfing. Curr Probl Pediatr 1993; 23:322–326.
42. Smith MM, Lifshitz F. Excessive fruit juice consumption as a contributing factor in nonorganic failure to thrive. Pediatrics 1994; 93:438–443.
43. Hyams JS, Etienne NL, Leichtner AM, Theuer RC. Carbohydrate malabsorption following fruit juice ingestion in young children. Pediatrics 1988; 82:64–68.
44. Lifshitz F, Ament ME, Kleinman RE, Klish W, Lebenthal E, Perman J, Udall JN Jr. Role of juice carbohydrate malabsorption in chronic nonspecific diarrhea in children. J Pediatr 1992; 120:825–829.
45. Nobigrot T, Chasalow FI, Lifshitz F. Carbohydrate absorption from one serving of fruit juice in young children: Age and carbohydrate composition effects. J Am Coll Nutr 1997; 16:152–158.
46. Campbell M, Lofters WS, Gibbs WN. Rastafarianism and the vegans syndrome. Br Med J Clin Res Ed 1982; 285:1617–1618.
47. Roberts IF, West RJ, Ogilvie D, Dillon MJ. Malnutrition in infants receiving cult diets: A form of child abuse. Br Med J 1979; 1:296–298.
48. Sanders TA, Reddy S. Vegetarian diets and children. Am J Clin Nutr 1994; 59(suppl):1176S–1181S.
49. Ramsay M, Gisel EG, Boutry M. Non-organic failure to thrive: Growth failure secondary to feeding-skills disorder. Dev Med Child Neurol 1993; 35:285–297.

50. Dobbing J. Vulnerable periods in developing brain. In: Dobbing J, ed. Brain, Behavior and Iron in the Infant Diet. New York: Springer-Verlag, 1990.

51. Pollitt E, Oh S. Early supplementary feeding, child development, and health policy. Food Nutr Bull 1994; 15:208–214.

52. Wachs TD. Relation of mild-to-moderate malnutrition to human development: Correlational studies, J Nutr 1995; 125 (suppl):2245S–2254S.

53. Idjradinata P, Pollitt E. Reversal of developmental delays in iron-deficient anemic infants treated with iron. Lancet 1993; 341:1–4.

54. Walravens PA, Hambidge KM, Koepfer DM. Zinc supplementation in infants with a nutritional pattern of failure to thrive: A double blind controlled study. Pediatrics 1989; 83:532–538.

55. Bithoney WG. Elevated lead levels in children with nonorganic failure to thrive. Pediatrics 1986; 78:891–895.

56. Chatoor I, Egan J. Nonorganic failure to thrive and dwarfism due to food refusal: A separation disorder. J Am Acad Psychoanal 1983; 22:294–301.

57. Chatoor I, Egan J, Getson P, Menielle E, O'Donnell R. Mother-infant interactions in infantile anorexia nervosa. J Am Acad Child Adolesc Psychiatry 1988; 27:535–540.

58. Lifshtiz F, Finch NM, Lifshitz JZ. Failure to thrive, In: Children's Nutrition. Boston: Jones & Bartlett, 1991, pp 253–270.

59. Berwick DM, Levy JC, Kleinerman R. Failure to thrive: Diagnostic yield to hospitalisation. Arch Dis Child 1982; 57:347–351.

60. Benjamin DR. Laboratory tests and nutritional assessment: Protein-energy status. Pediatr Clin North Am 1989; 36:139–161.

61. Figueroa-Colon R. Clinical and laboratory assessment of the malnourished child. In: Suskind RM, Lewinter-Susking L, eds. Textbook of Pediatric Nutrition, 2nd ed. New York: Raven Press, 1992, pp 191–205.

62. Abdenur JE, Pugliese MT, Cervantes C, Fort P, Lifshitz F. Alterations in spontaneous growth hormone in children with nonorganic nutritional dwarfing. J Clin Endocrinol Metab 1992; 75:930–939.

63. Lifshitz F, Friedman S, Smith M, Cervantes C, Recker B, O'Connor M. Nutritional dwarfing: A growth abnormality associated with reduced erythrocyte Na+, K+-ATPase. Am J Clin Nutr 1991; 54:997–1004.

64. Carrillo A, Rising R, Tverskaya R, Lifshitz F. Effect of exogenous recombinant human growth hormone on an animal model of suboptimal nutrition. J Am Coll Nutr 1998; 17:276–281.

65. Abdenur JE, Solans CV, Smith MM, Carman C, Pugliese MT, Lifshitz F. Body composition and spontaneous growth hormone secretion in normal and short stature children. J Clin Endocrinol Metab 1994; 78:277–282.

66. Singer L. Long-term hospitalization of failure to thrive infants: Developmental outcome at three years. Child Abuse Neglect 1986; 10:479–486.

67. Fryer GE. The efficacy of hospitalization of nonorganic failure-to-thrive children: A meta-analysis. Child Abuse Neglect 1988; 12:375–381.

68. Casey PH, Wortham B, Nelson JY. Management of children with failure to thrive in a rural ambulatory setting: Epidemiology and growth outcomes. Clin Pediatr 1984; 23:325–330.

69. World Health Organization. Energy and protein requirements. Report of a joint FAO/WHO/UNU Expert Consultation. WHO Technical Report Series No. 724. Geneva: World Health Organization: 1985.

70. Sentongo TA, Tershakovec AM, Mascarenhas MR, Watson MH, Stallings VA. Resting energy expenditure in young children with failure to thrive. J Pediatr 2000; 136: 3:345–350.

71. Cole C, Rising R, Hakim A, Danon M, Mehta R, Choudhury S, Sundaresh M, Lifshitz F. Comprehensive assessment of the components of energy expenditure in infants using a new infant respiratory chamber. J Am Coll Nutr 1999; 18:233–241.

72. Ramsay M, Zelazo PR. Food refusal in failure to thrive infants: Nasogastric feeding combined with interactive-behavioral treatment. J Pediatr Psychol 1988; 13:329–347.

73. Murray CA, Glassman MS. Nutrient requirements during growth and recovery from failure to thrive. In: Accardo PJ, ed. Failure to Thrive in Infancy and Early Childhood. Baltimore: University Park Press, 1981.

74. Angeles IT, Schutnick WJ, Matulessi P, Gross R, Sastroamidjojo S. Decreased rate of stunting among anemic Indonesian preschool children through iron supplementation. Am J Clin Nutr 1993; 58:339–342.

75. Rosado JK, Lopez P, Munoz E, Martinez H, Allen LH. Zinc supplementation reduced morbidity, but neither zinc nor iron supplementation affected growth or body composition of Mexican preschoolers. Am J Clin Nutr 1997; 65:160–161.

76. Whitehead RG, Biol FI. Protein and energy requirement of young children living in the developing countries to allow for catch-up growth after infections. Am J Clin Nutr 1977; 30:1545–1547.

77. Reeds PJ, Jackson AA, Picou D, Poulter N. Muscle mass and composition in malnourished infants and children and changes seen after recovery. Pediatr Res 1978; 12:613–618.

78. Fjeld CR. Energy Metabolism and Body Composition During Catch-up Growth in Malnourished Children. Chicago: University of Chicago Press, 1987.

79. Kabir I, Malek MA, Rahman MM, Khaled MA, Mahalanabis D. Changes in body composition of malnourished children after dietary supplementation as measured by bioelectrical impedance. Am J Clin Nutr 1994; 59:5–9.

80. Chatoor I. Infantile anorexia nervosa: A developmental disorder of separation and individuation. J Am Acad Psychoanal 1989; 17:43–64.

81. Sturm L, Dawson P. Working with families—An overview for providers. In: Kessler DB, Dawson P, eds. Failure to Thrive and Pediatric Undernutrition—A Transdisciplinary Approach. Baltimore: Paul H Brookes, 1999.

82. Porter B, Skuse D. When does slow weight gain become failure to thrive? Arch Dis Child 1991; 66:905–906.

83. Solans CV, Lifshitz F. Body weight progression and nutritional status of patients with familial short stature with and without constitutional delay in growth. Am J Dis Child 1992; 146:296–302.

84. Albertsson-Wickland K, Karlberg J. Natural growth in children born small for gestational age with and without catch-up growth. Acta Pediatr (Suppl) 1994; 339:64–70.

85. Kelleher KJ, Casey PH, Bradley RH, Pope SK, Whiteside L, Barret KW, Swansom

ME, Kirby RS. Risk factor and outcomes for failure to thrive in low birth weight preterm infants. Pediatrics 1993; 91:941–948.

86. Davies DP. Growth of ''small-for-dates'' babies. Early Hum Dev 1981; 5:95–105.
87. Low JA, Galbraith RS, Muir D, Killen H, Pater B, Karchmar J, Campbell D. Intrauterine growth retardation: A study of long-term morbidity. Am J Obstet Gynecol 1978; 130:534–545.
88. Westwood M, Kramer MS, Munz D, Lovett JM, Watters GV. Growth and development of full-term nonasphyxiated small-for-gestational-age newborns: Follow-up through adolescence. Pediatrics 1983; 71:376–382.
89. Arisake O, Arisaka M, Kiyokawa N, Shimizu T, Nakayama Y, Yabuta K. Intrauterine growth retardation and early adolescent growth spurt in two sisters. Clin Pediatr 1986; 25:559–561.
90. Botero D, Lifshitz F. Intrauterine growth retardation and long-term effects on growth. Curr Opin Pediatr 1992; 11:340–347.
91. Sheard NF. Growth patterns in the first year of life: What is the norm? Nutr Rev 1993; 52:54.
92. Salmenpera L, Perheentupa J, Simes MA. Exclusively breast fed healthy infants grow slower than reference infants. Pediatr Res 1985; 19:307–312.
93. Dewey KG, Heining MJ, Nommsen LA, Peerson JM, Lonnerdal B. Growth of breast-fed infants from 0 to 18 months: The DARLING Study. Pediatrics 1992; 89:1035–1041.
94. Oates RK, Peacock A, Forrest D. Long-term effects of nonorganic failure to thrive. Pediatrics 1985; 75:36–40.
95. Singer L. Long term hospitalization of nonorganic failure-to-thrive infants: Patient characteristics and hospital course. J Dev Behav Pediatr 1987; 8:25–31.
96. Birch LL, Johnson SL, Andresen G, Peters JC, Schulte MC. The variability of young children's energy intake. N Engl J Med 1991; 324:232–235.
97. Casey PH. Diagnostic coding of children with failure to thrive. In: Kessler DB, Dawson P, eds. Failure to Thrive and Pediatric Undernutrition—A transdisciplinary approach. Baltimore: Paul H Brookes, 1999, pp 281–286.
98. Hess CA. Managed care as part of family-centered service systems. In: Kessler DB, Dawson P, eds. Failure to Thrive and Pediatric Undernutrition—A Transdisciplinary Approach. Baltimore: Paul H Brookes, 1999, pp 287–305.

13

Feeding Disorders

Carlos H. Lifschitz
USDA/ARS Children's Nutrition Research Center, Baylor College of
Medicine, and Texas Children's Hospital, Houston, Texas

1 INTRODUCTION

Although it is difficult to provide accurate data, it would seem that the incidence
of feeding disorders in children is increasing (1) and is as high as 80% in developmentally delayed children. Feeding is only one manifestation of the many important ways in which parents nurture their infants and children. When parents are
overly concerned about feeding, they can exacerbate temporary feeding difficulties and misbehaviors by inappropriate responses to the child's behavior (2). Early
detection might reduce the likelihood that minor feeding disturbances will develop into severe feeding problems. Behavior management strategies and a pleas-
ant social context for mealtimes can improve children's eating and mealtime behavior. Impairments in the parent-infant relationship may lead to serious feeding problems, which may make referrals to appropriate support services necessary.

This chapter discusses the diagnostic and therapeutic approaches to infants
and children with specific feeding problems that, if not addressed, would adversely affect the child's nutrition and growth. It does not, however, address in
detail problems that are primarily behavioral in nature or a result of parental
misperception. Feeding problems can cause a disruption in family dynamics. In
order to assess such problems accurately and intervene therapeutically, a team

approach is recommended. The professional members of the feeding team should include a gastroenterologist, an occupational therapist, speech therapist, dietitian, psychologist, nurse, and sometimes a social worker (3). In cases of pediatric patients with neurological disabilities, the evaluation should encompass the child's ability to suck, masticate, and swallow and control head and trunk as well as his or her nutritional and neurological status and the family's desires and expectations in regard to the child's feeding capabilities.

2 ETIOLOGY

At particular risk of late development of feeding problems are small preterm infants, particularly those who received tracheal intubation for a prolonged period and/or had a complicated neonatal course. Often, these infants are managed with prolonged orogastric intubation for feeding purposes, and they may develop a hyperactive gag reflex or even a complete feeding aversion. Other times, the problem is less severe, and the infants are successfully fed by mouth by experienced nurses before being discharged home. After hospital discharge, however, when parents are expected to continue the feeding, this is not always feasible: fatigue, gagging, or simply interruption of sucking can lead to frustration by the caretakers. Regurgitation and vomiting can result in insufficient caloric intake, the consequences of which may not be discovered for several weeks. When parents become aware of the infant's increased nutritional needs, they may intentionally or unintentionally force-feed the infant, who progressively develops a feeding aversion that worsens the situation. Regurgitation can lead to esophagitis and irritability, resulting in diminished nutrient intake, which can ultimately lead to a complete refusal of the breast or bottle. Although it may be necessary to use a nasogastric tube to administer all feedings or feeding supplements, the extended presence of a tube in the nasal cavity can lead to middle ear dysfunction (4). In addition, the tube's passage through the lower esophageal sphincter may cause gastroesophageal reflux, particularly if it is one of the larger tubes (5). Infants, who were born before term—especially those with bronchopulmonary dysplasia, cardiac problems (6), neurological impairment, craniofacial dysmorphisms, or genetic syndromes—often have associated feeding and swallowing difficulties (7). Feeding disorders in children usually present a complex problem. A review of the reports from a feeding-team evaluation of 103 children aged 4 months to 17 years indicated that 38% of the children studied had a history of prematurity, and 74% presented evidence of developmental delay (8). The following five categories or combinations were coded most frequently: structural-neurological-behavioral (30%), neurological-behavioral (27%), behavioral (12%), structural-behavioral (9%), and structural-neurological (8%). Overall, behavioral issues were coded more often (85%) than neurological conditions (73%), structural abnormalities (57%), cardiorespiratory problems (7%), or metabolic dysfunction

(5%). The authors concluded that the majority of children in this sample had a behavioral component to their complex feeding problem regardless of concurrent physical factors.

2.1 Symptoms

Common problems affecting feeding include *tongue thrusting*, prolonged/exaggerated *bite reflex*, abnormally increased/decreased *gag reflex*, *tactile hypersensitivity*, and *drooling* (9). *Coughing* and chronic wheezing and/or bronchitis can be secondary to aspiration during swallowing or from *gastroesophageal reflux*.

Recurrent episodes of wheezing; coughing, particularly during or immediately after meals; and/or chronic bronchitis, which may be the result of aspiration, are of particular relevance. A history of recurrent otitis media and/or hoarseness may also indicate alterations in the swallowing mechanism, causing nasopharyngeal regurgitation. Other issues on which to gather information are the existence of symptoms such as excessive crying, irritability, refusal to eat, interruption of feeding before the meal is completed, or waking up in the middle of the night, which may be indicative of *esophagitis*. In neurodevelopmentally impaired children, caretakers may report changes in feeding abilities or behavior which may be too subtle to be detected by health care providers not familiar with the child.

Whenever a growing child experiences lack of weight gain for a substantial period of time, weight loss, loss of acquired feeding skills, frequent episodes of coughing or choking, or recurrent pneumonia, evaluation by specialized professionals is required. In a retrospective study of 142 children referred for a swallow function study, aspiration was identified in 44% (10). A history of pneumonia within 1 year of the videofluoroscopic contrasted swallow function study (VFS) was found in 35%. Aspiration, gastroesophageal reflux, and age 1 year or less were significant risk factors for pneumonia. Children with traumatic brain injury were at less risk for pneumonia than all other children with suspected dysphagia.

3 CLINICAL EVALUATION

The assessment of the feeding of a child suspected of having a problem begins with a complete medical history, emphasizing the postnatal course, the concerns of the family and/or primary or referring physician, and any previous evaluations or tests that have been performed (11). An occupational therapist or speech therapist with feeding expertise should perform an assessment of the child's development and environment, followed by a clinical feeding evaluation that includes an examination of the oral musculature, posture control, and respiration. The evaluation location must be quiet, comfortable, spacious, and devoid of interference.

Knowledge of the child's development is important because this provides information about the child's cognition and psychosocial and physical status— information that is imperative to have in order to decide how to interact with the child, plan the intervention, and set goals. The child's cognition and psychosocial status is usually gained through an interview, clinical observations, and a review of the medical history. Any history or evidence of vomiting or regurgitation during or after feeding is relevant to a complete assessment of the scope of the problems involved. In dealing with a patient with a suspected or confirmed neuro-developmental problem, it is important to assess muscle tone. For example, in children with cerebral palsy, changes in muscle tone usually relate to the types of feeding problems that are seen; these will require specific management (12). Oromotor evaluation and a clinical feeding assessment can provide valuable information regarding the oral phase of swallowing, while a videofluoroscopic study (VFS) may help to identify disorders in the pharyngeal and esophageal phases of swallowing and/or aspiration. In many cases, the presence of a feeding difficulty may not be completely apparent (Table 1).

3.1 Nutritional Assessment

A dietitian should perform an assessment of nutritional status; if it proves deficient, an estimation of the child's energy needs should be made. Energy requirement for catch-up growth can be calculated as follows:

$$\text{Kcal/kg/day} = \frac{\text{IBW for age (kg)} \times \text{kcal/kg/day (for weight/age)}}{\text{Actual weight (kg)}}$$

where IBW = ideal body weight.

TABLE 1 Criteria for Swallow Evaluation Referral

Choking with feeds
Coughing with feeds
Apnea with feeds
Brady/tachycardia during feeds
Audible respiration
Wet, gurgling vocal quality
Refusal to eat
Excessive drooling/inability to handle secretions
Recurrent upper respiratory infections, pneumonia, congestion, asthma
Poor weight gain
Nasal regurgitation
Frequent emesis
Failure to thrive
Feeding longer than 30 min

3.2   Dietary Needs of the Child with Cerebral Palsy

It is difficult to accurately determine the energy needs of a child with cerebral palsy or another cause of neurodevelopmental delay. Estimation of energy needs can be made from a history of long-term growth and weight gain, dietary history, basal energy expenditure, or various calculations (13). Anthropometric measurements are sometimes of limited value in nutrition assessment because of varying growth patterns in children with cerebral palsy, genetic syndromes, or other causes of severe neurodevelopmental impairment compared to children without such problems (14). Many of these children tend to be underweight and short based on standard references for growth. The National Child Health Statistics standard reference scale can be useful to follow long-term growth and to make assessments, but it should not be used to evaluate growth based on the normal pediatric population (15,16). Height measurements in severely spastic children are also difficult to obtain. For more details on feeding problems in children with developmental disabilities, see Refs. 17 and 18.

3.3   Psychosocial Evaluation

An assessment of the interactions between the child and caregivers will indicate the emotional support being provided for the child. Feelings of guilt, manipulation of the caretaker by the child, or unusual demands by other members of the family on a tacitly designated caretaker may create situations that require the intervention of a psychotherapist. Information on the availability of resources within the home and immediate community is helpful in planning the necessary intervention strategies. The assistance of a social worker may be required.

3.4   Radiological Evaluation of Swallow Function

The aim of the VFS contrasted swallow function study—also known as the modified barium swallow study, swallow function study, or oropharyngeal motility study (19,20)—is to objectively evaluate the oral preparatory/oral transit phase and the pharyngeal phase of the swallow. Many patients show no clinical signs of swallowing difficulty, such as coughing and choking, but have recurrences of pneumonia, upper respiratory infection, or chronic congestion. Such children may have *"silent" aspiration* (no protective cough reflex), and a swallow function study may identify the problem (21). The swallow function study, however, provides a limited amount of information regarding the esophageal phase of the swallow. For more thorough information regarding the esophageal phase, an upper gastrointestinal series should be performed and interpreted by a radiologist. The swallow function study per se is performed by a radiologist and a speech therapist trained in the evaluation of dysphagia, following a protocol described by Logeman (22). This protocol consists of a systematic checklist with which to evaluate the oral and pharyngeal phases of swallowing. Modifications in positioning are often made with the child positioned in an upright, seated position. Infants are positioned on their sides, lying at a semireclined angle to best mimic a normal feeding position. In general, lateral radiographic views of the swallowing mechanism are obtained. Various food and/or liquid consistencies are given, depending on the age and/or ability of the child. Information regarding the consistencies that are easy or difficult for the child to swallow should be obtained during the clinical feeding evaluation and utilized during the swallow study. Food and liquids are mixed with liquid barium or barium paste. Approximately three swallows of each food or fluid consistency are administered.

Swallow study results have been used to alter the diet; to eliminate certain food of fluid consistencies secondary to aspiration; and to change positioning for optimal feeding. A child's swallowing ability should be monitored at periodic intervals with VFS data as well as clinical observation in order to make appropriate changes in dietary textures and to determine whether oral feedings can either be initiated or continued safely.

There is a relatively small number of published investigations regarding VFS assessment of dysphagia in children; the information that exists mainly concerns children with cerebral palsy (20,23,24). In a report by Griggs et al., 70% of children with cerebral palsy aspirated during a swallow function study, 60% of whom had "silent" aspiration (24). Because of these statistics, a VFS swallow function study should be performed on a child with cerebral palsy if his or her medical history is suspect.

Rogers conducted a retrospective review of clinical evaluations and swallow function studies performed on 90 children with cerebral palsy (20). He found that while all had abnormal oral and pharyngeal phases of swallowing, 97% demonstrated a delayed initiation of the swallow reflex and 58% had pharyngeal residue after the swallow. Of the 38% who aspirated during and/or after the swallow, 97% displayed "silent" aspiration. The consistency most commonly aspirated was that of liquid.

3.5 Other Medical Evaluation

The evaluation of children with choking or coughing spells while eating or drinking and those with recurrent pneumonia may require a *bronchoscopy* when a swallow function study fails to demonstrate an abnormality. The finding of lipid-laden macrophages in bronchial washings (25) and/or chronic bronchial inflammation diagnosed by bronchoscopy may support the diagnosis of aspiration. Direct visualization of the epiglottis by nasolaryngoscopy while the patient swallows a colored liquid has been a successful diagnostic tool in adults but is hard to perform in young children.

Recurrent *otitis media* and/or *hoarseness* may also be secondary to the misdirection of liquids while swallowing. In this case, consultation with an otorhinolaryngologist may help make the diagnosis. Patients who are reported to have experienced a change in behavior—such as onset of excessive crying, irritability, refusal to eat, interruption of feedings before the meal is completed, or waking up in the middle of the night—may have esophagitis secondary to gastroesophageal reflux (see Chap. 19).

Studies that may be indicated include upper endoscopy, 24-hr esophageal pH monitoring, esophageal manometry, and/or determination of upper esophageal sphincter pressure and function.

4 INTERVENTION

A patient with feeding problems may benefit from several types of intervention, among which we can mention those related to suck, gastroesophageal reflux, nutritional status, psychosocial, posture, tone, and other aspects.

4.1 Occupational Therapy Intervention

In making recommendations, it is important to evaluate the child's eating environment. An optimal environment includes appropriate physical and emotional support for the child. The physical environment should include appropriate positioning and seating and eating surfaces for the older child. Rules for feeding times, between-meal snacks, and overall behavior may be necessary for some families. For children with neurodevelopmental problems, the feeding specialist's intervention plan may include manipulation of posture and positioning to elicit more normal tonal patterns, provision of oral exercises to improve oral motor skills, prescription of adaptive aids as compensatory measures, and/or education of others regarding developmentally appropriate eating behaviors and patterns (26). Throughout the process, the feeding specialist works with the child and family as part of the team.

Feeding a child with a severe feeding problem becomes a challenging, time-consuming process and overwhelms parents. As some parents report, the child may provide few cues as to hunger or fulfillment and as a result may not be provided with an appropriate quantity of food (27). Specific intervention with the caregiver may be necessary and could include relaxation techniques, time management, or arranging respite for the caregivers of children with severe neurodevelopmental impairment.

4.2 Medical Intervention

Patients with suspected or proven gastroesophageal reflux may undergo a therapeutic trial with a combination of drugs such as antacids, mucosal surface protectors such as sucralfate, prokinetics, and/or medications to temporarily increase the tone of the lower esophageal sphincter, and H_2 or acid pump inhibitors. When medical therapy to treat gastroesophageal reflux fails, a *fundoplication* is warranted. However, parents should be advised that recurrent pneumonia, bronchitis, or reactive airway disease due to aspiration of secretions will not necessarily be resolved by a fundoplication and at best will be improved by diminishing the gastroesophageal reflux component.

In patients with poor nutritional status who are unlikely to meet their energy needs by mouth, a *gastrostomy* should be recommended. Many parents are reluctant to accept a gastrostomy; the benefits must be clearly explained to the family while keeping their wishes in mind. Even in cases when children are successfully fed by mouth at the expense of the almost full-time dedication of the caretaker (usually the mother), a gastrostomy may shorten the feeding time. This will allow more time for caretakers to attend to the other children in the family and themselves and will diminish the stress imposed from the difficult task of giving feedings successfully.

4.3   Dietary Intervention

In children with disabilities, energy needs and losses can vary widely depending on the severity and type of disability (28,29). Children with severe hypertonia and athetoid movements can expend energy far in excess of perceived needs and current intake (30). Children with spastic cerebral palsy can have energy needs below the recommended dietary allowances, leading to a risk for obesity. Poor feeding skills can increase energy needs and losses in any child with cerebral palsy.

After a patient has had an assessment of energy needs, a feeding plan can be implemented. A patient may need only an addition of high-calorie foods to his or her diet or a change in food textures and consistencies, switching from a solid to a thick or thin puree, in order to increase energy intake.

Many children with long-standing failure to thrive, with or without a feeding impairment, will need supplemental or full feedings via nasogastric, gastrostomy, or jejunostomy tubes (31,32). After the evaluation has been completed, high-calorie products can be attempted, but sufficient energy intake for catch-up growth may require *force-feeding*—a situation to be avoided at all costs. Supplemental feedings may have to be adjusted, depending on formula tolerance and weight gain. Nasogastric feedings should be used for a limited time only; they may be indicated in the newborn period, but prolonged use may lead to aversive oral behaviors. The term *prolonged*, however, is difficult to define and could be considered as being more than 8 to 10 weeks. Nasogastric feedings can be indicated to provide additional calories for catch-up growth in a patient who is recovering from another illness or surgery, who is expected to return to the basal level of intake, or who has a respiratory illness and is transiently unable to take enough volume by mouth. Nasogastric feedings could also be used to determine whether a patient can handle appropriate amounts of bolus feeds and in that way determine whether a fundoplication will be necessary or if a gastrostomy (percutaneous or surgical) will suffice. Transition to oral feeds is a gradual process (33). In the child over the age of 1 year, it is often difficult to keep a nasogastric tube in place without having the child pull it out. Arm restraints may be required, but this option is generally not well accepted by parents of older children.

4.4 Treatment for Gastroesophageal Reflux and Esophagitis

Empirical treatment with an antacid, an H_2 blocker, and an anti–gastroesophageal reflux medication can be attempted as a noninvasive way to support the diagnosis of esophagitis (see Chap. 19). If such treatment fails, referral to a gastroenterologist for possible endoscopy is warranted. A recent report has linked esophagitis, which is not responsive to these measures, to hypersensitivity to cow's milk protein (34). Semielemental diets (such as Nutramigen, Pregestemil, Alimentum, or Alfare) have resulted in improvement of symptoms of esophagitis. Small doses of corticosteroids have also been employed successfully (35).

The decision to perform a fundoplication is not always easy, and it is even more complex in a patient with neurodevelopmental delay. Many of these patients swallow large amounts of air; after the fundoplication, they may be unable to burp the air out, becoming bloated and uncomfortable. Patients with impaired neurological function also have a greater tendency than neurologically normal patients to develop postprandial retching—a problem that exasperates many parents and is quite difficult to resolve. Dumping syndrome can also complicate a fundoplication (36).

4.5 Psychosocial Issues

The disruption of the usual family dynamics caused by a child with a severe medical condition may result in a wide range of psychosocial and financial problems. In our experience, feeding problems can result in feelings of poor parenting and inadequacy. Often, because feeding by mouth is the only skill that some children with neurodevelopmental problems can demonstrate, the child's parents will insist on oral feeding despite lengthy, difficult feeding sessions and recurrent episodes of aspiration pneumonia. At times, this situation can become challenging to manage, particularly when school personnel refuse to administer oral feedings to a child, because of the risk of aspiration, while the parents insist that the child handles oral feedings well at home. Frustration and anger are not unusual in a family dealing with a child with a severe illness, particularly if the patient loses previously acquired skills such as eating. A psychotherapist may help in these situations. A social worker may be needed in order to identify and organize the services that the community has available to meet the needs of an individual patient. Behavior problems, child developmental skills, home environment, and parent emotional distress were compared among 50 families of children aged 11 to 70 months with differing etiologies of feeding disorders (37). Results showed that psychosocial functioning differed across feeding disorder classifications. Children whose feeding disorders stemmed from nonorganic causes had more behavioral problems than those with problems of strictly organic causes. Children with primarily or solely organic feeding disorders displayed lower developmental skills (and their parents experienced greater emotional distress) than children with primarily nonorganic feeding problems. High levels of parental distress was associated with older children who had poor feeding skills, less positive disciplinary practices, and higher social status.

5 CONCLUSION

It is important for children with feeding difficulties to undergo a feeding evaluation, because inadequate feeding skills, dysphagia, and/or excess feeding time can contribute significantly to poor weight gain and growth, parental exhaustion, and the disruption of family life. Gastroesophageal reflux can lead to inadequate weight gain and growth. Parents need to be educated as to the nature of the problems, the potential solutions, and the likelihood of resolving the problems. In our experience, even minor improvements in feeding are received with gratitude by the caretakers of children with feeding difficulties.

ACKNOWLEDGMENTS

This work is a publication of the USDA/ARS, Children's Nutrition Research Center, Department of Pediatrics, Baylor College of Medicine and Texas Children's Hospital. Funding has been provided in part from the USDA/ARS Cooperative Agreement No. 58-6258-6001. The contents of this publication do not necessarily reflect the views or policies of the U.S. Department of Agriculture, nor does mention of trade names, commercial products, or organizations imply endorsement by the U.S. government. The author thanks Leslie Loddeke, B.J., for editorial assistance.

REFERENCES

1. Manikam R, Perman JA. Pediatric feeding disorders. J Clin Gastroenterol 1999; 30: 34–46.
2. Finney JW. Preventing common feeding problems in infants and young children. Pediatr Clin North Am 1986; 33:775–788.

3. Babbitt RL, Hoch TA, Coe DA, Cataldo MF, Kelly KJ, Stackhouse C, Perman JA. Behavioral assessment and treatment of pediatric feeding disorders. J Dev Behav Pediatr 1994; 15:278–291.

4. Vento BA, Durrant JD, Palmer CV, Smith EK. Middle ear effects secondary to nasogastric intubation. Am J Otol 1995; 16:820–822.

5. Noviski N, Yehuda YB, Serour F, Gorenstein A, Mandelberg A. Does the size of nasogastric tubes affect gastroesophageal reflux in children? J Pediatr Gastroenterol Nutr 1999; 29:448–451.

6. Thommessen M, Heiberg A, Kase BF. Feeding problems in children with congenital heart disease: the impact on energy intake and growth outcome. Eur J Clin Nutr 1992; 46:457–464.

7. Cruz MJ, Kerschner JE, Beste DJ, Conley SF. Pierre Robin sequences: secondary respiratory difficulties and intrinsic feeding abnormalities. Laryngoscope 1999; 109: 1632–1636.

8. Burklow KA, Phelps AN, Schultz JR, McConnell K, Rudolph C. Classifying complex pediatric feeding disorders. J Pediatr Gastroenterol Nutr 1998; 27:143–147.

9. Arvedson JC. Management of swallowing problems. In: Arvedson JC, Brodsky L, eds. Pediatric Swallowing and Feeding; Assessment and Management. San Diego, CA: Singular Publishing Group, 1993, pp 364–365.

10. Taniguchi MH, Moyer RS. Assessment of risk factors for pneumonia in dysphagic children: significance of videofluoroscopic swallowing evaluation. Dev Med Child Neurol 1994; 36(6):495–502.

11. Kramer SS, Eicher PM. The evaluation of pediatric feeding abnormalities. Dysphagia 1993; 8:215–224.

12. Trier E, Thomas AG. Feeding the disabled child. Nutrition 1998; 14(10):801–805.

13. Krick J, Murphy PE, Markham JFB, Shapiro BK. A proposed formula for calculating energy needs of children with cerebral palsy. Dev Med Child Neurol 1992; 34:481–487.

14. Spender QW, Cronk CE, Charney EB, et al. Assessment of linear growth of children with cerebral palsy: use of alternative measures for height or length. Dev Med Child Neurol 1989; 31:206.

15. Feucht S. Assessment of growth. Nutr Focus 1989; 4:1–8.

16. Krick J, Murphy-Miller P, Zeger S, Wright E. Pattern of growth in children with cerebral palsy. J Am Diet Assoc 1996; 96:680–685.

17. Admunson JA, Sherbondy A, Van Dyke DC, et al. Early identification and treatment necessary to prevent malnutrition in children and adolescents with severe disabilities. J Am Diet Assoc 1994; 94:880–883.

18. Lifschitz C, Browning K, Linge I, McMeans AR, Turk C. Feeding disorders in children with cerebral palsy. In: Miller G, ed. The Cerebral Palsies. Newton, MA: Butterworth and Heinemann, 1998, pp 309–319.

19. American Speech, Language, and Hearing Association. Instrumental diagnostic procedures for swallowing. ASHA 1991; 33:67–73.

20. Rogers B, Arvedson J, Buck G, Smart P, Msall M. Characteristics of dysphagia in children with cerebral palsy. Dysphagia 1994; 9:69–73.

21. Arvedson J, Rogers B, Buck G, Smart P, Msall M. Silent aspiration prominent in children with dysphagia. Int J Pediatr Otorhinolaryngol 1994; 28(2–3):173–181.

22. Logeman JA. Appendix B—Videofluorographic worksheet. In: Logeman JA. Manual for the Videofluorographic Study of Swallowing. Austin, TX: PRO-ED, 1993, pp 157–162.

23. Mirrett PL, Riski JE, Glascot J, et al. Videofluoroscopic assessment of dysphagia in children with severe cerebral palsy. Dysphagia 1994; 9:174–179.

24. Griggs CA, Jones PM, Lee RE. Videofluoroscopic investigation of feeding disorders in children with multiple handicaps. Dev Med Child Neurol 1989; 31:303–308.

25. Nussbaum E, Maggi JC, Mathis R, Galant S. Association of lipid-laden alveolar macrophages and gastroesophageal reflux in children. J Pediatr 1987; 110:190–194.

26. Crane S. Feeding the handicapped child—a review of intervention strategies. Nutr Health 1987; 5(3–4):109–118.

27. Krieger I. Nutrition and the Central Nervous System: Pediatric Disorders of Feeding, Nutrition, and Metabolism. New York: Wiley, 1982, pp 156–157.

28. Azcue MP, Zello GA, Levy LD, Pencharz PB. Energy expenditure and body composition in children with spastic quadriplegic cerebral palsy. J Pediatr 1996; 129:870–876.

29. Stallings VA, Zemel BS, Davies JC, Cronk CE, Charney EB. Energy expenditure of children and adolescents with severe disabilities: a cerebral palsy model. Am J Clin Nutr 1996; 64:627–634.

30. Bandini L, Patterson B, Ekvall SW. Cerebral palsy. In: Ekvall SW, ed. Pediatric Nutrition in Chronic Disease and Developmental Disorders. New York: Oxford University Press, 1993, pp 165–172.

31. Lifschitz CH. Enteral feeding in children. Ann Nestle 1988; 46:73–81.

32. Marin OE, Glassman MS, Schoen BT, Caplan DB. Safety and efficacy of percutaneous endoscopic gastrostomy in children. Am J Gastroenterol 1994; 89:357–361.

33. Schauster H, Dwyer J. Transition from tube feedings to feedings by mouth in children: preventing eating dysfunction. J Am Diet Assoc 1996; 96:277–281.

34. Walsh SV, Antonioli DA, Goldman H, Fox VL, Bousvaros A, Leichtner AM, Furuta GT. Allergic esophagitis in children: a clinicopathological entity. Am J Surg Pathol 1999; 23:390–396.

35. Liacouras CA, Wenner WJ, Brown K, Ruchelli E. Primary eosinophilic esophagitis in children: successful treatment with oral corticosteroids. J Pediatr Gastroenterol Nutr 1998; 26:380–385.

36. Samuk I, Afriat R, Horne T, Bistritzer T, Barr J, Vinograd I. Dumping syndrome following Nissen fundoplication, diagnosis, and treatment. J Pediatr Gastroenterol Nutr 1996; 23:235–240.

37. Budd KS, McGraw TE, Farbisz R, Murphy TB, Hawkins D, Heilman N, Werle M, Hochstadt NJ. Psychosocial concomitants of children's feeding disorders. J Pediatr Psychol 1992; 17:81–94.

14

Carbohydrate Malabsorption

Jan Dekker and Alexandra W. C. Einerhand
Erasmus University Rotterdam, Rotterdam, The Netherlands

Hans A. Büller
Erasmus University Medical Center and
Sophia Children's Hospital, Rotterdam, The Netherlands

1 INTRODUCTION

Dietary carbohydrates can be absorbed through the intestinal epithelium only in the form of monosaccharides. Yet free monosaccharides are scarce in the human diet, and most sugars are ingested in the form of disaccharides and polysaccharides. To this end, the small intestinal epithelium contains several glycohydrolases that are essential in degrading the more complex carbohydrates into absorbable monosaccharides. The resulting monosaccharides are absorbed by the small intestinal epithelium via specific transporters and subsequently released into the blood to build and maintain the body. The term *carbohydrate absorption* therefore encompasses the digestion of sugars to monosaccharides, the uptake of these into the epithelium of the intestine, as well as the transport of the monosaccharides into the blood.

Absorption of carbohydrates is essential to allow a child to grow and thrive. In newborns, lactose in milk forms the sole form of carbohydrate. This disaccharide is hydrolyzed into glucose and galactose by lactase in the small intestine.

After several months, other disaccharides and polysaccharides, particularly starch, become the predominant carbohydrate sources. These compounds are degraded in the small intestine primarily by sucrase-isomaltase, in concert with α-amylase present in saliva and in pancreatic secretions. Degradation of starch yields glucose, whereas the degradation of sucrose yields equimolar amounts of glucose and fructose. The resulting monosaccharides—glucose, galactose, and fructose—are transported into the epithelium and then into the blood by specific transporters. Therefore, this chapter concentrates primarily on the two crucial enzymes in carbohydrate digestion, lactase and sucrase-isomaltase, and on three sugar transporter proteins, designated sodium-dependent glucose transporter-1 (SGLT1), glucose transporter-2 (GLUT2), and glucose transporter-5 (GLUT5), which are pivotal for the absorption of the monosaccharides into the enterocytes and their release into the blood.

Carbohydrate malabsorption is a symptom that can be caused by many potential malfunctions, which can hamper diagnosis. That the system of degradation and uptake of sugars is essential to the survival of the child appears most dramatically from the severely affected phenotypes of the children with mutations in the genes coding for the key proteins in this system, mentioned above. Particularly, defects in the genes coding for lactase, sucrase-isomaltase, or SGLT1 are lethal unless the child is properly treated. These defects are referred to as *primary deficiencies*, i.e., the gene coding for one of these proteins is mutated, so that activation of the gene yields an inactive protein or none. These defects are heritable traits but are also very rare. Far more common are secondary deficiencies, which are caused by damage to the small intestinal epithelium that harbors these proteins. These deficiencies usually have other underlying causes, and most often these are diseases affecting the integrity of the small intestine. For diagnosis as well as treatment, it is very important to understand the background of primary and secondary deficiencies.

This chapter highlights the most important dietary carbohydrates and the enzymes and transporter proteins needed to degrade sugars and transport the monosaccharides into the body. It describes some of the molecular details of these proteins and the physiology of the small intestinal epithelium in order to provide a basis for the understanding of the malfunctions that may result in clinical symptoms of carbohydrate malabsorption. Finally, it provides a basis for the diagnosis of the various causes of carbohydrate malabsorption and for therapeutic management. Many fundamental aspects of intestinal function and various aspects of carbohydrate digestion and absorption are reviewed in the excellent book edited by Leonard Johnson (1).

2 DIETARY CARBOHYDRATE AND ITS DIGESTION

The actions of carbohydrate-degrading enzymes toward their respective substrates are closely related to the types of chemical bonding of the monosaccharide units within their substrates. This subdivision is related to the conformation of the C1 carbon atom of the monosaccharide that is released by a particular enzyme. The hydroxyl group of the C1 atom is in either an α or β conformation, and the respective bonds between two monosaccharides are referred to as α-glycosidic and β-glycosidic bonds (Fig. 1). It is important to realize that all enzymes discussed here are able to split sugars bound by either α- or β-glycosidic bonds—i.e., none of the discussed α-glycohydrolases are able to split β-bound sugars, and vice versa. Another type of subdivision of these hydrolytic enzymes relates to the monosaccharide that they release—e.g., lactase is a β-glycohydrolase with specificity toward substrates containing β-linked glucose and galactose. Therefore, lactase is a β-glucosidase as well as a β-galactosidase. Sucrase-isomaltase, on the other hand, is a complex of two α-glycohydrolases, which have similar but not identical activities toward substrates containing α-glycosidically linked glucose. Therefore, each of these subunits is considered an α-glucosidase. The nomenclature and enzyme specificity of the relevant enzymes is given in Tables 1 and 2.

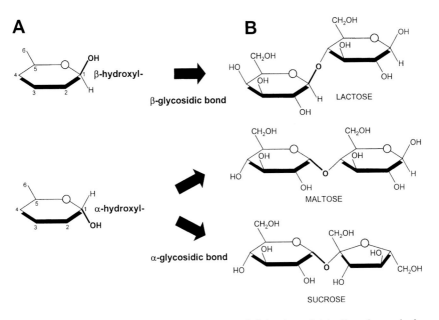

Figure 1 The distinction between α- and β-hydroxyl binding in carbohydrates. Panel A shows the simplified carbon skeleton of two hexose monosaccharides, in which the numbering of the six individual carbon atoms is indicated. The difference between α- and β-hydroxyl bonds is due to conformation at the C1 atom of the monosaccharide, as indicated. Panel B shows some of the most relevant examples of α- and β-glycosidic bonds in disaccharides, namely in lactose (β-glycosidic bond) and maltose and sucrose (both α-glycosidic bonds).

TABLE 1 The Glycohydrolases of the Human Gastrointestinal Tract

Preferred name	EC number(s)	Synonym(s)	Source
α-Amylase	3.2.1.1	—	Saliva
α-Amylase	3.2.1.1	—	Pancreas
Lactase	3.2.1.23,-45,-46,-62	Lactase-phlorizin hydrolase	Small intestine
		Lactase-glycosylceramidase	
		β-Glycosidase complex	
Sucrase-isomaltase	3.2.1.10,-48	Sucrase-α-dextrinase	Small intestine
Maltase-glucoamylase	3.2.1.4,-20	α-Limit dextrinase	Small intestine
		Glucoamylase complex	
		γ-Amylase	
Trehalase	3.2.1.28	α,α'-Trehalose-1-α-glucohydrolase	Small intestine

TABLE 2 Enzymatic Specificities and Natural Substrates of Intestinal Brush-Border Glycohydrolases[a]

Enzyme and constituting subunits		General specificity	Natural substrates
Lactase		β (1-4) glycosyl bonds	Lactose, phlorizin, cellobiose, cellotriose, cellotetrose, cellulose, glucosylceramide, galactosylceramide, lactosylceramide.
Sucrase-isomaltase	Sucrase	α (1-4) glycosyl bonds	Sucrose, maltose, maltotriose
	Isomaltase	α (1-6) glucosyl bonds	Isomaltose, maltose, maltotriose
Maltase-glucoamylase		α (1-4) glucosyl bonds	Maltose, maltohexose, maltooctanose, amylopectin, glycogen, starch, amylose (low on isomaltose)
Trehalase		α,α'-trehalose	Trehalose

[a] Lactase and maltase-glucoamylase each contain two active sites but are present in the human small intestinal brush border as single transmembrane enzymes (compare Figs. 3 and 4). Therefore their enzymatic specificities are given for the molecules as an entity. Sucrase-isomaltase is composed of two subunits that are the proteolytic cleavage products of a single pro–sucrase-isomaltase protein (Figs. 3 and 4). As the individual enzymatic specificities of these subunits could be experimentally determined, these are listed separately.

2.1 Starch and Glycogen

Starch, which constitutes a natural mixture of amylose and amylopectin, is the major carbohydrate source in the human diet after the lactation period; it is found in potatoes, rice, and wheat and consequently in plant-based daily products like bread and pasta. Starch consists of very large glucose polymers in which the glucose residues are linked by α(1-4) glucosidic bonds in amylose as well as in amylopectin (Fig. 2). Next to these bonds, amylopectin also contains branch points formed by α(1-6) glucosidic bonds between glucose residues (Fig. 2). Animal-based polysaccharides are of much less importance to human nutrition;

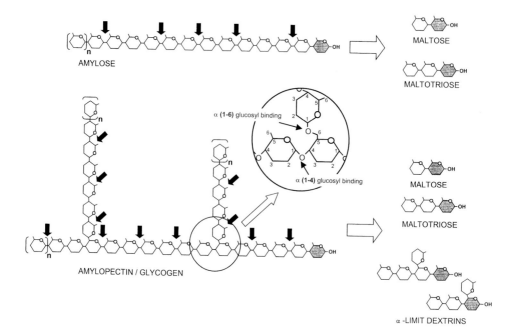

FIGURE 2 Digestion of the major polymeric carbohydrates by α-amylase. The α-amylases from saliva and pancreas digest the polymeric carbohydrates in the diet, particularly amylose, amylopectin, and glycogen. Notice that the chemical structure of amylopectin and glycogen is identical. Amylose consists of very long linear polymers of glucose, bound by α(1-4)glucosidic bonds. These bonds are attacked by the α-amylases from saliva and pancreas, as indicated by the black arrows, which results in a mixture of largely maltose and to a lesser degree maltotriose. Amylopectin and glycogen are similar to amylose but contain additional branching points consisting of α(1-6)glucosidic bonds. One of these branching points is shown in a blown-up version to highlight the two different types of glycosidic bonds. Indicated in this blowup are the numbers of the individual carbon atoms, analogous to Fig. 1A. The α(1-6)glucosidic bonds are not attacked by α-amylase; therefore the branching points remain intact and give rise to a group of molecules, designated α-limit dextrins, that contain the carbohydrate remnants with at least one such branching point. The prevailing products of amylopectin and glycogen digestion by α-amylase are, however, maltose and maltotriose, and only small amounts of α-limit dextrins. Indicated to the right of the carbohydrate molecules (gray shading) are the so-called reducing saccharide groups at the ends of the carbohydrate molecules. Basically, this reducing group consists of the free OH-group present on the C1 atom of the terminal monosaccharide. The presence of these reducing groups can be measured in feces and is used diagnostically (see Sec. 6.4). Notice, in this respect, that the amount of reducing groups increases drastically upon digestion of these polymeric carbohydrates. An increase in the amount of these "reducing substances" can be taken as evidence that the carbohydrates are not absorbed by the intestine.

only glycogen is present in sufficient amounts to contribute to the human carbohydrate intake. Glycogen is also a glucose polymer, which has an identical branched structure as amylopectin, although the number of branch points is usually much higher than in amylopectin. The branched structure of amylopectin and glycogen makes the molecules more compact and more difficult to digest than amylose. Starch consisting of a high percentage of amylopectin is often referred to as resistant starch.

Starch and glycogen are partly digested by salivary and pancreatic α-amylase, which hydrolyzes only the $\alpha(1\text{-}4)$ glucosidic bonds in starch (Fig. 2). The α-amylase liberates the glucose constituents only in units of two or three, resulting in production of large amounts of maltose and maltotriose, respectively, and to relatively small amounts of the "α-limit dextrins." Alpha-limit dextrins comprise a complex mixture containing at least one $\alpha(1\text{-}6)$ glucosidic branch point originating from glycogen or the amylopectin component of starch (Fig. 2).

2.2 Fiber

Fibers are defined as polymeric carbohydrates that cannot be degraded in the small intestine. Normally, dietary fiber consists primarily of plant-based cellulose. Biochemically, cellulose consists of very large polymers of glucose residues, which are linked by $\beta(1\text{-}4)$ glucosidic bonds. This β-bond cannot be hydrolyzed by humans. Fibers like cellulose, pectins, and inulins are passed through the small intestine undegraded but are rather efficiently fermented in the colon by the normally present bacteria into short-chain fatty acids. After a starch-rich meal, some residual starch will also reach the colon to be fermented in a similar way as the fibers. In a way, starch, particularly the more resistant types with high contents of amylopectin, can be categorized as "fiber." It is estimated that, in normal individuals, about 5 to 20% of consumed starch reaches the colon undegraded. The resulting short-chain fatty acids are very important for the normal functioning of the colonic epithelium, and their absorption constitutes a major form of rescuing energy from these dietary sugar polymers.

2.3 Disaccharides

The disaccharide lactose is found exclusively in mammalian milk and is the most important carbohydrate source for neonates and young children. It is exclusively hydrolyzed by small intestinal lactase (Tables 2 and 3). Lactose consists of a galactose and a glucose residue, joined by a $\beta(1\text{-}4)$ glycosidic bond (Fig. 1). A second important dietary disaccharide is sucrose, which is found in many fruits and some vegetables. It consists of a glucose and a fructose residue, joined by an $\alpha(1\text{-}4)$ glucosidic bond (Fig. 1) and is hydrolyzed exclusively by small intestinal sucrase subunit of the sucrase-isomaltase enzyme complex (Tables 2 and 3).

TABLE 3 Molecular Forms and Processing of Dietary Poly- and Disaccharides

Saccharide	Molecular form of substrate	Organ(s)	Enzyme (-complex)
Carbohydrate polymers:			
Amylose[a]	Linear glucose-polymer, α (1-4) bonds	Mouth Pancreas Small intestine	α-Amylase α-Amylase Sucrase-isomaltase Maltase-glucoamylase
Amylopectin[a]	Branched glucose-polymer, α (1-4) bonds with α (1-6) branch points	Mouth Pancreas Small intestine	α-Amylase α-Amylase Sucrase-isomaltase Maltase-glucoamylase
Glycogen	Branched glucose-polymer, α (1-4) bonds with α (1-6) branch points	Mouth Pancreas Small intestine	α-Amylase α-Amylase Sucrase-isomaltase Maltase-glucoamylase
Cellulose	Linear glucose-polymer, β (1-4) bonds	Colon	Bacteria
Disaccharides:			
Lactose	Glucosyl-β (1-4) galactose	Small intestine	Lactase
Sucrose	Glucosyl-α (1-4) fructose	Small intestine	Sucrase-isomaltase[b]
Maltose	Glucosyl-α (1-4) glucose	Small intestine	Maltase-glucoamylase[c] Sucrase-isomaltase[c]
Trehalose	Glucosyl-α,α′-glucose	Small intestine	Trehalase

[a] Starch is a natural mixture of amylose and amylopectin.
[b] Only the sucrase-subunit of sucrase-isomaltase has sucrase activity.
[c] Both subunits of maltase-glucoamylase as well as sucrase-isomaltase have maltase activity.

Maltose is not present in the regular diet in significant amounts. Yet it is increasingly used as syrup for sweetening industrially processed foods and beverages. Free maltose is further present in malted products like beer. Most dietary maltose and maltotriose result from starch digestion by α-amylase (Fig. 2). The starch-derived products of α-amylase digestion are further degraded by combined actions of the maltase-glucoamylase and sucrase-isomaltase enzyme complexes, each containing two different active sites (Tables 2 and 3). Each of the two subunits in these two complexes has maltase and maltotriase activity, hydrolyzing α(1-4) glucosidic bonds. The sucrase-isomaltase and the maltase-glucoamylase enzyme complexes liberate free glucose from their dimeric and oligometric substrates. In humans, the sucrase-isomaltase is far more abundant than the maltase-glucoamylase and is therefore responsible for about 80% of the maltase (and maltotriase) activity in the small intestine (2). The α(1-6) glucosidic bonds in limit dextrins, also resulting from starch (and glycogen) digestion, are almost exclusively hydrolyzed by the isomaltase subunit of sucrase-isomaltase, thereby liberating the α(1-6) glucosidically bound glucose residues from these dextrins (Table 2). Both subunits of maltase-glucoamylase also have this isomaltase activity (Table 2), but are generally thought to play only marginal roles in humans in in vivo hydrolysis of these bonds.

3 THE SMALL INTESTINAL EPITHELIUM

3.1 Cell Types and Tissue Homeostasis

The small intestinal epithelium harbors four major cell types: enterocytes, goblet cells, enteroendocrine cells, and Paneth cells (Fig. 3). The enterocytes are the most predominant cell type and the only relevant one for carbohydrate absorption. Morphologically, the small intestinal epithelium is made up of characteristic villi and the crypts of Lieberkühn. All cell types of the epithelium arise from pluripotent stem cells located near the bottom of the crypts. After cell division, the daughter cells either migrate upward to the villus tip or to the bottom of the crypt. Moving deeper into the crypt, they differentiate into Paneth cells. While moving toward the tip of the villus, they differentiate into a mixture of mostly enterocytes, about 5% goblet cells, and 1% enteroendocrine cells (Fig. 3). The stem cells in the crypt continuously generate new epithelial cells at a great pace. The speed of proliferation is closely matched with removal of cells from the epithelium by programmed cell death (apoptosis) and/or exfoliation. The migration of the epithelial cells, from the moment of cell division to the villus tip, takes about 3 days in rodents and about 5 days in humans.

Apoptosis (or regulated cell death) was recently recognized as a potent and general mechanism to regulate cell turnover and plays a prominent role in epithelial homeostasis. First, apoptosis functions to restrict the number of proliferating

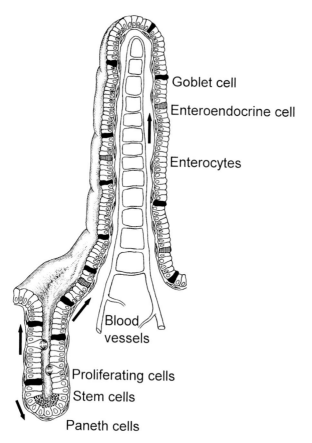

Goblet cell

Enteroendocrine cell

Enterocytes

Blood vessels

Proliferating cells

Stem cells

Paneth cells

FIGURE 3   Basic architecture of the small intestinal epithelium. The epithelium is composed of invaginations, the crypts of Lieberkühn, and finger- or leaf-like structures, the villi. The four differentiated cell types of the epithelium are indicated: black, goblet cells; cross-hatched, enteroendocrine cells; granular, Paneth cells. All other white cells are enterocytes. The stem cells, which are responsible for the production of all differentiated cell types, are located close to the bottom of the crypt. By cell division, these stem cells give rise to a class of proliferative cells, which undergo several additional cell cycles before differentiating into one of the four cell types mentioned above. A small number of cells migrate deeper into the crypt, giving rise to Paneth cells. Most of the cells, during and after proliferation, migrate to the villi and are committed to develop into enterocytes, goblet, or enteroendocrine cells. The migration rate of the epithelial cells on the villus is about 1 to 2 cell positions per hour, resulting in their removal by either extrusion or apoptosis at the villus tips. The whole epithelium is renewed every 5 days. The arrows indicate the migration directions of the cells in the epithelium. (From Ref. 3.)

cells in the crypts. Second, apoptosis occurs at the top of the villus to remove cells from the epithelium. It is generally accepted that the removal of epithelial cells by either shedding or apoptosis does not leave gaps in the epithelial layer. Thus, the epithelium manages to remove cells without disrupting the occluding functions of the tight junctions, which is very important to maintain an effective barrier. The high proliferative capacity of the intestinal epithelium is very important in the repopulation of the epithelium after damage; this is especially relevant in secondary glycohydrolase and transporter deficiencies.

The ability of intestinal stem cells to produce the full repertoire of daughter cells is already present within the epithelium of the embryonic gut. Nevertheless, the epithelium displays a surprising flexibility under specific conditions. The flexibility of the epithelium and its stem cells is best displayed under conditions of villus atrophy. When the intestinal mucosa is severely damaged, due to toxic or noxious substances or infectious disease, the stem cells, which lie in the crypts, appear to be spared. When the cause of the insult disappears, the stem cells are able to restore the epithelial architecture within a few days.

3.2 Structure of the Enterocyte

Intestinal villus enterocytes have a pivotal role in the degradation and subsequent absorption of nutrients. Only small quantities of nutrients are used within the enterocytes; most of these are passed into the blood and via the portal vein to the liver and the rest of the body (see Chaps. 1 and 3). Enterocytes are highly specialized, polarized cells. The apical and basolateral plasma membrane domains are separated by tight junctions, which form diffusion barriers for the membrane components of both domains. All specialized functions associated with degradation and uptake of nutrients are located in the apical plasma membrane, which lines the intestinal lumen. Figure 4 gives an outline of the villus enterocyte and the most important proteins for the digestion and absorption of sugars are indicated.

Although basically representing the same cell type, enterocytes in either the crypt or villus epithelium have distinct functions. In the crypts, the secretory functions of the enterocytes predominate, whereas the enterocytes of the villi have mainly hydrolytic and absorptive functions. Thus, crypt enterocytes are, for example, responsible for the secretion of water and chloride ions in diarrhea (i.e., the secretory response in many diseases) and IgA-secretion as part of the mucosal defense. Villus enterocytes are responsible for the degradation and uptake of nutrients. Like other enterocytes, following their primary differentiation in the crypt they migrate progressively toward the villus tip and undergo a functional switch at the crypt-villus junction. A number of crypt-specific proteins are down regulated, while villus-specific proteins are switched on. Mature enterocytes develop an intricate and specialized apical microvillar membrane, essential in the degradation and uptake of nutrients: the brush-border membrane, a very closely

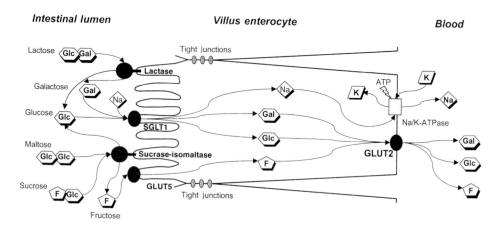

FIGURE 4 Important steps in carbohydrate absorption in the small intestine. Schematic representation of a small intestinal enterocyte showing the most important compounds of the carbohydrate hydrolysis and absorption system. The enterocyte is shown with its apical membrane (the brush-border membrane) to the left and the basolateral membrane to the right. These plasma membrane domains are separated by the tight junctions, which also serve to seal off the intestinal luminal compartment from the body's interior. Indicated are the two most important glycohydrolases, lactase and sucrase-isomaltase, and the three most important monosaccharide transporter proteins, SGLT1, GLUT2, and GLUT5. Also indicated is the sodium-potassium ATPase (Na/K-ATPase) that is responsible for the sodium (and potassium) gradient over the apical brush-border membrane, which is essential for the active uptake of galactose and glucose over this membrane. Glc, glucose; Gal, galactose; F, fructose; Na, sodium; K, potassium.

packed array of microvilli, which contains the glycohydrolases, like lactase and sucrase-isomaltase, and monosaccharide transporters, particularly SGLT1 and GLUT5.

4 INTESTINAL BRUSH-BORDER GLYCOHYDROLASES

The glycohydrolases are present in the brush-border membrane of villus enterocytes. They are membrane-bound proteins protruding from the cells into the lumen of the gut. They perform the last essential steps in the hydrolysis of sugars to absorbable monosaccharides, primarily during the degradation of lactose, sucrose, maltose, maltotriose, and α-limit dextrins. The structures, synthesis, and enzymatic functions of the brush-border glycohydrolase family of proteins, lactase, sucrase-isomaltase, trehalase, and maltase-glucoamylase are described in greater detail in a previous review (3).

4.1 Lactase

Lactase is found in virtually all mammals and is the sole enzyme capable of degrading lactose present in milk. It is thus essential during the first phase of mammalian life, when milk is the only nutrition, and lactose in milk constitutes the only carbohydrate source. Besides its enzymatic specificity toward lactose, which is by far its most important function, lactase has also catalytic activities toward hydrophobic substrates, like phlorizin (a rare plant product) (Tables 1 to 3). Classically, this enzyme complex carried a double name, lactase-phlorizin hydrolase (Table 1), suggesting that there would be a lactose as well as a phlorizin hydrolyzing subunit. In fact, the mature lactase has two active sites but consists of only one polypeptide. We demonstrated that there is most likely one major active site, which is capable of hydrolyzing both lactose as well as hydrophobic substrates, and a minor active site with residual activity toward hydrophobic substrates (4). We refer to the enzyme as lactase, in view of its main function.

Lactase is a protein of 1927 amino acids and is produced in a prolactase form in enterocytes as a 220-kDa precursor protein, prolactase (Fig. 5). During the transport of this prolactase to the brush-border membrane, the precursor is proteolytically cleaved into its mature form of 160 kDa, which becomes inserted into the brush-border membrane, and a propeptide. This propeptide has no enzymatic activity but it is crucial in the proper folding, transport, and processing of lactase within the cells (5). A single hydrophobic domain was identified at the C-terminus of the protein, which functions as a transmembrane anchor domain. During biosynthesis, lactase forms dimers, which is the functional form of the enzyme in the brush border (Fig. 6). In in vivo experiments in adult rats, the mean residence time of lactase in the brush border of enterocytes was estimated to be 7.8 h (6). The sequence of lactase revealed a fourfold internal homology (designated as domains L1 to L4 in Fig. 5), most likely due to two independent duplication events of the gene during evolution. The domains L2–L4 of lactase show homologies of about 50%. Although there are functional similarities, there is no sequence homology between lactase and the lysosomal β-galactosidase.

Lactase is capable of hydrolyzing many β-glycosidic compounds, which can be summarized as follows (Table 2): lactose, cellobiose and cellodextrins (i.e. small fragments of cellulose, not occurring in the normal diet), several naturally occurring hydrophobic substances such as phlorizin and β-glycosylceramides (very scarce in the normal diet), and a large number of (hydrophobic) test substrates, such as *ortho*-nitrophenyl-β(1-4)-galactopyranoside (ONP-gal; Table 4). There is no activity to any α-glycosidic compound (e.g., maltase or sucrase).

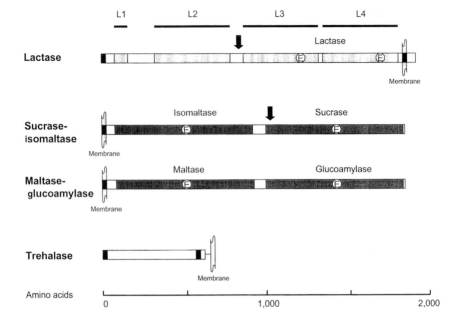

FIGURE 5   Primary structures of the sugar hydrolyzing enzymes of the small intestine. Depicted are the four known glycohydrolases that are collectively responsible for the essential final steps in the hydrolysis of dietary sugars into absorbable monosaccharides. Lactase and sucrase-isomaltase are essential, whereas maltase-glucoamylase and trehalase have only auxiliary roles. The proteins are indicated in the form of their primary polypeptide sequence with their N-terminal sequences to the left and their C-termini to the right. The lactase protein consists of four similar (homologous) regions, indicated by the four light-gray boxed areas, designated L1 through L4. Only the regions L3 and L4 contain enzymatically active sites, whereas the N-terminal regions L1 and L2 are cleaved off intracellularly during biosynthesis and are not part of the mature, functional enzyme. As indicated, lactase is inserted into the enterocyte's membrane through a hydrophobic transmembrane sequence at its C-terminal part. The overall structures of sucrase-isomaltase and maltase-glucoamylase are highly similar. Both proteins consist of two very similar (homologous) regions, each with its separate enzymatic activity. Not only the two parts of the same protein (e.g., sucrase and isomaltase) but also the regions among the proteins (e.g., isomaltase and maltase) are highly similar. The latter are indicated by the dark-shaded boxes. Both protein are inserted into the plasma membrane through a hydrophobic sequence at their extreme N-terminal ends. Sucrase-isomaltase is proteolytically split into separate subunits that, however, remain attached by noncovalent bonds. A difference is that maltase-glucoamylase is not split into separate subunits and that the protein is present on the cells as a single protein. Trehalase is not structurally related to the other three proteins; it is attached to the membrane by a separate hydrophobic structure that is coupled to the protein at its C-terminus (a so-called GPI-anchor). The black-boxed areas indicate highly hydrophobic peptide sequences; E indicates the enzymatic active site within each subunit, and the arrows indicate proteolytic cleavage sites. The size of the protein is indicated by the number of amino acids.

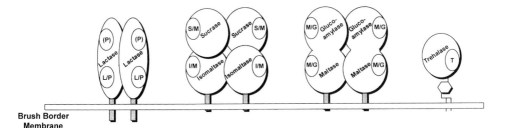

FIGURE 6 The sugar hydrolyzing enzymes on small intestinal enterocyte. Lactase, sucrase-isomaltase, and maltase-glucoamylase are present in the plasma membrane of the enterocytes as dimers—i.e., functional units that contain four enzymatically active sites. Functional trehalase is present as a monomer. The enzyme activities of the respective enzymatic sites are indicated. P, phlorizin hydrolase; L, lactase; S, sucrase; I, isomaltase; M, maltase; G, glucoamylase; T, trehalase. Enzymatic sites with two activities are indicated, separated by a slash (e.g., S/M). The marginal phlorizin hydrolase activity is indicated by brackets (P).

The mature functional lactase consists only of regions L3 and L4. Based on the lactase sequence, two enzymatic active sites were identified in lactase, one in each of the regions L3 and L4 (Figs. 5 and 6). The function of these two sites was explored in our laboratory by a technique that replaces amino acids within the protein by other amino acids of choice (4). Making alterations in the active site of lactase region L3 hardly affected the enzymatic activity. Only the

TABLE 4 Specific Test Substrates to Determine the Individual Activities of the Brush Border Glycohydrolases

Enzyme (complex)	Subunit	Substrate	Enzymatic activity tested
Lactase	—	Lactose ONP-gal[a]	Lactase-phlorizin hydrolase complex
Sucrase- isomaltase	Sucrase Isomaltase	Sucrose Isomaltose	Sucrase Isomaltase
Maltase- glucoamylase	—	Amylose Amylopectin	Maltase- glucoamylase complex
Trehalase	—	Trehalose	Trehalase

[a] ONP-gal, *ortho*-nitrophenyl-β(1-4)-galactopyranoside.

hydrolysis of hydrophobic substrates like ONP-Gal was reduced to 75%, while the lactose hydrolysis was not affected at all. In contrast, changes in the active site of region L4 abolished all activity toward lactose, as well as about 75% of the activity towards hydrophobic substrates. Thus, we concluded that all the lactase activity as well as most of the activity toward hydrophobic substrates is confined to the active site in region L4, whereas the site in region L3 only displays minor activity toward the hydrophobic substrates.

4.2 Sucrase-Isomaltase

Sucrase-isomaltase is an enzyme complex containing two separate polypeptides, each with an enzymatically active site. This enzyme complex represents quantitatively the most important maltase activity in humans. It further contains all intestinal sucrase activity, which is essential for the digestion of sucrose. In fact, the enzyme complex is most specifically detected by its sucrase activity, which is unique to this complex and distinguishes it from the maltase-glucoamylase complex (Table 4).

Human sucrase-isomaltase is produced as a pro–sucrase-isomaltase, which consists of 1827 amino acids (Fig. 5). The sequence shows twofold internal sequence homology in the sucrase and isomaltase regions. A sequence at the N-terminus of pro–sucrase-isomaltase comprises the only hydrophobic region, which serves as a transmembrane anchor. The pro–sucrase-isomaltase is transported to the brush-border membrane, where it is proteolytically cleaved into its mature form by pancreatic proteinases in the gut lumen, yielding a 120-kDa sucrase subunit and a 140-kDa isomaltase subunit. Only the isomaltase subunit is directly associated with the membrane, while the sucrase subunit interacts noncovalently with the isomaltase subunit but not with the membrane. In the brush border of enterocytes, sucrase-isomaltase is present as dimers (Fig. 6). In fetal rat—which has not yet developed a functional pancreas—only pro–sucrase-isomaltase is produced in the intestine. The mean residence time in vivo of rat sucrase-isomaltase in small intestinal brush border membrane is 5.8 h (6). The sequence of sucrase-isomaltase shows remarkable similarities to human lysosomal α-glucosidase. The human lysosomal (acid) α-glucosidase (EC 3.2.1.20) is able to hydrolyze lysosomal glycogen and demonstrates homology of about 26% to the sucrase as well as the isomaltase subunits of rabbit, rat, and human sucrase-isomaltase. This shows that these enzymes are not only related in function but may also have a common origin in evolution.

Sucrase-isomaltase accounts for about 80% of the maltase activity in the small intestine. Both sites of sucrase-isomaltase possess maltase activity, but the enzyme complex exhibits only very limited activity toward larger glucose polymers. The two active sites within the complex have overlapping substrate specificity. However, the sucrase subunit is responsible for all of the sucrase activity in the small intestine. The activity of the isomaltase subunit can be distinguished from the activity of the sucrase subunit by the fact that it does not display any sucrase activity but instead displays isomaltase activity, which is not exhibited by the sucrase subunit (Table 4). The substrate specificity of the intact enzyme complex and its individual subunits can be summarized as follows (Tables 2 and 3). The sucrase subunit hydrolyzes sucrose but not compounds containing $\alpha(1\text{-}6)$ glucosidic bonds. The isomaltase subunit hydrolyzes $\alpha(1\text{-}6)$ glucosidic bonds, as in isomaltose, but not sucrose. Both subunits hydrolyze maltose and maltotriose (i.e., their primary function), and both subunits hydrolyze hydrophobic aryl-α-glucopyranosides (which do not occur naturally in the diet) to some extent. The complex shows no activity toward polymeric glucose, such as starch, and both subunits show only minor activity towards small α-limit dextrins. Compared to sucrase-isomaltase, the specific activity of maltase-glucoamylase toward degradation of α-limit dextrins is much higher, although the α-limit dextrins represent only a small part of the nutritionally important carbohydrates.

4.3   Trehalase and Maltase-Glucoamylase

There are two additional glycohydrolases in the brush border of the enterocytes, maltase-glucoamylase and trehalase (Tables 1 to 3; Figs. 5 and 6). Their particulars are covered elsewhere (3). Although in themselves very interesting, both enzymes have only auxiliary functions in the human small intestine. This is best illustrated by the fact that they are not able to cover the functions of lactase or sucrase-isomaltase under circumstances when either of these enzymes is absent (as in primary lactase or sucrase-isomaltase deficiency; see Sec. 6). The presence of trehalase is curious in itself, as its natural substrate, trehalose, is very scarce in the human diet (insects and mushrooms) and of seemingly little nutritional importance. Maltase-glucoamylase is an α-glucosidase and is very similar in structure and function to sucrase-isomaltase (Tables 1 to 3; Figs. 5 and 6). However, it accounts only for 20% of the maltase activity in the human small intestine. And although it has a clearly identified role in the digestion of several nutritionally important sugars, its relative rarity means that it cannot substitute sucrase-isomaltase in absence of the latter (see also Sec. 6.2.3). Noteworthy in this respect is the glucoamylase activity that is displayed by both the maltase and the glucoamylase subunit of this enzyme complex (Fig. 6; Tables 2 and 3). This refers to the ability to degrade medium-length glucose polymers and α-limit dextrins, which appear during the (partial) digestion of starch. Both the maltase and glucoamylase subunits also have the ability to degrade polymeric amylose and amylopectine, although not very efficiently. Yet, this activity distinguishes this enzyme complex from sucrase-isomaltase (Table 4).

4.4   Lactase and Sucrase-Isomaltase Levels Are Regulated by the Activity of the Genes

The tissue-specific expression of lactase and sucrase-isomaltase is very similar. Both enzymes are confined to the brush-border membranes of the enterocytes of the small intestinal villi. However, the expression of lactase and sucrase-isomaltase during development is different and in some respects even completely opposite. Lactase is strongly up-regulated before birth and declines during weaning (only in some Caucasian populations does lactase remain high; see Sec. 6.2.2), remaining low during adulthood, while sucrase-isomaltase is not present at high levels until weaning but thereafter remains at high levels during adult life. These phenomena are genetically imprinted into the development of the intestine and cannot be influenced to any large extent by external factors, like hormones or sugars.

It is widely accepted that the regulation of lactase and sucrase-isomaltase expression is primarily transcriptional (e.g., Refs. 7 to 11). This means that the turning on and off of these genes determines the level of production of the respective functional enzymes. From the very different developmental expression patterns of both enzymes, as observed in humans as well as animals, it appears that the various mechanisms of regulation of lactase and sucrase-isomaltase genes operate quite independently. In recent years, the structure of the lactase and sucrase-isomaltase genes has been analyzed, enabling detailed studies of the spatial and temporal expression of these enzymes (e.g., Refs. 12 to 15). As expected, it was found that the location of the genes in the genome and the structure and regulation of the genes was very different.

4.5   Lactase and Sucrase-Isomaltase Levels Are Hardly Influenced by the Presence of Sugars

The levels of expression of brush-border glycohydrolases are developmentally imprinted. Nevertheless, there is still a minor role for some carbohydrate substrates in the regulation of the level of the individual enzymes. However, since the early observations by Plimmer in 1906, in adult rabbits and rats, it has become clear that lactase is not inducible by the presence of milk or lactose in the diet (16). Whereas only a slight inhibitory effect on lactase activity has been shown for glucose, administration of lactose does not elevate lactase-specific activity (17). The independence of lactase expression from substrate supply is emphasized by the fact that lactase expression is increased tremendously prior to birth—i.e., in the complete absence of lactose. In humans, neither prolonged ingestion of lactose nor elimination of lactose from the diet altered lactase activity (18,19). Thus, all evidence suggests that the level of lactase activity is genetically determined and only minor control may be exerted by glucose, but no regulation is exerted by lactose.

Sucrase-isomaltase is somewhat more prone to substrate regulation than lactase (reviewed in Ref. 20). Starvation had different effects on jejunal glycohydrolases: lactase activity remained virtually unchanged, while sucrase-isomaltase activity increased (21). Dietary sucrose is able to increase the activity of sucrase-isomaltase. This up-regulation of sucrase-isomaltase by dietary sucrose was clearly a specific process that increased the amount of active enzymes per cell, as sucrose did not in any way change the cell migration rate, the number of enterocytes, or the crypt-villus ratio (22).

5 MONOSACCHARIDE TRANSPORTERS

The monosaccharides resulting from the actions of lactase and sucrase-isomaltase—i.e., glucose (primarily from lactose and starch), galactose (primarily form lactose), and fructose (primarily from sucrose)—are absorbed into the epithelium through transporter proteins (Fig. 4). The apical plasma membrane contains the sodium-dependent glucose (and galactose) transporter-1 (SGLT1). Fructose is transported over the apical membrane by the glucose transporter-5 (GLUT5). All three monosaccharides are transported over the basolateral membrane to enter the blood via the glucose transporter-2 (GLUT2). The transporters SGLT1 versus GLUT2 and GLUT5 are members of separate transporter protein families that show very little structural resemblance. The transport of glucose and galactose via SGLT1 is energy-dependent, whereas the GLUT-type proteins transport their substrates energy independently.

5.1 Uptake of Glucose and Galactose: Sodium-Dependent Glucose Transporter 1

The uptake of galactose and glucose from the intestinal lumen depends on the 664 amino acids–long sodium-dependent glucose transporter-1 (SGLT1) protein. The SGLT1 protein is incorporated into the brush-border membrane of villus enterocytes of the small intestine, and it transverses this membrane 14 times (Fig. 7). The transport of glucose and galactose is energy-dependent, but in an indirect manner. During each cycle of transport, either one glucose or one galactose molecule is transported from the lumen into the cell together with two sodium ions, hence its name. The 14 membrane-spanning domains form a selective pore that allows entry of one molecule of glucose or galactose together with two sodium ions. The enterocyte, like all cells, possesses a sodium-gradient over its cell membrane, with relatively high concentrations of sodium outside the cell. This gradient is generated through the action of the sodium/potassium-ATPase in the basolateral membrane of the enterocytes (Fig. 4), which pumps sodium out of the cell and potassium into the cell at the expense of ATP. Therefore, the maintenance of the sodium gradient is at the expense of cellular energy. SGLT1 functions

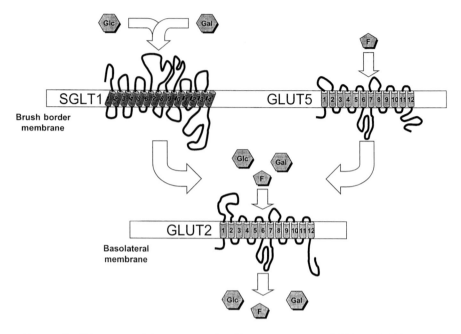

FIGURE 7 The essential monosaccharide transporters SGLT1, GLUT5, and GLUT2. The glucose and galactose resulting from dietary di- and polysaccharide digestion is transported by the SGLT1 transporter. Per round, one monosaccharide—i.e., either glucose or galactose—is transported into the enterocyte's cytosol. Dietary fructose is uniquely transported into the enterocyte by the GLUT5 transporter. All three monosaccharides are transported from the enterocyte to the blood by the GLUT2 transporter. Notice that the SGLT1 transporter has a structure that is not related to the GLUT-type transporters. SGLT1 has 14 membrane-spanning domains, whereas each of the GLUT proteins have 12 such domains. Both GLUT-type transporters have a similar structure, but distinct differences do exist, consistent with their different functions and localization in the plasma membrane of the enterocytes.

only in the presence of a sodium gradient and is therefore energy-dependent, but in an indirect manner. The gain of this system is that the glucose or galactose can be taken up by the cells even in the presence of concentration gradients that would normally slow down their uptake by diffusion or even force the diffusion of the monosaccharides in the other direction. The uptake of glucose together with sodium ions is also an important mechanism of water transport from the intestinal lumen into the body. It was calculated that with each round of action of SGLT1, 260 water molecules enter the enterocyte, and that this may be responsible for the absorption of 5L of water per day in humans (23). This water transport associated with the action of SGLT1 forms the basis for the application of oral rehydration solution in the rehydration of patients in acute diarrhea (see also Sec. 6.3).

5.2 Uptake of Fructose: Glucose Transporter 5

Intestinal fructose is absorbed through the glucose transporter-5 (GLUT5), which very specifically mediates entry of fructose into the cell (Fig. 4). Its name, which is somewhat confusing, originates in the fact that GLUT5 belongs to a family of very similar proteins, which all (i.e., except GLUT5) transport glucose over plasma membranes (1). This 501–amino acid protein is, like SGLT1, also present in the brush border of villus enterocytes in the small intestine, where it spans the plasma membrane 12 times (Fig. 7). Although there is a superficial resemblance between SGLT1 and GLUT5, their detailed structures and amino acid sequences are very different. This is also reflected in the transport mechanisms. The function of GLUT5 is ranked under facilitated transport, which is driven by the concentration gradient of fructose over the apical plasma membrane. The 12 membrane-spanning domains form a highly selective pore, allowing passage of fructose but not of glucose or galactose or any other physiologically relevant monosaccharide. Unlike SGTL1, which functions as a one-way system (facing inward), GLUT5 functions as a two-way pore, which could in principle also allow efflux of fructose to the lumen. This implies that the uptake of fructose is less efficient than that of glucose and galactose by SGLT1. This may be one of the underlying mechanisms responsible for the fact that the uptake of fructose is easily saturated. This means that high amounts of fructose (as present, for example, in processed apple juice) may lead to malabsorption symptoms and may be one of the causes of "toddler's diarrhea" (see also Sec. 6.2.6).

5.3 Release of Monosaccharides from the Enterocytes into the Blood: Glucose Transporter-2

Glucose transporter-2 (GLUT2) belongs to the same protein family as GLUT5 and has a similar structure and working mechanism. This 525–amino acid protein also spans the plasma membrane 12 times, forming a pore, working very much in the same way as in GLUT5 (Fig. 7). In contrast to GLUT5, the pore of GLUT2 is not very selective, as it transports glucose, galactose, and fructose. Also in contrast to GLUT5, GLUT2 is present in the basolateral membrane, facilitating exit of the mentioned monosaccharides from the enterocytes into the blood (Fig. 4).

5.4 Regulation of Expression of the Monosaccharide Transporters

SGLT1 and GLUT2 are already expressed in the intestinal epithelium during gestation. From day 0 after birth, these transporters are needed to transport glucose and galactose resulting from lactose-digestion by lactase. Also GLUT5 is apparently present at birth, as neonates with SGLT1 deficiency can survive on a fructose diet that is free from lactose, glucose, and galactose (see also Sec. 6.2.5).

The levels of monosaccharide transporters are usually reversibly and rapidly regulated by the monosaccharides they transport (1). This is in contrast to the glycohydrolases, which are not regulated to any large extent by the presence of their substrate (Sec. 4.5). This adaptation of the levels of the transporters has two main components. First, there is a relatively slow adaptation (over days) to changes in the carbohydrate diet, which depends on increased activation of the respective genes, leading to increased production of the transporter proteins. Second, there is a much more rapid mechanism (over minutes) to enhance the presence of transporter protein in the plasma membrane. It appears that large amounts of the transporter proteins are present in small vesicles in the enterocytes, which can fuse rapidly to the plasma membrane (exocytosis) upon stimulation by the presence of their cognate sugar. It therefore appears that there is a very fast reaction of the enterocytes to increase the amount of transporter proteins by exocytosis of preexisting proteins (i.e., shortly after a meal). If the daily presence of these sugars becomes more structural (change of diet), the enterocytes are stimulated to produce more transporter protein on a regular basis.

6 CARBOHYDRATE ABSORPTION DISORDERS

Carbohydrate malabsorption is a clinical finding with many potential causes, which are usually subdivided into primary and secondary disorders (Table 5). Primary disorders relate to genetic (congenital) defects in any of the genes responsible for the production of one of the essential enzymes or transporters, as described above (Secs. 4 and 5). Secondary malabsorption signifies the inability to degrade and/or absorb sugars as a result of damage to the intestinal epithelium. Primary malabsorption, like most genetic disorders, is very rare. Secondary malabsorption occurs rather frequently as a result of gastrointestinal diseases. Primary disorders have one unequivocal cause and one unambiguous (primary) result; for example, primary lactase deficiency leads to the inability to degrade lactose. Secondary disorders may affect many more functions of the intestine apart from the carbohydrate absorption and often also affects degradation and uptake of other nutrients, but it may also compromise the epithelial integrity, leading, for instance, to inflammatory processes. However, the clinical symptoms

TABLE 5 Carbohydrate Malabsorption[a]

Disease	Age of onset	Symptoms[b]	Due to	Diagnostic characteristics	Treatment
Primary deficiencies					
Congenital lactase deficiency	Birth	Chronic	Lactose in diet	Positive H_2-breath test with lactose Normal duodenal biopsy Absence of lactase by enzyme assay	Replace lactose by glucose polymer (1:1). Use lactase enzyme preparations.
Adult type hypolactasia	3–11 years	Chronic	Lactose in diet	Positive H_2-breath test with lactose Normal duodenal biopsy Low/absent lactase by enzyme assay	Use lactase enzyme preparations. Low-lactose diet (e.g., yogurt).

TABLE 5 Continued

Disease	Age of onset	Symptoms[b]	Due to	Diagnostic characteristics	Treatment
Sucrase-isomaltase deficiency	3 months, introduction of sucrose and/or starch in diet	Chronic	Sucrose or starch in diet	Positive H_2-test with sucrose Normal duodenal biopsy Absence of sucrase by enzyme assay	Omit sucrose, reduce starch.
GLUT2 deficiency	Birth	Chronic	Carbohydrate in diet	Liver disease Normal duodenal biopsy	None.
SGLT1 deficiency	Birth	Chronic	Glucose or galactose in diet	Positive H_2-breath test with glucose or galactose Normal duodenal biopsy	Replace all carbohydrate by fructose.
Fructose malabsorption	Any age, often 1–2 years	Recurrent with fructose ingestion	High fructose diet	Positive H_2-breath test with fructose Normal duodenal biopsy	Reduce amount of dietary fructose.

Secondary deficiencies (the most frequent cause is listed first)

Gastroenteritis (infectious)	0–2 years (e.g., rotavirus)	Acute	e.g., Rotavirus other viruses	Serology/feces positive for virus, bacterium or parasite	Rehydrate if necessary. Nonspecific therapy.
Food intolerance	Age 0–1 years	Chronic	Specific nutrient hypersensitivity (milk, eggs)	Eosinophilia Villus damage in duodenal biopsy	Omit nutrient from diet.
Celiac disease	Any age	Chronic	Gluten hypersensitivity	Characteristic villus atrophy in duodenal biopsy	Omit gluten from diet.
Crohn's disease	Any age	Intermittent	Inflammation of small intestine	Focal inflammation in duodenal biopsy	Treat inflammation.
Short-bowel syndrome	Neonatal	Chronic	Surgical intervention	Not applicable	Give enteral or parenteral nutrition.
Radiation	Any age	Acute	Radiation	Not applicable	None.
Chemotherapy	Any age	Acute	Chemotherapeutic drugs	Not applicable	None.

[a] This table indicates the most frequent causes of primary and secondary carbohydrate malabsorption. Particularly, the list for the causes of secondary deficiencies is not complete, as there are many causes of intestinal damage that may result in carbohydrate malabsorption.

[b] Symptoms are described in Section 6.1.

of primary (Sec. 6.2) and secondary (Sec. 6.3) malabsorption are often quite similar, and distinguishing these disease entities needs careful analysis.

6.1 Symptoms of Carbohydrate Malabsorption

Carbohydrate malabsorption results from the inability to degrade or absorb one or more carbohydrates from the diet. Clinical symptoms of this type of malabsorption have two major causes. The first is associated with the consequences of the lack of carbohydrate, a very important energy source. Malabsorption often leads to malnutrition, which may result in weight loss and failure to thrive (see Chap. 12). The second cause of symptoms is associated with the fate of the unabsorbed carbohydrate, which enters the colon, where it is fermented mainly into small organic acids and gas, such as H_2. Part of these organic acids can be absorbed into the system; in cases of excess production, however, accumulation in the colon—together with the carbohydrate that cannot be fermented—leads to diarrhea. Accumulation of gases leads to flatulence. The diarrhea results in dehydration, and the concomitant loss of fluid and electrolytes further contributes to weight loss. Also, the decreased passage time of food through the intestine negatively affects the degradation and uptake of other nutrients. Further, the patients suffer from discomfort, anorexia, and general malaise.

Particularly in children, the combination of malnutrition and dehydration will affect growth and development. It must be noted that the combination of these symptoms during prolonged periods of time can lead to a negative spiral, which can easily result in a chronically deficient condition. As explained in Sec. 3, the intestinal epithelium has a very high turnover, with a very high energy expenditure. If, as result of primary or secondary carbohydrate malabsorption, the energy requirements of the body cannot be met, the body will no longer be able to sustain the renewal of the intestinal epithelium. The reduced ability of the intestine to absorb nutrients results in a vicious circle of cause and consequence which leads the patient to deteriorate more and more. Therefore, under these conditions, it is very important to carefully consider the feeding options (see Chaps. 3, 4, 15, 16, and 17).

6.2 Primary Disorders: Congenital Carbohydrate Malabsorption

Genetic or primary disorders, in which any of the glycohydrolases or sugar transporter proteins are either missing or not functional, are rare. Nevertheless, defects in the genes coding for lactase, sucrase-isomaltase, or SGLT1 are lethal unless they are properly treated. In may appear surprising that these key proteins for the sugar absorption process have no natural backup in the intestine. Yet there are only a few related proteins with similar functions, but these are unable to take over the tasks of the enzymes and transporters discussed above. All primary deficiencies in glycohydrolases and transporters are autosomal recessive disorders, which means that the deficiency becomes clinically apparent only when both alleles of the respective genes in an individual are not functional. This explains why these disorders appear most frequently in closed communities and in consanguineous relationships. An exception is late-onset lactase deficiency adult-type hypolactasia (see below), which is due to the turning off or at least down-regulation of lactase production.

6.2.1 Primary Lactase Deficiency Is Very Rare

Congenital lactase deficiency is very rare, and only a few families in whom lactase activity was completely absent have been described (24–26). Clinically, lactase deficiency becomes manifest immediately after birth, as the inability to digest lactose in mother's milk leads to diarrhea, malnutrition, and weight loss. If left untreated, it will lead to the death of the newborn within a few weeks. Treatment involves the use of lactose-free milk, in which glucose polymers are the carbohydrate. After weaning the child to adult-type food, gastrointestinal symptoms can be prevented by avoiding lactose-containing products (comparable to adult-type hypolactasia; see Sec. 6.2.2). It is important to realize that milk is an important source of calcium; therefore the avoidance of milk should be balanced with a sufficient calcium supply (see Chap. 7). It was very recently found that the ability to activate the lactase gene is determined by a segment of chromosome 2, close to but separate from the position of the lactase gene that is also located on chromosome 2. The properties of this part of chromosome 2, which lies at some distance from the actual lactase gene, determine the activation of the lactase gene (26).

6.2.2 Adult-Type Hypolactasia: Not Rare but Also Not a Disorder

Except for the very rare cases of primary lactase deficiency, all newborns and young children have the ability to digest lactose. Many children, however, around the age of 3 or 4 years, lose the ability to digest lactose. It appears that in most of the world's population, the level of lactase in the small intestine is down-regulated to low levels, a phenomenon often described as "late-onset lactase deficiency," "adult-type lactase deficiency," or "adult-type hypolactasia." We use the latter term to relate to this condition, in which the individuals develop gastrointestinal symptoms of lactose malabsorption upon ingestion of significant amounts of milk or other lactose-containing products. This down-regulation of lactase in the small intestine is genetically determined and occurs in members of nearly all races—i.e., some 75% of the human population—except in Caucasians. In fact, this condition should not be considered a disease or disorder, and using the term *deficiency* for this condition is a misnomer. The down-regulation of lactase during childhood, which persists into adult life, is the normal situation in most humans, as it is in all other mammals. This down-regulation of lactase is genetically imprinted and is not related to the ingestion of milk or lactose. Therefore, it is a primary, and not an acquired, phenotype.

Adult-type hypolactasia begins to play a role around the third or fourth year of life, with the down-regulation of lactase levels in non-Caucasians (11). It must be emphasized that lactase is never turned off completely and that all these children and adults display low but significant lactase activity. These low levels of lactase usually still allow modest ingestion of lactose (1 to 2 cups of milk a day) without malabsorption symptoms. As mentioned (Sec. 4.4), human lactase levels were shown to be regulated by the activity of the gene: low lactase activity in humans is strictly correlated with low activity of the gene, leading to low levels of functional enzyme (reviewed in Ref. 3). However, it was found that there were no differences in the human lactase genes of individuals with lactase persistence throughout life and adult-type hypolactasia (15). The mechanisms for the down-regulation of lactase at the molecular level in adult-type hypolactasia are poorly understood.

6.2.3 Primary Deficiency of Sucrase-Isomaltase

Primary sucrase-isomaltase deficiency is somewhat less rare than primary lactase deficiency; 2% of white American subjects may be heterozygous (27). Sucrase-isomaltase deficiency is also inherited as an autosomal recessive trait. Many different mutations that lead to either nonfunctional proteins or the complete absence of the protein were identified in the sucrase-isomaltase protein molecules in various subjects with sucrase-isomaltase deficiency (28). The symptoms of carbohydrate malabsorption arise somewhat later in life than do those of primary lactase deficiency, and they become apparent only after significant amounts of sucrase and/or starch have entered the diet, usually at the age of 3 months and beyond (29). Treatment is essential for the growth and development of the child and consists of a sucrose- and starch-restricted diet in which sufficient attention is paid to meeting energy requirements through the addition of other energy supplying nutrients. Sucrose is poorly tolerated by these patients, even in small quantities, as the sucrase subunit of this enzyme complex contains the only sucrase activity (Tables 2 and 3; Fig. 6). It is important to realize that maltase-glucoamylase in these sucrase-isomaltase–deficient patients is still capable of digesting modest amounts of starch (Sec. 4). Therefore, starch is still tolerated in small quantities even in the complete absence of sucrase-isomaltase.

6.2.4 Primary Trehalase and Maltase-Glucoamylase Deficiencies

As explained in Sec. 4, trehalase and maltase-glucoamylase are not essential enzymes for human survival. Although primary, congenital deficiencies were found for both enzymes, malabsorption symptoms normally remain subclinical (27,30). Therefore, these deficiencies seem clinically unimportant.

6.2.5 Primary SGLT1, GLUT5, and GLUT2 Deficiencies

Worldwide, about 200 patients have been diagnosed with primary SGLT1 deficiency (31). Many different molecular defects were found in these patients, each leading to a nonfunctional SGLT1 protein. As expected, this condition leads to very severe neonatal diarrhea and, if left untreated, to death within a few weeks. SGLT1 is essential for the handling of both glucose and galactose arising from lactose digestion; therefore, lactose should be omitted from the diets of these infants immediately after birth. As the GLUT5 is normally present in these patients, children with SGLT1 deficiency survive on fructose replacement formulas, although they may not thrive as well. These patients suffer a lifelong intolerance of glucose (and galactose) and therefore must rely on fructose as the main carbohydrate in their diets, avoiding starch and other carbohydrates that will liberate glucose or galactose upon digestion.

Primary GLUT2 deficiency has recently been shown to be the cause of the rare Fanconi-Bickel syndrome, with which some 82 patients have been diagnosed (32). These patients suffer from mild intestinal malabsorption and, as GLUT2 is also important in the liver, also suffer from glycogen accumulation and hepatomegaly. The deficiency is not fatal and patients seem to survive quite well, although their growth is severely stunted. As monosaccharides are apparently still transported over the basolateral plasma membrane of the enterocytes in the absence of GLUT2, it is very likely that there are other yet unknown but less efficient mechanisms for monosaccharides to pass this membrane. These mechanisms are not yet understood at the molecular level and therefore not accounted for in the outline of carbohydrate absorption in Figure 4. As GLUT2 plays a role in the transport of each of the important dietary monosaccharides—glucose, galactose, and fructose—dietary management of this disease is difficult and may not be very effective (see Ref. 32 for recommendations).

Thus far, no primary deficiency of GLUT5 has been reported. If these deficiencies exist, the symptoms may be subclinical, as normal ingestion of free fructose and sucrose (the main source of fructose) is not very high. However, with the increasing use of free fructose as a sweetener in, for example, soft drinks, it may well be that possible GLUT5-deficient patients may develop clinical symptoms and will be more readily identified in the future.

6.2.6 Fructose Malabsorption

Thus far only one ''disorder'' has been identified that is caused by the inability of the healthy intestine to absorb sufficient quantities of a particular carbohydrate. It appears that GLUT5 has only a limited capacity to absorb free fructose. Free fructose is only a minor constituent of the normal diet, but it is increasingly used in the industrial processing of food. Particularly, high-fructose corn syrup is used for sweetening soft drinks, because fructose can be produced quite easily from glucose and is about two times sweeter than glucose. The main "natural" source of free fructose is apple juice, which is sometimes given to children at 1 to 2 years in large volumes. Some of these toddlers develop "toddler's diarrhea," which resolves upon limiting the apple juice intake (33). One could argue that this is a primary "defect" and that this is a form of fructose "malabsorption." It is, however, far more realistic to suggest that fructose is not a major part of the natural diet of children or adults at any age, and that this form of malabsorption is primarily caused by the industrial processing of food. In fact, the free fructose from apple juice or other sources is absorbed quite well up to a certain point. Only if that limit is exceeded does fructose arrive in the colon, where it is fermented and gives rise to diarrhea. This, therefore, is probably best described as a nutritionally induced disorder (34).

6.3   Secondary Carbohydrate Malabsorption

Secondary deficiencies in sugar degradation or uptake occur frequently in diseases in which the small intestinal epithelium is damaged. In the more severe cases, such a deficiency is characterized by villus damage or atrophy (Table 5). Frequently, damage to the small intestinal epithelium leads to a decreased number of functional epithelial cells. Of course, during extensive damage to the epithelium, many more essential enzymes and transporters may be lost (not to mention the compromised epithelial integrity), leading often to a much broader spectrum of anomalies than the primary deficiencies of specific transporters and/or enzymes, as described above. As a result, it is much more difficult to manage these diseases clinically by merely adjusting the types and amounts of carbohydrate in the diet (see Chaps. 17 and 28). In general, however, if the carbohydrate intake exceeds the lowered capacity of the affected small intestine to degrade and absorb sugars, diarrhea will result. Secondary carbohydrate malabsorption can occur for many different reasons, and several of these are briefly described here (Table 5).

There are several chronic conditions that lead to secondary carbohydrate malabsorption. Microvillar inclusion disease constitutes a very rare primary disease that causes carbohydrate malabsorption. Patients with this heritable trait are unable to form a functional microvillar domain in their enterocytes and are therefore unable to absorb carbohydrates, amino acids, and many other essential nutrients. Signs of malabsorption often start immediately after birth, and the only treatment is total parenteral nutrition. Today the life expectancy of these patients is limited.

In contrast to microvillar inclusion disease, which affects the entire intestine, other chronic conditions may result in carbohydrate malabsorption depending on the extent of functional epithelial surface that is lost. In Crohn's diseases, chronically inflamed parts of the small intestinal mucosa are often found, leading to increased numbers of nonfunctional epithelial cells and to lesions in the epithelium (see Chap. 27). Depending on the extent on the affected mucosal surface, carbohydrate malabsorption can occur in these patients, which usually resolves upon treatment of the mucosal inflammation and subsequent restoration of mucosal architecture. Also hypersensitivity to specific nutrients such as milk or eggs usually affects the small intestinal epithelium. Patients with celiac disease, for example, are very likely to develop villus atrophy in the proximal small intestine, due to sensitivity to α-gliadin, a protein that is found in gluten (see Chap. 21). Like celiac disease, food intolerance may occur at any age, but it is more frequently seen in young children (see Chap. 25). Although celiac disease is a rather distinct disease entity, food intolerance resembles celiac disease in that the patients may show damage to the villus epithelial cells in response to particular food compounds, like cow's milk. The villus damage or atrophy and the ensuing carbohydrate malabsorption resolve upon the avoidance of gluten in the case of celiac disease or the other respective causative nutrient.

Surgical intervention in the small intestine, usually for intestinal atresia or necrotizing enterocolitis in newborns, also results in a decreased absorptive area. When the absorptive surface area of the remnant small intestine is too small to absorb enough nutrients to sustain the body, the patient is considered to have a short bowel syndrome and parenteral nutrition often becomes necessary (see Chap. 29). The small intestine has only limited potential to adapt to short bowel syndrome, and the resulting carbohydrate malabsorption often becomes chronic.

There are several more acute forms of secondary carbohydrate malabsorption. For example, rotavirus infection results in damage to small intestinal epithelium and also induces acute, secretory diarrhea by a separate mechanism. This infection is self-limited and often the whole cycle of infection, diarrhea, and recovery takes about a week. In developing countries, where fecal-to-oral infection sometimes occurs very frequently, it may have a recurrent character. Carbohydrate malabsorption during this type of diarrhea should not cause the patient long-lasting effects, as the period of poor nutrient intake is limited (see Chap. 15). However, the resulting dehydration is of much more concern and is often treated by ''oral rehydration solution,'' basically a physiological solution containing glucose and sodium chloride. The effectiveness of this solution depends on the action of SGLT1, which is able to transport the glucose together with the sodium ions into the enterocytes. The transport of glucose plus sodium also causes the uptake of large amounts of water (Sec. 5.1).

Therapeutic irradiation of the abdomen or chemotherapy leads to inhibition of cell proliferation in tumors but also of intestinal epithelial cells. Next to the bone marrow, the intestine is the organ that is most sensitive to these treatments; particularly with chemotherapy, the intestine is often the dose-limiting organ. The inhibition of cell proliferation may lead to small intestinal villus atrophy and secondary carbohydrate malabsorption. Both these therapeutic treatments and the intestinal damage last only for short periods, but treatments are often administered repeatedly, giving rise to prolonged periods of carbohydrate malabsorption. Therefore particular attention should be paid to the diet, with respect to carbohydrate malabsorption, in cancer patients who undergo these treatments.

6.4 Notes on the Diagnosis of Carbohydrate Malabsorption

Diagnosing carbohydrate malabsorption is not particularly easy. Below, we briefly describe the major options for diagnosis (see also Chap. 32). Diarrhea is the most prominent symptom, and one of the clinical clues is provided by the age of onset of diarrhea. Primary deficiencies in lactase and SGLT1 produce chronic diarrhea immediately after birth. Sucrase-isomaltase deficiency becomes apparent with the introduction of sucrose and starch to the diet, usually at about 3 months. These forms of carbohydrate malabsorption can be well diagnosed using either the noninvasive fecal sugar test or the noninvasive H_2-breath test (see below and Tables 4 and 5). The primary GLUT2 deficiency is rather difficult to diagnose by its intestinal symptoms, as carbohydrate malabsorption in the form of diarrhea is mild, although it occurs shortly after birth. This disorder is better diagnosed by its symptoms of liver disease (32). Some causes of secondary malabsorption, like celiac disease and particularly Crohn's disease, usually arise later in life and are very rarely seen within the first months of life. Food intolerance, particularly cow's milk intolerance, is generally not present at birth but often develops within the first months of life. Other causes of diarrhea are inflicted by therapy, as in short bowel syndrome, radiation, and chemotherapy, and are therefore self-evident. Toddler's diarrhea, caused by excessive fructose ingestion, is related to age, as the name suggests.

Stool examination in general is very useful in diagnosing carbohydrate malabsorption. Stool weights above 150 to 200 mg/m^2 of body surface per day can be taken as a quantitative measure for diarrhea. In malabsorption, intact carbohydrate molecules reach the colon with two likely conseqences: 1) The presence of reducing substances in the feces that are basically the free OH-groups at the C1 atom of the carbohydrates (Fig. 2) and 2) a drop in fecal pH below 6 due to the fermentation of the carbohydrates by bacteria to organic acids (primarily short chain fatty acids and lactate; see Sec. 2.2.). The fecal pH can be assessed by Nitrazine paper, and the presence of reducing substances can be estimated in children below the age of 2 using Clinitest tablets in the fresh watery portion of the stool. However, the presence of low fecal pH or reducing substances to diagnose carbohydrate malabsorption are valid only when 1) carbohydrate has been ingested, 2) intestinal transit time is rapid, 3) stools are collected fresh and assayed immediately, and 4) bacterial metabolism of carbohydrates is incomplete. The complete bacterial metabolism of dietary carbohydrates will lead to formation of CO_2, H_2, and H_2O, which does not affect fecal pH and annihilates any measurable reducing substances from the stool. Also the presence of fecal sucrose cannot be measured by Clinitest tablet directly. Sucrose does not possess a reducing group, as this disaccharide has no free OH-group on its C1 atoms. Therefore, sucrose can only be measured after the hydrolysis of fecal sucrose by boiling a stool sample in dilute HCl.

To diagnose carbohydrate malabsorption noninvasively, several breath tests have been developed. These are based on the formation of gases, particularly H_2, by the complete colonic fermentation of carbohydrates (see Chap. 32). Test solutions of a particular carbohydrate are given to the patient and the formation of H_2 in breath is measured several hours after ingestion. As baseline formation of H_2-production is very low, these tests provide a sensitive measure of carbohydrate malabsorption (17).

More invasive tests are based on obtaining small intestinal biopsies through duodenoscopy (35) (see Chap. 32). These small mucosal biopsies can be evaluated histologically to assess the extent of tissue damage (e.g., villus atrophy, signs of inflammation). The presence of particular enzymes can be demonstrated by immunohistochemistry, using specific antibodies to detect them, like lactase and sucrase-isomaltase (36). Also, these biopsies can be homogenized and specific glycohydrolase activities can be measured by enzyme assays, using the proper test substrates (Tables 4 and 5). Diagnosis of the infectious causes of gastroenteritis should also be performed on the serum or feces of patients to detect the causative organism. A combination of these tests is essential for establishing a final diagnosis.

REFERENCES

1. Johnson LR. Physiology of the Gastrointestinal Tract. 3rd ed. New York: Raven Press, 1994.
2. Semenza G. Anchoring and biosynthesis of stalked brush border membrane proteins: glycosidases and peptidases of enterocytes and renal tubuli. Annu Rev Cell Biol 1986; 2:255–313.
3. Van Beers EH, Büller HA, Grand RJ, Einerhand AWC, Dekker J. Intestinal brush border glycohydrolases: structure, function and development. Crit Rev Biochem Mol Biol 1995; 30:197–262.
4. Neele AM, Einerhand AWC, Dekker J, Büller HA, Freund JN, Verhave M, Grand RJ, Montgomery RK. Verification of the lactase site of rat lactase-phlorizin hydrolase by site-directed mutagenesis. Gastroenterology 1995; 109:1234–1240.

5. Naim NY, Jacob R, Naim H, Sambrook JF, Gething MJ. The pro-region of human intestinal lactase-phlorizin hydrolase. J Biol Chem 1994; 269:26933–26943.
6. Dudley MA, Hachey DL, Quaroni A, Hutchens TW, Nichols BL, Rosenberger J, Perkingson JS, Cook G, Reeds PJ. In vivo sucrase-isomaltase and lactase-phlorizin hydrolase turnover in the fed adult rat. J Biol Chem 1993; 268:13609–13616.
7. Escher JC, De Koning ND, Van Engen CGJ, Arora S, Büller HA, Montgomery RK, Grand RJ. Molecular basis of lactase levels in adult humans. J Clin Invest 1992; 89:480–483.
8. Rings, EHHM, De Boer PAJ, Moorman AFM, Van Beers EH, Dekker J, Montgomery RK, Grand RJ, Büller HA. Lactase gene expression during early development of rat small intestine. Gastroenterology 1992; 103:1154–1161.
9. Rings EHHM, Krasinski SD, Van Beers EH, Dekker J, Montgomery RK, Grand RJ, Büller HA. Restriction of lactase gene expression along the horizontal (proximal to distal) axis of rat small intestine during development. Gastroenterology 1994; 106: 1223–1232.
10. Krasinski SD, Estrada G, Yeh KY, Yeh M, Traber PG, Verhave M, Rings EHHM, Büller HA, Montgomery RK, Grand RJ. Lactase-phlorizin hydrolase and sucrase-isomaltase biosynthesis is transcriptional regulated during postnatal development in rat small intestine. Am J Physiol 1994; 267:G584–G594.
11. Wang Y, Harvey CB, Hollox EJ, Phillips AD, Poulter M, Clay P, Walker-Smith JA, Swallow DM. The genetically programmed down-regulation of lactase in children. Gastroenterology 1998; 114:1230–1236.
12. Tung J, Markowitz AJ, Silberg DG, Traber PG. Developmental expression of SI is regulated in transgenic mice by an evolutionarily conserved promoter. Am J Physiol 1997; 273:G83–G92.
13. Krasinski SD, Upchurch BH, Irons SJ, June RM, Mishra K, Grand RJ, Verhave M. Rat lactase-phlorizin hydrolase/human growth hormone transgene is expressed on small intestinal villi in transgenic mice. Gastroenterology 1997; 113: 844–855.
14. Markowitz AJ, Wu GD, Burkenmeier EH, Traber PG. The human sucrase-isomaltase gene directs complex patterns of gene expression in transgenic mice. Am J Physiol 1993; 265:G526–G539.
15. Boll W, Wagner P, Mantei N. Structure of the chromosomal gene and cDNAs coding for lactase-phlorizin hyrolase in humans with adult-type hypolactasia or persistence of lactase. Am J Hum Genet 1991; 48:889–902.
16. Plimmer RHA. On the presence of lactase in the intestine of animals and on the adaptation of the intestine to lactose. J Physiol 1996; 35:81–96.
17. Rings EHHM, Van Beers EH, Krasinski SD, Verhave M, Montgomery RK, Grand RJ, Dekker J, Büller HA. Lactase; origin, gene expression, localization, and function. Nutr Res 1994; 14:775–797.
18. Kogut MD, Donnell GN, Shaw KNF. Studies of lactose absorption in patients with galactosemia. J Pediatr 1967; 71:75–81.
19. Gilat T, Russo S, Gelman-Malachi E, Aldor TAM. Lactase in man, a non-adaptable enzyme. Gastroenterology 1972; 62:1125–1127.
20. Henning SJ. Ontogeny of enzymes in the small intestine. Annu Rev Physiol 1985; 47:231–245.

21. Holt P, Yeh KY. Effects of starvation and refeeding on jejunal disaccharidase activity. Dig Dis Sci 1992; 37:827–832.
22. Ferraris RP, Villenas SA, Diamond J. Regulation of brush-border enzyme activities and enterocyte migration rates in the mouse small intestine. Am J Physiol 1992; 262:G1047–G1059.
23. Loo DD, Zeuthen T, Chandy G, Wright EM. Cotransport of water by the Na^+/glucose cotransporter. Proc Natl Acad Sci USA 1996; 93:13367–13370.
24. Savilahti E, Launiala K, Kuitunen P. Congenital lactase deficiency: a clinical study on 16 patients. Arch Dis Child 1983; 58:246–252.
25. Mobassaleh M, Montgomery RK, Biller JA, Grand RJ. Development of carbohydrate absorption in the fetus and neonate. Pediatrics 1985; 75:160–166.
26. Järvilä I, Enattah SN, Kokkonen J, Varilo T, Savilathi E, Peltonen L. Assignment of the locus for congenital lactase deficiency to 2q21, in the vicinity of but separate from the lactase-phlorizin hydrolase gene. Am J Hum Genet 1998; 63:1078–1085.
27. Welsh JD, Poley JR, Bhatia M, Stevenson DE. Intestinal disaccharidase activities in relation to age, race, and mucosal damage. Gastroenterology 1978; 75:847–855.
28. Louvard D, Kedinger M, Hauri HP. The differentiating intestinal epithelial cell. Annu Rev Cell Biol 1992; 8:157–195.
29. Treem W R. Congenital sucrase-isomaltase deficiency. J Pediatr Gastroenterol Nutr 1995; 21:1–14.
30. Lebenthal E, Khin-Maung U, Zheng BY, Lu RB, Lerner A. Small intestinal glucosamylase deficiency and starch malabsorption: a newly recognized alpha-glucosidase deficiency in children. J Pediatr 1994; 124:541–546.
31. Wright EM. Genetic disorders of membrane transport: I. Glucose galactose malabsorption. Am J Physiol 1998; 275:G879–G882.
32. Santer R, Schneppenheim R, Suter D, Schaub J. Steinman B. Fanconi-Bickel syndrome—the original patient and his natural history, historical steps leading to the primary defect, and a review of the literature. Eur J Pediatr 1998; 157:783–797.
33. Hoekstra JH, van den Aker JH, Ghoos YF, Hartemink R, Kneepkens CM. Fluid intake and industrial processing in apple juice induced chronic non-specific diarrhea. Arch Dis Child 1995; 73:126–130.
34. Corpe CP, Burant CF, Hoekstra JH. Intestinal fructose absorption: clinical and molecular aspects. J Pediatr Gastroenterol Nutr 1999; 28:364–374.
35. Van Beers EH, Einerhand AWC, Taminiau JAJM, Heymans HSA, Dekker J, Büller HA. Pediatric duodenal biopsies: mucosal morphology and glycohydrolase expression do not change along the duodenum. J Pediatr Gastroenterol Nutr 1998; 26:186–193.
36. Van Beers EH, Rings EHHM, Taminiau JAJM, Heymans HSA, Einerhand AWC, Dekker J, Büller HA. Lactase and sucrase-isomaltase gene expression in the duodenum during childhood. J Pediatr Gastroenterol Nutr 1998; 27:37–46.

15

A Rational Approach to Feeding Infants and Young Children with Acute Diarrhea

Kenneth H. Brown
University of California, Davis, Davis, California

1 INTRODUCTION

Diarrhea is a clinical syndrome characterized by the frequent passage of loose or watery stools due to abnormally increased fecal excretion of electrolytes and water (1). For purposes of epidemiological surveillance, *diarrhea* is usually defined operationally as the excretion of three or more unformed stools per day, although a higher cutoff for stool frequency may be applied for young breast-fed infants, whose bowel movements are ordinarily looser and more frequent than those of non-breast-fed infants (2). Episodes of diarrhea can be classified according to both the appearance of the stool and the duration of illness. *Watery diarrhea* refers to stools of loose, liquid, or ''rice-water'' consistency, while the term *dysentery* indicates diarrhea that is accompanied by the excretion of blood and mucus in the feces. *Acute diarrhea* is defined as episodes that last less than 2 weeks; *persistent diarrhea* refers to those episodes that last more than 14 days. The latter may occur because of an unusually long duration of infection, complications of that infection, or exposure to multiple sequential infections that are superimposed and therefore appear clinically to be a single prolonged illness.

Noninfectious diseases—such as underlying metabolic conditions, protein sensitivity, or others—may also produce prolonged illness.

Acute childhood diarrhea is generally caused by infection and may be accompanied by nausea, vomiting, abdominal cramping and/or pain, fever, dehydration, and metabolic acidosis. Diarrheal episodes can also be complicated by anorexia, malabsorption, and depletion of those nutrients that are lost along with the blood excreted in dysenteric stools, all of which can produce secondary malnutrition. At the global level, the World Health Organization estimates that approximately 80% of all episodes of diarrhea are acute, watery diarrhea; 10% are acute dysentery; and 10% are persistent diarrhea. Diarrhea is a leading cause of death among children in low-income countries, resulting in an estimated 4 million deaths each year (3). Childhood diarrhea is also an important cause of physician visits, lost days of parental employment, and hospital admissions in the United States (4) and other industrialized countries, thereby having an enormous economic impact in these settings.

There are three major components of therapy for patients with diarrhea: fluid and electrolyte replacement, appropriate antimicrobial agents for susceptible organisms such as *Shigella* and *Vibrio cholerae*, and dietary therapy. This chapter focuses primarily on the dietary management of children with acute diarrhea. Appropriate fluid and electrolyte management and antimicrobial therapy have been described previously in detail (1,5). Evaluation and treatment of chronic diarrhea is discussed elsewhere in this text (Chap. 28).

1.1 Pathophysiology of Diarrhea

In simplest terms, diarrhea can be considered to be the result of an imbalance between gastrointestinal secretion and intestinal absorption. Specific microbial toxins produced by *V. cholerae*, selected strains of *Escherichia coli*, and similar organisms are capable of inducing excessive secretion of electrolytes by intestinal crypt cells and secondary fluid loss into the intestinal lumen, resulting in "secretory diarrhea." Other pathogens, such as certain viruses, produce diarrhea by disrupting the normal absorptive function of the villus enterocyte, causing incomplete absorption of dietary components and secondary "osmotic diarrhea." Dysentery results from both the immunological response that occurs when organisms like shigellae invade the mucosa of the distal ileum or colon and from the cytotoxins secreted by these organisms.

1.2 Etiology

It is possible to identify pathogenic organisms in the stool of about 75% of diarrhea patients assessed at clinical facilities that are capable of identifying the full range of enteropathogens, including toxigenic organisms and viruses (6). Mixed infections occur about 10 to 20% of the time in hospitalized patients. Selected bacterial, viral, and parasitic agents that are important causes of acute diarrhea and dysentery are shown in Table 1. Some agents, such as *V. cholerae* and nontyphoid *Salmonella*, may have limited geographic distribution, while others, such as rotavirus, occur more universally, albeit in selected age groups.

1.3 Nutritional Consequences of Diarrhea

Diarrhea affects children's nutritional status primarily through its impact on dietary intake and intestinal function, each of which is discussed briefly in the following sections.

1.3.1 Effect of Diarrhea on Dietary Intake

The effects of illness on children's dietary intakes have been examined in clinical studies of hospitalized children (7) and during longitudinal, community-based observations (8). Most of these studies identified some reduction of energy intake during illness, although the quantitative impact of infection varies according to the severity of illness and usual child feeding practices. In particular, children with more severe diarrhea, dehydration, and/or acidosis have a greater reduction in dietary intake (7). On the other hand, breast-fed infants are partially protected from illness-related anorexia (8).

1.3.2 Effects of Diarrhea on Intestinal Function and Nutrient Absorption

Diminished intestinal absorption during diarrhea results from 1) damage to enterocytes and their nutrient transport pathways, caused either directly by patho-

TABLE 1   Major Pathogens That Cause Acute Diarrhea or Dysentery

Type of pathogen	Examples of organisms	Usual type of diarrhea
Bacteria	Enterotoxigenic and enteropathogenic *Escherichia coli*	Watery
	Salmonella (nontyphoid)	Watery
	Vibrio cholera	Watery
	Campylobacter jejuni	Watery or dysentery
	Shigella	Dysentery
Virus	Rotavirus	Watery
	Norwalk agent	Watery
	Enteric adenovirus	Watery
Parasite	*Cryptosporidium*	Watery
	Giardia lamblia	Watery
	Entamoeba histolytica	Dysentery

gens and the immune responses that they induce or by their release of toxins; 2) aberrations of intestinal motility; and 3) increased fecal loss or bacterial hydrolysis of bile acids. The effects of enteric infections on macronutrient absorption have been reviewed previously (9,10). Briefly, abnormalities of digestion and/ or mucosal transport of carbohydrates, protein, and fat occur frequently during diarrhea. Maldigestion of carbohydrates is of particular nutritional and clinical importance for several reasons: 1) the superficial location of brush-border carbohydrases makes them particularly vulnerable, so carbohydrate malabsorption is relatively common; 2) a large proportion of dietary energy is provided by sugars and starch, so incomplete absorption can represent a sizable loss of dietary energy; 3) the osmotic force that is generated by unabsorbed carbohydrates can further accentuate intraintestinal fluid accumulation and fecal loss; and 4) bacterial fermentation of intracolonic carbohydrate can contribute to metabolic acidosis (see Chap. 14). Maldigestion of lactose is of particular concern during the management of childhood diarrhea for several reasons. First of all, the beta-galactosidase (lactase) enzyme seems to be the most vulnerable brush-border hydrolytic enzyme following mucosal injury. Second, lactose, or milk sugar, is a major component of the diets of breast-fed infants and of infants and children who receive milk-based infant formulas and other dairy products.

Research has also shown that intestinal permeability to test sugars is altered during and after diarrhea (11,12). Importantly, studies in West Africa have found a strong association between abnormal intestinal permeability and impairment of children's growth (13). Thus, diarrhea may continue to affect nutritional status adversely through subclinical malabsorption, even after the more obvious symptoms of illness subside. Several studies suggest that continued feeding during illness and supplementation with specific nutrients, such as zinc, may reduce the frequency and duration of abnormal intestinal mucosal permeability following diarrhea (11,14). These results may have important implications, not only for longer-term nutritional outcomes (13) but also for the risk of sensitization to dietary proteins and future occurrence of food allergy (11).

Several studies have also found increased fecal excretion and net negative balances of selected micronutrients during diarrhea. For example, Chilean investigators reported negative balances of zinc and copper during the early stage of acute diarrhea that were directly proportional to the severity of stool losses (15). Decreased absorption of B vitamins has also been described.

1.3.3 Effect of Diarrhea on Physical Growth

Most investigators who have attempted to quantify the cumulative impact of diarrhea on children's weight gain and linear growth have documented a negative relationship between diarrheal prevalence and growth increments, although the magnitude of this relationship varies considerably across studies. Reports have described a modifying effect of diet on the relationship between diarrhea and growth. For example, it appears that diarrhea exerts less of a negative effect on the growth of breast-fed infants than on non-breast-fed infants (16), possibly due in part to the aforementioned protective effect of breast-feeding on diarrhea-induced anorexia and to the reduced severity of infection in breast-fed infants or the beneficial nutritional components of breast milk. Some investigators have also found that growth impairment secondary to diarrhea is reduced among children who receive food supplements (17) and among those whose usual dietary intake is greater between episodes of illness. Thus, it appears that an adequate diet can provide some protection from the nutritional complications of diarrhea.

2 DIETARY MANAGEMENT OF CHILDREN WITH DIARRHEA—GENERAL ASPECTS OF TREATMENT

Two general treatment strategies for reducing the nutritional complications of diarrhea have been proposed: 1) continued feeding of sufficient amounts of food during illness to avoid any nutritional deficiencies or 2) increased feeding between episodes to permit compensatory growth after the illness has resolved. Although continued feeding during illness might seem more reasonable from a nutritional perspective, clinicians have raised the concern that incomplete digestion of food consumed during diarrhea might augment stool output, thereby increasing the risk of dehydration and acidosis (9). Thus, until recently, the optimal timing for the introduction of dietary treatment during diarrhea has been somewhat controversial. As described in the following section, however, there now appears to be a general consensus on the advisability of continued feeding during illness.

During the past decade, a number of clinical trials have been completed in different regions of the world to examine particular aspects of dietary therapy, including the appropriate timing of feeding in relation to onset of illness, the risks and benefits of feeding milk-containing diets, the effects of providing commonly available staple foods versus refined infant formulas, the impact of dietary fiber, and the importance of specific micronutrients. In all cases, carefully defined diets were prepared, and the children's dietary intake and stool output were monitored. Nutritional outcomes included net absorption of nutrients of interest, changes in body weight and other anthropometric indicators, and in some cases biochemical measures of protein or micronutrient status. These studies provide useful information for the rational design of dietary therapy, as discussed in the following sections.

2.1 Optimal Timing of Introduction of Foods During Treatment of Diarrhea

Several studies have compared the effects of continued versus interrupted feeding during acute diarrhea (Table 2). In one of these, four different feeding regimens were provided to randomly assigned groups of mildly undernourished Peruvian

TABLE 2 Recent Clinical Trials of Early Versus Later Feeding for the Management of Children with Acute Diarrhea

Author, year (ref.)	Country	Patients	Dietary treatments	Outcomes
Brown, 1988 (18)	Peru	Inpatients, <3 years	1) complete lactose-free formula, 2) diluted formula, 3) ORS,[a] or 4) intravenous solution	No difference in treatment failure rates; no difference in stool output among groups treated orally; increased energy absorption and weight gain in groups treated with greater oral intakes.
Sandhu, 1997 (19)	Europe	Inpatients, < 3 years	1) Usual diet or 2) ORS for 24 hr, then usual diet	No difference in clinical complications; greater weight gain with early introduction of usual diet.
Gazala, 1988 (20)	Israel	Outpatients, 1–12 months	1) ORS for 6 hr, then usual diet, or 2) ORS for 24 hr, then usual diet	No differences in clinical complications, duration of illness, or weight gain.
Margolis, 1990 (21)	United States	Outpatients, <1 year	1) Usual formula or 2) ORS for 24 hr, then usual formula	No differences in complications or severity of diarrhea; greater adherence to treatment in group fed early.

[a] Oral rehydration solution.

patients (18). One group received a formula diet prepared from casein (milk protein), sucrose, and vegetable oil at a concentration of 73 kcal/dL immediately following rehydration therapy, while a second group received the same formula diluted by half with water for 2 days prior to introduction of the undiluted formula. The third and fourth groups received only glucose-electrolyte solution for the first 48 hr of therapy, either orally or intravenously in the respective groups, and then the half- and full-strength formulas during subsequent 2-day periods. The children in all dietary groups were similar initially, and there were no differences in the treatment failure rates by study group. Stool outputs by children who received nothing by mouth were significantly less during the first 2 days of treatment, but there were no differences among the three groups of children who received any of the oral diets or solutions (Fig. 1). Moreover, once all children were receiving oral feedings, on the third day of the study, there were no differences in fecal excretion rates by treatment group. In other words, stool outputs of the children who consumed anything by mouth were similar regardless of whether their diets were nutritionally adequate formulas, diluted formulas, or just glucose-electrolyte solutions.

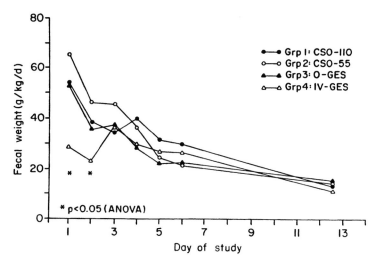

FIGURE 1   Mean stool output (g/kg body weight per day) by day of treatment and amount and type of dietary intake. (Data from Ref. 18.) CSO-110, casein-sucrose-vegetable oil diet, provided at level of 110 kcal/kg body weight per day; CSO-55, casein-sucrose-vegetable oil diet, provided at level of 55 kcal/kg body weight per day; O-GES, oral glucose-electrolyte solution; IVG-GES, intravenous glucose-electrolyte solution. See text for description of dietary management by day of study.

The children's apparent absorption of energy varied directly in relation to the amount of energy consumed. Thus, children who received the full-strength diet at the start of the period of treatment had significantly greater net energy and nutrient absorption than those who received the diluted diet or the rehydration solutions. These differences in absorption were also reflected in the increments in body weight (Fig. 2). While children who received the full-strength formula gained weight continuously throughout the period of observation, those who received any of the more dilute diets lost weight progressively until the day after they began receiving the nutritionally complete formula. Even after 2 weeks of treatment, significant differences between dietary groups persisted. These results indicate that lactose-free-formula diets can be provided continuously to patients with acute diarrhea to protect against nutritional deterioration without increasing the risk of clinical complications.

Two hundred thirty young children with acute diarrhea and mild to moderate dehydration, who were generally well nourished, were enrolled in a recently completed, multicenter, randomized trial of early versus late feeding (19). The children were admitted to one of 12 hospitals in 11 European countries. Following initial evaluation and a 4-hr period of rehydration, approximately half the patients

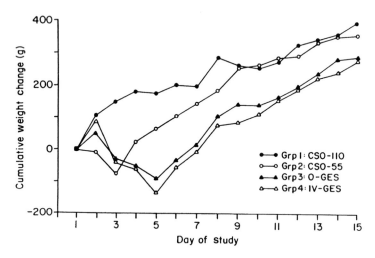

FIGURE 2   Mean cumulative changes in body weight by day of treatment and amount and type of dietary intake. (Data from Ref. 18.) CSO-110, casein-sucrose-vegetable oil diet, provided at level of 110 kcal/kg body weight per day; CSO-55, casein-sucrose-vegetable oil diet, provided at level of 55 kcal/kg body weight per day; O-GES, oral glucose-electrolyte solution; IV-GES, intravenous glucose-electrolyte solution. See text for description of dietary management by day of study.

were assigned to receive their usual diets, while the remaining children were given only oral glucose-electrolyte solution for one day before being allowed to resume their usual feeding regimens. Breast-fed patients were allowed to continue nursing regardless of their assigned treatment group. There were no differences in the frequency of unscheduled intravenous therapy or other complications by treatment group. During the first day of hospitalization, total fluid intake did not differ by treatment group, but children who continued to receive their usual diets gained approximately 100 g more weight. Differences in cumulative weight gain disappeared by day 4 of treatment. The authors concluded that, as had been shown previously in undernourished children, continued feeding is also advantageous for well-nourished children during acute diarrhea.

Other studies have been completed among ambulatory patients who were randomly assigned to early or later feeding during treatment of acute diarrhea (20,21) (Table 2). As with the previous studies, there were no differences in the rate of clinical complications with the early-feeding regimen. On the other hand, those patients who were fed early in the course of treatment tended to gain more weight, and they appeared to be more comfortable. Moreover, parental adherence to the treatment guidelines was greater with the early-feeding program.

2.2 Amount of Food Energy and Frequency of Feeding

In theory, the amount of food given to patients during diarrhea should be sufficient both to provide their usual energy and nutrient needs and to replace any excessive losses due to vomiting, intestinal malabsorption, and/or the increased catabolism associated with fever. However, it is not possible to predict a particular patient's nutritional needs because of interindividual variation in energy and nutrient requirements and the difficulty in assessing the magnitude of diarrhea-imposed nutrient losses. Nevertheless, in practice, it is the patient's appetite that determines how much food is actually consumed, so the clinician's responsibility is simply to assure that a sufficient amount of food is made available to allow the child to satisfy his or her nutrient needs to the extent that the appetite allows. As a minimum, the age-specific recommended energy intakes should be offered; if the patient consumes all the food that is offered and still appears hungry, additional increments of food energy can be provided. According to the U.S. Recommended Dietary Allowances, average energy needs are 108 kcal/kg body weight per day for infants less than 6 months of age, 98 kcal/kg body weight per day for those between 6 and 11 months, and 102 kcal/kg body weight per day for children from 1 to 3 years of age (22). In general, even if patients experience anorexia initially, their appetite returns within 1 to 2 days with repair of acidosis and dehydration and control of infection. Thus, there should be no need for tube feeding during the first few days of treatment of acute diarrhea.

There is evidence from studies of infants with persistent diarrhea that fecal output is reduced and the net balance of nutrients is greater when a formula diet is delivered by continuous infusion than by intermittent bolus feeding (23), probably because the former provides a more favorable relationship between the amount of food entering the intestine per unit time and the amount of available digestive enzymes and mucosal absorptive surface. These conclusions are supported by the results of a recently published randomized trial completed in Chinese infants with acute diarrhea who received the same total amount of milk divided into either 6 or 12 feedings per day (24). Infants who were fed more frequently had a significantly shorter duration of diarrhea and reduced fecal output. Extrapolating from these two sets of observations, it seems reasonable to recommend more frequent feeding of smaller amounts of food during illness. Again, specific guidelines are elusive because of individual variation in appetite, sleep patterns, and the time available to the child's caregiver.

2.3   Type of Food and Food Components

Recommendations on child feeding during illness must consider not only the amount of food and frequency of feeding but also the specific types of food to be provided. The latter depends, of course, on the usual diet of the patient prior to illness. A number of studies have been carried out to examine the safety and nutritional efficacy of a broad range of mixed diets and food components for children with diarrhea. Specific information is provided in the following sections for breast-fed and non-breast-fed infants and young children of different ages.

2.3.1   Breast Milk

There are multiple theoretical benefits of continued breast feeding during diarrhea. For example, in addition to its nutritional components, human milk contains anti-infective properties that may limit the duration of infection and growth factors that may promote more rapid recovery of the intestinal mucosa following enteric infections. Indeed, several epidemiological studies indicate that not only are breast fed infants more resistant to infection but their illnesses tend to be of shorter duration when they occur. These theoretical advantages of breast-feeding must be balanced against the potential risk imposed by the relatively high lactose content of human milk. The results of one clinical trial are of particular interest with regard to this uncertainty. In this study, hospitalized breast-fed infants with acute diarrhea were randomly assigned to receive either continued breast-feeding and oral glucose-electrolyte solution or only the rehydration solution during the first 24 hr of treatment (25). Notably, the group that was breast-fed continuously had reduced stool output during the first day of hospitalization compared with those whose breast-feeding was interrupted. Thus, continued breast-feeding seems advantageous for both nutritional and clinical reasons, and has the added benefit of maintaining maternal lactation capacity.

2.3.2   Nonhuman Milks

In view of the frequent occurrence of lactose maldigestion by children with diarrhea, particular concern has been raised about the appropriateness of feeding lactose-containing, milk-derived diets during diarrhea. Because incompletely absorbed lactose passes into the colon, where it draws more water into the colonic lumen, milk feeding could conceivably increase the severity of diarrhea.

The results of clinical trials that have been completed to examine the use of nonhuman milks during diarrhea are inconsistent. A metanalysis of these trials was therefore carried out to compare the outcomes in children who were treated with either lactose-containing or lactose-free diets (26). Of the 10 suitable studies that were identified, which included a total of nearly 1000 patients, 5 found significant increases in treatment failure rates with lactose-containing diets. Pooled data from all studies indicated an overall treatment failure rate of approximately 22% among children who received dietary regimens that included lactose-containing milks compared with a treatment failure rate of about 11% among those who were given lactose-free diets. Notably, however, when the studies were disaggregated according to the patients' initial severity of dehydration, only those studies that included children who were moderately or severely dehydrated on admission found an increased risk of treatment failure with the lactose-containing diets (Fig. 3). There were no differences in the risk ratios by dietary group in those studies that enrolled only children with mild or no dehydration. Thus, the vast majority of children with acute diarrhea who have undetectable or mild dehydration can safely continue receiving undiluted, lactose-containing nonhuman

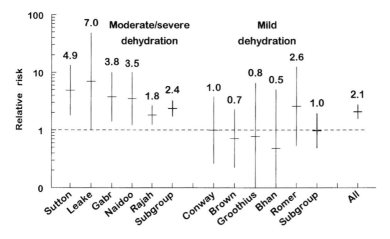

FIGURE 3   Risk of treatment failure in groups that received either lactose-containing or lactose-free dietary regimens, by individual study and initial degree of dehydration. (Data from Ref. 26.)

milks. Children with more severe diarrhea and dehydration may have a slightly excess treatment failure rate if they receive undiluted lactose-containing milk. Therefore, these patients should be managed under close supervision or with dietary regimens that have a reduced lactose content.

It is worth reemphasizing that diets with reduced lactose content can be prepared without sacrificing total energy and nutrient intakes, even in infants who receive milk-based formulas exclusively when free from illness. A broad range of nutritionally complete, lactose-free infant formulas are commercially available. Even in settings where these formulas are too expensive or not readily available, it is possible to mix a milk-based formula with the local staple, so that each provides approximately half the energy intake. For example, liquid formulas based on locally available evaporated milk and cooked noodles have been used successfully to treat children with acute diarrhea in Peru (27). The use of reduced-lactose yogurt as an alternative diet will be discussed below.

2.3.3 Mixed Diet

Information is also available from several regions of the world on the suitability of a variety of mixed diets prepared from locally available foods for children with diarrhea. For example, Alarcon et al. (28) compared two formulations of locally available Peruvian foods—a toasted wheat and pea flour mixture and a potato and milk mixture—with a standard, commercially available, lactose-free, soy-protein-isolate formula. During the first 2 days of therapy, when diarrhea was most severe, there were no differences in total stool output by treatment group, and there were no differences in treatment failure rates by study diet. During subsequent days, those children who received the staple food diets had higher stool weights than those receiving the soy formula. This result is not unexpected, however, because indigestible components of these staple foods induce greater stool weights even in diarrhea-free children. On the other hand, the median duration of diarrhea, as defined by continued excretion of liquid stool, was only 60 hr in the two groups of children receiving common foods, compared with a median duration of 144 hr in those who received the soy formula. The changes in body weights during the 1-week period of observation were extremely variable and not statistically different by treatment group.

Other studies of mixed diets have been completed in Venezuela (29), Nigeria (30), Mexico (31), and elsewhere (Table 3). These studies have consistently found that children could be managed successfully with the cheaper and presumably more accessible local food mixtures. The study from Mexico was particularly interesting because the investigators found that the treatment failure rate due to recurring dehydration was significantly less when a mixture of rice, chicken, and other common foods was used instead of a soy–protein isolate infant formula (31). All of the studies noted a reduced duration of diarrhea, as defined above, when the mixed diets were compared with the fiber-free infant formulas.

TABLE 3 Recent Clinical Trials of Mixed Diets Versus Milk or Infant Formulas for the Dietary Management of Children with Acute Diarrhea

Author (ref.)	Year	Study diet(s) (control diet)	Results
Brown (27)	1991	Wheat noodles, milk (milk)	Decreased treatment failure rate, reduced fecal output and reduced duration of illness with noodles-and-milk diet.
Alarcón (28)	1991	Wheat, peas, carrots, oil; Potato, milk, oil (soy formula)	No difference in treatment failure rate or fecal output on days 1 and 2 of therapy. Fecal output reduced with soy formula on days 5 and 6, but longer duration of diarrhea with soy formula.
Romer (29)	1991	Plantain-chicken-oil (milk)	Reduced fecal output and reduced duration of illness with mixed diet.
Grange (30)	1994	Maize, cowpea, oil, sugar (soy formula)	No difference in treatment failure rate or fecal output on days 1 to 5 of therapy. Fecal output was reduced with soy formula on day 6, but duration of diarrhea was longer with soy formula.
Maulén (31)	1994	Rice, chicken, beans, carrots, oil (soy formula)	Decreased treatment failure rate and reduced duration of illness with mixed diet.

2.3.4 Dietary Fiber

Because of the foregoing observations regarding the reduced duration of diarrhea among children who received mixed diets composed of fiber-containing staple foods, a study was carried out to assess whether these differences may have been due to the effect of dietary fiber. Peruvian children with acute diarrhea were treated with a soy–protein isolate formula with or without added soy polysaccharide as a source of fiber (32). There were no differences in stool output by dietary group or in the increments in body weight during therapy. However, there was a substantial reduction in the median duration of liquid stool excretion among those children who received the fiber-supplemented diet. Thus, it appears that the presence of fiber in the diet contributes to reduced diarrheal duration.

2.3.5 Micronutrients

Perhaps the most active area of current research on nutritional aspects of diarrhea treatment concerns the role of specific micronutrients in therapeutic regimens. Available studies have focused primarily on the potential benefits of supplementation with zinc, vitamin A, and folic acid, although other vitamins and minerals may also be of interest. An early trial of zinc supplementation of East Indian patients with acute diarrhea found no significant differences in clinical outcomes by treatment group when all patients were considered (33). However, when the investigators restricted their analysis to those children who were defined as zinc-depleted on the basis of a reduced zinc concentration in baseline rectal mucosal biopsy specimens, they found decreased stool frequency and duration of diarrhea in the zinc-supplemented group.

Since that initial report, several publications have described a beneficial effect of zinc supplementation on diarrheal severity and duration. For example, Sazawal and colleagues (34) conducted a randomized, community-based trial of 937 urban Indian children 6 to 35 months of age with acute diarrhea. The children received a multivitamin preparation either with or without 20 mg of elemental zinc provided as zinc gluconate, and they were visited periodically thereafter to determine the severity and duration of the presenting episode. The probability of diarrhea continuing on any particular day of observation was reduced by 23% in the zinc-supplemented group. Among the subset of children who began treatment within 3 days of onset of diarrhea and after controlling for potential confounding variables, there was a 26% reduction in the proportion of episodes lasting more than 7 days. The impact of zinc supplementation on diarrheal duration was greater among children who were either wasted or stunted, but there was no modifying effect of initial plasma zinc concentration on the duration of illness. The mean daily frequency of excretion of watery stools was reduced by 39% in the zinc-supplemented group.

Other studies, completed in Bangladesh (35) and Peru (36), found similarly beneficial effects of zinc supplementation for children with diarrhea (Table 4). In summary, it is notable that each of the aforementioned studies identified a positive impact of zinc supplementation on diarrheal duration and/or severity, and a recent pooled analysis of these trials confirmed that the results are highly statistically significant (37). It is important to recognize, however, that all the cited studies were conducted in populations where zinc deficiency is likely to be common because of limited intake of animal products and/or consumption of grains with high levels of phytic acid, which can inhibit zinc absorption. Because the mechanism for the observed effects of zinc is unknown, it is uncertain whether these results are due to the impact of zinc on the host's nutritional status or

TABLE 4 Results of Therapeutic Trials of Zinc Supplementation for Treatment of Children with Diarrhea

Author, year (ref.)	Country	Patients	Treatment	Outcome
Sachdev, 1988 (33)	India	Children 6–18 months old hospitalized for acute diarrhea	20 mg zinc or placebo	Decreased duration of diarrhea and stool frequency in zinc-treated subgroup with low initial rectal mucosal zinc concentration.
Sazawal, 1995 (34)	India	Ambulatory patients 6–35 months old with acute diarrhea	ORS[a] and multivitamins with or without 20 mg zinc	Decreased duration of diarrhea and frequency of liquid stool excretion in zinc-treated group.
Roy, 1997 (35)	Bangladesh	Children 3–24 months old hospitalized for acute diarrhea	Vitamins and minerals with or without 20 mg zinc	Decreased duration of diarrhea and less stool output in zinc-treated group.
Penny, 1999 (36)	Peru	Community-based study of children 6–35 months old with persistent diarrhea	20 mg zinc or placebo	Decreased duration of post-treatment illness in zinc-treated group; no effect on stool frequency.

[a] Oral rehydration solution.

whether zinc may exert some pharmacological effect on the host or may inhibit the survival or proliferation of enteric pathogens. Thus, it is not known whether similar results would occur in better-nourished patients. Another issue still to be resolved is the importance of the timing of initiation of zinc therapy. Although one study found that the effect of zinc was greater when treatment was initiated earlier during the course of the episode, results of one trial conducted among children with persistent diarrhea also indicated some advantage of zinc supplementation, even though this was introduced relatively late in the course of the illness.

Several trials have also been conducted to study the effect of large doses of vitamin A on the severity and duration of acute diarrhea. Henning and colleagues (38) completed a randomized trial of 83 hospitalized Bangladeshi children with acute, watery, noncholera diarrhea, most of whom were breast-fed. There was no detectable benefit of vitamin A treatment on total stool output or duration of illness. More recently, Bhandari et al. (39) reported the results of a randomized, community-based trial in which either 60 mg retinol equivalents (RE) of vitamin A or a placebo was given to 900 Indian children 1 to 5 years of age with acute diarrhea. When all children were considered, there was no significant effect of vitamin A on mean diarrheal duration or severity, although the proportion of children whose episode persisted more than 14 days was reduced by 70% in the vitamin A–treated group. Notably, among the subgroup of non-breast-fed children, there was a significant 16% reduction in the mean duration of illness and a 27% reduction in the mean number of stools excreted. By contrast, there was no significant effect of vitamin A therapy in breast-fed children. Thus, it appears that vitamin A may be a useful adjunct to therapy in those populations with a high likelihood of subclinical vitamin A deficiency, particularly in non-breast-fed children.

In another brief report from South Africa, 76 preschool children with acute diarrhea, most of which was associated with rotavirus, were allocated to a group that received 5 mg of folic acid every 8 hr during hospitalization or to an untreated control group (40). The duration of diarrhea was significantly reduced by more than half in the group that was supplemented with folic acid. These results have yet to be confirmed in other settings.

In summary, a growing number of studies have found that supplementation with specific micronutrients can reduce the duration and/or severity of diarrhea. Additional research is still needed to determine which populations are most likely to benefit from including micronutrient supplements in standard therapeutic regimens and whether supplementation with multiple micronutrients is as effective as providing specific single micronutrients.

2.3.6 Probiotics

Biotherapeutic agents, or ''probiotics,'' are viable bacteria that benefit the host by interfering in some way with the function or survival of potential pathogens (see Chap. 5). Although these biotherapeutic organisms are not truly foods or nutrients per se, they are often incorporated into foods and are therefore considered briefly in this review. For example, certain bacteria and yeasts can be introduced into dairy products to prolong their shelf life and enhance specific organoleptic characteristics of the foods. If the organisms that are inoculated are capable of fermenting lactose, the cultured milk products may have a reduced lactose content (41). Moreover, if the products are not pasteurized, the organisms may survive in the gut and continue to produce beta-galactosidase, which can hydrolyze lactose that has not been previously digested in vitro (42). There is some evidence indicating that children with diarrhea may tolerate yogurt better than milk (43).

The specific mechanisms of action of probiotics are unknown, but in addition to their possible modification of selected components of the diet, it is conceivable that they may interfere with the ability of pathogens to colonize the gut by altering the gut milieu (e.g., pH), competing for intraluminal nutrients, secreting antibiotic "bacteriocins," interfering with adherence to intestinal mucosal binding sites, or enhancing the host's immune function (44,45). Specific probiotic agents that have been studied recently for the treatment or prevention of diarrhea include *Lactobacillus casei* sp. strain GG, *Lactobacillus reuterii*, and *Bifidobacterium bifidum*, among others (45). *Lactobacillus casei* sp. strain GG was reported to reduce the duration and/or severity of acute watery diarrhea associated with rotavirus in Finland and with nonrotaviral agents in Pakistan and Thailand, but did not seem to affect the clinical course of dysentery in the latter two sites. *Lactobacillus reuterii* was effective in reducing the duration of diarrhea and frequency of vomiting and excretion of watery stool among Finnish children hospitalized with acute illness, which was associated mainly with rotavirus.

Several groups of experts have recently reviewed the efficacy of biotherapeutic agents for the treatment and prevention of diarrhea (45,46). Both groups concluded that additional studies are needed to test these agents under different clinical and field conditions. Specific questions remain concerning the impact of probiotics on individual etiological agents of disease, the proper dose of these biotherapeutic agents, and whether they are particularly useful for the treatment or prevention of diarrhea or both.

3 SUMMARY OF RECOMMENDED TREATMENT AND DISCUSSION OF WHAT CAN GO WRONG

An algorithm for the approach to dietary management of young children with acute diarrhea was developed on the basis of the results of the clinical trials reviewed herein (Fig. 4). Critical factors in planning a dietary treatment regimen are the age of the child, the preillness feeding practices, and the severity of diarrhea and dehydration. In all cases, breast-fed infants should continue to receive breast milk during their illness, not only to provide adequate energy and nutrient

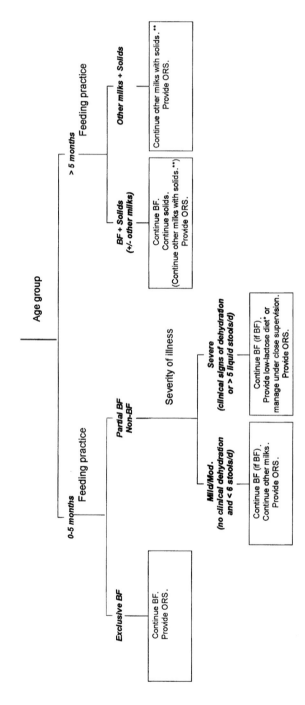

FIGURE 4 Recommended dietary management of children with acute diarrhea, according to age group, preillness feeding practices, and severity of diarrhea. BF, Breast-feeding; ORS, oral rehydration solution; *low lactose-diet, see text; **see text for discussion of how to combine other milks with solids.

intakes and to assist with the control of infection and early clinical recovery, but also to protect maternal lactational capacity, which depends on continued expression of milk. In young infants who are being fed exclusively with lactose-containing, nonhuman milk prior to illness, continuation or modification of the usual diet depends on the severity of illness, as described above. In older children who are receiving complementary foods in addition to breast milk or other milk-based diets, these foods can be given along with the respective milk. The amount of complementary food that is provided should be sufficient to meet theoretical energy and nutrient requirements for age, which have been reviewed recently by the World Health Organization and UNICEF (47). Children with a high risk of deficiency of specific micronutrients should receive appropriate supplements.

Feeding frequency should be increased to the extent possible, considering child sleep patterns and any limitations of available caregiver time. In addition to clinical assessment of stool output and hydration status, dietary intake and body weight should be monitored daily during inpatient treatment as simple indicators of the nutritional response to therapy. In all cases, a follow-up evaluation should be scheduled several weeks after the acute illness to confirm complete nutritional recovery. The vast majority of patients with acute diarrhea can be managed successfully with the therapeutic regimens described herein. In a limited number of cases, however, problems of anorexia, malabsorption, or persistent illness may undermine therapeutic efforts. These latter conditions are described briefly, as follows.

3.1 Anorexia

As indicated above, anorexia usually occurs due to metabolic abnormalities imposed by dehydration and acidosis, so appetite generally returns fairly rapidly with appropriate rehydration therapy. Even in the patient with anorexia, it is important to continue offering food frequently, so the return of appetite can be recognized promptly. There is generally no need to provide gastric feedings during the first few days of illness unless the patient is severely malnourished or at risk for hypoglycemia. However, hydration status should be monitored closely in case anorexia and/or vomiting precludes successful oral rehydration therapy. Persistent anorexia may signal other systemic or gastrointestinal disease, such as septicemia or intestinal obstruction, so appropriate diagnostic evaluation and treatment may be needed.

3.2 Malabsorption

Intestinal malabsorption leading to osmotic diarrhea and secondary dehydration is another potential concern. Symptomatic malabsorption is most commonly caused by maldigestion of carbohydrates, which can be detected by the presence of stools with low pH (<6.5) and/or positive reducing substances if reducing sugars, like lactose, are being consumed in the diet. Appropriate treatment of carbohydrate malabsorption is to reduce intake of the specific carbohydrate or remove it entirely from the diet. This can be accomplished without altering the total daily energy intake, either by replacing the offending carbohydrate with one that is better tolerated or by substituting another macronutrient source, like dietary fat, for some of the carbohydrate. Subclinical malabsorption is usually detected by poor weight gain following illness, hence the need for follow-up examination.

3.3 Persistent Diarrhea

In the unusual case that diarrhea persists beyond 2 weeks, further evaluation may be indicated to rule out other causes of persistent illness. The reader is referred to Chapter 28 for a complete discussion of these issues.

REFERENCES

1. World Health Organization. A Manual for the Treatment of Diarrhoea. (WHO/CDD/SER/80.2). Geneva: World Health Organization. 1990.
2. Weaver LT, Ewing G, Taylor LC. Bowel habit of milk-fed infants. J Pediatr Gastroenterol Nutr 1988; 7:568–571.
3. Claeson M, Merson MH. Global progress in the control of diarrheal diseases. Pediatr Infect Dis J 1990; 9:345–355.
4. Ho M, Glass RI, Pinsky PF, Young-Okoh N, Sappenfield WM, Buehler JW, Gunter N, Anderson LJ. Diarrheal deaths in American children. JAMA 1988; 260:3281–3285.
5. Santosham M, Brown KH, Sack RB. Oral rehydration therapy and dietary therapy for acute childhood diarrhea. Pediatr Rev 1987; 8:273–278.
6. Black RE. Epidemiology of diarrhoeal disease: implications for control by vaccines. Vaccine 1993; 11:100–106.
7. Brown KH, Perez F. Determinants of dietary intake during childhood diarrhea and implications for appropriate nutritional therapy. Acta Paediatr Suppl 1992; 381:127–132.
8. Brown KH, Stalings RY, Creed de Kanashiro H, Lopez de Romanã G, Black RE. Effects of common illnesses on infants' energy intakes from breast milk and other foods during longitudinal community-based studies in Huascar (Lima), Peru. Am J Clin Nutr 1990; 52:1005–1013.
9. Brown KH, MacLean WC Jr. Nutritional management of acute diarrhea: an appraisal of the alternatives. Pediatrics 1984; 73:119–125.
10. O'Loughlin EV, Scott RB, Gall DG. Pathophysiology of infectious diarrhea: changes in intestinal structure and function. J Pediatr Gastroenterol Nutr 1991; 12:5–20.
11. Isolauri E, Untunen M, Wiren S, Vuorinen P, Koivula T. Intestinal permeability changes in acute gastroenteritis: effects of clinical factors and nutritional management. J Pediatr Gastroenterol Nutr 1989; 8:466–473.
12. Goto K, Chew F, Torun B, Peerson JM, Brown KH. Epidemiology of altered intes-

tinal permeability to lactulose and mannitol in Guatemalan infants. J Pediatr Gastroenterol Nutr 1999; 28:282–290.

13. Lunn PG, Northrup-Clewes CA, Downes RM. Intestinal permeability, mucosal injury, and growth faltering in Gambian infants. Lancet 1991; 338:907–910.

14. Roy SK, Behrens RH, Haider R, Akramuzzaman SM, Mahalanabis D, Wahed MA, Tomkins AM. Impact of zinc supplementation on intestinal permeability in Bangladeshi children with acute diarrhoea and persistent diarrhoea syndrome. J Pediatr Gastroenterol Nutr 1992; 15:289–296.

15. Castillo-Duran C, Vial P, Uauy R. Trace mineral balance during acute diarrhea in infants. J Pediatr 1988; 113:452–457.

16. Rowland MGM, Goh Rowland SGJ, Cole TJ. Impact of infection on the growth of children from 0 to 2 years in an urban West African community. Am J Clin Nutr 1988; 47:134–138.

17. Lutter CK, Mora JO, Habicht J-P, Rasmussen KM, Robson DS, Sellers SG. Nutritional supplementation: effects on child stunting associated with diarrhea. Am J Clin Nutr 1989; 50:1–8.

18. Brown KH, Gastañaduy AS, Saavedra JM, Lembcke J, Rivas D, Robertson AD, Yolken R, Sack RB. Effect of continued oral feeding on clinical and nutritional outcomes of acute diarrhea in children. J Pediatr 1988; 112:191–200.

19. Sandhu BK, Isolauri E, Walker-Smith JA, Banchini G, Van Caillie-Bertrand M, Dias JA, Guandalini S, Hoekstra JH, Juntunen M, Kolacek S, Marx D, Micetic-Turk D, Razenberg MCAC, Szajewska H, Tarminiau J, Weizman Z, Zanacca C, Zetterstrom R. Early feeding in childhood gastroenteritis. J Pediatr Gastroenterol Nutr 1997; 24: 522–527.

20. Gazala E, Weitzman S, Weizman Z, Gross J, Bearman JE, Gorodischer R. Early vs. late refeeding in acute infantile diarrhea. Israel J Med Sci 1988; 24:175–179.

21. Margolis PA, Litteer T, Hare N, Pichichero M. Effects of unrestricted diet on mild infantile diarrhea. Am J Dis Child 1990; 144:162–164.

22. Food and Nutrition Board, National Research Council. Recommended Dietary Allowances, 10th ed. Washington, DC: National Academy Press, 1989.

23. Parker P, Stroop S, Greene H. A controlled comparison of continuous versus intermittent feeding in the treatment of infants with intestinal disease. J Pediatr 1981; 99:360–364.

24. Wan C, Phillips MR, Dibley MJ, Liu Z. Randomised trial of different rates of feeding in acute diarrhoea. Arch Dis Child 1999; 81:487–491.

25. Khin-Maung-U, Nyunt-Nyunt-Wai, Myo-Khin, Mu-Mu-Khin, Tin-U, Thane-Toe. Effect on clinical outcome of breast feeding during acute diarrhoea. BMJ 1985; 290: 587–589.

26. Brown KH, Peerson JM, Fontaine O. Use of nonhuman milks in the dietary management of young children with acute diarrhea: a meta-analysis of clinical trials. Pediatrics 1994; 93:17–27.

27. Brown KH, Perez F, Gastañaduy AS. Clinical trial of modified whole milk, lactose-hydrolyzed whole milk, or cereal-milk mixtures for the dietary management of acute childhood diarrhea. J Pediatr Gastroenterol Nutr 1991; 12:340–350.

28. Alarcon P, Montoya R, Perez F, Dongo JW, Peerson JM, Brown KH. Clinical trial of home available, mixed diets versus a lactose-free, soy-protein formula for the

dietary management of acute childhood diarrhea. J Pediatr Gastroenterol Nutr 1991; 12:224–232.

29. Römer H, Guerra M, Piña JM, Urrestarazu MI, Garcia D, Blanco ME. Realimentation of dehydrated children with acute diarrhea: comparison of cow's milk to a chicken-based formula. J Pediatr Gastroenterol Nutr 1991; 13:46–51.

30. Grange AO, Santosham M, Ayodele B, Lesi A, Stallings RY, Brown KH. Evaluation of a maize-cowpea-palm oil diet for the dietary management of Nigerian children with acute, watery diarrhea. Acta Paediatr 1994; 83:825–832.

31. Maulen I, Brown KH, Acosta MA, Fernandez-Varela H. Comparison of a rice-based, mixed diet versus a lactose-free, soy-protein isolate formula for young children with acute diarrhea. J Pediatr 1994; 125:699–706.

32. Brown KH, Perez F, Peerson JM, Fadel J, Brunsgaard G, Ostrom KM, MacLean WC Jr. Effect of dietary fiber (soy polysaccharide) on the severity, duration, and nutritional outcome of acute, watery diarrhea in children. Pediatrics 1993;92:241–247.

33. Sachdev HPS, Mittal NK, Yadav HS. A controlled trial on utility of oral zinc supplementation in acute dehydrating diarrhea in infants. J Pediatr Gastroenterol Nutr 1998; 7:877–881.

34. Sazawal S, Black RE, Bhan MK, Bhandari N, Sinha A, Jalla S. Zinc supplementation in young children with acute diarrhea in India. N Engl J Med 1995; 333:839–844.

35. Roy SK, Tomkins AM, Akramuzzaman SM, Behrens RH, Haider R, Mahalanabis D, Fuchs G. Randomized controlled trial of zinc supplementation in malnourished Bangladeshi children with acute diarrhea. Arch Dis Child 1997; 77:196–200.

36. Penny ME, Peerson JM, Marin M, Duran A, Lanata CL, Lönnerdal B, Black RE, Brown KH. Randomized, community-based trial of the effect of zinc supplementation, with and without other micronutrients, on the duration of persistent childhood diarrhea in Lima, Peru. J Pediatr 1999; 135:208–217.

37. Bhutta ZA, Black RE, Brown KH, Meeks Gardner J, Gore S, Hidayat A, Khatun F, Martorell R, Ninh NX, Penny ME, Rosado JL, Roy SK, Ruel M, Sazawal S, Shankar A. Therapeutic effects of oral zinc in acute and persistent diarrhea in children in developing countries: pooled analysis of randomized controlled trials. Am J Clin Nutr 2000; 72:1516–1522.

38. Henning B, Stewart K, Zaman K, Alam AN, Brown KH, Black RE. Lack of therapeutic efficacy of vitamin A for non-cholera, watery diarrhea in Bangladeshi children. Eur J Clin Nutr 1992; 46:437–443.

39. Bhandari N, Bahl R, Sazawal S, Bhan MK. Breast-feeding status alters the effect of vitamin A treatment during acute diarrhea in children. J Nutr 1997; 127:59–63.

40. Haffejee IE. Effect of oral folate on duration of acute infantile diarrhoea. Lancet 1988; 2:334–335.

41. Savaiano DA, Abou El Anouar A, Smith DE, Levitt MD. Lactose malabsorption from yogurt, pasteurized yogurt, sweet acidophilus milk, and cultured milk in lactase-deficient individuals. Am J Clin Nutr 1984; 40:1219–1223.

42. Kolars JC, Levitt MD, Aouji M, Savaiano DA. Yogurt–an autodigesting source of lactose. N Eng J Med 1984; 310:1–3.

43. Boudraa G, Touhami M, Pochart P, Soltana R, Mary JY, Desjeux JF. Effect of feed-

ing yogurt versus milk in children with persistent diarrhea. J Pediatr Gastroenterol Nutr 1990; 11:509–512.
44. Saavedra JM. Microbes to fight microbes: a not so novel approach to controlling diarrheal disease. J Pediatr Gastroenterol Nutr 1995; 21:125–129.
45. Elmer GW, Surawicz CM, McFarland LV. Biotherapeutic agents: a neglected modality for the treatment and prevention of selected intestinal and vaginal infections. JAMA 1996; 275:870–876.
46. Sanders ME. Summary of conclusions from a consensus panel of experts on health attributes of lactic cultures: significance to fluid milk products containing cultures. J Dairy Sci 1993; 76:1819–1828.
47. Brown KH, Dewey KG, Allen LH. Complementary feeding of young children in developing countries: a review of current scientific knowledge. Geneva, Switzerland: World Health Organization, 1998.

16

Nutritional Support of the Chronically Ill Child

Harland S. Winter
Harvard Medical School and MassGeneral Hospital for Children,
Boston, Massachusetts

Jacqueline Madden
MassGeneral Hospital for Children, Boston, Massachusetts

1 INTRODUCTION

Children with chronic illness are particularly vulnerable to nutritional deficiencies. Not only are metabolic needs increased, but also utilization and absorption of nutrients may be impaired. All these factors may contribute to poor growth, delayed maturation, and exacerbation of the underlying chronic illness. Once undernutrition or malnutrition develops, growth and development may be impaired and lead to progression of the underlying disease, specific nutrient deficiencies, immune compromise, and/or an increased incidence of infections. Nutritional support in a child with a chronic illness should restore or maintain normal growth and maturation as well as contribute to the improvement of the child's quality of life. For many chronic illnesses, nutritional support may modify the progression of the illness. For example, in inflammatory bowel disease and sickle cell anemia, the provision of adequate nutrition may decrease the number of exacerbations of disease. In this chapter, general causes of growth failure are discussed, followed by management of specific chronic diseases of the cardiovascular, renal, pulmonary, hepatobiliary, and immune systems.

2 PATHOPHYSIOLOGY OF GROWTH FAILURE
IN CHRONIC DISEASES

Pediatricians must distinguish growth failure from short stature disease (see Chap. 12). Growth failure is always associated with a pathological process, whereas short stature may not be associated with disease. The definition of growth failure is a height velocity less than 10% of the growth velocity curve of the reference population. Short stature is defined as a height below the 3% of the height growth chart. The weight in relation to height, as calculated by the body mass index (BMI), is another measurement that can be used to assess growth failure. P_{50} refers to the 50th percentile for age and gender.

$$\text{The relative BMI is: } 100 \times \frac{\text{wt(kg)}/\text{ht}^2(\text{m})}{\text{wt}_{P_{50}}/\text{ht}^2_{P_{50}}}$$

If the relative BMI is less than 90%, the child is underweight. If the relative BMI is less than 80%, the child is malnourished. Children with chronic diseases associated with malabsorption or inadequate caloric intake will usually have a BMI below 90%, because weight gain is affected more than linear growth. Conversely, in children with growth delay from endocrine or genetic diseases,

TABLE 1 Causes of Nutritional Compromise

Causes of decreased food intake
  Esophagitis
  Gastritis
  Duodenitis
  Difficulty chewing
  Nausea
  Pancreatitis
  Zinc deficiency
  Dementia
  Depression/despair
  Pain
Causes of increased metabolic requirements
  Fever
  Altered metabolism
  Cytokine production
Causes of increased loss of nutrients
  Vomiting
  Diarrhea
  Steatorrhea
  Enteric infection
  Lactose malabsorption

height will be more affected than weight, resulting in a normal or above-normal BMI.

In chronic illness, nutritional compromise may result from decreased nutrient intake, increased metabolic requirements, and increased loss of nutrients. Symptoms and diseases that result in each of these problems are listed in Table 1. Neurological disorders such as cerebral palsy are often associated with undernutrition, in part because of problems related to chewing and swallowing (see Chap. 13). Children with extensive burn injuries will require intense nutritional support to provide the additional calories needed to heal the skin but also to compensate for metabolic abnormalities based upon the increased demands from fever and possible pulmonary compromise. Children with inflammatory bowel disease may have malabsorption resulting in a loss of both calories and, if the terminal ileum is involved, specific nutrients such as vitamin B_{12} (see Chap. 27). Nutritional compromise results in growth delay, which—if not reversed—carries implications that persist into adulthood.

3 CARDIAC DISEASE

Growth failure commonly accompanies congenital heart disease. Cyanotic lesions such as transposition of the great arteries, tetralogy of Fallot, tricuspid atresia, truncus arteriosus, total anomalous venous return, pulmonary atresia, Ebstein's anomaly, and hypoplastic left heart syndrome are more commonly associated with delayed weight gain and growth; whereas acyanotic lesions—such as atrial septal defect, ventricular septal defect, patent ductus arteriosus, common arteriovenous canal, pulmonic stenosis, and coarctation of the aorta—affect weight more severely than height. In children with cyanotic congenital heart disease, the severity of growth failure and delay in skeletal maturation is directly related to the degree of hypoxemia. Pulmonary hypertension is the most important factor resulting in malnutrition and growth failure (1). Correction of the structural abnormality and improved hemodynamic function often results in increased growth velocity. Congestive heart failure causes decreased cardiac output and reduced renal and mesenteric blood flow. This may result in impaired absorption, altered intestinal motility and delayed gastric emptying, and tolerance of smaller quantities of feedings. The cause for decreased volume of feedings may also be related to medications such as digitalis, renal disease, or tachypnea. In children with acyanotic congenital heart disease—such as ventricular septal defects—no difference in resting energy expenditure and energy intake was noted in comparison to healthy, age-matched controls. However, total energy expenditure was higher in the children with heart disease, suggesting that they have an elevated energy cost of physical activity. Their poor weight gain may be a result of their inability to meet their increased caloric requirements (2).

Children who have had a Fontan procedure may develop protein-losing enteropathy. Although loss of albumin results in decreased oncotic pressure, mucosal edema, and malabsorption, other proteins and nutrients—such as transferrin, ceruloplasmin, fibrinogen, lipoproteins, alpha-1 antitrypsin, trace minerals, calcium, and iron—may be lost from the gastrointestinal tract. Edema, ascites, and lymphopenia may result from venous and lymphatic obstruction. A stool with an elevated alpha-1 antitrypsin level supports the diagnosis. Treatment includes dietary therapy with increased protein and decreased long-chain fat with supplements containing medium-chain triglycerides. Calcium and fat-soluble vitamins may need to be replaced as well. Medications used to treat congenital heart disease may affect nutrient utilization, as summarized in Table 2.

The nutritional assessment of congenital heart disease includes determination of the type of lesion. Cyanotic conditions and onset at birth greatly affect the ability to feed. Diaphoresis during feeding suggests that the cardiac output is not sufficient for the stress of eating. Tachypnea may impair oral intake and require the placement of a nasogastric or gastrostomy tube to achieve adequate caloric intake (see Chap. 17). Clubbing and cyanosis associated with poor suck or swallow indicate insufficient cardiac output and desaturation. To estimate the energy needs of an infant with congenital heart disease, the provider should add 30 to 60 kcal/kg/day to the recommended daily allowance (RDA) (3).

Enteral support should be avoided in children with 1) poor cardiac output or unstable medical management; 2) a lesion dependent on a patent ductus arteriosus with poor mesenteric blood flow (e.g., interrupted aortic arch, coarctation of the aorta, single ventricle); 3) a recent resuscitation; 4) junctional ectopic tachycardia; 5) bowel obstruction; or 6) gastrointestinal bleeding. Parenteral support may be the only means to provide sufficient nutrition for these children.

Successful nutritional support can be achieved by maximizing cardiac function either by direct intervention or medical treatment, correcting iatrogenic abnormalities of pharmacotherapy, avoiding nutritional deficiencies, and providing sufficient energy either by enteral or parenteral means. Practical suggestions for managing the nutritional needs of children with congenital heart disease are listed in Table 3 (4). Trying to sort out the cardiac and behavior issues contributing to poor growth is frequently a challenge. Careful monitoring of intake and observation of feeding often help to define the problem (5).

Nutritional issues are frequently cited as important in the prevention of coronary heart disease. These problems are associated with hyperlipidemia and are discussed more completely in Chapter 11. Recent studies evaluating which lifestyle parameters are relevant in the prediction of high risk during adulthood suggest that cardiopulmonary fitness is directly related to physical activity. Although eating a balanced diet is important, it is no substitute for regular exercise (6). The Bogalusa Heart Study data suggest that being overweight is associated with risk factors in childhood that, if corrected, could reduce the adult incidence of cardiovascular disease, hyperlipidemia, and hypertension. Nutritional therapy has a role not only

TABLE 2 Effects of Medications Used to Treat Patients with Heart Disease

Medication	Anorexia	↓K⁺	↓Na⁺	↓Cl⁻	↓Mg²⁺	Nausea	Diarrhea	Other
Furosemide	+	+	+	+		+		
Captopril								↓K⁺
Digoxin	+	+			+	+		
Chlorothiazide	+	+					+	
Propanolol					+			↓Mg, riboflavin Hypoglycemia

Source: Adapted from Ref. 32.

TABLE 3 Suggestions for Nutritional Support for Children with Congenital Heart Disease

1. Increase energy requirements from maintenance of 75–120 kcal/kg/day by 20 to 100% with stress, surgery, or growth delay.
2. Provide high-calorie foods by decreasing water content, increasing protein (8–10%), carbohydrate (35–65%), and fat—either LCT or MCT (35–50%) content.
3. Limit fluid intake.
4. Restrict sodium to 2.2–3 mEq/kg/day.
5. Monitor electrolytes, especially potassium (2–3 mEq/kg/day).
6. Maintain urine osmolarity below 400 mosm/L.

in restoring and maintaining growth in children with known cardiac disease but also in preventing cardiac disease that develops later in adulthood.

4 RENAL DISEASE

Children with chronic renal failure experience many nutritional and metabolic abnormalities; these are listed in Table 4. The tempo of the disease and the ultimate outcome of chronic dialysis or renal transplantation should be considered in constructing a care plan. Assessment of blood urea nitrogen, creatinine, sodium, potassium, glucose, phosphate, calcium, magnesium, bicarbonate, hematocrit, triglyceride, and cholesterol—as well as the severity of the renal impairment—determine the need for replacement of vitamins and minerals. Protein and energy requirements are based on the RDA for height age. Although protein intake may have to be restricted because of renal dysfunction, there is no evidence in children

TABLE 4 Nutritional and Metabolic Consequences of Chronic Renal Failure

Acidosis
Salt loss
Protein/energy malnutrition
Osteodystrophy
Hyperkalemia
Hypermagnesemia
Loss of water soluble vitamins
Anemia
Edema
Oxalate stones
Growth retardation

TABLE 5 Formulas for Children with Renal Disease

	Manufacturer	Kcal/mL	Protein g/L (sources)	Fat g/L (sources)	Carbohydrate g/L (sources)	Na/K (meq/L)	Ca/P (mg/L)	mosm/kg Water
Similac PM 60/40	Ross Products	0.67	16 (whey, caseinate)	38 (soy, coconut)	69 (lactose)	7/15	380/190	250
Amin-aid	R & D Laboratories	2.0	19 (free amino acids)	46 (partially hydrogenated soybean oil, soy lecithin, mono- and diglycerides)	365 (maltodextrin, sucrose)	<15/<15	–/–	700
Suplena	Ross Products	2.0	30 (caseinates)	96 (high oleic safflower and soy oil, soy lecithin)	255 (maltodextrin, sucrose, cornstarch)	34/29	1430/730	600
Renalcal Diet	Nestle Clinical Nutrition	2.0	34 (essential L-amino acids, select non-essential amino acids, whey protein concentrate)	82 (MCT oil, canola oil, corn oil, soy lecithin)	290 (maltodextrin, modified cornstarch)	–/–	–/–	600
Nepro	Ross Products	2.0	70 (caseinates)	69 (high oleic safflower and soy oil)	213 (corn syrup, sucrose, FOS)	37/27	1370/685	665

that a reduction in protein intake will alter the progression of end-stage renal disease.

Fluid restriction—determined by fluid allowance, metabolic status, and glomerular filtration rate—requires calorically dense formula feedings for infants. Because increasing the concentration of formula results in increased renal solute load, the use of carbohydrate and fat is an effective means of increasing caloric density. Excretion of electrolytes is impaired and must be monitored as renal function changes. Specific formulas and nutritional supplements are listed in Table 5. If caloric requirements for growth cannot be met by oral supplements, tube feedings must be considered. The volume that can be tolerated is determined by the child's renal function. If total parenteral nutrition is required, potassium, magnesium, and phosphate should be withheld initially until the level of excretion is established. Both vitamin A and selenium are excreted by the kidneys and should be monitored. The management of nutritional and metabolic problems in children with chronic renal failure is summarized in Table 6.

About two-thirds of children receiving dialysis receive peritoneal dialysis

TABLE 6 Management of Nutritional and Metabolic Problems in Children with Chronic Renal Failure

Poor caloric intake and delayed growth	Nutritional supplements, nasogastric tube feedings, total parenteral nutrition, growth hormone. Start with RDA and increase as tolerated until growth starts.
Acidosis	Provide additional $NaHCO_3$ and bicitra.
Loss of salt	Increase salt intake.
Renal osteodystrophy	Restrict phosphate intake, bind phosphate with calcium carbonate or calcium acetate.
Potassium retention	Restrict intake, sodium polystyrene sulfonate (Kayexalate), correct acidosis.
Elevated magnesium	Restrict intake by avoiding Mg-containing antacids or cathartics.
Hypertension or edema	Restrict sodium intake.
Anemia of chronic disease	Erythropoietin and iron supplementation.
Loss of water-soluble vitamins	Nephrocaps or Nephrovites.
Increased homocysteine levels	Supplement with folic acid, vitamin B_6, and vitamin B_{12}.
Increased vitamin A	Avoid ingestion of liver and stop supplementation with vitamin A.
Oxalate stones	Avoid vitamin C supplementation and foods such as spinach.

(7). The loss of protein in the dialysis effluent may potentiate protein-calorie malnutrition. The use of intradialytic parenteral nutrition to provide a supplemental source of amino acids is being evaluated (8,9). Gastrostomy tube feedings are also effective in improving weight gain and growth in children receiving chronic peritoneal dialysis (10). For children receiving hemodialysis, using more frequent dialysis in combination with adequate nutrition can normalize growth (11). Renal transplantation restores normal renal function and should reverse the nutritional and metabolic problems caused by chronic renal failure. However, these changes may require time, and other problems may result from immonosuppression related to the transplant itself. Medications such as prednisone can cause increased appetite, hypertension, or gastritis.

Children with chronic renal disease have the potential to be cured by receiving a kidney transplant. The age at which renal function is restored will determine growth potential. Nevertheless, the provision of maximal nutritional support throughout the course of the chronic illness (12) will enhance the child's ability to achieve his or her genetic potential.

5 LIVER DISEASE

The liver plays a central role in the synthesis of lipids, proteins, and carbohydrates; for that reason, any disease that impairs hepatic function ultimately affects absorption and utilization of nutrients (13). Biliary tract diseases in which the common bile duct is obstructed or stenotic are associated with decreased bile in the intestinal lumen, resulting in malabsorption of lipids. Because of the high caloric value of fats, steatorrhea may result in poor weight gain. Diseases that injure the hepatic parenchyma—such as biliary atresia (14), autoimmune hepatitis, and chronic infectious hepatitis—impair not only bile acid synthesis but also the synthesis of protein and complex carbohydrates (15). Total parenteral alimentation, especially in the neonate, can injure the liver, resulting in cirrhosis and hepatic failure (16,17). Nutritional support for children with chronic progressive liver disease or hepatic transplantation (18,19) requires careful monitoring (20). The reader is referred to Chapter 30, on liver disease, for more details on issues that relate to problems encountered by children with hepatic failure or hepatobiliary tract obstruction.

Children with chronic liver disease require between 100 to 150% of the RDA to maintain growth. Protein should be restricted only in situations in which hepatic encephalopathy limits the quantity of protein. In these situations, the use of branched chain amino acids may beneficial, but their use remains controversial. Infants are usually given Portagen (Mead Johnson), Pregestimil (Mead Johnson) or Alimentum (Ross Products) because they contain 85, 55, and 50% of medium-chain triglyceride respectively. For children over one year of age, the elemental products Peptamen Junior (Nestle Clinical Nutrition) and Vivonex Pediatric (Sandoz Nutritional Co.) contain medium-chain triglycerides and should be used. For adolescents, products designed for the adult can be used. These include Hepatic Aid (McGaw), NutriHep Diet (Nestle Clinical Nutrition), Vital HN (Ross Products), Vivonex TEN (Sandoz Nutrition Co.) and Peptamen (Nestle Clinical Nutrition).

Although the underlying liver disease may have a great effect on utilization of nutrients, many of the medications used to treat complications of hepatic dysfunction may themselves affect nutritional status. Cholestyramine, used in children with pruritus secondary to cholestasis, binds bile acids and impairs absorption of fat, especially fat-soluble vitamins. Children taking cholestyramine may require additional fat-soluble vitamins and supplemental medium-chain triglyceride as a source of fat. Phenobarbital, given to increase the flow of bile, alters vitamin D metabolism and, with prolonged administration, can potentiate rickets if not monitored. Patients with hepatic encephalopathy may be treated with neomycin, which can injure the small intestinal mucosa, resulting in steatorrhea, carbohydrate malabsorption, and vitamin B_{12} deficiency. Medium-chain triglycerides and supplemental vitamin B_{12} may be needed. Lactulose, also used to treat hepatic encephalopathy, causes an osmotic diarrhea requiring monitoring of sodium and potassium losses in the stool.

The recommended doses for supplementation with vitamins and minerals are listed in Table 7. Children with biliary atresia or hepatic injury that begins shortly after birth require early intervention, as nutritional deficiencies may develop rapidly. An important factor in the management of these children is frequent reevaluation and close monitoring. Sudden changes in hepatic function may

TABLE 7 Vitamin and Mineral Supplementation for Children with Chronic Liver Diseases

Fat soluble vitamins	
Vitamin A	5000–25,000 IU/day
Aquasol A (emulsified)	
Vitamin D	3–5 μm/kg/day
Vitamin D_3 (Calderol)	
Vitamin E	15–25 IU/kg/day (31)
d-α-tocopherol polyethylene glycol-1000 succinate (TPGS, Liqui E)	
Vitamin K_1	2.5–5 mg/day
Mephyton	
Minerals	
Zinc sulfate	1 mg/kg/day
Calcium (elemental)	25–100 mg/kg/day
Phosphorus (elemental)	25–50 mg/kg/day

result in increased prolongation of the protime and bleeding (21). Monitoring serum albumin, 25-hydroxy vitamin D, and protime in addition to standard nutritional parameters, is an important aspect of the care of the child with chronic liver disease. Additional information can be obtained at the American Liver Foundation web site (www.liverfoundation.org).

6 CHRONIC PULMONARY DISEASES

Cystic fibrosis, a pulmonary disorder in children, requires nutritional intervention in part because of the pancreatic insufficiency that is part of the disease. Mutations in the gene that encodes for the CF transmembrane conductance regulator (CFTR) result in a protein responsible for chloride transport. Patients with the mutation have thick, viscous mucus, especially in the lungs and pancreas. This mucus blocks the airways and the pancreatic ducts, resulting in chronic obstructive lung disease and pancreatic insufficiency. A detailed discussion of cystic fibrosis can be found in Chapter 31. In this section, aspects of nutritional management are presented.

For the 30,000 individuals in the United States who live with cystic fibrosis, nutritional management is a critical aspect of care. Growth in the child with cystic fibrosis is complicated by increased resting energy expenditure from the chronic cough, recurrent pulmonary infections, and impaired oxygenation. Nutrient losses are related to the pancreatic insufficiency, decreased bile acid pool and emesis related to cough. Furthermore, caloric intake may be decreased because of muscle wasting and fatigue, anorexia, and depression; but when they are not acutely ill, children with cystic fibrosis consume more calories than age-matched controls (22). All these factors contribute to putting the growing child with cystic fibrosis at risk for malnutrition and delayed growth. Nutritional management of the child with cystic fibrosis is based upon compensation for malabsorption. Enzyme replacement therapy is discussed in Chapter 31, but specific nutrient and vitamin requirements are listed in Table 8.

Human breast milk with enzyme supplementation is optimal for infants with cystic fibrosis. For mothers who choose to use prepared formula, either soy- or cow's milk–based preparations are equivalent alternatives that will sustain growth (23). All formulas, even hydrolysates, require pancreatic enzyme supplementation. Elemental formulas are not needed unless there are concomitant illnesses requiring this type of nutritional intervention. The controversy between Toronto and Boston over the restriction of fat in the diet has been convincingly settled in favor of the Canadian approach to encourage normal fat intake. Improved nutritional support and better control and prevention of infection have resulted in a much longer life expectancy for these children. The Cystic Fibrosis Foundation maintains a web site (www.cff.org) offering information about achieving optimal nutrition.

TABLE 8 Nutritional Management of Cystic Fibrosis

	0–6 Months	7–12 Months	1–5 Years	6–10 Years	>10 Years
Calories	120–200% of the RDA				
Protein	RDA for age				
Fat	40% of total calories, 3–5% of total calories as essential fatty acids				
Sodium (may increase in hot weather)	2 mmol/kg/day as NaCl	1 mmol/kg/day as NaCl	10 mmol/day (300 mg NaCl bid)	20 mmol/day (600 mg NaCl bid)	30–40 mmol/day (600 mg NaCl tid-qid)
Vitamin A	1500 IU/day		1–2 years: 1500–3000 IU/day 2–8 years: 5000 IU/day >8 years: 5000–10,000 IU/day		
Vitamin D	400–1000 IU/day				
Vitamin E	25 IU/day	50 IU/day	100 IU/day	100–200 IU/day	200–400 IU/day
Vitamin K	2.5 mg/week (2 twice weekly if on antibiotics)		5 mg twice weekly		
Water soluble vitamins	Twice the RDA for age				
Zn, Fe, Ca	RDA for age				

7 HIV DISEASE

Children with HIV disease experience altered growth and nutritional deficiencies that begin early in childhood. The reasons for these problems are multifactorial but in part are probably related to the immunoregulatory dysfunction. The relationship between immune deficiency, enteric infection, malabsorption, and malnutrition-induced immune deficiency complete a self perpetuating cycle that causes progressive deterioration of the immune function and the development of opportunistic infection, wasting, and malignancy. The goals of nutritional management in the HIV-infected child are to preserve lean body mass, maintain normal growth and development, provide sufficient caloric intake, and control symptoms of malabsorption. Early intervention with calorically dense formulas and supplements plays a critical role in the care of the HIV-infected child. Fevers and recurrent infection increase the metabolic demands and should be treated. At the first signs of loss of lean body mass (24), slow weight gain, or delayed linear growth, nutritional evaluation should be initiated.

Nutritional assessment for the HIV-infected child should include anthropometric measurements including height, weight, head circumference, triceps skinfold thickness, and midarm circumference. In addition, a detailed dietary history is needed to determine not only if the child is ingesting enough calories but also if the family has the resources to purchase the food. Protein status can be determined by measuring prealbumin and retinol binding protein; if malnutrition is suspected, specific micronutrients can be quantified. Assessment of body composition by bioelectrical impedance analysis, dual emisson x-ray apsorptometry (DEXA) scan, or computed tomography may be of benefit in following an individual child's response to therapy. The causes of malnutrition in HIV-infected children are listed in Table 9.

Decreased oral intake is one of the most common causes of malnutrition in HIV-infected children and the cause is often difficult to identify. Specific nutritional deficiency is uncommon in developed countries but is common in communities in which malnutrition is endemic. Assessment of the availability of food for the family is a crucial part of the evaluation. If the responsible adult in the home is HIV-infected and unable to shop or prepare food, children will not thrive. Assessment of caloric intake using diet recall or a diary will help distinguish decreased intake from malabsorption. Children with HIV disease appear to develop lactase deficiency earlier than predicted by genetic background. Therefore, if a child is experiencing diarrhea or increased gas, restriction of lactose might ameliorate the symptoms. Lactose intolerance is usually not associated with weight loss or poor growth (25). If the cause of the malnutrition or delayed growth cannot be corrected, enteral supplements can be provided either orally or via nasogastric/gastrostomy tube (26,27). In rare situations in which the intestinal mucosa is so injured that enteral support is not feasible, parenteral nutrition

TABLE 9   Causes of Malnutrition in HIV-Infected Children

Decreased oral intake
  Oral ulcers
  Esophagitis
  Gastritis
  Duodenitis
  Anorexia
  Depression
  Despair
  Pain
  Neurological impairment
  Altered taste (drug-induced, zinc deficiency)
  Food not available
  Aversion to food (behavioral, nausea)
Increased nutrient loss
  Vomiting
  Diarrhea
  Pancreatitis
    Drug-induced: ddI, ddC, d4T, pentamidine
    Infectious: cytomegalovirus, *Mycobacterium avium* complex
  Malabsorption
    Lactose
    Steatorrhea: usually related to mucosal injury or pancreatitis
Increased nutrient requirements
  Fever
  Infection
  Cytokine production
  Endocrine disease
    Thyroid
    Adrenal
    Growth hormone

---

should be used. More extensive guidelines for nutritional support for the HIV-infected child are available (28,29).

Maintenance of growth is one of the most important aspects of management for an HIV-infected child. Even though children may appear to be well nourished because of increased fat mass, they may have decreased lean body mass and not be growing at the expected rate (30). During adolescence, short stature and delayed sexual maturation are at the top of the list of concerns expressed by children entering puberty. Early nutritional intervention may prevent these growth issues later in life. Studies are currently ongoing to assess the role of early nutritional therapy on growth and body composition.

TABLE 10   What Can Go Wrong in Nutritional Therapy in Children
with Chronic Disease

1. The underlying chronic condition may not respond to management.
2. Assessment of nutritional status may be inadequate.
3. Initiation of nutritional intervention may be delayed.
4. Treatment plan may fail to be modified as the child grows and
   develops.

8   CONCLUSION

The role of nutritional therapy in the management of chronic diseases depends
on the impact of the underlying disorder on digestion and nutrient absorption.
In most patients, improving the function of the diseased organ system will decrease the need for ongoing nutritional support. Problems that the clinician may
face are listed in Table 10. However, in many children, this goal cannot be
achieved and clinicians are left to manage situations in which ongoing nutritional
support and evaluation are necessary.

REFERENCES

1. Varan B, Tokel K, Yilmaz G. Malnutrition and growth failure in cyanotic and acyanotic congenital heart disease with and without pulmonary hypertension. Arch Dis
   Child 1999; 81:49–52.
2. Ackerman II, Karn CA, Denne SC, Ensing GJ, Leitch CA. Total but not resting
   energy expenditure is increased in infants with ventricular septal defects. Pediatrics
   1998; 102:1172–1177.
3. Gaedeke NMK, Hill CS. Nutritional issues in infants and children with congenital
   heart disease. Crit Care Nurs Clin North Am 1994; 6:153–163.
4. Forchielli ML, McColl R, Walker WA, Lo CL. Children with congenital heart disease: a nutritional challenge. Nutr Rev 1994; 52:348–353.
5. McGrail K. Nutritional considerations for infants and children with congenital heart
   disease. Top Clin Nutr 1997; 13:62–68.
6. Twisk JW, Kemper HC, van Mechelen W, Post GB. Which lifestyle parameters
   discriminate high- from low-risk participants for coronary heart disease risk factors.
   Longitudinal analysis covering adolescence and young adults. J Cardiovasc Risk
   1997; 4:393–400.
7. Edefonti A, Picca M, Damiani B, Loi S, Ghio L, Giani M, Consalvo G, Grassi MR.
   Dietary prescription based on estimated nitrogen balance during peritoneal dialysis.
   Pediatr Nephrol 1999; 13:253–258.
8. Brewer ED. Pediatric experience with intradialytic parenteral nutrition and supplemental tube feeding. Am J Kidney Dis 1999; 33:205–207.

9. Qamar IU, Secker D, Levin L, Balfe JA, Slotkin S, Balfe JW. Effects of amino acid dialysis compared to dextrose dialysis in children on continuous cycling peritoneal dialysis. Perit Dial Int 1999; 19:237–247.
10. Ramage IJ, Geary DF. Harvey E, Secker DJ, Balfe JA, Balfe JW. Efficacy of gastrostomy feeding in infants and older children receiving chronic peritoneal dialysis. Perit Dial Int 1999; 19:231–236.
11. Tom A, McCauley L, Bell L, Rodd C, Espinosa P, Yu G, Yu J, Girardin C, Sharma A. Growth during maintenance hemodialysis: impact of enhanced nutrition and clearance. J Pediatr 1999; 134:464–471.
12. Warady BA, Alexander SR, Watkins S, Kohaut E, Harmon WE. Optimal care of the pediatric end-stage renal disease patient on dialysis. Am J Kidney Dis 1999; 33: 567–583.
13. Novy MA, Schwarz KB. Nutritional considerations and management of the child with liver disease. Nutrition 1997; 13:177–184.
14. Kaufman SS, Murray ND, Wood P. Nutritional support for the infant with extrahepatic biliary atresia. J Pediatr 1987; 110:679–686.
15. Protheroe SM. Feeding the child with chronic liver disease. Nutrition 1998; 14:796–800.
16. Quigley EMM, Marsh MN, Schaffer JL, Martin RS. Hepatobiliary complications of total parenteral nutrition. Gastroenterology 1993; 104:286–301.
17. Pereira GR. Hyperalimentation-induced cholestasis. Am J Dis Child 1981; 135:842–845.
18. Sutton M. Nutritional support in pediatric liver transplantation. Diet Nutr Suppl News 1989; 11:1–3.
19. Roggero P, Cataliotti E, Ulla L, Stuflesser S, Nebbia G, Bracaloni D, Lucianetti A, Gridelli B. Factors influencing malnutrition in children waiting for liver transplants. Am J Clin Nutr 1997; 65:1852–1857.
20. Maes M, Sokal E, Otte JB. Growth factors in children with end-stage liver disease before and after liver transplantation: a review. Pediatr Transplant 1997; 1:171–175.
21. Rashid M, Durie P, Andrew M, Kalnins D, Shin J, Corey M, Tulllis E, Pencharz PB. Prevalence of vitamin K deficiency in cystic fibrosis. Am J Clin Nutr 1999; 70: 378–382.
22. Stark LJ, Mulvihill MM, Jelalian E, Bowen AM, Powers SW, Tao S, Susan Creveling, Passero MA, Harwood I, Light M, Lapey A, Hovell MF. Descriptive analysis of eating behavior in school-age children with cystic fibrosis and healthy control children. Pediatrics 1997; 99:665–671.
23. Reilly JJ, Evans TJ, Wilkinson J, Paton JY. Adequacy of clinical formulae for estimation of energy requirements in children with cystic fibrosis. Arch Dis Child 1999; 81:120–124.
24. Fontana M, Zuin G, Plebani A, Bastoni K, Visconti G, Principi N. Body composition in HIV-infected children: relations with disease progression and survival. Am J Clin Nutr 1999; 69:1282–1286.
25. Miller TM, Orav EJ, Martin SR, McIntosh K, Winter HS. Malnutrition and carbohydrate malabsorption in children with vertically transmitted human immunodeficiency virus 1 infection. Gastroenterology 1991; 100:1296–1302.
26. Henderson RA, Saavedra JM, Perman JA. Effect of enteral tube feeding on growth

on children with symptomatic human immunodeficiency virus infection. J Pediatr Gastroenterol Nutr 1994; 18:429–434.

27. Miller TL, Awnetwant EL, Evans S, McIntosh K. Gastrostomy tube supplementation for HIV infected children. Pediatrics 1995; 96:696–702.

28. Heller LS. Nutritional support for children with HIV/AIDS. AIDS Reader 2000; 10: 109–114.

29. Task Force on Nutrition Support in AIDS. Guidelines for nutrition support in AIDS. Nutrition 1989; 5:39–46.

30. Miller TL, Evans SJ, Orav EJ, McIntosh K, Winter HS. Growth and body composition in children infected with the human immunodeficiency virus-1. Am J Clin Nutr 1993; 57:588–592.

17

Enteral and Parenteral Nutrition

Robert J. Shulman and Sarah Phillips
Baylor College of Medicine, Houston, Texas

1 INTRODUCTION

Nutritional support in critically or chronically ill children can blunt the catabolic response to trauma and severe illness and often rehabilitate those who are malnourished. Done appropriately, it will minimize the risk of infection and other complications.

The delivery of appropriate nutritional support begins with assessment of the following: (1) nutritional status of the patient, (2) functional status of the gastrointestinal (GI) tract, (3) chewing and swallowing ability, (4) behavioral factors, and (5) underlying disease.

Nutritional status is the first consideration, because those patients who are significantly malnourished will require a more aggressive approach to rehabilitation that can, in turn, influence initial nutritional support decisions. For example, the severely malnourished patient is at risk for development of the refeeding syndrome, which, if left untreated, can result in death. The degree of malnutrition can also influence decision regarding the rate at which enteral and/or parenteral feeds are delivered and tolerated (1).

The functional status of the GI tract is the next consideration. This includes an assessment of the child's ability to take oral feedings. Even when a child is able to take some or all feedings orally, consideration must still be given to its ability to chew and swallow, how tired the child gets with feeding, and his or her mental status. Oral (ideally) or enteral (directly into the GI tract) nutrition is always preferable to parenteral (intravenous) nutrition. Oral and enteral nutrition are recognized as providing benefits over parenteral nutrition for a number of reasons. Oral feeding preserves feeding skills that, in the young infant, can be lost within weeks of disallowing oral intake [i.e., making them "nil per os" (NPO)]. If oral feedings are not feasible, the main decision is whether nutrition can be provided enterally or parenterally.

Even if enteral feedings can be used, GI function must be assessed to determine how and what type of feeding can be used. For example, dysmotility of the GI tract can influence the location of feeding (gastric versus small intestinal), rate of delivery, and/or volume. The absorptive capacity of the small intestine is frequently a limiting factor as to whether the patient can be fed enterally or parenterally and is also important in formula selection.

Part of the benefit of enteral nutrition is its ability to preserve GI mucosal integrity (2). The intestine has an important role in immune function as a defense against intestinal pathogens and toxins. The presence of luminal nutrients helps maintain intestinal mucosal integrity and function, thereby potentially minimizing the risk of bacterial translocation. Some oral or enteral nutrition is better than none. Used in conjunction with parenteral nutrition, it can still be beneficial in reducing the risk of parenteral nutrition–associated complications. Parenteral nutrition is important for providing nutritional support in patients who are physically and/or medically unable to tolerate enteral feedings.

The decision to feed a patient enterally or parenterally may seem straightforward at first glance (Fig. 1) but is often influenced more by convention and

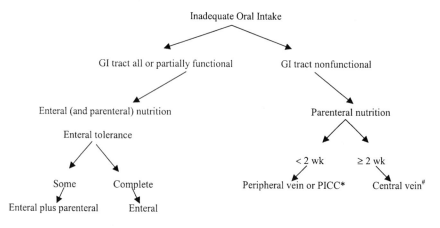

FIGURE 1 Algorithm for enteral and parenteral nutrition. *Peripherally inserted central catheter; # surgically placed central vein catheter.

perception than medical need. While it is generally accepted that enteral feeding is optimal for most patients, parenteral nutrition is frequently administered because it is perceived to be convenient and easy. This is especially true in the pediatric population, where parents and practitioners can be reluctant to place nasogastric or gastrostomy tubes. Although parenteral nutrition can provide nutrients and promote healing and growth, it is associated with more complications and expense. Thus, decisions to feed enterally or parenterally require careful assessment by the medical team.

2 ENTERAL NUTRITIONAL SUPPORT

Consider enteral nutritional support for the child who is either unable or unwilling to consume an amount orally that is sufficient to support adequate growth and development. Indications for enteral feedings in the pediatric population are listed in Table 1 (3). Commonly, the primary problem is inadequate intake secondary to a medical or behavioral problem. This usually manifests as poor weight gain. Often, several attempts at supplementing the diet or concentrating the caloric density of feedings have been unsuccessful. This lack of success at increasing intake may be related to several factors. For example, in children with mental retardation or cerebral palsy, oral feedings require an inordinate amount of time and effort by caregiv-

TABLE 1 Indications for Enteral Nutrition Support

Problem	Medical condition	Indications for support
Inadequate Intake	Congenital anomalies Neurologic disorders Cancer Psychological disorders Short-bowel syndrome	1. Child consumes <50–60% of nutritional needs 2. Requires feeding time of greater than 4–6 hr/day
Malabsorption	Chronic diarrhea Inflammatory bowel disease Cystic fibrosis	3. Severe wasting: less than 70% of expected weight
Increased requirements	Burns Congenital heart disease Bronchopulmonary dysplasia Sepsis and trauma	4. Depressed linear growth 5. Suboptimal weight gain for 3 months 6. Weight loss over 3-month period 7. Weight-for-height <2 standard deviations from mean

Source: Adapted from Ref. 3.

ers or may place the patient at risk for aspiration pneumonia (see Chap. 13). Other children may fail to consume sufficient nutrients due to anorexia of disease, as is often seen in cancer (4). Often, a child's underlying disease results in increased metabolic requirements or losses that are so large that the child is unable to meet the nutritional demands orally. Such situations are found in children with heart disease, severe gastroesophageal reflux (see Chap. 19), short bowel syndrome (see Chap. 29), renal disease, and cancer (see Chap. 16) (5–7). Abnormal feeding behaviors that result in food refusal, volitional vomiting, or severely limited food choices also may necessitate enteral feeding support.

2.1 Indications for Enteral Nutritional Support

Enteral feedings may be the sole source of nutrition or used in combination with oral intake and/or parenteral nutrition. These feedings may be delivered by tube via the stomach or small intestine. The formula used is determined by the ability of the GI tract to digest and absorb nutrients. Feedings can be divided into several boluses throughout the day or delivered continuously by infusion pump feedings throughout the day and/or night (see below). General guidelines for establishing enteral nutritional support are shown in Figure 1.

2.2 When to Initiate Enteral Nutritional Support

In the chronically ill child, enteral nutritional support ideally should be initiated soon enough to preclude the development of immune dysfunction or growth failure. In order to do so, it is important to follow the weight gain (or lack thereof) and be aware of the nutritional intake history. Although it is dependent upon the record keeping abilities of the parent or caretaker, a 5-day diet diary (kept prospectively) can be helpful in identifying when inadequate intake is becoming manifest.

In critically ill or injured patients, enteral nutrition should be initiated as soon as they are hemodynamically stable and electrolyte abnormalities have been corrected. In severely injured patients, hypomotility is common, and this may preclude enteral feeding for some period.

Although bowel sounds are used to reflect GI function, they are a poor indicator. The absence of bowel sounds does not necessarily bar the use of enteral feedings. Passage of gas per rectum is a good indicator of the return of motility after surgery or injury. However, the potential for gut ischemia and necrosis is increased with the use of inotropic and/or vasopressor medications. They are a contraindication to feedings directly into the small bowel.

2.3 Route of Administration

The route of administration of enteral nutrition depends upon the functional status of the gastrointestinal tract, absorptive capacity of the small intestine, and whether enteral feeding is to be used for short-term rehabilitation or long-term nutritional management. Feeding routes and indications are outlined in Table 2. Enteral feedings can be delivered into the stomach or through the pylorus (i.e., transpylorically) into the small intestine.

Gastric feedings most closely simulate the normal physiological and hormonal responses to oral intake (8). Additionally, gastric feedings allow for delivery of greater osmotic loads and larger volumes than do feedings directly into the small intestine. As a consequence, feedings can be delivered as boluses. On the other hand, gastric feedings also can be used if enteral feedings need to be given continuously because of poor motility or absorption. Gastric feedings are relatively easy to administer and can be done by parents or other caretakers. Nasogastric tubes or gastrostomy tubes (or buttons) can be used to deliver feedings into the stomach. Generally, nasogastric tubes are indicated for short-term rehabilitation (weeks to a few months) and gastrostomy tubes for longer-term management. For nasogastric tube insertion, air can be injected and the end of the tube auscultated at the presumed site of the opening to ensure that the tube is not located in the airways.

While gastric feedings are preferable in most instances, many patients are not candidates for this method. Transpyloric feedings, or feedings directly into the small bowel, are indicated when feedings via the gastric route cannot be administered safely or effectively. For example, some patients with severe gastroesophageal reflux can be at risk for aspiration when gastric feedings are used. Individuals with gastroparesis (poor gastric emptying) and ventilated and sedated patients may also be candidates for transpyloric feedings.

2.3.1 Feeding Tubes

Feeding tubes are made from polyurethane, silicone rubber, polyethylene, and polyvinyl chloride. Polyurethane and silicone tubes are soft, cause little discomfort, and do not stiffen, even over many weeks to months. Polyethylene and polyvinyl chloride are easier to introduce than the softer tubes. However, they harden quickly and have been reported to cause gastrointestinal perforation unless they are changed frequently (3 to 5 days). For tubes positioned in the small bowel, radiological confirmation is useful.

Placement of a transpyloric feeding can be accomplished at the bedside using a nasoenteric tube that uses a tip with a pH sensor (Zinetics, Inc.) (9). It provides a real-time pH readout, enabling the tube to be advanced into the duodenum by recognition of pH changes. Weighted tubes can also be used. Long-term small intestinal feeding in patients with poor gastric function can also be accomplished using a gastrostomy with a transpylorically placed tube or by using a surgically placed jejunostomy tube.

2.4 Formula Selection

Feedings available for the pediatric patient consist of human milk, infant formulas, pediatric enteral formulas, blenderized feedings, or adult formulas adapted

TABLE 2 Enteral Feeding Methods and Indications

Site	Delivery route	Indications	Disadvantages
Stomach	Orogastric	Prematurity	Aspiration
	Nasogastric	Short-term nutritional support	Choking if gag reflex present
		Inadequate oral intake due to increased needs or anorexia of chronic disease	May exacerbate gastroesophageal reflux and problems with impaired GI motility
		Refusal to eat	
		Nocturnal feedings	
		Inability to suck or swallow	
	Gastrostomy	Long-term tube feeding	Surgical or percutaneous endoscopic gastrostomy placement
		Upper GI congenital anomalies	May exacerbate gastroesophageal reflux
		Esophageal injury/obstruction	
Small bowel	Transpyloric	Congenital upper GI anomalies	Jejunostomy not appropriate for patients at operative risk
	Nasojejunal	Inadequate gastric motility	
	Gastrojejunal	After upper GI surgery	
	Jejunostomy	High aspiration risk	
		Severe gastroesophageal reflux	
		Functioning intestinal tract with esophageal or gastric obstruction	

Source: Adapted from Ref. 3.

to the pediatric patient. The selection of an appropriate formula for the pediatric patient can be daunting in light of the numerous formulas available and the limited ability of many hospital formularies to stock such a wide array of products. The choice of an appropriate feeding depends upon the age, underlying disease, absorptive capacity, and nutritional needs of the child. Guidelines for formula selection are given in Table 3.

In general, formulas are designed for four basic age groups: preterm infants (<37 weeks), infants (0 to 1 year of age), children (1 to 10 years), and older children and adults (11 years and older). Within each age group formulas are divided into several subgroups (Table 4) depending on the protein source, degree of protein hydrolysis, and whether they are intended for oral or tube feedings.

TABLE 3   Guidelines for Formula Selection

1. Identify appropriate age category:
    Preterm
    Infant: 0–1 year
    Pediatric: 1–10 years
    Older child and adult: ≥ 11 years
2. Identify protein source required:
    Cow's milk–based: sodium caseinate, whey
    Soy: soy protein isolates
    Hydrolyzed protein: peptides
    Synthetic amino acids: free amino acids
3. Determine absorptive capacity:
    Polymeric formula
    Hydrolyzed protein or elemental (free amino acids)
4. Determine fat source required:
    Long-chain fats
    Medium-chain triglycerides (MCT)
5. Evaluate nutritional requirements
    Fluids: potential restriction
    Calorie: assess for catchup growth or obesity
    Protein: assess need for catchup or ongoing losses
    Vitamin: assess in cases of fluid restriction and when using adult
        formulas
6. Consider need for modular additives to meet nutritional requirements
    Formula concentration
    Fat: long-chain triglycerides, medium chain triglycerides
    Carbohydrate: glucose polymers, dextrose, fructose
    Protein: casein, soy
7. Evaluate need for fiber: long-term therapy and/or neurologically
    impaired
8. Evaluate osmolality and renal solute load

TABLE 4 General Formula Composition

	Description				
	Protein	Carbohydrate	Fat	Indications	Examples
Preterm Cow's milk–based	Nonfat milk Whey protein concentrate	Lactose Corn syrup solids Glucose polymers	MCT[a] Vegetable	Neosure and Enfamil 22 may be used post-discharge	Enfamil Premature Similac Special Care NeoSure Enfamil 22
Infant: 0–1 year Cow's–milk based	Intact casein/whey	Lactose	Vegetable	Infants with normal GI function	Enfamil Similac Gerber Good Start
Soy-based	Soy protein iso-late	Sucrose Corn syrup solids Sucrose	Soy Vegetable Coconut	Infants with allergies or after diarrhea	Alsoy Isomil Prosobee

	Protein	Carbohydrate	Fat	Indication	Products
Hydrolyzed casein	Casein hydrolysate	Lactose-free corn syrup solids Dextrose	MCT Vegetable	Malabsorption Allergies	Pregestimil Nutramigen Alimentum
Elemental	Free amino acids	Lactose-free corn syrup solids Dextrose	Vegetable	Malabsorption Allergies	Neocate
Pediatric: 1–10 years					
Cow's milk-based	Intact casein/whey	Hydrolyzed corn-starch, sucrose	Vegetable MCT	Supplement or sole source of nutrition	Pediasure Kindercal Resource Just for Kids
Hydrolyzed	Enzymatically hy-drolyzed whey	Maltodextrins, cornstarch	MCT Vegetable	Metabolically stressed Impaired GI function	Peptamen Jr.
Elemental	Free amino acids	Corn syrup solids, sucrose	MCT Vegetable	Malabsorption Allergy	Elecare Neocate 1+ Vivonex Pediatric

a Medium-chain triglycerides.

Probably the most important factor discriminating between formulas is the degree to which the protein component is intact. Polymeric formulas contain intact proteins. Hydrolyzed formulas have the protein component predigested to varying degrees. In some formulas the protein component may consist of large protein fragments, whereas in others it may be in the form of amino acids and small peptides. Elemental formulas contain amino acids with no intact protein component. Indications for these three types of formula are shown in Table 4. In general most patients will do well on a polymeric formula. The hydrolyzed formulas are reserved for patients with protein sensitivity (i.e., allergy). The elemental formulas are for patients with such a severe degree of protein sensitivity that they will react even to the small peptides found in the hydrolyzed formulas.

Formulas also may differ based upon the carbohydrate (Table 4). Sugars used in formulas include lactose (usually only found in infant formulas), sucrose (enhances palatability), and starch (usually in the form of glucose polymers or corn syrup solids). Starch offers the advantage of a lower osmolality compared with disaccharides such as lactose and sucrose. This can be helpful in patients with impaired carbohydrate digestion due either to low enzyme activity (e.g., lactose intolerance) or injury to the small intestinal mucosa (e.g., chronic diarrhea in infants, radiation enteritis).

The third component that differentiates formulas is the fat content. Fat sources may include long-chain triglycerides or a combination of long- and medium-chain triglycerides (MCT). Long-chain triglycerides are a necessary component of formulas because the essential fatty acids, linoleic and linolenic, are long-chain and therefore found only in long-chain triglycerides. Medium-chain triglycerides offer the theoretical advantage of being absorbed with little need for bile acids or pancreatic lipase (10). Additionally, there is evidence that they are also absorbed in the colon (11). In patients with liver disease or terminal ileal disease, where bile acid deficiency may exist, the presence of medium-chain triglycerides may offer some advantage over long-chain triglycerides alone. On the down side, medium chain triglycerides are expensive and not very palatable. Coconut oil is an alternative, as it is rich in medium-chain triglycerides.

In addition to selecting the type of protein, carbohydrate, and fat, one must also select the concentration of these nutrients. In general, protein concentrations are in the range of 2 to 4% (2 to 4 g/dL). Carbohydrate concentration can vary widely, from 7 to 14% or more. The higher the concentration, the greater the osmolality and the more likely it is that it will induce discomfort from colonic bacterial degradation of carbohydrate to gas or outright diarrhea if the degree of carbohydrate malabsorption exceeds that which can be salvaged by the colonic bacterial flora (12).

Although there are a dizzying array of products, it may be difficult to find a formula that contains the components needed in the concentration desired. In selecting a product, it is important to be sure that all the components (protein, carbohydrate, fat) are the suitable type and in the appropriate concentration. The decision as to which product to use is based upon the patient's underlying condition (with reference to gastrointestinal tolerance) and factors such as nutritional and fluid status. For example, fluid restriction may necessitate the use of calorically dense formulas in patients with cardiac, pulmonary, or renal problems. Formulas may be concentrated by adding less water to the concentrate or by adding more powder.

Another method for altering the composition of a formula is by adding modular components such as additional protein, fat, or carbohydrate. These can be added to increase the amount of a specific component. In preterm infants, formula concentrations greater than 24 kcal/mL require close monitoring of renal solute load, fluid balance, and electrolytes. In older children, caloric densities greater than 30 kcal/mL may induce cramping and/or diarrhea.

2.5 Method of Delivery

Enteral nutrition can be delivered continuously or intermittently (bolus). The delivery method is dependent upon the route (gastric versus transpyloric) and the functional status of the gastrointestinal tract. Enteral feeding methods are outlined in Table 5.

2.5.1 Bolus Feeding

Bolus feedings are given intermittently, as meals or in conjunction with meals, and are generally not given via pump. They are usually administered over 15 to 30 min by gravity drip. These feedings generally require more time and patient monitoring than do continuous feeds (thus their unpopularity with nursing staff). They can be useful in the patient who takes some but not all nutrition orally. The patient can eat and the remainder given via a bolus feeding through a nasogastric tube or gastrostomy tube or button.

Bolus feedings should be used only in patients who are at low risk of aspiration. Patients with cerebral palsy or heart disease are candidates for bolus feeds because they tire quickly or eat slowly. Bolus feedings may not be appropriate for children with delayed gastric emptying, those at risk for aspiration, or those with significantly diminished intestinal absorptive capacity (e.g., short-bowel syndrome).

Bolus feedings can also be administered via infusion pump over 30 min to 1 hr. These feedings are appropriate for patients with some degree of gastrointestinal impairment who are unable to tolerate bolus feedings over 10 to 15 min but are not ill enough to require continuous infusions (see below). This method also may be needed in patients with formulas that contain increased concentrations of energy or protein, because the thickness of the feeding may increase its viscosity to the point that it infuses too slowly.

TABLE 5 Enteral Feeding Methods

Type	Potential indications	Advantages	Disadvantages
Bolus	Alert patients Functional GI tract Low risk of aspiration Formulas with modular components	Physiological Mimics normal feeding Patient mobility May not require infusion pump	Time-consuming for care-giver May not be indicated in patients with reflux, aspiration, delayed gastric emptying, or malabsorption
Continuous	Critically ill (intubated or sedated) Decreased absorptive capacity Transpyloric feedings Malabsorption	Less risk for aspiration Fewer mechanical complications Better tolerated in patients with impaired GI function	Increased risk of formula contamination Less physiological Requires an infusion pump Modular components may separate

2.5.2   Continuous Feeding

Continuous feedings are delivered at a constant rate over an extended period of time (usually 12 to 24 hr) via an infusion pump. Patients, who are critically ill, have decreased digestive or absorptive capacity, or are being fed transpylorically are candidates for continuous feedings. Compared with bolus feedings, continuous feedings enhance nutrient digestion and absorption in patients with significant malabsorption (e.g., cystic fibrosis, chronic diarrhea of infancy) (13). They are useful in patients with gastric or esophageal disease, such as those with severe gastroesophageal reflux (14). Cyclic feedings also can be instituted during the transition from tube to oral feedings, especially in children at risk for nutritional depletion.

Continuous feedings are particularly suited for overnight infusion (usually over 10 to 18 hr). This regimen is useful for supplementing nutritional intake while minimizing the impact on oral intake and appetite during the day. Continuous feedings are often used in combination with parenteral nutrition in patients who can tolerate some enteral intake.

Formulas to which additional fat has been added as a modular component may not be delivered optimally via continuous infusion. The fat can rise to the top of the bag and adhere to the bag and tubing, diminishing the amount delivered to the patient.

Initiation and Advancement.   The initiation and advancement of enteral feedings depends on the age of the patient, the functional state of the gastrointestinal tract, and the method of delivery (i.e., bolus versus continuous) (Table 6).

TABLE 6   Initiation and Advancement of Enteral Feedings

	Bolus	Continuous
Initiate	Full strength if ≤ 300 mOsm ½ or ¾ strength if >300 mOsm 1–5 mL/kg per feeding every 2–4 hr	Full strength if 300 mOsm ½ or ¾ strength if >300 mOsm 0.5–2.0 mL/kg/hr
Advance	1–10 mL/kg every 2–3 hr Increase rate or caloric density	0.5 mL–1.0 mL/hr every 8–24 hr Increase rate or caloric density
Goal	Infants: 5–8 feedings per day Children: 4–6 feedings per day Adolescents: 3–5 feedings per day	Maximize nutritional intake, digestive and absorptive function with smallest impact on oral intake

However, there remains considerable disparity between institutions in the method of initiating enteral feedings. In general, enteral feedings can be initiated at full strength and the administration rate increased gradually as tolerated (every 8 to 12 hr to every day). However, in preterm infants, there are data to suggest that half-strength feedings are better tolerated than full-strength feedings (15,16) (see Chap. 8). Sometimes patients will tolerate an increase in rate but not concentration or vice versa. In order to ascertain if feeding intolerance is the result of alterations in infusion rate or concentration, changes in these parameters should occur independently of each other.

2.6 Feeding Transitions

The ease of transition from enteral to oral, continuous to bolus or oral, or parenteral to enteral or oral is dependent upon several factors. These include age of the patient, underlying disease, and medical treatments being given (e.g., chemotherapy). The only rule is that there are no rules. A child who has been on parenteral nutrition for months can be switched to full oral feedings immediately if he or she is hungry and the GI tract is functional. The patient should be given the benefit of the doubt and the transition made rapidly unless and until the patient demonstrates intolerance.

The most important point to remember in transitioning from one feeding route to another is to ensure that the nutritional intake continues to be adequate. Central-strength parenteral nutrition that includes intravenous lipid provides more energy per milliliter than do most enteral formulas. Hence, if enteral or oral feedings are being advanced at the same rate that the parenteral nutrition is being decreased, less energy is being provided. This also can be true in the case of the preterm infant who is being transitioned from peripheral parenteral nutrition to breast milk (see Chap. 6).

Particularly in infants, if long term nonoral feeding has been required, the child is at risk for developing mouth sensitivities, oral defensive behaviors, and other abnormal feeding behaviors (see Chap. 13) (17). This can make the transition to oral feedings difficult and frustrating for both parents and the health care team. The risk of oral aversion underlines the importance of providing oral stimulation to infants who are NPO (nil per os). This can be accomplished by providing occupational therapy. In patients who will tolerate small amounts orally, even these quantities may be enough to obviate feeding aversion.

2.7 Monitoring of Enteral Nutrition

The close monitoring of the patient's response to treatment can ameliorate many complications associated with enteral tube feedings. Monitoring the response to enteral tube feedings involves assessing tolerance to the feedings, the metabolic effects of the feedings, the adequacy of nutrients provided, and mechanical problems (Table 7).

2.7.1 Tolerance

Assessing patient tolerance to tube feedings requires checking the patient for the presence of abdominal distention, vomiting, gastric residuals, and the number and consistency of stools. In patients with malabsorption, it may be necessary to monitor stool pH and glucose with each stool or at intervals through the day. Stool pH < 6 or the presence of glucose or other reducing sugars signifies carbohydrate malabsorption. If left unchecked, this can increase stool losses and result in acidosis (12). Daily checks for the presence or absence of abdominal distention, emesis, and stool frequency should occur until tolerance clearly is established.

Metabolic Tolerance. Metabolic and biochemical parameters warrant close monitoring in the malnourished child. Signs and symptoms of fluid overload, refeeding syndrome, and electrolyte and mineral imbalances should be checked for daily until the patient is stable. Malnourished children (<75% of

TABLE 7 Monitoring Enteral Feedings

Problem	Prevention/Intervention
Diarrhea/abdominal cramping	Decrease delivery rate Decrease carbohydrate content Consider lactose-free or fiber-containing products
Vomiting, nausea, bloating	Change to a formula with medium-chain triglycerides or lower percentage of fat Formula should be at room temperature prior to tube feedings Monitor for correct tube placement
Hyperglycemia	Reduce carbohydrate content Reduce flow rate Consider insulin administration
Constipation	Change to a product containing fiber Increase free water intake
Gastric retention of formula	Monitor for correct tube placement Position patient on right side Consider continuous or transpyloric feeding
Clogged feeding tube	Flush tubing with water every 6 to 8 hr Check appropriateness of tube size for high caloric density or fiber formulas

expected weight for height) are at risk for hypophosphatemia, potassium shifts, and hypomagnesemia (i.e., the refeeding syndrome) and need to be monitored particularly closely (18,19). These conditions are most likely to occur in the first 2 to 3 weeks of nutritional therapy. If they are left unchecked, the refeeding syndrome can result in death (18,19).

2.7.2 Adequacy

Monitoring of anthropometric and growth parameters assesses the nutritional adequacy of feedings. After the goal volumes and rates have been achieved, evaluate changes in weight gain weekly. Finally, evaluate for appropriate weight gain for age and catch-up needs. For patients on long-term support, changes in height should be assessed monthly. Triceps skin fold and midarm muscle circumference can be measured every 2 to 4 weeks in the short term and every 1 to 3 months long term. Serum albumin can provide information regarding the adequacy of protein intake over a 2- to 3-week period. Prealbumin (transthyretin) can be used to assess protein intake sufficiency over 24 to 48 hr. However, interpretation of these measures is complicated in the presence of significant liver disease, protein-uria, or enteric protein loss (i.e., protein-losing enteropathy) (20). Blood urea nitrogen (BUN) can also be used to appraise short-term protein intake but requires normal renal function.

2.7.3 Mechanical Complications

Mechanical complications related to tubes and tube placement are common. Placement should be checked prior to every feeding for bolus or intermittent feeds and every shift for continuous feeds (this requirement will vary by institutional policy).

2.8 Complications and Problems

Most enteral feeding complications can be divided into four major categories: infectious, gastrointestinal, metabolic, and mechanical. Complications of enteral feeding are listed in Table 7.

3 PARENTERAL NUTRITIONAL SUPPORT

Parenteral nutrition can be lifesaving in patients who are unable to tolerate adequate amounts of nutrients enterally. However, because of its disadvantages, the decision to use it should be made judiciously.

3.1 Indications for Parenteral Nutrition Support

Parenteral nutrition is indicated in cases where enteral intake is not adequate to support weight gain and growth (Fig. 1). Examples include patients with short-bowel syndrome and severe pseudo-obstruction. Except in the preterm infant, parenteral nutrition is not indicated if it is to be used for less than 1 week. Generally it should be used only if a trial of enteral feeding into the stomach or small intestine has failed (21).

3.2 When to Initiate Parenteral Nutrition Support

If it is likely that the patient will be unable to meet nutritional requirements enterally for more than a week (infants), 10 days (older infants), or 2 weeks (children), the use of parenteral nutrition should be considered (Fig. 1). Often, the decision as to when to use parenteral nutrition is more of an educated guess based on the likely course of the patient than it is a clear-cut decision. In significantly malnourished patients who do not tolerate adequate amounts of energy and protein enterally, parenteral nutrition should be used.

3.3 Route of Administration

Generally, the peripheral route of administration is preferable (Table 8). If the peripheral line is changed before the vein is damaged (i.e., every 48 hr) it is possible to maintain a patient on peripheral parenteral nutrition for weeks. On the other hand, unless a topical anesthetic is used, repeated changing of intravenous catheters is unkind to patients. An alternative is the use of a midline or peripherally inserted central catheter (PICC) (22,23). These catheters can be placed at the bedside by a specially trained team (e.g., nurses). A PICC is advantageous compared with a midline because it is less likely to occlude and can be used to infuse higher-concentration solutions.

3.4 Components

3.4.1 Carbohydrates

Dextrose (glucose) is the carbohydrate used in parenteral nutrition solutions. It supplies 3.4 kcal/g (5% dextrose = 5 g/dL = 50 g/L = 278 mOsm). Glucose infusion rates of 6 to 13 mg/kg per minute are generally well tolerated. At these rates the liver oxidizes most of the glucose for energy. Delivery of greater than 14 mg/kg/min can result in hyperglycemia, hypertriglyceridemia, fatty liver, or excessive CO_2 production (24,25).

3.4.2 Protein

Protein is provided as free amino acids. They supply 4 kcal/g (3% amino acids = 3 g/dL = 30 g/L = 300 mOsm). Protein requirements can range from the recommended daily allowance (RDA) for age to twice the RDA for catch-up growth and repletion. Excess amino acid infusions (more than twice the RDA) can result in azotemia.

TABLE 8 Choice of Access for Parenteral Nutrition

Anticipated need	Peripheral (solutions < 1000 mOsm)	Comments
<7–10 days	Peripheral IV	Change site on a routine basis
7–21 days	Midline	Peripherally placed Cannot be used to draw blood
	Central (solutions > 1000 mOsm)	
14 days–1 month	Peripherally inserted central venous catheter (PICC)	Percutaneously placed, usually in the basilic vein Single or double lumen catheters
>1 month	Nonimplanted	Surgically placed Single-, double-, or triple-lumen catheters Not recommended for home use
>1 month	Implanted (tunneled)	Surgically placed Single-, double-, or triple-lumen catheters Good for long-term home use
>1 month	Totally implanted venous access system (TIVAS) ("port")	Surgically placed Single- or double-lumen catheters Not indicated for continuous TPN[a] infusions

[a] Total parenteral nutrition.
Source: Adapted from Ref. 3.

3.4.3 Fat

Fat is provided as an emulsion. It supplies 2 kcal/mL (20% = 20 g/dL = 280 mOsm). Lipid may be delivered up to 4 g/kg/day (20 mL/kg/day) but should not exceed 60% of calories or 500 mL per day. Essential fatty acids represent approximately 40% of the solution. It is necessary to provide at least 3 to 4% of energy as essential fatty acids, which works out to be approximately 0.5 g/kg/day of intravenous fat emulsion (26,27).

3.5   Ordering Parenteral Nutrition

There are general guidelines as to the concentration of nutrients that are used in parenteral nutrition solutions (Table 9). It should be recognized that these are starting points and that the composition of the solution may have to be individualized based upon nutrient requirements, existing (e.g., hypoproteinemia) or anticipated (e.g., hypophosphatemia secondary to refeeding syndrome) deficiencies, or ongoing losses (e.g., diarrhea, ostomy output).

In general there are two major methods of ordering parenteral nutrition depending on the preference of the institution. In *method 1*, the physician orders or checks off the final concentration of nutrients desired on a standard order form similar to that in Table 9. In *method 2*, the physician also must calculate the amount of each nutrient (e.g., milliliters of dextrose, sodium, etc.) to be added per unit of parenteral nutrition solution.

TABLE 9   Parenteral Nutritional Solutions

	Peripheral strength (0.5 kcal/mL)			
Components*	Preterm	Infant (0–1 year)	Child (>1–10 years)	Adolescent (>10 years)
Dextrose (g)	12.5	12.5	12.5	12.5
Amino acids (g)	2.4	2.2	2.2	2.2
NaCl (mEq)	2.6	2.6	2.6	4.0
K_2HPO_4 (mmol)	1.5	1.2	0.6	0.5
Ca^2 gluconate (mmol)	1.5	1.2	0.5	0.5
$MgSO_4$ (mEq)	0.5	0.5	0.8	1.0
KCl (mEq)	0.2	0.2	0.8	2.0
Heparin (units)	10	10	10	10
	Central strength			
	0.5 kcal/mL	0.5 kcal/mL	0.8 kcal/mL	0.8 kcal/mL
Dextrose (g)	12.5	12.5	20	20
Amino acids (g)	2.4	2.2	3.0	3.0
NaCl (mEq)	2.6	2.6	3.8	6.0
K_2HPO_4 (mmol)	1.5	1.2	1.0	0.5
Ca^2 gluconate (mmol)	1.5	1.2	0.9	0.5
$MgSO_4$ (mEq)	0.5	0.5	0.9	1.0
KCl (mEq)	0.2	0.2	1.3	3.0
Heparin (units)	10	10	10	10

* Expressed per 100 mL of solution.

TABLE 10 Recommended
Intravenous Amino Acid Intakes

Age (years)	Amino acid (g/kg/day)
0.0–0.5	2.2
0.5–1.0	1.6
1–3	1.2
4–6	1.1
7–10	1.0
11–14	1.0
15–24	1.9

3.5.1 Method 1

The first step is to determine the amino acid intake. The more malnourished the patient, the greater the amino acid intake should be (see below). Use Table 10 to determine the minimum amount of amino acids to be provided. For patients who are normally nourished, use their actual weight (kg). For those who are underweight or obese, use their ideal weight for height (i.e., weight at the 50 percentile for their height).

$$\text{Protein } (g \cdot kg^{-1} \cdot d^{-1}) \times \text{weight (kg)} = \text{total g/day}$$

or

$$\text{Protein } (g \cdot kg^{-1} \cdot d^{-1}) \times \text{ideal weight (kg)} = \text{total g/day}$$

The second step is to ascertain the appropriate energy intake (see Table 11). For patients who are normally nourished, use their actual weight (kg). For those who

TABLE 11 Intravenous
Energy Intakes

Age (years)	Energy (kcal/kg/day)
0.0–0.5	95–110
0.5–1.0	90–100
1–3	85–95
4–6	80–90
7–10	70–80
11–14	60–70
15–24	45–55

are underweight or obese, use their ideal weight for height (i.e., weight at the 50th percentile for their height).

Energy (kcal/kg/day) $\times$ weight (kg) = total kcal/day

or

Energy (kcal/kg/day) $\times$ ideal weight (kg) = total kcal/day

Step 3 is to determine the contribution to total daily energy from amino acids, dextrose, and fat. The usual distribution is 70% from amino acids/dextrose and 30% from fat. It is necessary to provide at least 3 to 4% of energy as essential fatty acids, which works out to be approximately 0.5 g/kg/day of intravenous fat emulsion (26,27). Do not administer more than 60% of calories as fat so as to avoid ketosis. Therefore, presuming a 70:30 distribution, use the total energy value from Table 11 to calculate the proportion of energy from fat.

Total energy (kcal/day) $\times$ 0.7
= energy from dextrose/amino acids (kcal/day)
Total energy (kcal/day) $\times$ 0.3 = energy from fat (kcal/day)

From this, the volume and rate of lipid administration can be calculated (step 4).

Energy from fat (kcal/day) $\div$ 2 = mL/day of lipid

mL/day of lipid $\div$ 24 hr = rate of infusion

The amount of lipid infused must be increased stepwise over a few days. This is particularly important in preterm infants or in patients who are likely to have existing hypertriglyceridemia (e.g., stressed, steroid-treated). Administer one-third the rate on the first day; two-third the second day; and the full rate on the third day.

Step 5 is to determine the volume of amino acid/dextrose solution to be administered. The amino acids, dextrose (glucose), electrolytes, minerals, and vitamins are administered in a single solution. From Table 12, choose the concentrations of amino acids and dextrose that are desired. Commonly, for peripheral administration 2% amino acids and 12% dextrose are used, and for central administration 3% amino acids and 20% dextrose are used. Calculate the volume of solution to administer based upon total energy from amino acids and dextrose to be provided per day and the energy density of the solution to be used. From step 2 obtain the value for the total energy intake (kcal/day); from step 3 obtain the value for the amount of energy from amino acids and dextrose (kcal/day).

Energy from amino acids and dextrose (kcal/day)
$\div$ energy density of solution
= mL/day of amino acid/dextrose solution to be administered
mL/day of amino acid/dextrose solution to be administered $\div$ 24 hr
= rate of administration (mL/hr)

TABLE 12 Caloric Density of Amino Acid/Dextrose Solutions (kcal/mL)

	Amino acids, %								
	1.0	2.2	2.5	2.7	3.0	3.5	4.0	5.0	6.0
Dextrose, %									
7.5	0.30	0.35	0.36	0.37	0.38	0.40	0.42	0.46	0.50
10.0	0.38	0.43	0.44	0.45	0.46	0.48	0.50	0.54	0.58
12.5	0.47	0.52	0.53	0.54	0.55	0.57	0.59	0.63	0.67
15.0	0.55	0.60	0.61	0.62	0.63	0.65	0.67	0.71	0.75
20.0	0.72	0.77	0.78	0.79	0.80	0.82	0.84	0.88	0.92
25.0	0.89	0.94	0.95	0.96	0.97	0.99	1.01	1.05	1.09
30.0	1.04	1.09	1.1	1.11	1.12	1.14	1.16	1.20	1.24
35.0	1.23	1.28	1.29	1.30	1.31	1.33	1.35	1.39	1.43
40.0	1.40	1.45	1.46	1.47	1.48	1.50	1.52	1.56	1.60

Step 6 is to ascertain if the nutritional goals will be met. From the step 5 calculation, obtain the mL/day of amino acid/dextrose solution to be administered. Compare with the value from step 1 and adjust the concentration as necessary to meet the step 1 goal.

$$\text{mL/day of amino acid/dextrose solution} \times \% \text{ amino acid} \div 100$$
$$= \text{g/day amino acids}$$

Step 7 is to ensure that fluid requirements will be met. Although maintenance fluid requirements almost always are met with standard administration of parenteral nutrition, this can be checked easily. Add the volume of amino acid/dextrose (mL/day from step 5) to the volume of lipids (mL/day from step 4) and compare the sum to maintenance fluid requirements.

By body surface area, fluid requirements are 1600 mL/m^2 per day:

$<$5 kg: weight (kg) $\times$ 0.05 + 0.05 = m^2
5–10 k: weight (kg) $\times$ 0.04 + 0.1 = m^2
10–20 kg: weight (kg) $\times$ 0.03 + 0.2 = m^2
20 kg: weight (kg) $\times$ 0.02 + 0.3 = m^2

By body weight, fluid requirements per day are as follows:

1–10 kg: 100 mL/kg
11–20 kg: 1000 mL + 50 mL/kg for each kg $>$ 10 kg
$>$20 kg: 1500 mL + 20 mL/kg for each kg $>$ 20 kg

Step 8 is to determine the appropriate amount of electrolytes, minerals, and trace minerals to be added to the amino acid/dextrose solution. The total daily

TABLE 13 Electrolyte and Mineral Requirements (mEq/kg/day)

	Neonatal	Child/Adolescent
Sodium (as NaCl)	2.0–6.0	3.0–5.0
Potassium (as KCl)	2.0–3.0	1.0–2.0
Chloride	2.0–3.0	2.0–3.0
Phosphorus (as K_xPO_x)	2.0–2.6	0.65–2.0
Magnesium (as Mg_2SO_4)	0.15–0.32	0.13–0.5
Calcium (as Ca gluconate)	4–5.2	0.3–2

electrolyte, mineral, and trace mineral needs are calculated similarly to those of protein (see step 1). Determine the daily requirement from Table 13 (electrolytes and minerals) and Table 14 (trace minerals). This amount of electrolyte and mineral is added to the total volume of amino acid/dextrose solution to be administered per day (mL/day) (from step 5). If the amount of electrolyte or mineral must be expressed per 100 mL or 1000 mL, calculate as follows:

$$\text{Amount of Nutrient/day} \times 100 = \text{amount to add per 100 mL}$$
$$\text{mL/day of amino acid/dextrose solution}$$
$$\text{Amount of nutrient/day} \times 1000 = \text{amount to add per 1000 mL}$$
$$\text{mL/day of amino acid/dextrose solution}$$

See step 5.

3.6 Calcium and Phosphorus

Calcium and phosphorous solubility in parenteral nutrition solutions depends on their concentration, the Ca/P ratio, pH, temperature, the amino acid concentration, and the type of commercial amino acid product used (28). Cysteine may be added to preterm and infant parenteral solutions (30 to 40 mg cysteine per gram of amino acid) to increase the solubility of calcium and phosphorous by lowering the pH of the solution. The addition of cysteine can decrease the serum

TABLE 14 Recommended Intravenous Trace Mineral Intakes

Mineral	Zn	Cu	Cr	Mn	Se
Infants <2.5 kg (µg/kg/day)	400	40	0.4	10	2
Infants >2.5 kg (µg/kg/day)	100	10	0.1	2.5	1.5
Adolescents (µg)	4000	1600	16	400	80

TABLE 15 Maximal Calcium and Phosphorus
Concentrations[a]

	2% Amino acids	
	Calcium meq/L	Phosphorus mmol/L
Without cysteine	26	12
	35	30
With cysteine[b]	30	15
	10	30

[a] This table is intended as a general guideline and is
not to be used in lieu of a qualified pharmacist's verification of the compatibility of the admixture. Modifications to formulations, method, and order of preparation will result in differences in calcium/phosphate
compatibility.
[b] 30 mg/g amino acids.

bicarbonate of the infant (29). The maximum recommended calcium and phosphorus concentrations are shown in Table 15.

3.7 Vitamins

Vitamins are supplied in commercial preparations. These preparations contain
the vitamins in fixed amounts. Table 16 shows the vitamin content of the most
commonly used preparations. Suggested dosing is shown in Table 17.

TABLE 16 Intravenous Vitamin Preparations

Vitamin (per vial)	A (IU)	D (IU)	E (IU)	C (mg)	Thiamin (mg)	Riboflavin (mg)	Niacin (mg)
MVI Pediatric	2300	400	7	80	1.2	1.4	17
MVI-12	3300	200	10	100	3.0	3.6	40

Vitamin (per vial)	B_6 (mg)	Folacin (μg)	B_{12} (μg)	K (μg)	Biotin (μg)	Pantothenate (mg)
MVI Pediatric	1	140	1	200	20	5
MVI-12	4	400	5	200	60	15

Source: Adapted from Ref. 3.

TABLE 17 Suggested Intravenous Vitamin Dosing

Patient	Amount	Product
1 kg	30% of a vial (1.5 mL)[a]	MVI-Pediatric
1 kg–3 kg	65% of a vial (3.25 mL)[a]	MVI-Pediatric
>3 kg–11 years	100% of a vial (5 mL)	MVI-Pediatric
>11 years	100% of a vial (10 mL)	MVI-12 plus 20 μg/day vitamin K

[a] Per kg/day.

3.8 Trace Minerals

Trace minerals also are available in commercial preparations, usually containing fixed amounts. Table 14 shows recommended intakes for trace minerals.

3.8.1 Method 2

In method 2, the specific volume of nutrient that must be added from a stock solution must be given. For example, the volume of a stock 70% (g/dL) dextrose solution needed to produce a final concentration of 20% must be provided. To do this, calculate the parenteral nutrition order as outlined in method 1, then use Tables 18 to 23 to assist with the calculations.

3.9 Compatibilities and Solubilities

Acidosis may require the addition of base to parenteral nutrition. Bicarbonate should *never* be added because it will result in precipitation of calcium and phosphorus. If base is required, it should be administered as Na or K acetate. Electrolytes can be balanced by replacing NaCl, KPhos, or KCl with the acetate.

Many drugs are incompatible with parenteral nutrition solutions (30,31). Check with your pharmacist when administering other drugs intravenously through the same catheter that is used to deliver parenteral nutrition.

3.10 Monitoring

The frequency of monitoring primarily depends upon the stability of the patient. General guidelines are given in Table 24. To determine the adequacy of the amino acid intake in the short term, either the blood urea nitrogen (BUN) or prealbumin can be measured. Both reflect changes in amino acid intake with 24 to 48 hr. Because the BUN reflects urea synthesis from protein, it should be between 12 mg/dL (i.e., enough amino acids are being provided) and 20 mg/dL (i.e., not enough to cause azotemia) presuming normal renal function. Prealbumin (trans-

TABLE 18 Fluid, Energy, and Protein Requirements from Birth to 3 Years

Body weight kg	Maintenance fluid requirements		Total energy requirements			Protein RDA[a]		
	Per 1600 mL/m² mL	By body weight mL	Birth-6 months kcal/day	6-12 months kcal/day	1-3 years kcal/day	Birth-6 months g/day	6-12 months g/day	1-3 years g/day
1	160	120	110			2		
2	240	240	220			4		
3	320	300	330			7		
4	400	400	440			9		
5	480	500	550	500		11	10	
6	544	600	630	600		13	12	
7	608	700	735	700	665	15	14	13
8	672	800	800	760	760	18	16	14
9	736	900	900	855	855	20	18	16
10	800	1000	1000	950	950	22	20	18
11	848	800	1100	1045	990	24	22	20
12	896	850	1200	1140	1080	26	24	22
13	944	900		1170	1170		26	23
14	992	950		1260	1260		28	25
15	1040	1000		1350	1350		30	27
16	1088	1050			1360			29
17	1136	1100			1445			31
18	1184	1150			1530			32
19	1232	1200			1615			34
20	1280	1250			1700			36

[a] If patient is undernourished, either use ideal body weight or add up to 100% for replenishment.

TABLE 19 Fluid, Energy, and Protein Requirements from 3 Years to 18 Years

Body weight kg	Maintenance fluid requirements		Total energy requirements				Protein RDA[a]			
	Per 1600 mL/m² mL	By body weight mL	3–6 years kcal/day	6–10 years kcal/day	10–14 years kcal/day	14–18 years	3–6 years[a] g/day	6–10 years[a] g/day	10–14 years[b] g/day	14–18 years[b] g/day
15	1040	1250	1275	1200			17	15		
16	1088	1300	1360	1200			18	16		
18	1184	1400	1530	1350			20	18		
20	1120	1500	1600	1500			22	20	20	
25	1280	1600	2000	1875	1400		28	25	25	
30	1440	1700	2400	2250	1750		33	30	30	27
35	1600	1800	2800	2625	2100	1925	39	35	35	32
40	1760	1900		2800	2275	2200		40	40	36
45	1920	2000		3150	2600	2475		45	45	41
50	2080	2100		3500	2925	2500		50	50	45
60	2400	2300		4200	3000	3000		60	60	54
70	2720	2500		4900	3600	3500		70	70	63
80	3200	2700			4200	3600			80	72
90	3360	2900			4800	4050				81
100	3680	3100				4500				90

[a] If patient is undernourished, either use ideal body weight or add up to 100% for replenishment.
[b] If patient is undernourished, either use ideal body weight or add up to 150% for replenishment.

TABLE 20   Volume and Energy
Content of a 10% Amino Acid Solution

Grams	mL	Calories
1	10	4
2	20	8
3	30	12
4	40	16
5	50	20
6	60	24
7	70	28
8	80	32
9	90	36
10	100	40
11	110	44
12	120	48
13	130	52
14	140	56
15	150	60
16	160	64
17	170	68
18	180	72
19	190	76
20	200	80
22	220	88
24	240	96
26	260	104
28	280	112
30	300	120
35	350	140
40	400	160
45	350	180
50	450	200
55	550	220
60	600	240
65	650	260
70	700	280
75	750	300
80	800	320
85	850	340
95	950	380
100	1000	400
105	1050	420
110	1100	440
115	1150	460
125	1200	480
120	1250	500
130	1300	520
140	1400	560
150	1500	600

TABLE 21 Volume and Energy
Content of a 70% Dextrose Solution

Grams	mL	Calories
14.7	21.0	50
29.4	42.0	100
44.1	63.0	150
58.8	84.0	200
73.5	105.0	250
88.2	126.1	300
102.9	147.1	350
117.6	168.1	400
132.4	189.1	450
147.1	210.1	500
161.8	231.1	550
176.5	252.1	600
191.2	273.1	650
205.9	294.1	700
220.6	315.1	750
235.3	336.1	800
250.0	357.1	850
264.7	378.2	900
279.4	399.2	950
294.1	420.2	1000
308.8	441.2	1050
323.5	462.2	1100
338.2	483.2	1150
352.9	504.2	1200
367.6	525.2	1250
382.4	546.2	1300
397.1	567.2	1350
411.8	588.2	1400
441.2	630.3	1500
470.6	672.3	1600
500.0	714.3	1700
529.4	756.3	1800
558.8	798.3	1900
588.2	840.3	2000
647.1	924.4	2200
705.91	1008.4	2400
764.7	1092.4	2600
823.5	1176.5	2800
882.4	1260.5	3000
941.2	1344.5	3200
1000.0	1428.6	3400
1058.8	1512.6	3600
1117.6	1596.6	3800
1176.5	1680.7	4000
1235.3	1764.7	4200
1294.1	1848.7	4400

TABLE 22   Electrolyte Concentrations

Electrolyte	Composition per mL
Sodium chloride	4 mEq Na
Sodium acetate	2 mEq Na
Potassium chloride	2 mEq K
Potassium acetate	2 mEq K
Potassium phosphate	3 mmol P, 4.4 mEq K
Calcium gluconate	0.465 mEq Ca
Magnesium sulfate	4 mEq Mg

TABLE 23   Conversion Factors

Electrolyte	Mg	mEq	mmol
Na	23	1	1.0
K	39	1	1.0
Cl	35	1	1.0
P	31	1	1.0
Mg	12	1	0.5
Ca	20	1	0.5

TABLE 24   Laboratory Monitoring During Parenteral Nutrition

	Neonate		Child/Adolescent	
	Initial	Follow-up	Initial	Follow-up
Intake/output	Daily	Daily	Daily	Daily
Urine glucose	Every void	Every shift	Every void	Every shift
Electrolytes, BUN	2–3 times/wk	Weekly	2–3 times/wk	Weekly
Ca, P, Mg	Weekly	Every other wk	Weekly	Every other wk
Albumin	Baseline	Every other wk	Baseline	Every other wk
Triglycerides	4 hr after infusion started	4 hr after a rate increase	4 hr after infusion started	4 hr after a rate increase
ALT (SGPT)	Baseline	Monthly	Baseline	
Bilirubin (D/I)	Baseline	Every other wk	Baseline	Monthly

thyretin) can be used similarly but can be affected by liver disease, zinc deficiency, and renal disease.

Triglycerides are often elevated in patients with sepsis, pancreatitis, renal disease, or diabetes. It is prudent to check a baseline level in these patients before starting lipids in order to interpret the 4 hr infusion level.

Low albumin concentrations will result in an artifactually lowered calcium concentration. Therefore, check the ionized calcium concentration when total serum calcium levels are low because of a decreased albumin concentration.

Zinc concentrations are often decreased in patients with gastrointestinal losses (e.g., diarrhea, ostomy output), inflammatory bowel disease, cystic fibrosis, or fistulas. Anticipate these losses and provide adequate replacement as well as maintenance amounts.

3.11 Transition to Enteral Feedings

Most enteral diets are less energy-dense than parenteral nutrition. Consequently, to provide the same energy intake a greater volume of enteral feeding is required than of parenteral nutrition. If the GI tract can tolerate the volume, there is no need to wean the patient from parenteral nutrition. To avoid hypoglycemia, central-strength parenteral nutrition should never be abruptly stopped in young infants unless they are receiving oral or enteral feedings during that time.

Parenteral nutrition diminishes appetite in proportion to the amount administered (32–34). This effect may last for 1 to 2 days after decreases in parenteral nutrition intake. This should be taken into account when transitioning from parenteral to enteral feedings. Although appetite is suppressed, the sensation of hunger is not removed completely.

3.12 Cyclic Parenteral Nutrition

Administering parenteral nutrition for less than 24 hr has a number of advantages. First, it offers greater mobility for patients and families. By allowing some hours where the patient is not bound to the infusion pump, some degree of normality is restored to the patient and family. Second, if the patient is receiving some oral feeding and the time off parenteral nutrition is sufficient, the patient's appetite can be stimulated to some degree. Third, it has been argued that administering parenteral nutrition cyclicly is more physiological and less likely to cause liver disease and other adverse effects (35,36,37).

Particularly in patients who are not being fed at the time, it is important to decrease the infusion of parenteral nutrition gradually to prevent hypoglycemia. The rate of parenteral nutrition solution infusion should be decreased by 50% at 30 min prior to discontinuation of the infusion. In infants less than 1 year of age, the rate may need to be decreased 50% beginning 60 min and then again at 30 min prior to discontinuation. Generally, there is no reason to increase the rate gradually when restarting the infusion unless the patient has exhibited intolerance (i.e., glycosuria) in the past.

3.13 Pitfalls to Avoid

Because of its central role in preserving immune integrity, be sure to provide adequate protein and, secondarily, enough energy. Remember that energy cannot substitute for protein.

Anticipate the "refeeding syndrome" (life-threatening hypophosphatemia and hypokalemia) in patients who are moderately or severely malnourished by providing at least 20 to 50% more phosphorus and potassium (18,19). The refeeding syndrome is most likely to occur in the first to second week of parenteral nutrition therapy presuming that the energy intake is adequate. Consequently, monitor serum phosphorous and potassium daily or every other day for at least the first week of parenteral nutrition.

Catheter obstructions generally are preventable. Check with the pharmacy before coadministering drugs through the same catheter as the parenteral nutrition. Observe compatibility guidelines for administration of calcium and phosphorus. *Never* put bicarbonate in a parenteral nutrition solution.

3.14 Complications

The list of complications related to parenteral nutrition is extensive. They generally fall into three categories: metabolic, infectious, and mechanical. Some of the more common ones are listed in Table 25. As noted above, most of these are preventable with close attention to detail and adherence to standard protocols, including the use of a multidisciplinary nutritional support team (38,39).

TABLE 25 Complications of Parenteral Nutrition Administration

Infectious	Metabolic	Mechanical
Local	Nutrient derangements	Catheter occlusion
Systemic	Decreases (e.g., hypoglycemia)	Central vein thrombosis
	Increases (e.g., hyperphosphatemia)	Cardiac arrhythmia
	Fluid derangements	Air embolus
	Overload	
	Dehydration (e.g., secondary to osmotic diuresis from hyperglycemia)	
	Liver disease	
	Cholestasis (mostly infants)	
	Fatty liver (mostly older children)	

REFERENCES

1. deWitt, RC and Kudsk, KA, General nutritional therapeutic issues: Enteral nutrition. Gastroenterology Clin 1998; 27:371–386.
2. Buchman AL, Moukarzel AA, Bhuta S, Belle M, Ament ME, Eckhert CD, Hollander D, Gornbein J, Kopple JD, Vijayaroghavan SR. Parenteral nutrition is associated with intestinal morphologic and functional changes in humans. J Parenter Enter Nutr 1995; 19:453–460.
3. Conkin CA et al., eds. The Baylor Pediatric Nutrition Handbook for Residents. Nestle, Inc. 1999.
4. Nelson KA. The cancer anorexia-cachexia syndrome. Semin Oncol 2000; 27:64–68.
5. Vanderhoof JA, Hofschire PJ, Baluff MA, Guest JE, Murray ND, Pinsky WW, Kugler JD, Antonson DL. Continuous enteral feedings: an important adjunct to the management of complex congenital heart disease. Am J Dis Child 1982; 136:825–827.
6. Vanderhoof JA, Langnas AN. Short-bowel syndrome in children and adults. Gastroenterology 1997; 113:1767–1778.
7. Kuizon BD, Nelson PA, Salusky IB. Tube feeding in children with end-stage renal disease. Miner Electrolyte Metab 1997; 23:306–310.
8. Lucas A, Bloom SR, Aynsley-Green A. Postnatal surges in plasma gut hormones in term and preterm infants. Biol Neonate 1982; 41:63–67.
9. Botoman VA, Kirtland SH, Moss RL. A randomized study of a pH sensor feeding tube vs a standard feeding tube in patients requiring enteral nutrition. J Parenter Enter Nutr 1994; 18:154–158.
10. Velazquez OC, Seto RW, Rombeau JL. The scientific rationale and clinical application of short-chain fatty acids and medium-chain triacylglycerols. Proc Nutr Soc 1996; 55:49–78.
11. Jeppesen PB, Mortensen PB. Colonic digestion and absorption of energy from carbohydrates and medium-chain fat in small bowel failure. J Parenter Enter Nutr 1999; 23(suppl):S101–S105.
12. Kien CL. Digestion, absorption, and fermentation of carbohydrates in the newborn. Clin Perinatol 1996; 23:211–228.
13. Parker P, Stroop S, Greene H. A controlled comparison of continuous versus intermittent feeding in the treatment of infants with intestinal disease. J Pediatr 198; 99:360–364.
14. Ferry GD, Selby M, Pietro TJ. Clinical response to short-term nasogastric feeding in infants with gastroesophageal reflux and growth failure. J Pediatr Gastroenterol Nutr 1983; 2:57–61.
15. Sarna MS, Saili A, Pandey KK, Dutta AK, Mullick DN. Premature infant feeding: role of diluted formula. Indian Pediatr 1990; 27:829–833.
16. Currao WJ, Cox C, Shapiro DL. Diluted formula for beginning of feeding of premature infants. Am J Dis Child 1988; 142:730–731.
17. Dello Strologo L, Principato F, Sinibaldi D, Appiani AC, Terzi F, Dartois AM, Rizzoni G. Feeding dysfunction in infants with severe chronic renal failure after long-term nasogastric tube feeding. Pediatr Nephrol 1997; 11:84–86.
18. Solomon SM, Kirby DF. The refeeding syndrome: a review. J Parenter Enter Nutr 1990; 14:90–97.
19. Brooks MJ, Melnik G. The refeeding syndrome: an approach to understanding its complications and preventing its occurrence. Pharmacotherapy 1995; 15:713–726.

20. Louay Omran M, Morley JE. Assessment of protein energy malnutrition in older persons: Part II. Laboratory evaluation. Nutrition 2000; 16:131–140.
21. Frosta P, Biharia D. The route of nutritional support in the critically ill: physiological and economical considerations. Nutrition 1997; 13:58S–63S.
22. Hogan MJ. Neonatal vascular catheters and their complications. Radiol Clin North Am 1999; 37:1109–1125.
23. Chung DH, Ziegler MM. Central venous catheter access. Nutrition 1998; 14:1119–1123.
24. Quigley EM, Marsh MN, Shaffer JL, Markin RS. Hepatobiliary complications of total parenteral nutrition. Gastroenterology 1993; 104:286–301.
25. Talpers SS, Romberger DJ, Bunce SB, Pingleton SK. Nutritionally associated increased carbon dioxide production: excess total calories vs high proportion of carbohydrate calories. Chest 1992; 102:551–555.
26. Jeppesen PB, Hoy CE, Mortensen PB. Essential fatty acid deficiency in patients receiving home parenteral nutrition. Am J Clin Nutr 1998; 68:126–133.
27. Gutcher GR, Farrell PM. Intravenous infusion of lipid for the prevention of essential fatty acid deficiency in premature infants. Am J Clin Nutr 1991; 54:1024–1028.
28. Porcelli PJ, O'Shea TM, Dillard RG. A linear regression model to predict the pH of neonatal parenteral nutrition solution. J Clin Pharm Ther 2000; 25:55–59.
29. Laine L, Shulman RJ, Pitre D, Lifschitz CH, Adams J. Cysteine usage increases the need for acetate in neonates who receive total parenteral nutrition. Am J Clin Nutr 1991; 54:565–567.
30. Niemiec PW Jr, Vanderveen TW. Compatibility considerations in parenteral nutrient solutions. Am J Hosp Pharm 1984; 41:893–911.
31. Trissel LA, Gilbert DL, Martinez JF, Baker MB, Walter WV, Mirtallo JM. Compatibility of parenteral nutrient solutions with selected drugs during simulated Y-site administration. Am J Health Syst Pharm 1997; 54:1295–1300.
32. Stratton RJ, Elia M. The effects of enteral tube feeding and parenteral nutrition on appetite sensations and food intake in health and disease. Clin Nutr 1999; 18:63–70.
33. Shulman RJ. Does parenteral nutrition suppress appetite? J Pediatr Gastroenterol Nutr 1992; 15(4):463–464.
34. McCutcheon NB, Tennissen AM. Hunger and appetitive factors during total parenteral nutrition. Appetite 1989; 13:1239–1241.
35. Fleming CR. Hepatobiliary complications in adults receiving nutrition support. Dig Dis 1994; 12:191–198.
36. MacFie J. Cyclic parenteral nutrition. Nutrition. 1997; 13:46–48.
37. Collier S, Crough J, Hendricks K, Caballero B. Use of cyclic parenteral nutrition in infants less than 6 months of age. Nutr Clin Pract 1994; 9:65–68.
38. Meadows N. Monitoring and complications of parenteral nutrition. Nutrition 1998; 14:806–808.
39. Wesley JR. Nutrition support teams: past, present, and future. Nutr Clin Pract 1995; 10:219–228.

18

Nutrition in Disorders of Amino Acid Metabolism

Marcello Giovannini, Carlo Agostoni, and Enrica Riva
University of Milan and San Paolo Hospital, Milan, Italy

1 INTRODUCTION

Inborn errors of amino acid metabolism occur when sequentially altered base pairs affect proteins or enzymes in such a way that they are unable to carry out their specific biochemical functions. The resulting enzymatic block leads to substrate accumulation within the cell. Some of this material is shunted toward alternative metabolic pathways. While metabolites that occur prior to the enzymatic block accumulate, substances normally catalyzed downstream of the block will be decreased. Thus, an inborn error of amino acid metabolism may be detected when increased amounts of substrate or decreased amounts of common products are found in the urine, blood, or tissues. A more complete description of the underlying mechanisms of these disorders can be found in Scriver et al. (1). Early detection of an inborn error of metabolism is necessary to prevent severe mental deficiency, chronic disease, or even death. In the future, management could be approached through enzyme replacement and gene therapy. Genetic counseling and dietary treatment, however, remain essential to the prevention and care of all genetic disorders. Two main areas of intervention can be contemplated. The first is to alter the dietary amino acid pattern to achieve a balance between circulating adequate levels of essential amino acids and prevention of plasma accumulation of nonessential amino acids. The second is to decrease total nitrogen intake when toxic protein by-products threaten to accumulate while plasma amino acid levels remain within the norm. Patients on semisynthetic diets should receive the recommended dietary allowance of essential amino acids, essential polyunsaturated fatty acids, minerals, and vitamins. Energy and nitrogen supplies should also be sufficient for normal growth and development. The relevance of energy to maximize nitrogen utilization should be stressed in these regimens, given the narrowness of the therapeutic window, the toxicity of nitrogen compounds, and risks of oversupply or malnutrition.

1.1 General Principles of Treatment

In practice, dietary restrictions to correct dietary imbalances in metabolic disorders require the use of elemental diets. Chemically well-defined foods are used in limited and calculated amounts to provide all amino acids except those that are not allowed by the regimen. On the other hand, natural foods containing the full complement of amino acids seldom supply more than 25% of the patient's protein requirements. Furthermore, nitrogen-restricted and chemically defined products supply a narrow range of nutrients. Besides the crucial amino acids, the dietary essentiality and adequate amounts of sufficient dietary components must be demonstrated through long-term use, as in total parenteral nutrition. The definition of dietary essentiality, or the nonavailability of a chemical compound from endogenous sources, is today extended to include the specific contribution of a food to psychophysical health (2). Nutrients that fall within this secondary definition were once defined as semiessential.

1.2 Essential Nutrients

While the intake of certain nutrients such as amino acids may be restricted in patients with inborn errors of amino acid metabolism, minimum levels must be maintained in order to allow for protein synthesis during growth. All essential amino acids must be administered and a positive nitrogen balance achieved to allow catabolic events to predominate over anabolic processes. Thus preformed amino acids are supplied and closely monitored to prevent excess or deficits. A rapidly changing tissue like the skin provides early warning signs of essential nutrient deficit. Acrodermatitis-like syndromes have been described in patients suffering from the less common forms of amino acid disorders, in which dietary essential branched chain amino acids are reduced to minimal levels (3). These syndromes are akin to the clinical events triggered by a deficiency of essential fatty acids (4) or by a zinc deficit (5). Even with the increasing availability of enriched foods intended for patients with a metabolic disorder, infants on semi-synthetic diets are particularly prone to nutritional deficiencies. The first sign of scaling dermatitis localized to the face and limbs should always induce suspicion of a deficient diet. Patients with a poor nutritional status may be lethargic and anorectic and fail to gain weight or height. In these stages combined enteral and parenteral support is required to maximize recovery.

1.3 Semiessential Nutrients

A second-line intervention is to provide nutrients to promote specific metabolic pathways and improve the nutritional outcome. Avoidance of whole natural foods may expose a child to secondary nutrient deficits of trace elements and minerals. While the lack of essential nutrients can have serious consequences for patients in the acute phases of the disorder, the need for semiessential nutrients may be increased in patients undergoing long-term dietary treatment or those on a recovery diet. Evidence is growing that some inborn errors of amino acid metabolism should be treated for life to prevent functional consequences, especially on the central nervous system. There is a need to supply the whole range of essential nutrients to women of childbearing age with hyperphenylalaninemia, for instance; but preventing high blood phenylalanine levels at conception has been associated with an embryofetopathic syndrome that has become a challenge for nutrition. Some nonessential amino acids, such as carnitine and long-chain polyunsaturated fatty acids, are among those compounds that may have to be supplied throughout life (5). Trials on the effects of supplementation with arachidonic acid and/or docosahexaenoic acid in hyperphenylalaninemia are currently in progress. Not only are these nutrients usually absent from the diet provided to these patients, but also the hypothesis of additional benefits for brain and tissue development remains to be put to the test.

1.4 Management Problems

The association between clinical status and metabolic activity becomes very relevant during infections, when muscle catabolism is increased, upsetting the amino acid balance. Septic events may also impair intestinal nutrient absorption. Any infection in these patients should be promptly diagnosed and adequately treated, and the exact composition of the prescribed course of medication should be known. During short infective episodes, patients should receive nutritional support by increasing fluid and carbohydrate intake with fruit juices and high-carbohydrate protein-free soft drinks of known composition. Misunderstandings about managing the diet of patients with inborn errors of metabolism may be frequent even on the part of caregivers. Additional efforts in parental and patient education must be undertaken. The prospect of lifelong nutritional support should be stressed at the onset of therapy, and parents and child should be reminded at intervals. With age, this becomes even more necessary as the child comes under peer pressure and the influence of school and the community. Children should be given sound reasons and advice geared to give them a sense of personal responsibility about avoiding certain foods and thus maintaining good health. Parents and children themselves may benefit from sharing experiences, participating in an association, and, with self-help, maintain the closest possible compliance with dietary schedules. Literature on alternative methods of preparation, mixing compatibility, and recipes experimenting with the allowed foods represents a further opportunity to promote self-control in a positive, enabling way.

1.5 Aims of the Dietary Intervention

Chronic therapy and follow-up should aim to secure development and quality of life by preventing acute attacks and protecting against functional damage, especially adverse neurochemical reactions. With the advances of treatment in terms of longer life expectancy and improved quality of life, emphasis has shifted toward the protection of pregnancy. With gestation, the mother requires complex dietary adjustments in response to her changing physiological requirements. This, however, is not without consequences to the fetus, as the placenta lacks a selective mechanism against an excess of amino acids or buildup of other material. When this happens, the growing infant's neural tissues may suffer from permanent damage. There is evidence of major fatty acid imbalance as the primary cause of these structural disturbances. While enzyme or gene therapy does not currently provide definitive answers to inborn errors of amino acid metabolism, dietary intervention now reaches out well beyond childhood and adolescence to include the reproductive age and improve prospects for both patients and their children in terms of health maintenance and quality of life.

2 HYPERPHENYLALANINEMIA

Hyperphenylalaninemia (HPA) is defined as plasma phenylalanine (Phe, an essential amino acid) concentrations above 120 μmol (2 mg/dL) and is caused by a disorder of the phenylalanine hydroxylation, which leads to the synthesis of tyrosine (Tyr). This may be the consequence of deficient phenylalanine hydroxylase (PAH) activity or a disturbance of the metabolism of tetrahydrobiopterin (BH4), a cofactor of the PAH enzyme. Both diseases are autosomal recessive. In PAH deficiency, both a genetic defect and ingestion of Phe are necessary for overt symptoms to develop. In the case of BH4 deficiency, mutation alone is the primary cause of the disease. The overall incidence of PAH deficiency among Caucasians is estimated to be around 100 cases per 1,000,000 live births. Wide geographic and ethnic variations of the various forms of the disease coexist. BH4 deficiency prevalence is estimated to be around 1 to 2 cases per million live births. While BH4 deficiency requires pharmacological intervention, PAH deficiency forms are amenable to dietary alterations. Although heterogeneous in presentation, PAH deficiency has been classified by consensus into four types, which are recognized by combining individual tolerance to dietary Phe and the pretreatment Phe plasma levels. Classic phenylketonuria (PKU) is characterized by the complete absence of PAH activity, while the milder forms are subdivided into moderate and mild PKU and mild HPA (or MHP), respectively (Table 1). In classic PKU, the accumulated Phe is shifted toward other biochemical pathways leading to the abnormal synthesis of metabolites such as phenylacetic, phenylpiruvic, and phenyllactic acids. The buildup of Phe causes neuron dysfunction and mental deficiency in the classic PKU type and, to a lesser extent, also in the milder PKU forms. The pathogenetic mechanisms of neurological damage in PKU are not fully understood, but two major hypotheses have been put forward: 1) an altered metabolism of the protein and lipid components of myelin with an accelerated myelin turnover directly caused by high Phe plasma levels (6) and 2) a depressed protein and neurotransmitter synthesis in the brain due to competitive mechanisms between Phe and other large neutral amino acids for passage through the blood-brain barrier (7). The debate on the origin of the damage and the implications for therapy, however, remains open (8).

2.1 Genetics

PAH deficiency is caused by mutation in the gene encoding PAH, which is located on chromosome 12. The different forms of PAH deficiency are allelic. More than 300 different mutations have been reported and account for the genetic heterogeneity of types of PAH deficiency. Each mutation has a particular influence on the enzyme activity and some mutations may suppress all PAH activity,

TABLE 1 Classification of PAH Deficiency Forms[a]

PAH deficiency form	Dietary Phe tolerance		Pretreatment blood Phe	
	mg/kg/day	mg/day	µmol/L	mg/dL
Classic PKU	<20	250–350	1200	20
Moderate PKU	20–25	350–400	600–1200	10–20
Mild PKU	25–50	400–600	600–1200	10–20
MHP	normal diet		<600	<10

[a] Because of rapid growth, definition of individual Phe tolerance must be assessed at least by the end of the second year.

while others still are associated with residual function in vitro in the range of 2 to 70%. Combinations of different mutations result in a spectrum of metabolic phenotypes, ranging from more severe forms requiring strict dietary management to milder hyperphenylalaninemia (MHP), in which dietary restriction of Phe is not necessary. Some studies have suggested a correlation between the PAH genotype and its metabolic phenotype, reporting associations of particular mutation combinations with peculiar phenotypes (9). However, the high number of mutations and the different methods and criteria used for diagnosis and classification in the different studies has resulted in an inability to predict the occurrence of the phenotype based on genotype evidence. This particular issue is currently being investigated, as a linear correlation between genotype and metabolic phenotype would be crucial for the diagnosis and implementation of dietary intervention. Regional programs of genetic screening have been initiated to detect heterozygous forms in countries where the heterogeneity of PAH mutations has a narrow range. In northern European countries, a few mutations include almost all mutant alleles (10).

2.2 Diagnosis

The diagnosis of HPA currently relies on the result of the Guthrie test, where levels of blood Phe below 120 μmol/L are considered normal. Routine diagnostic procedures include direct dosage of Phe plasma and Tyr, the evaluation of the Phe plasma response to oral BH4, and the analysis of urinary pterin metabolites to correctly assign a patient to a diagnostic category distinguishing between forms due to PAH or BH4 deficiency. Whenever a BH4-dependent form is suspected, direct determination of the three enzymes involved is recommended.

2.3 Clinical Outcome

The threat of biochemical damage to the brain persists throughout life (6). Follow-up of early-treated children with PKU has shown that diet discontinuation during childhood exposes a patient to cognitive and emotional deficits in a substantial number of adolescents and young adults (11,12). The extent of these disabling conditions include low IQ, dysfunctional mental processes, learning difficulties and anxiety, and personality disorders. In addition, neuron deterioration has been reported. Moreover, an embryofetopathic syndrome associated with high maternal Phe plasma levels in the periconceptional period is now well characterized (13). In our current understanding of PKU, diet compliance throughout adolescence and the reproductive age is recommended. The common experience is that once dietary restriction has been relaxed, it is quite difficult to go back to the original strict metabolic control. Most centers are extending this into a "diet-for-life" policy. In spite of these recommendations, even early-treated subjects—not just a poorly managed minority—exhibit some degree of intellectual deficit in childhood, well before there is any hope of relaxing or discontinuing treatment (14). Several studies have shown that structural changes in the brain (15) and abnormalities of visual function (16) occur in these patients. Thus the possibility remains that some unknown dietary factors affect the development of treated HPA patients (17). To overcome these impairments, modification of the composition of amino acid supplementation and the lipid quota by enriching diets with long-chain polyunsaturated fatty acids has been proposed.

2.4 Amino Acid Supplementation

Large neutral amino acids (LNAAs), including Phe, compete for transport across the blood-brain barrier via the L-type amino acid carrier. Accordingly, elevated Phe plasma levels impair the uptake of other LNAAs by the brain of patients with PKU. The direct effects of elevated brain Phe and depleted LNAAs are probably major causes of disturbed brain development and function in PKU (7). Carrier competition might conversely lower Phe buildup when plasma concentrations of all other LNAAs are increased. Concurrent LNAA supplementation blocks Phe influx, as magnetic resonance spectroscopy shows, but without slowing of the brain's electrical activity (18). Earlier findings have shown the positive effects of supplementing branched-chain amino acids (BACA), the major determinants of the LNAA quota (19). Also at issue is the hypothesis that the major determinant of mental deficit in treated patients with PKU could be the low availability of tyrosine. There are studies on the functional effects of tyrosine supplementation, but the results are still controversial (20). In sum, high Phe levels could displace LNAAs other than Phe and diet enrichment with specific amino acids could displace Phe in tissues and metabolic reactions, thus improving functional outcome. Studies to test these hypotheses are in progress.

2.5 The Lipid Approach to Diet in HPA

HPA allows a different approach to the dietary treatment of inborn errors of amino acid metabolism. The consequences of dietary protein deprivation extend their adverse effects to general tissue growth and development. Other nutrients must thus be included and/or manipulated to afford a measure of protection to the developing nervous system and also to relieve the potential consequences of other marginal nutritional deficiencies. The recent approach of providing preformed long-chain polyunsaturated fatty acids (LCPUFAs) shows some promise. Since treated HPA patients are denied the lipids of animal fats, they do not receive moieties such as arachidonic acid (AA) and docosahexaenoic acid (DHA) (21). The retina and the rod receptors are particularly rich in DHA and its deprivation may lead to a lower content in photosensitive structures. Thus the assessment of visual function has been considered a first step to evaluate the fatty acid status from a functional viewpoint, as clearly shown in studies assessing the visual acuity of artificially or breast-fed infants (both preterm and full-term) (22). An improvement of the response at visual stimulation, assessed with the visual evoked potential, has been demonstrated in older children with HPA who were given these lipids in their diet (23). Positive effects of dietary AA and DHA in pregnant women with PKU and in their children merit further investigation. AA and DHA enrichment, therefore, could be extended to many other diseases with potential brain involvement.

2.6 Maternal PKU

Maternal hyperphenylalaninemia is considered a high-risk factor for embryopathic and fetopathic syndromes that may affect the infant (24). Clinical manifestations include microcephaly, developmental delay, and intrauterine growth retardation in most cases, and, less often, congenital alterations of the heart, gastrointestinal system, and maxillary bones. Poor reproductive outcome has also been observed in women with PKU when dietary treatment was started late in pregnancy or when Phe plasma concentrations remained elevated. The following recommendations have been issued on the basis of multicenter studies (25):

Maintain Phe plasma levels between 120 and 360 μmol/L throughout pregnancy.

Begin strict dietary control in the preconceptional period, and, in any case, within the first 8 to 10 weeks of pregnancy.

Keep an adequate energy and protein intake while controlling for Phe plasma levels.

A clinical history of stillbirths, congenital malformations, and/or mental retardation should prompt the testing of women of reproductive age for their Phe blood levels.

2.7 Dietary Treatment—Principles and Follow-Up

The changing requirements of the growing organism, closely related to the varying growth rates and the maturation of the enzyme system, explain the subdivision of the type of dietary intervention into four major periods:

Infancy
Weaning
From 12 months to adolescence
Adulthood (major challenge: maternal PKU)

2.7.1 Infancy

Before weaning, the only dietary source of Phe is human milk or formula in amounts that are established on the basis of the individual Phe tolerance. The

TABLE 2 Range of Phe Plasma
and Suggested Dietary Supply
for Each Value

Plasma Phe		Dietary Phe, mg/kg
μmol/L	mg/dL	
<600	<10	70
600–1200	10–20	55
1200–1800	20–30	45
1800–2400	30–40	35
>2400	>40	25

final dietary balance is reached through Phe-free products, vegetable fats (e.g., olive oil) and carbohydrate-based products (e.g., maltodextrins). Phenylalanine (Phe) requirements vary among patients and according to the residual activity of the Phe-hydroxylase (PHA) enzyme. Also age, growth rate, and energy/protein intake and concurrent infections alter individual Phe requirements. The suggested values of Phe intake at the beginning of dietary treatment depend on the maximum Phe plasma levels (Table 2). On the basis of the Phe plasma levels, the necessity of a dietary program is carefully evaluated. If Phe plasma levels are below 600 μmol/L (10 mg/dL) mothers are allowed to freely breast-feed their infants. A daily breast-milk supply of around 100 mL/kg may be allowed with frequent monitoring of the Phe plasma levels, and (if necessary) minimal amounts of a Phe-free formula may be introduced to complement breast-feeding and control Phe plasma peaks. Breast-feeding may be permitted in infants with HPA (26)

TABLE 3 Phenylalanine Content of Milks[a]

Product	Content per 100 g			
	Protein, g	Phe, mg	Energy	
			kJ	kcal
Mature human milk	1.1	54	288	69
Cow's milk	3.3	170	269	64
Casein-based formula	1.9	100	275	65
Whey-based formula	1.5	56	275	65

[a] Values reported are indicative, given the variability of composition.
Source: Ref. 45.

if Phe plasma levels remain stable below 600 μmol/L (or ideally in the 200- to 500-μmol/L range). Breast milk intakes could also be varied more frequently in response to Phe plasma levels, and this may be achieved by altering the quantity of the Phe-free protein substitute supplied and by adjusting the duration of breast-feeding. In practical terms, this could be achieved by offering the infant complementary food prior to breast-feeding. Human milk offers many benefits in terms

TABLE 4 Examples of Dietary Schedules After Diagnosis and Definition of Phe Contents

Schedule 1	Phe "0" diet (blood Phe levels > 20 mg/dL at diagnosis)	
	Age: 20 days	Weight: 3050 kg
Phe-free formula (PKU 1 mix)	63 g	
Maltodextrins	34 g	
Per kilogram daily intakes: energy 135 kcal, protein 2.6 g		
Schedule 2	Phe: 50 mg/kg/day, milder form (180 mg/day)	
	Age: 1 month	Weight: 3600 kg
Human milk	150 g	
Standard infant formula	32 g	
Phe-free formula (Maxamaid XP1)	25 g	
Per kilogram daily intakes: energy 105 kcal, protein 2.3 g		
Schedule 3	Phe: 20 mg/kg/day (70 mg/day)	
	Age: 1 month	Weight: 3500 kg
Human milk	150 g	
Phe-free formula (Maxamaid XP1)	41 g	
Maltodextrins	10 g	
Olive oil	5 g	
Per kilogram daily intakes: energy 110 kcal, protein 2.1 g		
Schedule 4	Phe: 20 mg/kg day (70 mg/day)	
	Age: 1 month	Weight: 3500 kg
Human milk	150 g	
Phe-free formula (PKU 1 mix)	63 g	
Maltodextrins	5 g	
Per kilogram daily intakes: energy 127 kcal, protein 2.2 g		

of immunity and nutrition, which include central nervous system (CNS) protection factors such as the long-chain PUFAs. These nutritional properties have been put forward to explain the advantage in terms of later achievement among PKU infants who had been breast-fed instead of formula-fed in their first weeks of life before the institution of a dietary regimen (27). Even if the Phe content of mature breast milk may vary, its Phe content is lower than that of other infant formulas (Table 3). In the case of Phe, if plasma levels increase (within the 1200 μmol/L limit), it is advisable to increase amounts of Phe-free formula while decreasing the supply of breast milk up to reestablishment of Phe plasma levels within the allowed limits. Examples of standard formula schedules with a protein content within the lower limits and a Phe-free formula are reported in Table 4. In order to facilitate dietary complementation, nutritionally complete products (i.e., including also fats of both vegetable and animal origin, carbohydrates, trace elements, and vitamins) without Phe are now becoming available commercially to HPA patients (Table 5).

TABLE 5 Composition of Phe-Free Preparations (per 100 g)

Preparation	Proteins	Sugars	Lipids	PUFA	Calories
Milupa Special Products					
PKU 1	50	20.3	0		282
PKU 1 mix	10.1	56.3	27.6	4.2	514
				(0.2 LCP)	
PKU 2	66.7	8.2	0		300
PKU 3	68	3.9	0		288
Ross Products Division					
Abbott Laboratories					
Maxamaid Xp1	15.5	54	23	4.4	462
Maxamaid XP2	77.7	4	0		326
Maxamaid XP3	25	61	<0.5		300
Maxamum XP	34	41	<1		329
Mead Johnson					
Lofenalac	15	60	18	9.1	456
Phenyl-free	29	52	5.4	2.45	370
Nutricia-SHS					
Analog LCP	13	54	23	10.5	475
				(0.2 LCP)	

Key: LCP, long-chain polyunsaturated fatty acids; PUFA, polyunsaturated fatty acids.

2.7.2 Weaning Period

Beginning with the fourth month of life, requirements of Phe per kilogram decrease, paralleling the decreased rate of growth of the body (Table 6). With the introduction of solid foods, attention should shift to daily total Phe intakes rather than the per kilogram intake. There is no reason to believe that the weaning process should take place in infants with PKU at a time or in a manner different from that of normal infants (28) except that a lesser dietary intake of Phe is absolutely essential.

TABLE 6 Dietary Schedules at Onset of Weaning for Infants with PKU

Schedule 1	Phe: 42 mg/kg/day (340 mg/day)	
	Age: 5 months	Weight: 8 kg
Standard infant formula	75 g	
Phe-free formula (Analog LCP)	20 g	
Maltodextrins	40 g	
No-protein infant pasta	20 g	
Potatoes	20 g	
Carrots	20 g	
Summer squash	20 g	
Puréed apples	100 g	
Olive oil	10 g	
Per kilogram daily intakes: energy 96 kcal, protein 1.5 g		
Schedule 2	Phe: 24 mg/kg/day (144 mg/day)	
	Age: 5 months	Weight: 6 kg
Human milk	150 g	
Phe-free formula (Maxamaid XP1)	30 g	
Carrots	20 g	
Potatoes	40 g	
Summer squash	20 g	
No-protein infant pasta	40 g	
Olive oil	5 g	
Maize/sunflower oil	5 g	
Per kilogram daily intakes: energy 107 kcal, protein 1.9 g		

2.7.3 From 12 Months to Adolescence

Once solid foods have replaced milk, a complete range of commercially available vegetable and low-protein foods should ensure dietary diversification. This is based on the system of weight equivalents in Phe content (Table 7). A diet for a 4-year-old child is reported in Table 8. For adolescents on such a diet, Table 9 shows two different schedules. The "diet for life" policy represents a major challenge to adolescents and their families. Metabolic control using the criteria applied during childhood is quite difficult to achieve with teenagers. Time constraints, social pressures, financial limitations, and growing independence from

TABLE 7 Ponderal Equivalents

10-mg Phe equivalents	
Milk-derived foods:	
Whole cow's milk	6 g
No-protein milk Sno-Pro	100 g
Whole yogurt	5 g
Yogurt with fruit	4.5 g
Cereals:	
Rice	2.5 g
No-protein pasta	33 g
No-protein bread	80 g
Cornflakes	3 g
20-mg Phe equivalents	
Vegetables:	
Carrots	65 g
Potatoes	20 g
Spinach	20 g
French beans	25 g
Lettuce	35 g
Summer squash	25 g
Tomatoes	80 g
Canned tomatoes	60 g
Fresh beans	1 g
Fresh peas	5 g
Capsicum	50 g
Fruit:	
Banana	60 g
Apple	220 g
Pear	85 g
Peach	110 g

TABLE 8 Dietary Schedule for a 3-Year-Old Child

Phe: 21 mg/kg/day (360 mg/day) Age: 4 years Weight: 17 kg	
Whole cow's milk	80 g
Phe-free formula (Maxamaid XP3)	92 g
Carrots	40 g
Potatoes	60 g
Summer squash	40 g
Olive oil	25 g
Maize/sunflower oil	20 g
No-protein biscuits	50 g
No-protein pasta	100 g
Summer squash	10 g
Canned tomatoes	65 g
Fruit juice	125 g
Apple	220 g
Banana	90 g
Per kilogram daily intakes: energy 99 kcal, protein 1.6 g	

the family combine to interfere with dietary control. Added to these difficulties are the biological changes of adolescence, which reduce phenylalanine tolerance (29). We have unpublished data from an ongoing study showing that a diet-treated patient with PKU older than 13 years has a 30% probability of having higher blood Phe levels than younger counterparts even after adjusting for tolerance and dietary compliance (OR = 1.3, 95% CI = 1.1 to 1.5). This finding may be affected by the biological changes of adolescence. The upper acceptable limit of Phe plasma levels at this age, however, could be set within 600 to 720 µmol/L. These limits already exceed those acceptable for the prevention of maternal PKU and are well above the accepted range for breaching the blood-brain barrier. Beyond mere metabolic control, social support for the diet and a positive perception of the treatment has been faulted, and this has led to the development of support programs for adolescents and young adults (particularly females) with PKU.

2.7.4 Adult PKU and PKU in Pregnancy

Although most specialists recommend dietary restriction into adulthood, data on dietary compliance is lacking at a time when the population amenable to the diet-for-life intervention is now entering adulthood. Products tailored to individual metabolic needs are now advocated, and the next few years should be fraught

TABLE 9 Dietary Schedules for Adolescents

Schedule 1	Phe: 16 mg/kg/day (720 mg/day)
	Age: 13 years Weight: 45 kg

Phe-free formulas:	
PKU 2	52 g (equivalent to 34 g protein)
Maxamaid XP3	55 g (equivalent to 13 g protein)
No-protein cereals	240 g
Milk products (yogurt)	125 g
Vegetables	600 g[a]
Fruit	420 g[a]
Vegetable oil	50 g

Per kilogram daily intakes: energy 44 kcal, protein 1.4 g

Schedule 2	Phe: 13 mg/kg/day (625 mg/day)
	Age: 16 years Weight: 48 kg

Phe-free formula (PKU 2)	79 g (equivalent to 52 g protein)
No-protein cereals	350 g
Vegetables	420 g[a]
Fruit	90 g[a]
Fruit juice	125 g
Sugar	15 g
Vegetable oils	55 g

Per kilogram daily intakes: energy 49 kcal, protein 1.3 g

[a] Servings for each specific item (potatoes, carrots, apples, bananas . . .) calculated as Phe equivalents.

with problems and questions raised by the beginning of dietary intervention in the treatment of these patients. The greatest scientific challenge of recent years has been dietary intervention for women with PKU during the periconceptional period or within the first weeks of pregnancy in an effort to prevent congenital malformations. The biochemical goal of 120 to 360 µmol/L Phe (monitored by the Guthrie test) is reached by directly controlling Phe supply (Table 10) and adjusting for age, rate of weight gain, trimester of pregnancy, adequacy of energy intake, and general state of health. The changing requirement of each patient is established by frequent monitoring of Phe plasma levels. Phe requirements usually increase at approximately 20 weeks' gestation; thus a strict dietary regimen is required up to this period. Examples of diet for a well-compensated PKU pregnant woman are listed in Table 11. Supplementation with LNAA and/or tyrosine and/or LCPUFA represents the ultimate dietary challenge to improve the dietary prevention of fetal damage in women with PKU (30).

TABLE 10   Recommended Daily Nutrient Intakes for Pregnant Women with PKU

Trimester and age	PHE (g/day)	Protein (g/day)	Energy (kcal/day)
First			
15 to <19	200–600	75	2000–3500
>19	200–600	70	2000–3000
Second			
15 to <19	200–800	75	2000–3500
>19	200–800	70	2000–3000
Third			
15 to <19	300–1200	75	2000–3500
>19	300–1200	70	2000–3000

TABLE 11   Dietary Schedule for a Pregnant, Well-Compensated and Normal-Weight Woman with PKU During the Second Trimester of Pregnancy, Expressed as Phe Equivalents

	Phe: 5.8 mg/kg/day (340 mg/day) Age: 30 years Weight: 58 kg
Phe-free formula:	
PKU 3	98 g (equivalent to 66.6 g proteins)
or	
Maxamum XP	170 g (equivalent to 66.6 g proteins)
No-protein cereals	4 Phe equivalents
Milk	16 Phe equivalents
Vegetables	6 Phe equivalents
Fruit	2 Phe equivalents
Olive oil	55 g

Per kilogram daily intakes: energy 36 kcal, protein 1.2 g

3 OTHER ERRORS OF AMINO ACID METABOLISM

The mainstay of dietary treatment of errors of amino acid metabolism is special diet of foods that lack the amino acids which are blocked in the metabolic pathway. High-energy, protein-free products are used to fulfill dietary requirements (Table 12). Native proteins may be added (in the first year of life, standard infant formulas or whey-hydrolysates are used, depending on the presence of gastrointestinal symptoms) as well as low-protein vegetable foods. Legumes and nuts, which have a relatively high protein content, are generally excluded. Specially processed low-protein cereals are used to increase the energy supply while maintaining a low protein intake. On the whole, this approach follows the same principles as the treatment of hyperphenylalaninemias, and schedules with standard exchange food lists for the controlled amino acids are also used. Regular metabolic checkups of the patient and dietary assessments should be carried out in order to test the adequacy of the dietary schedules with age.

TABLE 12 Products for the Treatment of Inborn Errors of Amino Acid and Protein Metabolism

Disorder	Products
Tyrosinemia	*Milupa Special*: Tyr 1, Tyr 1 Mix, Tyr 2 *Ross Lab*: Analog XPhen Tyr, XPhen Tyr Met, Maxamaid XPhen Tyr, XPhen Tyr Met *Mead Johnson*: Low-Phe/Tyr diet powder
MSUD	*Milupa Special*: MSUD 1, MSUD 1 Mix, MSUD 2 *Ross Lab*: Analog MSUD, Maxamaid MSUD, Maximum MSUD *Mead Johnson*: MSUD diet powder
Homocystinuria	*Milupa Special*: HOM 1, HOM 1 Mix, HOM 2
(Cys-β-synthase deficiency)	*Ross Lab*: Analog XMet, Maxamaid XMet, Maxamum XMet *Mead Johnson*: Low-Met diet powder
Organic acidemias	*Milupa Special*: OS 1, OS 2
Defects in urea cycle enzymes	*Milupa Special*: UCD 1, UCD 2 (essential amino acids)
Nitrogen-restricted diets	*Mead Johnson*: Protein-free diet powder,[a] Moducal *Ross Lab*: Polycose powder, Duocal

[a] Formula enriched with minerals and vitamins.

3.1 Tyrosinemias

Tyrosine (Tyr) in humans is derived from the diet and from the hydroxylation of both dietary and endogenous Phe deriving from protein catabolism. Hypertyrosinemic states depend mainly on congenital disturbance of Tyr metabolism, although some cases may be secondary to hepatocellular disorders. Fumarylacetoacetate hydrolase (FAH) deficiency (type I tyrosinemia or hepatorenal tyrosinemia) is characterized by a Fanconi-like renal syndrome, glomerulosclerosis, progressive liver failure, cirrhosis evolving into hepatocellular carcinoma, and peripheral nerve deficit. Acute porphyria-like episodes may develop from the impairment of δ-aminolevulinic acid dehydratase activity by succinylacetone, a toxic metabolite. High succinylacetone levels in plasma and urine are diagnostic, along with hypertyrosinemia and (in cases of a concomitant adjunctive enzymatic defect) high plasma methionine levels. In the tyrosine aminotranferase (TAT) deficiency (type II tyrosinemia or oculocutaneous tyrosinemia), corneal erosions and hyperkeratoses on the fingers as well as on the palms of hands and soles of feet are commonly found; and mental retardation may occur. Both disorders are transmitted in an autosomal recessive fashion. The objective of the dietary support for hereditary tyrosinemias is to provide a biochemical environment that allows for the normal growth and development of intellectual potential while also preventing pathophysiological changes. Since a large quantity of Phe is normally hydroxylated to form tyrosine, this amino acid also should be restricted in the diet of patients with tyrosinemia (Table 13). Dietary therapy requires an accurate diagnosis because of the different types of approach between the two hereditary forms. In type I tyrosinemia, treatment with a diet restricted in Phe and Tyr does not prevent progression of liver disease and development of hepatocellular carcinoma (31). The Phe and Tyr restriction is less severe and prognosis is excellent for type II. The calculated intake of Phe and Tyr is based on blood analyses indicating the child's requirement and/or tolerance for each amino acid. Phe requirements are higher for children with tyrosinemia than children with HPA, since, as a general norm for inborn errors of metabolism, the more distal the block is in the catabolic pathway, the less affected the amino acid requirement. The Tyr requirements of children with tyrosinemia vary with the metabolic state and the accumulation of succinylacetone. Because of the high plasma methionine levels observed in type I tyrosinemia, methionine restriction (50 mg/kg of body weight for a 15-month-old child) has also been recommended. If methionine restriction is implemented, L-cysteine supplementation should be considered. Particular attention to the total protein and energy intakes should be paid as well as to all the metabolic disorders in which L-amino acids products are used, in which a conversion factor is needed for the equivalence between amino acid and protein nitrogen. Protein sources containing 20 to 70 mg Phe and 60 to 80 mg Tyr per kilogram of body weight per day are required to prevent a catabolic phase with

TABLE 13 Dietary Schedule for Type-1
Tyrosinemia

Age: 6 years	Weight: 21 kg
Tyr + Phe-free formula (Tyr 2)	32 g
No-protein pasta	190 g
No-protein biscuits	60 g
Whole cow's milk	120 g
Potatoes	100 g
Canned tomatoes	60 g
Carrots	195 g
Summer squash	220 g
Bananas	45 g
Apricot marmalade	30 g
Olive oil	45 g
Sugar	20 g
Fruit juice	125 g

Per kilogram daily intakes: energy 88 kcal, total
protein 1.5 g

overproduction of toxic metabolites. As far as energy needs, 150 kcal/kg per day represents a recommended supply for infants up to 2 years of age. In childhood, the limit should be kept above 100 kcal/kg per day. The recent introduction of an inhibitor of 4-hydroxyphenylpyruvic acid dioxygenase (pHPPD), 2-(2-nitro-4-trifluoromethylbenzoly)-1,3-cyclohexanedione (NTBC) has led to an improvement of both hepatic and renal conditions in type-I tyrosinemia (32). Liver transplantation has been successfully performed in some cases. For type-II hypertyrosinemia, ocular and skin symptoms seem to be quite responsive to the dietary treatment.

3.2 Homocystinuria

The most common form of homocystinuria is caused by a deficiency of cystathionine β-synthase, inherited as an autosomal recessive disease. This disorder occurs with an incidence varying from 1 in 36,000 to 1 in 330,000 and is characterized by high levels of homocysteine and methionine (Met) and low levels of cysteine in cells and physiological fluids. In a large survey of patients with this form of homocystinuria, 13% were responsive to vitamin B_6, the cofactor of the enzymatic reactions. Other errors of the Met metabolism are due to failure to synthesize methylcobalamin from vitamin B_{12} or a deficiency in 5,10 methylenetetrahydrofolate reductase, coenzymes required in the remethylation of homocysteine to form Met. In this case normal or low Met plasma concentrations are present. If these biochemical alterations are not treated early, skeletal alterations, dislocated lenses, intravascular thromboses, osteoporosis, malar flushing, and—in some patients—mental retardation will occur. The increased production of homocysteic acid in homocystinuria enhances sulfate esterification of connective tissue proteoglycans, leading to structural changes of tissues such as bones, perilenticular tissues, and vascular walls. The changes observed in the vascular structure have suggested a high potential for damage due to the sulfurate amino acids, and the recent advent of an association between hyperhomocysteinemia and atherosclerotic events has extended interest in the potential damage of high homocysteine levels in plasma, contributing to the development of a homocysteine theory of atherosclerosis (33). Indeed, it has been estimated that up to one-third of individuals with atherosclerotic vascular disease are heterozygous for hyperhomocysteinemia. Diverse effects of homocysteine on proteoglycan conformation, cholesterol metabolism, platelet and endothelial function, and coagulation factor activity contribute to accelerated atherosclerosis and the thrombotic propensity in homocystinuria. For the treatment of homocystinuria due to cystathionine β-synthase deficiency, the response to high-dose (up to 1 g) oral pyridoxine should be tested on plasma Met and homocysteine levels. If the levels of these amino acids are reduced, a gradual adjustment of the vitamin B_6 dosage is carried out until the minimum dose necessary to maintain normal levels is reached. For unresponsive patients, treatment is based on a Met-restricted diet supplemented with L-cysteine, which becomes an essential amino acid in homocistinuria. Folate should also be supplemented because of the excess use in remethylating homocysteine to Met. In infants and children affected by this disorder, it is necessary to consider energy, protein, Met, cysteine, folate, vitamins B_6 and B_{12}, and fluid needs on the basis of different ages. Younger infants have a greater Met requirement (35 to 50 mg/kg per day) than older infants (5 to 10 mg/kg). Met may be supplemented to the young infant through the addition of infant formulas to the low-Met or Met-free medical foods. In the successive ages, the Met requirement is reduced and small amounts of solid foods can be permitted (Table 14). At all ages a soluble form of L-cysteine (calcium cystinate) should be supplemented (300 mg/kg in young infants, reduced to 200 mg/kg at 6 months of age and 100 mg/kg at 3 years of age, and so on). For pregnant patients, it has been reported that the fetal outcome is good in women whose disorder is responsive to vitamin B_6 therapy and poor in women whose disorder is unresponsive to therapy (34). Finally, it has also been suggested that the daily dose of pyridoxine and/or folate should be raised in the whole population in order to prevent the high homocysteine levels associated to cardiovascular modifications (35). Theoretically, this could be obtained with an increase in the dietary consumption of vegetable foods and a decrease in animal proteins. This simple recommendation also includes other changes (less cholesterol and saturated fats, more carbohydrates and fiber)

TABLE 14 Dietary Schedule for Homocystinuria

Age: 10 years	Weight: 39 kg
Methionine-free formula (HOM 2)	30 g
Whole cow's milk	200 g
Yogurt	125 g
Pasta	200 g
No-protein bread	70 g
No-protein biscuits	55 g
Olive oil	57 g
Apricot marmalade	30 g
Carrots	200 g
Potatoes	300 g
Summer squash	250 g
Bananas	200 g
Apples	200 g
Sugar	10 g
Per kilogram daily intakes: energy 66 kcal, total protein 1.6 g	

that have been positively associated with the prevention of cardiovascular damage.

3.3 Maple Syrup Urine Disease

MSUD is the prototype of disorders of organic acid metabolism and results from a defect in the metabolism of branched-chain amino acids [BBCAs: leucine (Leu), isoleucine (Ile), and valine (Val)] with accumulation of these amino acids and the corresponding keto acids in blood, urine, and cerebrospinal fluid. The first symptoms and signs, present in the first days of life, are not unlike those of neonatal sepsis in that metabolic acidosis is present and there is CNS dysfunction. Unless the diagnosis is made promptly, infants may die of respiratory failure. BBCA-free mixtures should be begun by the enteral route as soon as the diagnosis is made. If enteral feeding is not possible, a central venous line with dextrose and lipids should be undertaken for initial care during the neonatal period to maintain energy and caloric needs. A higher supply of proteins and calories per kg/body/weight through BCAA–free formulas and high-caloric, protein-free products is generally recommended. After the diagnosis, a rapid decline of plasma Ile and Val by feeding BCAA-free formulas is observed; then these two amino acids may be added as free amino acids to prevent their deficiency and elevation of plasma Leu concentrations as a function of muscle catabolism or decreased protein synthesis. Energy intakes of 140 to 170 kcal/kg of body weight during this period are recommended to prevent the catabolism of body proteins. Quotas of each BCAA must be included in the diet for infants' requirements (36). The requirements for BCAAs are provided by small amounts of natural foods (milk, low-protein fruits and vegetables) and must be carefully regulated (Table 15). An overt deficiency of any one of the three amino acids can, with accumulation of the other two, produce tissue catabolism. A plasma excess of any of these amino acids will result in the reappearance of clinical signs and symptoms. Plasma concentrations of Ile, Leu, and Val should be maintained (3 to 4 hr after a meal) within the limits of 40 to 90, 80 to 200, and 200 to 425 μmol/L respectively. Patients surviving the first attacks often have lower body weight and height values than reference populations. Long-term therapy for MSUD requires strict dietary compliance. Frequent adjustments of the dietary prescriptions are necessary, based on appetite, growth, development, and levels of plasma BCAAs and α-keto acids. Recommended energy intakes after the initial acute period, during which patients may require up to 170 kcal/kg per day, are the same as for normal infants and children. The recommended protein intake for infants with MSUD after the initial acute period is even slightly above the limits indicated for normal infants and children. The cases of pregnant MSUD patients reported so far are scattered, but it seems that keeping the maternal plasma levels of the BCAA between 100 and 300 μmol/L is consistent with the delivery of a normal infant (37). Some patients who have an intermediate form of the disease with delayed and more moderate clinical symptoms will respond to the oral administration of thiamine, 100 to 1000 mg daily.

TABLE 15 Dietary Schedule for a Growth-Retarded MSUD Infant

Age: 9 months	Weight 4.6 kg
BCAA-free formula (MSUD 1)	14 g
Standard whey-formula	18 g
High-energy, protein-free product	30 g
No-protein pasta	45 g
Carrots	20 g
Potatoes	40 g
Summer squash	20 g
Olive oil	10 g
Mashed apple	100 g

Per kilogram daily intakes: energy 132 kcal, total protein 2.05 g

3.4 Histidinemia

Histidinemia is an autosomal recessive disorder of histidine (His) metabolism with an incidence range of 1 per 10,000 (Japan), 1 per 14,000 (Massachusetts), and 1 per 37,000 (Sweden). It is characterized by elevated His levels in both blood and urine due to a deficiency of histidase activity, which converts histidine to urocanic acid. The diagnosis is based on finding an elevation of His in the urine. Some patients have a speech defect and/or cognitive disability, while others have normal development of speech and intelligence. According to the most recent findings, histidinemia may be a benign biochemical finding and not a disorder needing dietary treatment. Indeed, in a large survey that included 58 Austrian patients treated with a His-restricted diet (35 mg/kg) and good metabolic control, no favorable effects of dietary treatment were observed as compared with 43 untreated patients (38). Clinical symptoms were found both in treated and untreated patients and, paradoxically, significantly higher IQ scores were found among the untreated patients. Scattered clinical responses to diet have also been reported (39). If treatment is considered in this example of a biochemical variant more than a disease, the principles of management should be the same as for phenylketonuria: a low His nitrogen supplement, with added vitamins and minerals, can be used to maintain normal growth and development. Recently an encapsulated histidase has been developed within cellulose-nitrate artificial cells for potential use in enzyme replacement therapy.

3.5 Inborn Errors of Metabolism Requiring a Modification of the Protein Source

3.5.1 Organic Acidemias

The most frequently recognized organic acidemias are propionic acidemia (PA) and methylmalonic acidemia (MMA). Both disorders are due to an alteration of propionate metabolism. Propionyl CoA is formed from the catabolism of four essential amino acids (isoleucine, valine, methionine, threonine), cholesterol, and odd-numbered long-chain fatty acids and is also produced by the anaerobic flora through fermentation in the gut. Different studies using stable isotopes have suggested that propionate derives from amino acids, oxidation of odd-chain fatty acids, and gut fermentation in percentages of 50, 30, and 20% respectively. Propionyl CoA is metabolized by an enzymatic reaction to methylmalonyl CoA, which is then converted to succinyl CoA. The missing lacking enzymes at the origin of PA and MMA are propionyl CoA carboxylase, which requires biotin as a cofactor, and methylmalonyl CoA mutase, which requires a cobalamin coenzyme (adenosylcobalamin, or AdoCbl) respectively. The inherited deficiency of propionyl CoA carboxylase activity is due to four different genetic defects involving the synthesis of the two carboxylase subunits and the enzymes that attach and cleave biotin to the subunits, holocarboxylase synthetase and biotinidase respectively. The inherited deficiency of methylmalonyl CoA mutase activity results from several genetic alterations involving either the mutase subunits or the cobalamin metabolism. All the disorders of propionate and methylmalonate metabolism are inherited as autosomal recessive traits. Most affected subjects have early dramatic manifestations in the neonatal period with refusal to feed, vomiting, lethargy, and hypotonia caused by severe metabolic acidosis. Dehydratation, seizures, and hepatomegaly occur less often. In some cases the presentation of clinical signs is delayed and patients suffer from acute encephalopathy, episodic ketoacidosis, and/or development retardation. Subjects with severe forms have recurrent episodes of decompensation precipitated by intercurrent febrile illnesses and gastroenteritis. Pathological alterations may involve brain, pancreas, heart, and blood cell lines, with the necessity to resort to blood transfusions. Laboratory tests show an increase of the propionic and methylmalonic acid in plasma and urine respectively, hyperammonemia, and a characteristic hyperglycinemia with a secondary deficiency of carnitine. The plasma and erythrocyte levels of odd-numbered long-chain fatty acids represent a finding that is often underrated. After being synthesized from the blocked compound, propionyl CoA, these molecules, which are normally absent, may be incorporated into the adipose tissue and then released during episodes of lipid oxidation (prolonged fasting, energy depletion, acute catabolic episodes), thus contributing significantly to the production of abnormal metabolites in a vicious cycle. The monitoring of plasma odd-numbered long-chain fatty acids has been proposed for checking the dietary control in both propionic and methylmalonic acidemia (40). Feeding problems are common (41). Vomiting and gastroesophageal reflux are often present and continuous or intermittent feeding is required to prevent catabolic states and the subsequent mobilization from adipose tissue stores of odd-numbered long-chain fatty acids. To maintain a good nutritional status, it is almost invariably necessary to give feeds via nasogastric tube or even gastrostomy. This may allow for nocturnal dietary supplies, helping to prevent endogenous protein catabolism and mobilization of adipose tissue stores. Therefore not just *what* is supplied (Table 16) but also *how* it is supplied is relevant to the achievement of successful therapy. The final aim is to prevent the excess accumulation of propionic acid, whatever its origin (from dietary amino acids and endogenous synthesis). The synthetic activity of the colonic fermenting flora may be controlled through the addition of oral metronidazole, which seems to be beneficial in reducing propionate production and excretion of the urinary metabolite. Carnitine supplements (100 mg/kg/day) are also widely used, since patients frequently have low plasma and tissue concentrations of free and total carnitine, with an increased ratio of acyl to total carnitine. In propionic acidemia, supplementation of biotin (10 mg/day) may be undertaken, since some patients may improve after their diets are enriched with this cofactor.

TABLE 16 Dietary Schedule for an Infant with Propionic Acidemia

Age: 4 months	Weight: 4.2 kg
High-energy protein-free product	64 g
Thre-, Iso-, Val-, and Met-free formula (OS 1)	14 g
Low-degree hydrolysate formula	22 g
Olive oil	10 g
Per kilogram daily intakes: energy 133 kcal, total protein 2.03 g	

In methylmalonic acidemia, some patients have a good response to a dose of vitamin B_{12} at a dosage of 1 mg/day. The dietary treatment of these patients is a challenge (42). The combination of several products and routes of administration is necessary and knowledge of the biochemical pathways connecting proteins, lipids, and carbohydrates is required to prevent untoward complications.

3.5.2 Urea Cycle Disorders

In mammals, the urea cycle is the major pathway for the metabolism of waste nitrogen. This cycle, which consists of five biochemical reactions (Fig. 1), is important to prevent the accumulation of toxic nitrogenous products and for the synthesis of arginine ex novo. One gram of protein contains about 0.16 g of nitrogen, which will be converted to 5.7 mmol of urea after complete catabolization. In children, a protein intake of 1.25 g/kg leads to the excretion of about 50% of urinary nitrogen as urea. The sources of nitrogen for urea synthesis are intra- and extrahepatic. In tissues other than the liver, the most relevant ammonium source is glutamine, while in the liver other amino acids may besides glutamine (alanine, aspartate, glycine, histidine, tryptophan, threonine, and lysine) may also give rise to ammonium. Defects in the synthesis of each of the five enzymes of the urea cycle have been described, with interindividual genetic and phenotypic variants. Urea cycle defects are all associated with hyperammonemia and increased plasma glutamine levels. The metabolism of other amino acids is also altered depending on the site of the metabolic block. The plasma amino acid levels proximal to the enzyme defect are increased, whereas those beyond the block are decreased. Four of these five diseases (carbamoyl-phosphate synthase (CPS), ornithine transcarbamoylase (OTC), argininosuccinate synthase (AS), and argininosuccinate lyase (AL) deficiency) are characterized by signs and symptoms due to the accumulation of urea precursors. The most serious clinical presentation occurs in full-term infants who are normal for 24 to 48 hr and then present with vomiting, irritability, progressive lethargy, apnea, and hypothermia. These forms may present later in infancy, childhood, and adulthood with episodic alter-

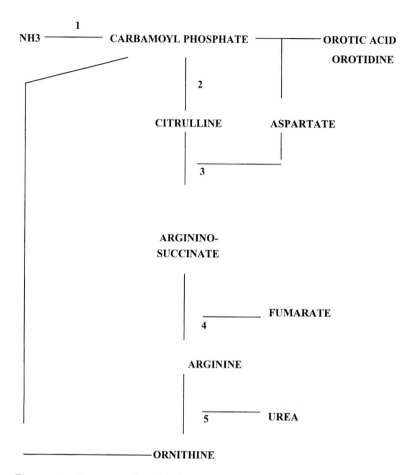

FIGURE 1 Enzymes involved in urea cycle disorders. (1) carbamoyl-phosphate synthase (CPS); (2) ornithine transcarbamoylase (OTC); (3) argininosuccinate synthase (AS); (4) argininosuccinate lyase (AL); (5) arginase.

ations of consciousness. The arginase deficiency is characterized by lower blood ammonium levels compared to other defects; the associated clinical picture consists of progressive spastic quadriplegia and mental retardation. Neurotoxicity has been attributed to high arginine levels. In the other enzymatic defects, the high concentrations of glutamine together with the associated increase in osmolality could be responsible for changes in the intracellular water content, leading to cerebral edema. It has also been suggested that some of the symptoms of hyperammonemia could be explained by an increase in brain serotonin secondary to a hyperammonemia-induced transport of tryptophan across the blood-brain barrier (43). All these defects are inherited as autosomal recessive traits except for the OTC deficiency, which is inherited as an X-linked disorder. Treatment aims to ensure that all nutritional needs are met while reducing the nitrogen flux through the urea cycle and utilizing alternative pathways of nitrogen excretion (44). When acute attacks develop, infants must be placed on a protein-free diet as a temporary measure. The same intervention is also recommended for the life-threatening conditions associated with the suspicion of an inborn error of protein metabolism. In the case of urea cycle disorders, a priority is to force the neonate into an anabolic phase with high-calorie feeds. Molecules facilitating the elimination of ammonium and nitrogen may be added (arginine, except for arginase deficiency, sodium benzoate, and phenylbutyric acid). Peripheral venous alimentation with glucose and lipids may be necessary. When gavage feeds are increased with protein-free products, peripheral alimentation should be decreased. After 4 to 5 days of no-protein, high-calorie, arginine- and benzoate-supplemented feeds, blood ammonia should revert to normal, and then a moderate addition of 1.0 to 1.5 g/kg/day of protein is necessary. The key issues of long-term therapy are reducing precursors of ammonia, correcting arginine deficiency, enhancing alternate mechanisms of waste nitrogen loss, and accelerating renal excretion of accumulated intermediates. Arginine deficiency, waste nitrogen, and accumulated intermediates are tackled by the same molecules used against acute attacks: L-arginine, sodium benzoate, and phenylbutyrate. The major dietary intervention is the reduction of ammonia precursors by protein restriction as well as prevention of body protein catabolism. Patients with severe forms of the disorder and those with marked protein aversion may need to be supplemented with essential amino acids (Table 17). Carnitine supplements may be necessary, as for any situation

TABLE 17   Dietary Schedule for a Case of Urea Cycle Disorder (Ornithine Carbamoyl Transferase Deficiency)

Age: 5 years; weight, 22.8 kg	
Essential amino acid mixture (UCD 2)	20 g
High-energy, protein-free product	80 g
No-protein pasta	170 g
No-protein biscuits	50 g
Whole cow's milk	130 g
Potatoes	180 g
Carrots	200 g
Apple	160 g
Olive oil	40 g
Per kg daily intakes: energy 88 kcal, protein 1.1 g	

in which protein-restricted diets are fed. Febrile episodes may precipitate life-threatening elevations in blood ammonia, requiring prompt diagnosis and treatment of the infection, decreased protein intake (even to zero), increased energy intake, and even peritoneal dialysis.

ACKNOWLEDGMENT

The help of Elvira Verduci, MD in preparing the manuscript is gratefully acknowledged.

REFERENCES

1. Scriver CR, Beaudet AL, Sly WS, Valle D. The Metabolic and Molecular Bases of Inherited Disease, 7th ed. New York: McGraw-Hill, 1995.
2. Koletzko B, Aggett PJ, Bindels JG, Bung P, Ferrè P, Gil A, Lentze MJ, Roberfroid M, Strobel S. Growth, development and differentiation: a functional food science approach. Br J Nutr 1998; 80(suppl 1):S5–S45.
3. DeRaeve L, De Meirleir L, Ramet J, Vandenplas Y, Gerlo E. Acrodermatitis enteropathic-like cutaneous lesions in organic aciduria. J Pediatr 1994; 124:416–420.
4. Hansen AE, Wiese HF, Boelsche AB. Role of linoleic acid in infant nutrition: clinical and chemical study of 428 infants fed on milk mixtures varying in kind and amount of fat. Pediatrics 1963; 31:171–192.
5. Mancini AJ, Tunnessen WW. Picture of the month. Acrodermatitis entreopatica-like rash in a breast-fed, full-term infant with zinc deficiency. Arch Pediatr Adolesc Med 1998; 152:1239–1240.
6. Hommes FA, Eller AG, Taylor EH. Turnover of the fast components of myelin and myelin proteins in experimental hyperphenylalaninemia: relevance to termination of dietary treatment in human PKU. J Inher Metab Dis 1982; 5:21–25.
7. Pardridge WM, Choi TD. Neutral amino acid transport at the blood-brain barrier. Fed Proc 1986; 45:2073–2078.
8. Bessman SP. Historical perspective: tyrosine and maternal phenylketonuria, welcome news. Am J Clin Nutr 1998; 67:357–358.
9. Guldberg P, Rey F, Zschocke J, Romano V, Francois B, Michiels L, Ullrich K, Hoffmann GF, Burgard P, Schmidt H, Meli C, Riva E, Dianzani I, Ponzone A, Rey J, Guttler F. A European multicenter study of phenylalanine-hydroxylase deficiency: classification of 105 mutations and a general system for genotype-based prediction of metabolic phenotype. Am J Hum Genet 1998; 63:71–79.
10. Zschocke J, Graham CA, Stewart FJ, Carson DJ, Nevin NC. Non-phenylketonuria hyperphenylalaninemia in Northern Ireland. Hum Mutat 1994; 4:114–118.
11. Smith I, Lobasher ME, Stevenson JE, Wolff OH, Schmidt H, Grubel-Kaiser S, Bickel H. Effect of stopping low-phenylalanine diet on intellectual progress of children with phenylketonuria. BMJ 1978; 2:723–726.
12. Seashore MR, Friedman E, Novelly RA, Bapat V. Loss of intellectual function in children with phenylketonuria after relaxation of dietary phenylalanine restriction. Pediatrics 1985; 75:226–232.

13. Levy HL, Waisbren SE. Effects of untreated maternal phenylketonuria and hyperphenylalaninemia on the fetus. N Engl J Med 1983; 309:1269–1274.
14. Smith I, Beasley MG, Wolff OH, Ades AE. Behavior disturbance in 8-year-old children with early treated phenylketonuria: report from the MRC/DHSS Phenylketonuria Register. J Pediatr 1988; 112:403–408.
15. Bick U, Fahrendorf G, Ludolph AG, Vasallo P, Weglage J, Ullrich K. Disturbed myelination in patients with treated hyperphenylalaninemias: evaluation with magnetic resonance imaging. Eur J Pediatr 1991; 150:185–189.
16. Korinthenberg R, Ullrich K, Fullenkemper F. Evoked potentials and electroencephalography in adolescents with phenylketonuria. Neuropediatrics 1988; 19:175–178.
17. Report of Medical Research Council Working Party on Phenylketonuria. Phenylketonuria due to phenylalanine hydroxylase deficiency: an unfolding story. BMJ 1993; 306:115–119.
18. Pardridge WM. Blood-brain barrier carrier-mediated transport and brain metabolism of amino acids. Neurochem Res 1998; 23:635–644.
19. Berry HK, Brunner RL, Hunt MM, White PP. Valine, isoleucine and leucine: a new treatment for phenylketonuria. Am J Dis Child 1990; 144:539–543.
20. Smith ML, Hanley WB, Clarke JT, Klim P, Schoonheit W, Austin V, Lehotay DC. Randomised controlled trial of tyrosine supplementation on neuropsychological performance in phenylketonuria. Arch Dis Child 1998; 78:116–121.
21. Galli C, Agostoni C, Mosconi C, Riva E, Salari PC, Giovannini M. Reduced plasma C-20 and C-22 polyunsaturated fatty acids in PKU children under dietary intervention. J Pediatr 1991; 114:562–567.
22. Uauy R, Peirano P, Hoffman D, Mena P. Birch D, Birch E. Role of essential fatty acids in the function of the developing nervous system. Lipids 1996; 31(suppl): S167–S176.
23. Agostoni C, Massetto N, Biasucci G, Basile I, Giovannini M, Riva E. Visual effects of long-chain polyunsaturated fatty acids in hyperphenylalaninemic children. Pediatr Res 1999; 45:911.
24. Levy HL, Ghavami M. Maternal phenylketonuria: a metabolic teratogen. Teratology 1996; 53:176–184.
25. Koch R, Levy HL, Matalon R, Rouse B, Hanley W, Azen C. The North-American Collaborative Study of maternal phenylketonuria: status report 1993. Am J Dis Child 1993; 147:1224–1230.
26. Smith I, Brenton DP. Hyperphenylalaninemias. In: Fernandes J, Saudubray JM, van der Berghe G, eds. Inborn Metabolic Diseases. 2nd ed. Berlin: Springer-Verlag, 1995, pp 147–160.
27. Riva E, Agostoni C, Biasucci G, Trojan S, Luotti D, Fiori L, Giovannini M. Early breastfeeding is linked to higher intelligence quotient scores in dietary treated phenylketonuric children. Acta Paediatr 1996; 85:56–58.
28. Cockburn F, Clark BJ. Recommendations for protein and amino acid intake in phenylketonuric patients. Eur J Pediatr 1996; 155(suppl 1):S125–S129.
29. Levy HL, Waisbren SE. PKU in adolescents: rationale and psychosocial factors in diet continuation. Acta Paediatr 1994; 407(suppl):92–97.
30. Rohr FJ, Lobbregt D, Levy HL. Tyrosine supplementation in the treatment of maternal phenylketonuria. Am J Clin Nutr 1998; 67:473–476.

31. Van Spronsen FJ, Thomasse Y, Smit GP, Leonard JV, Clayton PT, Fidler V, Berger R, Heymans HS. Hereditary tyrosinemia type I: a new classification with difference in prognosis on dietary treatment. Hepatology 1994; 20:1187–1191.

32. Holme E, Lindstedt S. Diagnosis and management of tyrosinemia type I. Curr Opin Pediatr 1995; 7:726–732.

33. Stamler JS, Slivka A. Biological chemistry of thiols in the vasculature and in vascular-related disease. Nutr Rev 1996; 1:1–30.

34. Koch R, Acosta PB, Williams JC. Nutritional therapy for pregnant women with a metabolic disorder. Clin Perinatol 1995; 22:1–14.

35. Cattaneo M. Hyperhomocysteinemia: a risk factor for arterial and venous thrombotic disease. Int J Clin Lab Res 1997; 27:139–144.

36. Gropper SS, Naglak MC, Nardella M, Plyler A, Rarback S, Yannicelli S. Nutrient intakes of adolescents with phenylketonuria and infants and children with maple syrup urine disease on semisynthetic diets. J Am Coll Nutr 1993; 12:108–114.

37. Van Calcar SC, Harding CO, Davidson SR, Barness LA, Wolff JA. Case reports of successful pregnancy in women with maple syrup urine disease and propionic acidemia. Am J Med Genet 1992; 44:641–646.

38. Widhalm K, Virmani K. Long-term follow-up of 58 patients with histidinemia treated with a histidine-restricted diet: no effect of therapy. Pediatrics 1994; 94:861–866.

39. Dyme IZ, Horwitz SJ, Bacchus B, Kerr DS. Histidinemia. A case with resolution of myoclonic seizures after treatment with a low-histidine diet. Am J Dis Child 1983; 137:256–258.

40. Wendel U. Abnormality of odd-numbered long-chain fatty acids in erythrocyte membrane lipids from patients with disorders of propionate metabolism. Pediatr Res 1989; 25:147–150.

41. Leonard JV. The management and outcome of propionic and methylmalonic acidemia. J Inher Metab Dis 1995; 18:430–434.

42. Van der Meer SB, Poggi F, Spada M, Bonnefont JP, Ogier H, Hubert P, Depondt E, Rapoport D, Rabier D, Charpentier C, Parvy P, Bardet J, Kamoun P, Saudubray JM. Clinical outcome and long-term management of 17 patients with propionic acidemia. Eur J Pediatr 1996; 155:205–210.

43. Bachmann C, Colombo JP. Increased tryptophan uptake into the brain in hyperammonaemia. Life Sci 1983; 33:2417–2424.

44. Feillet F, Leonard JV. Alternative pathway therapy for urea cycle disorders. J Inher Metab Dis 1998; 21(suppl 1):101–111.

45. Souci SW, Fachmann W, Kraut H. Food Composition and Nutrition Tables, 5th rev ed., Stuttgart, Germany: Medpharm Scientific Publishers, 1994.

19

Gastroesophageal Reflux

Colin D. Rudolph

Medical College of Wisconsin, Milwaukee, Wisconsin

Gastroesophageal reflux (GER) refers to the retrograde movement of gastric contents into the esophagus. Brief episodes of GER occur in normal infants, children, and adults. When refluxed material passes into the pharynx and out the mouth, then "spitting up" or vomiting occurs. In a small number of infants, GER may cause disease (GERD) characterized by chronic symptoms (Table 1). These include 1) malnutrition from inadequate caloric intake due to discomfort or from calorie loss due to vomiting, 2) esophageal symptoms of pain, inflammation and bleeding, and 3) airway symptoms of hoarseness and laryngitis, cough, apnea, and exacerbation of asthma or pneumonia. Establishing a clear relationship of any of these disorders to GER in an individual patient generally requires ruling out other potential causes of the disorder and subsequently demonstrating improvement following treatment of GER.

1 INCIDENCE OF GASTROESOPHAGEAL REFLUX

Half of all infants between 0 and 3 months of age and two-thirds of 4- to 6-month-old infants vomit at least once per day (1). The prevalence of vomiting decreases dramatically after 8 months of age. Typically infants with daily vom-

TABLE 1 Complications of Gastroesophageal Reflux

Disorders due to vomiting
Parental frustration
Iatrogenic weight loss due to limitations on feeding to prevent vomiting
Weight loss or inadequate weight gain from insufficient caloric intake
Disorders due to esophagitis
Dysphagia (may limit feedings, causing weight loss)
Chest pain, heartburn
Irritability and inconsolable crying in infants
Hematemesis, anemia, melena
Sandifer syndrome
Globus sensation
Barrett esophagus
Esophageal stricture
Respiratory disorders
Cough, hoarseness, stridor
Bronchospasm or wheezing
Apnea (especially obstructive)
Recurrent aspiration pneumonia or pulmonary fibrosis

---

iting outgrow this problem by 18 to 24 months of age and no evaluation or treatment is necessary (2). Clearly, all of these infants have gastroesophageal reflux, but the overwhelming majority of them are otherwise well and therefore do not have GERD.

The incidence of GER in normal children above 1 year of age is not known; however, some otherwise normal children continue to experience episodic vomiting with no other symptoms or problems. GER and esophagitis are rarely observed in normal children, but they are frequent in disabled children, with a prevalence of between 6 and 30% (3). Other patient groups with anatomic disorders such as tracheoesophageal fistula or laryngeal abnormalities may also be more prone to GERD due to either inadequate esophageal clearance or defective airway protective mechanisms.

2 PHYSIOLOGY OF GASTROESOPHAGEAL REFLUX

The lower esophageal sphincter (LES) is the major barrier that prevents reflux of gastric contents into the esophagus. It is composed of a specialized region of smooth muscle that is tonically contracted, maintaining a pressure barrier of 15 to 25 mmHg between the stomach and esophagus. Pressures are similar in the infant, older child, and adult. In the normal adult, this sphincter region is about 3 cm in length and is located at the level of the diaphragm. The crus of the diaphragm contributes an additional pressure barrier, contracting around the lower esophagus during inspiration (4). Thus, as intrathoracic pressure decreases and intraabdominal pressure increases during inspiration, the pressure barrier in the lower esophageal sphincter region increases. In the infant, the LES is located about 2 cm above the level of the diaphragm, so this additional diaphragmatic barrier function may be absent, increasing the propensity for GER.

When the stomach is distended, as after a meal, there are brief, transient episodes of lower esophageal sphincter relaxation. The gastric contents enter the esophagus and the upper esophageal sphincter contracts to prevent the gastric contents from entering the pharynx. The refluxate is then cleared from the esophagus by a series of peristaltic contractions that propel the contents back into the stomach. Residual acid is cleared from the esophageal wall during sequential swallows of saliva. The saliva contains bicarbonate, which dilutes and buffers the refluxed stomach acid. Although these episodes may occur many times each day, most individuals are unaware of them. Some individuals experience these episodes as painful, even in the absence of esophageal inflammation. If the mechanisms of esophageal clearance are ineffective, there is prolonged esophageal mucosal exposure to the caustic refluxed gastric contents, causing esophagitis (5).

When the esophageal wall is distended rapidly, the upper esophageal sphincter opens, allowing the gastric refluxate to pass into the pharynx. If air is refluxed from the stomach, belching occurs. When liquid or food is refluxed, spitting up or vomiting occurs. Prior to the opening of the upper esophageal sphincter, the vocal cords close, respiration ceases, and the larynx is pulled anteriorly as the epiglottis closes over the larynx (6). This laryngeal closure prevents aspiration of the refluxed material; if prolonged, however, it may cause apnea or laryngospasm with stridor. Following the episode of pharyngeal reflux, the material is cleared from the pharynx by either vomiting or swallowing, and breathing resumes. Abnormalities of these airway-protective mechanisms will potentially result in airway symptoms from inadvertent exposure of the larynx and airway to caustic materials. The small capacity of the esophagus and recumbent posture (lack of gravity) in the infant make it more likely that refluxed material will fill the esophagus and pass into the pharynx. Thus, the infant is more likely to regurgitate or vomit when GER occurs. If an infant lacks adequate airway-protective mechanisms, the more frequent reflux of gastric contents into the mouth makes the infant more likely to experience airway complications of GER than the adult.

3 DIAGNOSTIC TESTS FOR GASTROESOPHAGEAL REFLUX DISEASE

The differential diagnosis and diagnostic tests utilized for the evaluation of GER vary depending upon the presenting symptom. No test serves as the "gold stan-

TABLE 2 Strengths and Weaknesses of Diagnostic Tests for GERD with Different Symptom Presentations

Diagnostic test	Vomiting[a]	Esophageal disorders[b]	Airway disorders[c]
Upper GI contrast study	Defines other defects such as malrotation, achalasia, webs; GER observed in normal studies	Defines anatomic abnormalities; Rarely detects mucosal abnormalities	May detect aspiration but lacks sensitivity; May identify TEF[d], laryngeal cleft, vascular rings, other anatomic defects
Esophageal pH monitoring	Likely normal	Prolonged acid exposure correlates with risk for esophagitis; Cannot rule out presence of other types of esophagitis such as infection or eosinophilic esophagitis	Prolonged esophageal acid exposure may increase risk for GER-induced asthma; Laryngeal symptoms and airway symptoms may occur with normal results
Esophageal pH monitoring plus pneumogram	Not useful	Not useful	May establish relationship of GER and apnea or other pulmonary symptoms; Sensitivity is lacking so that symptoms may be related but study cannot prove causal effect
Nuclear scintigraphy	Can detect abnormalities of gastric emptying	Can demonstrate poor esophageal clearance but predictive value for esophagitis unclear	May detect episodes of aspiration but sensitivity unclear
Chest radiograph or CT scan	Not useful	Not useful	May show characteristic changes suggestive of aspiration but unable to determine if occurs with swallowing or GER

Bronchoscopy with lipid-laden macrophages	Not useful	Not useful	High numbers of lipid-laden macrophages suggest aspiration as cause of lung disease
Swallowing studies (videofluoroscopic or fiberendoscopic)	Not useful	Not useful	Can aid by demonstrating normal airway protection with swallowing, making GER more likely cause of aspiration; May demonstrate defective airway protective mechanisms indicating increased risk of aspiration when GER occurs
Laryngoscopy	Not useful	Not useful	May demonstrate laryngeal erythema, nodularity or swelling suggestive of GERD but sensitivity and specificity unclear
Empirical medical therapy	Not useful	Improvement suggests symptoms are due to GER; Disease severity and risk of sequelae are not evaluated; Empiric treatment doses not established in pediatric patients	Improvement suggests symptoms are due to GER; Empiric treatment doses not established in pediatric patients

a Vomiting may be associated with malnutrition and may occur in combination with esophageal or airway disorders.
b Esophageal disorders include pain, irritability, esophagitis, anemia, and Sandifer syndrome.
c Airway disorders include laryngeal inflammation with hoarseness or stridor and recurrent pneumonia.
d TEF, tracheoesophageal fistula.

dard'' for making a diagnosis of GERD. A series of tests may be required to determine if a particular disorder is being caused by GER. A detailed discussion of some of these tests is presented in Chapter 32. The following discussion and Table 2 briefly summarize the key pathophysiological questions relating to GER that are addressed by each test.

Radiographic imaging of the upper gastrointestinal tract (UGI) is useful to diagnose anatomic or physiological abnormalities that cause symptoms similar to those observed in GERD. A radiopaque dye (usually barium sulfate) is administered orally and the transit through the esophagus, stomach, and upper intestine is observed fluoroscopically. Anatomic disorders that may cause nonbilious vomiting—such as esophageal stricture, pyloric stenosis, or antral webs—can be identified. Disorders of esophageal motility such as achalasia may also be recognized. The UGI is not useful for diagnosis of GER because reflux of ingested radiographic contrast often occurs in normal individuals. However, many patients with potential complications from GER will require an UGI to rule out other potential causes of the presenting symptom.

Esophageal pH monitoring utilizes a pH sensor to record the number and duration of acid reflux episodes into the lower and/or upper esophagus (7). Prolonged esophageal mucosal exposure increases the risk for esophagitis; therefore this test is helpful to determine the risk of esophagitis. Apnea, aspiration pneumonia, and other complications of GER can occur in patients even when esophageal pH exposure is in the normal range, so that a ''normal'' pH probe result does not exclude GER as a possible causative factor. If the pH probe is combined with a pneumogram that measures oxygen saturation as well as chest wall and airflow movements, a clearer cause-and-effect relationship between some airway symptoms and episodes of GER may be evident. Unfortunately, these time-consuming and technically challenging tests often fail to clarify the relationship of airway symptoms and GER.

Nuclear scintigraphy evaluates the distribution of isotope-labeled formula or food following normal feeding. Episodes of GER are monitored for up to an hour after feeding. Since GER may occur in normal individuals, documentation of these episodes is of little pathophysiological significance. However, if aspiration into the lungs is detected, this provides a clear indication that airway protective mechanisms are deficient. No prospective trials have evaluated the value of nuclear scintigraphy for the evaluation of patients with possible GERD. The sensitivity and specificity of this test for any symptom presentation of GERD is unknown (8).

In children with recurrent pneumonia, thought possibly due to GER, a variety of other tests may be indicated. The *chest radiograph or computed tomography (CT)* examination may reveal changes suggestive of aspiration. Similarly, *bronchoscopy* can be combined with measurements of lipid-laden macrophage numbers in pulmonary washings to determine if aspiration has occurred. Although some lipid-laden macrophages are present in many normal infants and children, large numbers suggest likely aspiration. These tests cannot determine if aspiration is occurring with swallowing or following episodes of GER. Therefore, studies assessing airway protective mechanisms during swallowing may also be useful in managing patients with pulmonary disease thought to be possibly related to GER. A videofluoroscopic swallowing study (VSS) examines the flow of contrast material through the mouth and pharynx to evaluate the mechanics of swallowing (see Chap. 32). Similarly, a fiberendoscopic evaluation of swallowing (FEES) evaluates the movement of food through the pharynx. Exclusion of aspiration during swallowing suggests that aspiration occurs with GER. If aspiration does occur with swallowing, it is very likely that aspiration will also occur with episodes of GER. Thus, it is essential to evaluate the findings on each of these tests carefully, with management decisions being individualized.

Laryngoscopy can identify changes in laryngeal appearance, that may result from GER, including erythema, nodularity, and swelling. The specificity and sensitivity of these findings in relation to GER have not been well studied in children, but the response to GERD therapy can be followed relatively easily. Other disorders such as allergy likely cause similar changes in laryngeal appearance.

Empirical therapy with medications used to treat GER may also be considered a diagnostic test. Relief of pain or other symptoms following therapy with subsequent recurrence off therapy provides a reasonable indication that GER may be contributing to chronic symptom.

4 COMPLICATIONS OF GASTROESOPHAGEAL REFLUX: EVALUATION AND TREATMENT

The disorders associated with GER are best classified into three major categories: 1) vomiting with malnutrition, 2) esophageal disorders, and 3) airway or respiratory disorders (Table 1). Other atypical symptoms attributed to GER include recurrent otitis media, sinusitis, and dental erosion, but the relationship of these to GER in children is poorly documented. In an infant with none of these complications, GER should be considered a variation of normal and no therapy given. In older children, chronic or recurrent vomiting may be nonpathological but warrants investigation for associated disorders.

The differential diagnosis and diagnostic tests utilized for the evaluation of GER vary depending upon the presenting symptom. The use of these tests for varying symptom presentations is briefly discussed above. The following section focuses on the best strategy for the evaluation and treatment of specific symptom presentations in an individual patient. Treatment options may vary depending upon the type and severity of symptoms. A more in-depth discussion of various treatment approaches is provided later in the chapter.

4.1 Vomiting

The approach to the infant with chronic spitting up is outlined in Figure 1. The initial evaluation of an infant with vomiting focuses on excluding other possible anatomic, metabolic, and neurological causes of vomiting before assuming that simple GER is responsible for the vomiting. A history and physical exam is usually adequate to determine if other tests are required to rule out other causes of vomiting. Infants with bilious vomiting, hematemesis, forceful vomiting, abdominal distension, fever, lethargy or other neurological signs, or hepatosplenomegaly should never be assumed to be vomiting just from GER. Disorders such as pyloric stenosis and antral webs may present with nonbilious vomiting. Other anatomic disorders such as Hirschsprung disease, intussusception, and malrotation may also present with vomiting. Similarly, various infections—including meningitis, urinary tract infections, and even otitis media—may cause vomiting. Renal insufficiency, adrenal insufficiency, inborn errors of metabolism, and formula intolerances must also be considered as potential etiologies for chronic vomiting. Diagnostic tests may include an UGI, serum electrolyte studies, urinalysis, and a head CT scan, depending upon the exam and history. If the infant is an otherwise well, ''spitty'' baby that is growing steadily, evaluation and management should be limited to parental reassurance and education regarding the potential warning signs of GER complications.

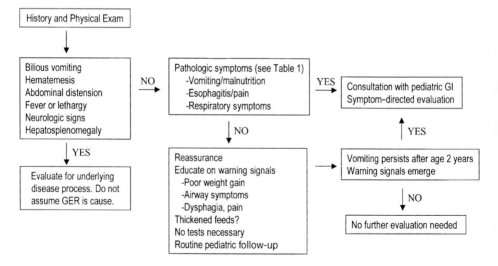

FIGURE 1   Evaluation of the infant with vomiting.

4.2 Malnutrition and Vomiting

Excessive vomiting due to GER is often cited as a cause of malnutrition in infants. However, in most cases, the poor weight gain is not caused by an inability of the infant to "keep down" adequate calories. Instead, the most common scenario is that the parent of a "spitty" baby reduces the volume and frequency of formula administered to the infant in an effort to reduce the amount of vomiting. The ensuing weight loss is the result of the restricted, inadequate intake and not of excessive vomiting. In these cases, treatment should focus on reassuring and educating the parents about the normal character and frequency of regurgitant vomiting in infants. Usually, no other intervention is required.

In some infants with malnutrition and vomiting, the parents offer adequate amounts of oral feeds but the infant ingests inadequate amounts of formula. Vomiting may not be a major contributing factor to poor growth so that other etiologies need to be considered (see Chap. 12). However, it is very difficult to exclude GER-induced esophagitis as a cause of pain and feeding refusal (9). Therefore, in these infants, an empirical trial of pharmacological therapy for GER may be considered. Alternatively, upper endoscopy with biopsy may be useful to rule out esophagitis as a cause of feeding refusal.

Rarely, severe GER is associated with enough vomiting to prevent growth despite adequate caloric consumption. In these infants, who eat vigorously and then vomit, "conservative" therapeutic measures are usually adequate. These include thickening of formula and/or increasing the caloric concentration of the formula, decreasing the volume of each feed and increasing the frequency of feeding (every 2 to 2 ½ hr), position changes, and possibly the use of prokinetic medications to improve gastric emptying and esophageal reflux. In very unusual cases, supplemental nasogastric nighttime drip feedings may be required to assure that adequate calories are delivered to the infant.

4.3 Esophageal Disorders

Poor esophageal clearance of refluxed gastric contents with prolonged exposure of the mucosal lining to acid causes mucosal inflammation or *esophagitis* (10). GER is the most common cause of esophagitis, but other etiologies—such as infection, allergy, or autoimmune disorders—can also cause esophagitis. In some individuals, acid exposure alone may cause pain even in the absence of inflammation, whereas in others there may be marked inflammation and no pain. In infants, irritability or feeding refusal may be the presenting symptom of esophagitis. Older children usually complain of chest pain or dysphagia. Some children may respond to the esophageal pain with repetitive stretching and arching movements, known as Sandifer syndrome, that are often mistakenly thought to be atypical seizures or dystonia.

More severe inflammation may cause chronic blood loss, presenting with anemia, hematemesis, or melena. If the inflammation is untreated, circumferential scarring or strictures may form, presenting with dysphagia. Chronic inflammation may also trigger mucosal replacement with a metaplastic, premalignant epithelium known as a Barrett esophagus. Diagnosis and treatment of esophagitis prior to the development of these chronic complications is desirable.

When milder symptoms of possible esophagitis, such as pain or irritability, occur in an otherwise normal child, it is reasonable to assess the response to a time-limited trial (2 to 3 months) of empirical medical therapy. More prolonged therapy should never be instituted without performing endoscopic evaluation of the esophagus to assess the degree of esophageal mucosal damage and risk of chronic complications. Empirical therapy is also contraindicated in any child with a potential predisposition to other causes of esophagitis, such as infection due to immunodeficiency. Upper endoscopy with biopsy is preferable to esophageal pH monitoring because it delineates the degree of mucosal damage (which does not correlate with the degree of abnormality on esophageal pH monitoring studies), and biopsies identify complicating lesions such as a Barrett esophagus as well as those due to other etiologies than GER (see Chap. 32). Usually, if GER is confirmed as the likely cause of esophageal symptoms, pharmacological therapy is instituted. Symptoms and mucosal healing should be monitored. Occasionally, surgical therapy is a reasonable alternative, although the potential complications must be balanced with the nuisance, risks, and cost of long-term administration of pharmacological therapy.

4.4 Airway Disorders

GER is associated with a variety of airway disorders including apnea, stridor, hoarseness, reactive airway disease, and recurrent pneumonia. Understanding the pathophysiology of the relationship of each disorder and GER helps to select appropriate diagnostic and treatment strategies. Symptoms result from either aberrant reflex protective events or from inflammation caused by exposure of the respiratory epithelium to the caustic gastric contents.

4.4.1 Apnea

Apnea may be associated with GER in infants. Typically, GER-related apnea occurs shortly after feeding in the awake infant (11). The infant often seems startled and exhibits respiratory efforts followed by mild cyanosis due to laryngospasm. Almost invariably, these episodes resolve spontaneously within seconds, with no sequelae, although they are frightening to the parent. Rarely, more severe episodes occur which are more prolonged, with more severe cyanosis. As the infant matures the episodes become less frequent, and they rarely recur by

6 to 8 months of age. No association of central apnea during sleep and GER has been demonstrated. Diagnostic testing may not be fruitful since the episodes often occur infrequently and may not occur during the test. Other causes of obstructive apnea, such as innominate artery airway compression, must be ruled out. In addition, apneic episodes can be confused with a seizure disorder or may occur with other central nervous system disorders. After excluding other potential causes of apnea, medical therapy with a combination of formula thickening, positioning, and pharmacological therapies (antisecretory and prokinetic) is usually adequate. In rare cases, the episodes are severe enough to warrant the risks of surgical therapy.

4.4.2   Asthma

Asthma or infant wheezing may be exacerbated by GER (12). Either esophageal acid exposure or microaspiration appears to stimulate vagal reflexes that cause airway constriction. Medical therapy, including newer proton-pump inhibitor therapies may improve asthma symptoms but do not appear to improve lung function (13). However, in selected patients with GER and asthma, surgical therapy appears to markedly decrease symptoms. Many previously steroid dependent asthmatics with GER improve following fundoplication (14). Unfortunately, there are no good tests to determine which patient will respond well to surgery. Patients with known esophagitis or prolonged acid exposure during esophageal pH monitoring appear to be more likely to improve with surgery.

4.4.3   Laryngeal Inflammation

Mucosal inflammation, granulation, vocal cord nodules, and stricture may result if gastric contents penetrate the laryngeal inlet. Clearance of acid from the larynx is very inefficient so that even infrequent episodes of laryngeal penetration by stomach acid may result in epithelial damage. Laryngeal symptoms such as *hoarseness* or *stridor* may be caused by GER, even in the absence of esophageal inflammation (15). The larynx appears erythematous and swollen. In contrast to asthma, GER-related laryngeal disease appears to respond well to aggressive medical therapy, but symptoms often recur when therapy is discontinued. GER may also impair healing following laryngeal surgery; therefore evaluation for GER prior to surgery may be useful.

4.4.4   Recurrent Pneumonia

Pneumonia with resulting chronic pulmonary fibrosis is the most serious airway complication of GER. The quantity of aspirated material required to cause pneumonia is unknown. As with laryngeal symptoms, GER-related aspiration pneumonia frequently arises in the absence of esophageal disease (16–18). Refluxed gastric contents enter the pharynx and inadequate airway protective mechanisms allow the caustic material to penetrate the larynx and pass into the lungs. Although aspiration of acid appears to be more damaging than aspiration of water, neutral buffering of the stomach contents may lead to a higher incidence of bacterial pneumonia, presumably because the reduced gastric acidity allows bacterial colonization of the stomach, so that aspiration of gastric contents, increases bacterial soiling of the lungs. The diagnostic evaluation differs from that for esophagitis, being more focused on the clinical history and on findings indicating aspiration, such as characteristic radiographic studies and high numbers of lipid-laden macrophages on pulmonary lavage (19). Studies of swallowing function may be helpful, since those children with documented disorders of airway protection during swallowing are more likely to have aspiration during GER episodes. Before invoking GER as the cause of recurrent pneumonia, other causes of recurrent pneumonia such as an anatomic abnormality (laryngeal cleft, tracheoesophageal fistula, vascular ring, pulmonary sequestration), aspiration during swallowing, foreign body, cystic fibrosis, or immunodeficiency must be ruled out. The role of medical therapy remains uncertain, but it is clear that surgical therapy is effective at preventing GER-related pneumonias.

5 TREATMENT OF GASTROESOPHAGEAL REFLUX DISEASE

A variety of different treatments are potentially useful for the treatment of gastroesophageal reflux disease (Table 3). The least aggressive therapy is conservative therapy requiring "lifestyle" changes. These involve changes in position and diet. Pharmacological therapy provides another option, usually being focused on either decreasing the number of GER episodes or on decreasing the acidity of refluxed gastric contents, thereby making them less caustic. Finally, surgical therapies, which are very effective for preventing GER, can be considered, but the high rate of complications mandates that surgical therapy be reserved for patients in whom medical therapy is not likely to prevent serious sequelae.

Selecting the approach to treatment depends upon the presenting symptom's type and severity. The clinical scenario dictates decisions regarding the urgency for initiating treatment and the aggressiveness of therapy. For example, in a child with mild pulmonary symptoms that may be a complication of GER, medical therapy would be considered. In contrast, in a child with severe pulmonary disease with GER as a potential contributing factor, surgical therapy may be selected. A dogmatic approach that escalates the type of therapy, regardless of the clinical scenario, is ill advised. The following section discusses each type of therapy. Table 3 summarizes the therapeutic options commonly used for treatment of GERD in children. Table 4 lists the medication doses commonly used to treat GERD in infants and children.

TABLE 3 Treatment of Gastroesophageal Reflux Disease

Conservative therapy/"lifestyle changes"
Positional changes
   Infant—supine position with head elevated
      (unless high risk from GER; then consider prone)
   Older child—head of bed elevated
Nutritional therapy
   Infant—
     Thicken feedings
      1 to 2 tbsp rice cereal/30 mL (1 oz) formula
      Commercial formulas with thickening agents
     Increase caloric density of formula with concentration
     Small frequent feeds (2.5 hr between feeds)
   Child—
     Avoid caffeinated beverages, peppermint, and chocolate
     Weight loss if obese
   Rarely, nasogastric or nasojejunal feeding may be required
Smoking cessation or decreased passive smoke exposure

Pharmacologic therapy
   Antacids
   Barrier agents
   Antisecretory agents
     H_2-receptor blockers
     Proton-pump inhibitors
   Prokinetic agents

Surgical therapy
   Nissen fundoplication
   Thal fundoplication
   Esophagogastric disconnection

5.1 Conservative Therapies

5.1.1 Lifestyle and Dietary Changes

In adults, changes in diet (avoidance of peppermints, chocolate, onions, fatty and spicy foods), avoidance of alcohol, weight loss, and smoking cessation are often recommended for treatment of GERD based on very limited data. In infants, one study showed a slight increase in GER when infants are exposed to passive smoking (20), but another showed no increase in GER in children with parents who smoke (18). Studies of the effects of other lifestyle factors on GERD have not been performed in children. Therefore, recommendations of weight loss, de-

TABLE 4 Pharmacological Treatment of Gastroesophageal Reflux Disease

Type of medication	Recommended oral dosage	Side effects/ precautions
H$_2$-receptor antagonists		
Cimetidine (Tagamet)	40mg/kg/day divided tid or qid (max 500 mg tid)	Rash, bradycardia, dizziness, gyneco-mastia, reduce hepatic metabolism of theophylline and other medications
Ranitidine (Zantac)	9 to 12 mg/kg/day divided tid (max 150mg tid)	Headache, dizziness, rash, constipation, diarrhea
Famotodine (Pepcid)	1 to 2 mg/kg/day divided bid (max 20 mg bid)	Headache, dizziness, constipation, diarrhea, nausea
Proton-pump inhibitors		
Omeprazole (Prilosec)	1 to 3.5 mg/kg/day divided qd or bid (max 20 mg qd)	Headache, diarrhea, abdominal pain, nausea
Lanzoprazole (Prevacid)	1.5 to 3.5 mg/kg/day divided qd or bid (max 30 mg qd)	Headache, diarrhea, abdominal pain, nausea
Rabeprazole (Aciphex)	Adult dose: 20 mg qd	Headache, diarrhea, abdominal pain, nausea
Prokinetic		
Cisapride (Propulsid)	0.8 mg/kg/day divided qid (max 10 mg qid or 20 mg bid)	Available only by limited access protocol due to safty concerns

creased smoking or smoke exposure, and avoidance of foods that may exacerbate GER are reasonable for other health-related reasons, but their efficacy as treatment of GERD is lacking.

In infants, dietary changes have been shown to decrease symptoms of GER and to improve weight gain. Thickening of formula decreases the number of episodes of vomiting but does not decrease the amount of time the esophagus is exposed to acid. In the United States, thickening has usually been achieved with the addition of rice cereal to formula (1 to 2 tbsp per ounce of formula) (21). Administration of this thick formula requires that the nipple be ''cross-cut'' to improve the flow rate. Newer formulas containing thickening agents such as carob flour and locust bean gum (Enfamil AR, Nutrilon AR) are now available and appear to be as effective (22). Furthermore, they do not require use of a cross-cut nipple. In infants with poor weight gain, simply increasing the caloric density of the formula may promote weight gain. Occasionally, administration of nighttime nasogastric feeding may be useful to supplement calories administered orally during the daytime. Rarely, nasojejunal feeding may be helpful as a temporary strategy to promote weight gain or prevent pulmonary complications of GER.

5.1.2 Positioning Changes

In adults, upright posture following meals and elevation of the head of bed during sleep has been shown to decrease the number of GER episodes. In children, similar recommendations are reasonable. Head-of-bed elevation is most easily achieved by placing a wedge under the mattress or by placing blocks under the legs at the head of the bed. An angle of 20 to 35 degrees is desirable but not always practical. In infants, prone positioning is effective to decrease GER episodes as compared with either the supine position or the supine upright (infant seat) position. However, concerns about the markedly increased risk of sudden infant death (SIDS) in the prone position versus supine position (14-fold increased risk) make the recommendation of prone positioning for treatment of GERD questionable (23). Left lateral positioning appears to be almost as effective as prone positioning for GER prevention, so that some authorities may recommend the use of side positioning (24). Unfortunately, it is difficult to maintain infants in this position and they are likely to roll over to the prone position. At this time, it seems reasonable to recommend that infants with GER be positioned in the supine position. Prone positioning should not be recommended except when the supine sleeping position results in adverse effects that outweigh the potential risk of SIDS. When prone positioning is necessary, it is recommended that parents be advised not to use sheepskin or other soft bedding, quilts, or pillows.

5.2 Pharmacological Therapy

Pharmacological therapies are directed to either reducing gastric acid secretion or reducing the amount and frequency of reflux by improving esophageal and gastric motility. A variety of agents have been used in the past, but there is little evidence to support the efficacy of many of these, as discussed below.

5.2.1 Antacids and Sodium Alginate

These agents have historically been used for the treatment of GER in both infants and adults. Antacids are difficult to administer in adequate amounts to infants and children. Limited information suggests that sodium alginate may decrease episodes of GER in infants, but the formulation utilized is unavailable in the United States (25). Therefore, neither of these agents is generally employed for the management of GERD in infants or children.

5.2.2 H₂-Receptor Antagonists (H₂RA)

These agents block the stimulatory effects of histamine on acid secretion by the gastric parietal cells. Numerous studies in adults demonstrate the efficacy of H_2RA therapy of heartburn and esophagitis, but there is only one randomized placebo-controlled trial that demonstrates efficacy in infants or children (26). Despite this lack of data, these agents are thought to be relatively effective if given in adequate doses. The doses recommended by manufacturers are generally less than that shown to be effective in the clinical setting (see Table 4). Aside from some differences in complication rates and drug interactions, no H_2RA seems to have greater efficacy than other agents in the class.

5.2.3 Proton-Pump Inhibitors

These agents inactivate the proton-pump that secretes gastric acid. There are no randomized controlled trials of proton pump inhibitors in infants or children. However, based on multiple case series of pediatric patients refractory to previous treatment regimens, omeprazole appears to be highly effective treatment for severe esophagitis, resulting in both symptomatic and endoscopic improvement while on treatment (27). However, prolonged therapy is necessary for treatment of esophagitis, with recurrence following cessation of therapy (28). The lack of dosing, efficacy and side effect information in infants and young children limits the use of these agents, but it is likely that they will supplant H_2RA's as the mainstay of anti-secretory therapy for GERD in children in the near future.

5.2.4 Prokinetic Therapy

These agents improve gastrointestinal motility, which theoretically should decrease vomiting and improve esophageal clearance. However, there is little evidence to support the efficacy of any of the agents currently available. Bethanechol has limited efficacy and a high rate of unacceptable side effects. Metoclopramide and domperidone have not been shown to be effective. Cisapride has been shown to reduce GER symptoms and promote healing of esophagitis in children (29). It also has been shown to be of some benefit in children with recurrent bronchopulmonary disease and in infants with repetitive short episodes of apnea (30). However, recent concerns about the safety of cisapride have resulted in its withdrawal from the marketplace. It is only available on a limited access protocol basis, making its use impractical in most circumstances.

5.2.5 Empirical Medical Therapy

To determine if a variety of symptoms are either caused or exacerbated by GER, a trial of aggressive medical therapy may provide the best and most cost effective diagnostic test. Alleviation of symptoms after the administration of high doses of proton-pump inhibitors and recurrence when medical therapy is discontinued has been shown to be cost effective for the evaluation of a relationship of GER and pain or laryngeal symptoms in adult patients. Empiric therapeutic trials have not been useful for establishing a relationship of GER and asthma in adults. Because the appropriate dose of proton-pump inhibitors are less well defined in pediatric patients, this approach may be more expensive (need to confirm adequate therapy in patients that fail treatment by doing esophageal pH monitoring) than in the adult population. However, it may remain the best single test to establish whether GER is contributing to symptoms such as pain or laryngeal symptoms.

5.3 Surgical Therapy

Surgical therapy is generally reserved for patients who are unresponsive to conservative medical therapy, lifestyle changes, and pharmacological therapy. The overwhelming majority of these patients have respiratory complications of GER. A smaller group of patients have severe esophagitis with stricture or Barrett esophagus. Various surgical approaches are available but none of these has been demonstrated to be superior in regard to complication rates or efficacy (33). Laparascopic fundoplication has gained popularity due to the more rapid postoperative recovery time, but there is no evidence that morbidity or outcome differs from the results of conventional surgical techniques (14).

Nissen fundoplication is by far the most popular procedure (see Chap. 33). The operative mortality is about 1%. Major complications occur in 10 to 15% of patients; they include breakdown of the fundoplication wrap, intrathoracic herniation of the wrap, slipping of the wrap over the body of the stomach, and bowel obstruction. Less serious complications that often profoundly affect a patient's comfort and life include gas bloat, dysphagia, dumping syndrome, gagging, and retching. Gas bloat with abdominal distention and postprandial discomfort occurs in about 30% of children following fundoplication. The symptoms resolve over time in many but not all patients. Dysphagia in the early postoperative period is seen in about one-third of patients. Dumping syndrome occurs occasionally after fundoplication, with symptoms of postprandial pallor, sweating, lethargy, and diarrhea (34). Children with dumping syndrome may refuse to feed because the negative experience of hypoglycemia is temporally associated with feeding. Gagging or retching occurs in about 10 to 15% of patients following fundoplication. Because of this high incidence of complications, some authorities advocate the use of a loose wrap or Thal procedure in all children. This approach may be particularly useful in children with disorders of esophageal motility, but overall complication rates appear to be similar. The incidence of all complications of Nissen fundoplication appears to be higher in children with neurological disorders; however, these children are most likely to require surgical therapy for GER due to their poor airway-protective mechanisms.

Some children have persistent symptoms of gas bloat, solid dysphagia, dumping syndrome, retching, or gagging. Because of these concerns, it is reasonable to assure that alternative medical therapies fail before recommending surgical therapy. When surgery is required, it is essential that the parents be made aware of the risk of these complications. Despite the potential complications, surgical intervention is very likely to prevent further GER-induced airway complications, which may prevent repeated episodes of airway disease, pulmonary failure, and even death.

An alternative approach to the prevention of gastroesophageal reflux that has been advocated for use in children with severe neurological disease is esophagogastric disconnection (35). This operation will prevent GERD but will also require a lifelong gastrostomy for venting and feeding. It should be considered only following failure of other medical and surgical treatment methods.

REFERENCES

1. Nelson SP, Chen EH, Syniar GM, Christoffel KK. Prevalence of symptoms of gastroesophageal reflux during infancy: a pediatric practice–based survey. Pediatric Practice Research Group. Arch Pediatr Adolesc Med 1997; 151:569–572.
2. Nelson SP, Chen EH, Syniar GM, Christoffel KK. One-year follow-up of symptoms of gastroesophageal reflux during infancy. Pediatrics 1998; 102(6):E67.
3. Del Giudice E, Staiano A, Capano G, Florimonte L, Miele E, Ciarla C, Campanozzi A, Crisanti AF. Gastrointestinal manifestations in children with cerebral palsy. Brain Dev 1999; 21307–21311.
4. Heine KJ, Dent J, Mittal RK. Anatomical relationship between crural diaphragm and lower esophageal sphincter: an electrophysiological study. J Gastrointest Motil 1993; 5:89–95.
5. Kawahara H, Dent J, Davidson G. Mechanisms responsible for gastroesophagal reflux in children. Gastroenterology 1997; 113:399–408.

6. Lang IM, Medda BK, Ren J, Shaker R. Characterization and mechanisms of the pharyngoesophageal inhibitory reflex. Am J Physiol 1998; 275:G1127–G1136.
7. Colletti RB, Christie DL, Orenstein SR. Indications for pediatric esophageal pH monitoring. J Pediatr Gastroenterol Nutr 1995; 21:253–262.
8. Fawcett H, Hayden C, Adams J, Swischuck L. How useful is gastroesophageal reflux scintigraphy in suspected childhood aspiration? Pediatr Radiol 1988; 18:311–313.
9. Mathisen B, Worrall L, Masel J, Wall C, Shepherd RW. Feeding problems in infants with gastro-oesophageal reflux disease: a controlled study. J Paediatr Child Health 1999; 35:163–169.
10. Black DD, Haggitt RC, Orenstein SR, Whitington PF. Esophagitis in infants: morphometric histological diagnosis and correlation with measures of gastroesophageal reflux. Gastroenterology 1990; 98:1408–1414.
11. Spitzer AR, Boyle JT, Tuchman DN, Fox WW. Awake apnea associated with gastroesophageal reflux: a specific clinical syndrome. J Pediatr 1984; 104:200–205.
12. Sheikh S, Stephen T, Howell L, Eid N. Gastroesophageal reflux in infants with wheezing. Pediatr Pulmonol 1999; 28:181–186.
13. Field SK, Sutherland, LR. Does medical antireflux therapy improve asthma in asthmatics with gastroesophageal reflux? A critical review of the literature. Chest 1998; 114:275–283.
14. Rothenberg SS, Bratton D, Larsen G, Deterding R, Milgrom H, Brugman S, Boguniewicz M, Copenhaver S, White C, Wagener J, Fan L, Chang J, Stathos T. Laparoscopic fundoplication to enhance pulmonary function in children with severe reactive airway disease and gastroesophageal reflux disease. Surg Endosc 1997; 11:1088–1090.
15. Gumpert L, Kalach N, Dupont C, Contencin P. Hoarseness and gastroesophageal reflux in children. J Laryngol Otol 1998; 112:49–54.
16. Tovar JA, Angulo JA Gorostiaga L, Arana J. Surgery for gastroesophageal reflux in children with normal pH studies. J Pediatr Surg 1991; 26:541–545.
17. Ahrens P, Heller K, Beyer P, Zielen S, Kuhn C, Hofmann D, Encke A. Antireflux surgery in children suffering from reflux-associated respiratory disease. Pediatr Pulmonol 1999; 28:89–93.
18. Blecker U, de PS, Hauser B, Chouraqui JP, Gottrand F, Vandenplas Y. The role of ''occult'' gastroesophageal reflux in chronic pulmonary disease in children. Acta Gastroenterol Belg 1995; 58:348–352.
19. Colombo JL, Hallber TK. Pulmonary aspiration and lipid-laden macrophages: in search of gold (standards). Pediatr Pulmonol 1999; 28:79–82.
20. Alaswad B, Toubas PL, Grunow JE. Environmental tobacco smoke exposure and gastroesophageal reflux in infants with apparent life-threatening events. J Okla State Med Assoc 1996; 89:233–237.
21. Orenstein SR, Magill HL, Brooks P. Thickening of feedings for therapy of gastroesophageal reflux. J Pediatr 1987; 110:181–186.
22. Borrelli O, Salvia G, Campanozzi A, Franco MT, Moreira FL, Emiliano M, Campanozzi F, Cucchiara S. Use of a new thickened formula for treatment of symptomatic gastrooesophageal reflux in infants. Ital J Gastroenterol Hepatol 1997; 29(3):237–242.
23. Kattwinkel J, Brooks J, Keenan ME, Malloy MD. Positioning and sudden infant

death syndrome (SIDS): update. Task Force on Infant Positioning and SIDS. Pediatrics 1996; 98:1216–1218.

24. Tobin JM, McCloud P, Cameron DJS. Posture and gastro-oesophageal reflux: as case for left lateral positioning. Arch Dis Child 1997; 76:254–258.

25. Buts JP, Barudi C, Otte JB. Double-blind controlled study on the efficacy of sodium alginate (Gaviscon) in reducing gastroesophageal reflux assessed by 24 h continuous pH monitoring in infants and children. Eur J Pediatr 1987; 146:156–158.

26. Cucchiara S, Gobio-Casali L, Balli F, Magazzu G, Staiano A, Astolfi R, Amarri S, Conti-Nibali S, Guandalini S. Cimetidine treatment of reflux esophagitis in children. J Pediatr Gastroenterol Nutr 1989; 8:150–156.

27. Israel DM, Hassall E. Omeprazole and other proton pump inhibitors: pharmacology, efficacy, and safety, with special reference to use in children. J Pediatr Gastroenterol Nutr 1998; 27:568–579.

28. Strauss RS, Calenda KA, Dayal Y, Mobassaleh M. Histological esophagitis: clinical and histological response to omeprazole in children. Dig Dis Sci 1999; 44:134–139.

29. Cucchiara S, Staiano A, Cappozzi C, Di Lorenzo C, Boccieri A, Auricchio S. Cisapride for gastro-oesophageal reflux and peptic oesophagitis. Arch Dis Child 1987; 62:454–457.

30. Saye Z, Forget P, Geukbelle F. Effect of cisapride on gastro-esophageal reflux in children with chronic bronchopulmonary disease: a double-blind cross-over pH-monitoring study. Pediatr Pulmonol 1987; 3:8–12.

31. Vandenplas Y, Belli DC, Benatar A, Cadranel S, Cucchiara S, Dupont C, Gottrand F, Hassall E, Heymans HS, Kearns G, Kneepkens CM, Koletzko S, Milla P, Polanco I, Staiano AM. The role of cisapride in the treatment of pediatric gastroesophageal reflux: the European Society of Paediatric Gastroenterology, Hepatology and Nutrition. J Pediatr Gastroenterol Nutr 1999; 28:518–528.

32. Shulman RJ, Boyle JT, Colletti RB, Friedman RA, Heyman MB, Kearns HG, Kirschner BS, Levy J, Mitchell AA, Van Hare G. The use of cisapride in children: the North American Society for Pediatric Gastroenterology and Nutrition. J Pediatr Gastroenterol Nutr 1999; 28:529–533.

33. Fonkalsrud EW, Bustorff-Silva J, Perez CA, Quintero R, Martin L, Atkinson JB. Antireflux surgery in children under 3 months of age. J Pediatr Surg 1999; 34:527–531.

34. Samuk I, Afriat R, Horne T, Bistritzer T, Barr J, Vinograd I. Dumping syndrome following Nissen fundoplication, diagnosis, and treatment. J Pediatr Gastroenterol Nutr 1996; 23:235–240.

35. Danielson PD, Emmens RW. Esophagogastric disconnection for gastroesophageal reflux in children with severe neurological impairment. J Pediatr Surg 1999; 34:84–86.

20

Peptic Ulcer Disease and Gastritis

Gisela Chelimsky and Steven J. Czinn
Case Western Reserve University School of Medicine and Rainbow Babies
& Children's Hospital, Cleveland, Ohio

Beverly Barrett Dahms
Case Western Reserve University School of Medicine and University
Hospitals of Cleveland, Cleveland, Ohio

1 INTRODUCTION

It has been estimated, during the past decade, that peptic ulcer disease affected
over 4 million people annually in the United States (1,2). For much of the last
century, the pathogenesis of gastroduodenal disease was thought to be due to a
number of predisposing factors, the most important one being hypersecretion of
gastric acid (3–5). Peptic ulcers were thought to develop at sites where the mucosa is particularly susceptible to damage by gastric acid. Gastric acid is secreted
by parietal cells, which possess specific H_2 receptors that regulate acid secretion.
According to the gastric acid paradigm of peptic ulcer formation, disease develops when an imbalance occurs between gastric acid and mucosal cytoprotective
mechanisms. That many patients with ulcers have normal levels of gastric acid
secretion indicates that gastric acidity is not sufficient to explain these disorders.
Factors such as genetic predisposition, diet, or the ingestion of medications or

agents directly toxic to the gastric mucosa (nonsteroidal anti-inflammatory drugs) may contribute to the development of peptic ulcer disease. Although medical treatments that were capable of curing the ulcer have been available for a number of years (6,7), the relapse rate of peptic ulcers following therapy with H_2-receptor antagonists and proton-pump inhibitors was as high as 85% (8).

2 GASTRITIS

The term *gastritis* is used by clinicians to define any type of inflammation in the stomach. More precisely, this term should be used only to describe a histologic diagnosis when evaluating gastric biopsies. The term *gastropathy* is more appropriately employed during endoscopy, indicating a condition that does not include histologic findings (9). In order to limit confusion, it is important to define terms commonly used in endoscopy reports. The term *erosion* refers to a mucosal break that does not penetrate the muscularis mucosa. An *ulcer*, on the other hand, extends through the muscularis mucosa into the submucosa. Erosions are often multiple and usually have white bases surrounded by a ring of erythema (9).

To maximize the value of an upper endoscopy performed in children, biopsies are routinely obtained to determine whether gastritis or other changes are present. A microscopically inflamed mucosa can appear visually normal on endoscopy; conversely, a red-appearing mucosa may be normal on histology (10).

Until recently, gastric inflammation was simply divided into superficial and atrophic gastritis. Chronic atrophic gastritis can be subdivided into two processes: (1) an autoimmune process in which much of the acid-secretory portion of the stomach is destroyed, leading to atrophy and hypochlorhydria (type A), and (2) the more common form of gastritis, involving only the antrum (type B). Type A gastritis is associated with pernicious anemia, achlorhydria, parietal cell antibodies, and/or antibodies against the H/K-ATPase component of parietal cells (11). Since the rediscovery of *Helicobacter pylori* and our understanding of the fundamental role this organism plays in the development of gastroduodenal disease, a number of newer and more complex grading systems have been proposed to characterize gastritis (9,12,13). The revised Sydney system (12) is a histological classification widely used in adult pathology, but many of the conditions described do not occur in children.

2.1 Classification of Gastritis and Gastropathy in Children

Recently, Dohil and collaborators (9,14) suggested a new classification of pediatric gastritis and gastropathies based on endoscopic appearance. They divided the gastritis into two groups: (1) erosive and/or hemorrhagic gastritis or gastropathies and (2) nonerosive gastritis or gastropathies (9).

2.1.1 Practical Considerations for the Evaluation of Gastritis and Ulcers in Children: Communication Between the Endoscopist and the Pathologist

Accurate clinicopathologic correlation of gastritis is achieved only when a detailed description is provided to the pathologist regarding the site of the biopsies, presence of focal lesions, and clinical presentation of the patient. In addition, a list of the medications taken by the subjects within the 2 months prior to the procedure is also helpful (NSAIDs, proton-pump inhibitors, nonprescription antacids, and antibiotics) (12).

2.1.2 Knowledge of Endoscopic Landmarks

Gastric disorders often have a predilection for certain areas in the stomach. Inaccurate landmark identification may result in erroneous or missed diagnoses. Briefly, the largest region of the stomach is the *gastric body* or *corpus*, which is endoscopically characterized by thick mucosal folds, or rugae. The *fundus* is immediately above the body and has a dome-shape configuration. The gastric body and fundus are composed of oxyntic (acid producing) mucosa with parietal and chief cells. The gastric *antrum* occupies the lower quarter or third of the stomach. The antrum ends in the pylorus and has mucous glands. The gastric *cardia* corresponds to a very short zone, immediately below the Z line, composed of mucous glands (9).

2.1.3 Recommendations for Gastric Biopsy Sampling in Children

In adults, five biopsy specimens are taken, two from the antrum (one from the distal lesser curvature and one from the distal greater curvature), two from the body (one from the lesser and one from the greater curvature) and one from the incisura angularis (12). The recommendations in children are less clear cut. Many authors obtain two biopsies from the prepyloric area and two from the greater curvature at the midbody (9). When *H. pylori* infection, Barrett's metaplasia, carditis due to gastroesophageal reflux or *H. pylori*, or mucosa-associated lymphoid tissue (MALT) lymphoma is suspected, additional biopsies immediately below the Z line should also be obtained. When a specific lesion is visualized, more specimens should be taken from the lesion or edge thereof (9). The purpose of this chapter is to review the pathogenesis, histological findings, and treatment of gastropathies and gastritis due to:

1. *Helicobacter pylori* infection
2. Gastritis associated with Crohn's disease
3. Eosinophilic/allergic gastritis
4. Gastritis due to NSAIDs
5. Gastritis due to use of proton-pump inhibitors

Helicobacter pylori Infection.   Over the last 100 years, there have been a number of reports suggesting that microbes may also play a role in the development of gastritis and peptic ulcers. In 1975, Steer and Colin-Jones used electron microscopy to observe bacteria under the mucous layer of the stomach in ulcer patients. This study resurrected the possibility that organisms infecting the gastric mucosa could play a role in the pathogenesis of gastritis and ulcer disease (15). However, it was not until *H. pylori* was successfully cultured by Marshall and Warren in 1982 that the association of infection with gastritis was accepted (16). *H. pylori* is a gram-negative, S-shaped rod, 0.5 by 3.0 μm in size. It has polar flagellae and produces enzymes including urease, catalase, and oxidase. This organism requires a microaerobic environment for culture, reflecting its environmental niche in the semipermeable mucous layer overlying the gastric epithelium.

Since 1983, many studies have correlated the presence of *H. pylori* with antral gastritis (17–19) and duodenal ulcers (20,21). Although all children infected with *H. pylori* develop histologically active chronic gastritis, the majority of children have apparently asymptomatic infections, which may never lead to clinically evident disease. Only a minority of children develop peptic ulceration or gastric cancer, the most severe manifestations of *H. pylori* infection.

Based on prevalence studies, *H. pylori* is among the most common bacterial infections in humans. Initial epidemiological studies confirmed that the prevalence of *H. pylori* increased with advancing age throughout the world. Recent reports from countries such as Gambia clearly demonstrate that colonization with *H. pylori* occurs very early in childhood, perhaps as early as 3 months of age (22,23). The method of acquisition and transmission is unclear. However, the most likely mode of transmission is fecal-oral. Evidence for this mechanism was demonstrated by isolation of viable *H. pylori* from the feces of children (24). Serological evidence of *H. pylori* in parents and siblings of children carrying the organism are consistent with intrafamilial spread (25). Finally, higher rates of infection also have been noted for institutionalized children (26). Risk factors such as minimal education and low socioeconomic status during childhood influence the prevalence (27,28).

Although the exact mechanism by which *H. pylori* produces gastric inflammation has not been established, a number of hypotheses have been proposed. One factor that may account for the gastric damage is the large amount of urease present in *H. pylori* (29). Urease hydrolyzes urea to ammonia and bicarbonate at the gastric mucosal surface. Ammonia can be directly toxic to epithelial cells, and the concomitant increase in the mucosal surface pH might interfere with gastric epithelial function, such as production of mucus (23). In addition to urease, *H. pylori* vacuolating cytotoxin has been the focus of intense investigation for several years. Cytotoxin-producing strains tend to be more virulent than toxin-negative ones (30).

The relationship between *H. pylori* and peptic ulcer disease is largely inferential. Specifically, nearly all cases of duodenal ulcers are associated with antral *H. pylori* gastritis (31). In addition, combinations of acid-suppressive drugs and antimicrobial agents not only eradicate *H. pylori* and heal duodenal ulcers but also markedly decrease the recurrence rate of duodenal ulcers. Twelve-month recurrence rates of <10% have been reported in patients successfully treated for *H. pylori* infection (8,32–34). In addition to the association of *H. pylori* with ulcers, a number of epidemiological studies have demonstrated that chronic *H. pylori* colonization can ultimately predispose an individual to a significantly increased risk of developing gastric adenocarcinoma (35–37) and/or mucosa-associated lymphoid tissue (MALT) lymphoma (38–40,41). These studies are so compelling that the World Health Organization has recently classified *H. pylori* as a human carcinogen (42).

The histological changes of *H. pylori* gastritis are best seen in the antrum, though all areas of the stomach are usually affected. The mucosa shows a moderate to severe diffuse chronic gastritis, with plasma cells and lymphocytes uniformly filling the lamina propria. Small foci of neutrophils may be seen within glandular epithelium and in the surrounding lamina propria, the "active" component. In the most severe cases, lymphoid follicles can be found; these often persist for some time even after successful treatment. If carefully sought, the organisms can be seen on routine hematoxylin and eosin–stained slides. They are present in the gastric mucous coat on the surface or within the superficial portions of the gastric pits. Many special stains have been advocated to enhance their recognition and are especially useful in cases where the organisms are few: Giemsa, Genta, Warthin-Starry, and immunoperoxidase stains (Fig. 1).

Based on numerous clinical and animal studies, treatment of peptic ulcer disease is now directed at eradicating *H. pylori*. Laboratory and clinical studies have confirmed that *H. pylori* is susceptible to numerous antimicrobial agents, including bismuth-containing compounds and the combination of H_2-receptor antagonists or proton-pump inhibitors with antimicrobial agents. Administration of single antibiotics or bismuth alone may transiently suppress infection but has little long-term impact on *H. pylori* colonization and associated pathology. The currently recommended therapies for eradication of *H. pylori* typically require combinations of two or three medications (33,43–45). Eradication rates of *H. pylori* as high as 90% have been achieved in clinical trials with various triple therapies such as a proton-pump inhibitor, clarithromycin, and metronidazole or omeprazole/lansoprazole, amoxicillin, and clarithromycin (46,47). However, drug therapies for the eradication of *H. pylori* from the gastrointestinal tract continue to have a number of limitations, including poor patient compliance, adverse side effects, and antimicrobial resistance. To date, no large controlled studies evaluating different therapeutic regimens to eradicate *H. pylori* infection in chil-

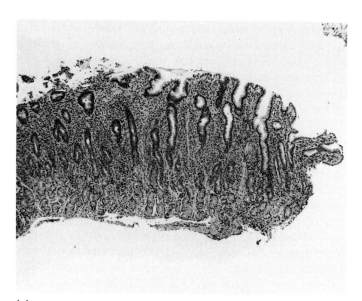

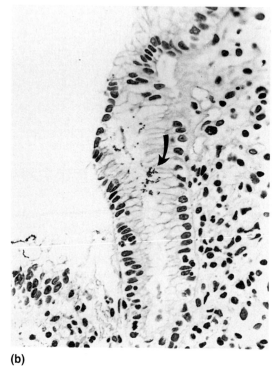

dren have been published. As in adults, eradication of *H. pylori* in children is very effective in the long-term healing of duodenal ulcers. Finally, as in adults, the treatment of asymptomatic *H. pylori*–positive children without evidence of peptic ulcer disease or MALT lymphoma remains controversial.

Information is lacking on issues such who to test, what test to use, who to treat, and how to treat in children.

The ability of *H. pylori* to persist in the human stomach despite the presence of a highly active immune response to the organism represents a remarkable adaptation of the organism to the host. Similarly, humans can carry *H. pylori* throughout life with little or no impairment of gastric function. An improved understanding of the relationship between *H. pylori*, the inflammation it induces, and the host response may lead to new treatment paradigms for persistent colonization with *H. pylori*.

2.2 Gastritis Due to Crohn's Disease

The reported prevalence of gastroduodenal involvement in Crohn's disease ranges from 0.5 to 8% of all cases (48) to 75% (49), 71% (50), and 80%. Studies limited to pediatric patients report an incidence of upper gastrointestinal involvement as high as 30% (13,51). Only 1% of these patients had disease limited to the upper gastrointestinal tract. Crohn's disease is the most common cause of granulomatous gastritis (13). Endoscopic and/or histological evidence of Crohn's disease of the stomach may occur in the absence of upper gastrointestinal symptoms and sometimes may precede the diagnostic features in the ileum or colon. The symptoms associated with upper gastrointestinal Crohn's disease include dysphagia, epigastric abdominal pain, nausea, and vomiting. Patients with upper gastrointestinal Crohn's disease also seem to have more severe weight loss than those with more distal disease (51). In many circumstances, histological upper endoscopic findings may help differentiate between Crohn's disease and ulcerative colitis (9,48), but it should be pointed out that gastritis may also be encountered in ulcerative colitis.

The histological diagnosis of Crohn's disease has traditionally relied on the presence of chronic inflammation and noncaseating (sarcoid) granulomas.

FIGURE 1 *Helicobacter pylori* gastritis. (a) Low magnification of an antral biopsy shows diffuse darkening of the lamina propria due to a dense infiltrate of chronic inflammatory cells—diffuse chronic gastritis. (Hematoxylin and eosin, ×63.) (b) High magnification shows the small bacilli in clusters in the superficial portion of a gastric pit (*arrow*). The immunostain used here enhances the appearance of the organisms against a pale background. (*H. pylori* immunoperoxidase stain, ×512.)

However, the incidence of granulomas in gastroduodenal Crohn's disease is only 10 to 15% in adult biopsy series (48,49) and up to from 30 to 39% in pediatric series (9). Granulomas are more commonly encountered in the stomach than in the duodenum.

In the past few years, it has been recognized that even in the absence of granulomas, gastric Crohn's disease has a number of distinctive histological features that often allow it to be distinguished from the many other causes of chronic gastritis, especially *H. pylori* gastritis. Gastric and duodenal Crohn's disease, as is true of Crohn's disease at other sites, is most often a focal chronic inflammatory process (48,49) (Fig. 2). By contrast, the chronic inflammation in *H. pylori* is characteristically diffuse. In addition, up to one-half of patients with gastric Crohn's disease demonstrate focal acute inflammation, usually centered around

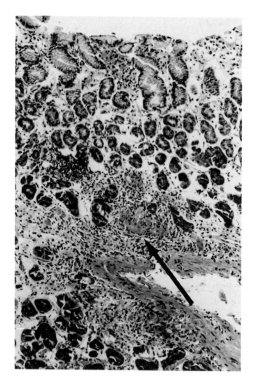

FIGURE 2   Gastric Crohn's disease. Small foci of chronic inflammation are characteristic of Crohn's disease. A granuloma is present in only one-third or fewer of these cases (arrow). Note the lack of inflammation in other areas of the lamina propria in comparison to Figure 1. (Hematoxylin and eosin, ×80.)

glands or foveolae (48,49). In the duodenum, the focal pattern of acute (active) and chronic inflammation is equally important in helping to distinguish Crohn's disease from the many other causes of chronic duodenitis (48).

2.3 Eosinophilic/Allergic Gastritis

Eosinophilic gastroenteritis is defined by three criteria: 1) the presence of gastrointestinal symptoms, 2) biopsies showing eosinophilic infiltration of one or more areas of the gastrointestinal tract from the esophagus to the colon, and 3) no evidence of parasitic or extraintestinal disease (52).

Eosinophilic gastritis is the gastric component of eosinophilic gastroenteritis. This is a chronic disease of unknown origin that can predominate in any of the layers of the intestinal wall (53). In a retrospective review of 40 cases of eosinophilic gastroenteritis, 23 had mucosal disease, only 12 had involvement of the muscularis layers, and 5 had evidence of subserosal disease (52).

The presentation of eosinophilic gastritis in children usually includes growth retardation as a major clinical feature and in many cases is associated with asthma, allergic rhinitis, or urticaria (54). Food allergies are commonly diagnosed in 50% of the patients with mucosal disease, compared with none of the subjects with muscularis or serosal involvement (52). Other nonspecific symptoms such as abdominal pain, vomiting, chronic diarrhea, dysphagia, and anemia have also been reported (52,54).

The histological findings in the gastric biopsies consist primarily of eosinophilic infiltration with necrosis and regeneration of the surface and glandular epithelium. The biopsies vary considerably. In the small intestine villi are usually normal or minimally altered. Increased eosinophils may be found in the lamina propria (54).

Corticosteroids are the mainstay of therapy in eosinophilic gastroenteritis, usually resulting in dramatic remission in all subjects with eosinophilic ascites and 75% remission in subjects with mucosal or muscularis involvement. The response to cromolyn in mucosal disease is equivocal. Dietary regimens are seldom useful for the treatment of eosinophilic gastritis but occasional responses to withdrawal of cow's milk may occur. In severe cases of muscle layer disease, pyloric outlet obstruction may occur, requiring surgery (52,54).

2.4 Gastric Changes Associated with Proton-Pump Inhibitor Therapy

Long-term suppression of gastric acid secretion may be necessary to treat severe reflux esophagitis or duodenal ulcer in pediatric patients. Proton-pump inhibitor therapy (omeprazole) is efficacious in these situations, but when used for periods longer than 12 months may induce distinctive changes in the acid producing (oxyntic) area of the stomach, the body and fundus. Polyps in the gastric body,

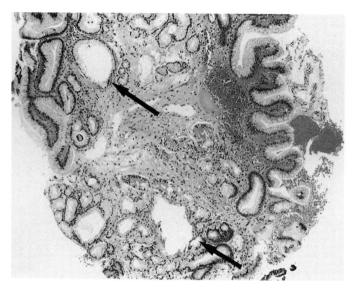

FIGURE 3   Proton-pump inhibitor–associated gastric polyp. This small sessile polyp is characterized by microcysts lined by mucous cells (arrows). (Hematoxylin and eosin, ×80.)

particularly on the greater curvature, have been found with prolonged use of proton-pump inhibitors. These polyps have most often been incidental findings during endoscopic examination and are usually less than 1 cm in diameter and sessile. If their etiology is not recognized, they may pose problems in differential diagnosis and may prompt consideration of a polyposis syndrome. Microscopically, these polyps are characterized by small cysts in the glandular layer lined by flattened parietal, chief, or mucous cells (Fig. 3). Occasionally dilated glands alone, without polyp formation, may be recognized on biopsy. These findings have been described in both pediatric and adult populations (55–58). Gastrin levels are only modestly increased after 2 years of omeprazole treatment (137 $\pm$ 11.5) compared to subjects on ranitidine (86 $\pm$ 7.2 pg/mL) ($p < 0.05$) (59). Efforts should be made to discontinue the use of proton-pump inhibitors in such patients.

2.5   Gastritis Associated with the Use of Nonsteroidal Anti-inflammatory Drugs (NSAIDs)

Prostaglandins enhance gastrointestinal mucosal protection. Aspirin and other NSAIDs are local irritants that produce gastric mucosal damage and, in addition, produce effects on gastric mucosa when administered systemically. The mechanisms underlying ulcer formation associated with the use of NSAIDs is not clear. The most studied effect is the inhibition of the enzyme cyclooxygenase and therefore a decrease in prostaglandin generation (60). The incidence of ulcers in adult subjects with rheumatoid arthritis taking NSAIDs is 20% (63,64). The risk of developing serious adverse gastrointestinal complications is very high in the elderly, but in children the incidence seems to be only slightly increased (61,65). In a study of children with juvenile rheumatoid arthritis, epigastric abdominal pain was the most common reason for referral to a gastroenterologist. Some 65% of the children had anemia, and 35% of this group had stools positive for occult blood. The association of anemia and abdominal pain was present in 47% of the cohort, which increased to 64% of the children with antral or duodenal erosions. The most common endoscopic finding in children with abdominal pain taking NSAIDs was gastritis or duodenitis, followed by gastric or duodenal ulcers (62). Lesions caused by NSAIDs are more commonly gastric than duodenal and usually involve the gastric antrum (9). Histologically, edema, vascular ectasia, super-

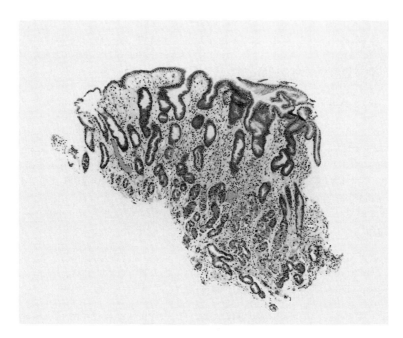

FIGURE 4 Gastropathy associated with nonsteroidal anti-inflammatory drug (NSAID) use. The lamina propria is edematous and congested. Foveolae (pits) are elongated and have a slightly serrated configuration. Inflammation is minimal to absent. (Hematoxylin and eosin, ×63.)

ficial erosions, and extravasated red blood cells are seen in the mucosa. Inflammation is sparse to absent unless ulceration is established. Regenerative epithelial changes with mucin depletion and nuclear enlargement may be seen during the healing phases after an erosion. The gastric pits may show hyperplasia and a characteristic sawtooth elongation with chronic ingestion of the drug(s) (Fig. 4).

Prevention of NSAID-induced ulcers is achieved with the use of misoprostol, a synthetic prostaglandin E_1 analog (61). In children, further studies are needed to support the use of misoprostol as a first line of preventive medication, but it may be useful in patients who do not respond to H_2-receptor antagonists (62). In adults, proton-pump inhibitors have protective effect against NSAID-related mucosal injuries in preventing both duodenal ulcers and gastric ulcers. Although H_2-receptor antagonists are commonly administered in association with NSAIDs, they have not been shown to prevent gastric ulcers, but they do prevent duodenal ulcers. Sucralfate has not been shown to be effective in preventing NSAID-related ulcers (61). In adults, the recommendations from the Ad Hoc Committee on Practice Parameters of the American College of Gastroenterology is that NSAID-induced ulcers should be treated by stopping the NSAID when the ulcer occurs. A proton-pump inhibitor is the drug of choice when the NSAIDs must be continued (61). More recently a new class of COX2 inhibitor NSAIDs have been approved, which may dramatically decrease the adverse gastrointestinal side effects associated with NSAID use. Further studies in pediatric patients are needed before recommendations can be made.

3 CONCLUSION

An improved understanding of the relationship between gastric inflammation, the host, immunological responses, and the various underlying etiologies is likely to lead to a better understanding of the pathophysiology behind gastritis. Such knowledge should lead to improved ways of preventing and treating the complications of gastritis and peptic ulcer disease.

REFERENCES

1. Elashoff J, Grossman M. Trends in hospital admissions and death rates for peptic ulcer disease in the United States. Gastroenterology 1980; 78:280–285.
2. Kurata J, Haile E, Elashoff J. Sex differences in peptic ulcer disease. Gastroenterology 1985; 88:96–100.
3. Blum A. Treatment of acid-related disorders with gastric acid inhibitors: The state of the art. Digestion 1990; 47(suppl 1):3–10.
4. Sachs G. Therapeutic control of acid secretion: pharmacology of the parietal cell. Curr Opin Gastroenterol 1990; 6:859–866.
5. Sachs G, Shin J, Besancon M, Gedda K. Receptors and pumps as targets in ulcer therapy. Digestion 1994; 55(suppl 2):1–62.

6. Feldman M, Burton M. Histamine2-receptor antagonist: standard therapy for acid-peptic diseases. N Engl J Med 1990; 323:1749–1755.

7. McTavish D, Buckley MM, Heel RC. Omeprazole. An updated review of its pharmacology and therapeutic use in acid-related disorders. Drugs 1991; 42:138–170.

8. Festen H. Prevention of duodenal ulcer relapse by long-term treatment with omeprazole. Scand J Gastroenterol 1994; 29(suppl 201):39–41.

9. Dohil R, Hassall E, Dimmick J. Gastritis and gastropathy of childhood. J Pediatr Gastroenterol Nutr 1999; 29:378–394.

10. Carpenter H, Talley N. Gastroscopy is incomplete without biopsy: clinical relevance of distinguishing gastropathy from gastritis. Gastroenterology 1995; 108:917–924.

11. Gleeson P, Toh B. Molecular targets in pernicious anaemia. Immunol Today 1991; 12:233–238.

12. Dixon M, Genta R, Yardley J, Correa P. Classification and grading of gastritis: the updated Sydney system. Am J Surg Pathol 1996; 20:1161–1181.

13. Dimmick J, Jevon G, Hassall E. Pediatric gastritis. Perspect Pediatr Pathol 1997; 20:35–76.

14. Dimmick JE JG, Hassall EG. Pediatric gastritis. Gastrointest Dis 1997; 20:35–76.

15. Steer H, Colin-Jones D. Mucosal changes in gastric ulceration and their response to carbenoxolone sodium. Gut 1975; 16:590–597.

16. Marshall B. Unidentified curved bacilli on gastric epithelium in active chronic gastritis. Lancet 1983:1273–1275.

17. Blaser M, Perez-Perez G, Kleanthous H, et al. Infection with *Helicobacter pylori* strains possessing cagA associated with risk of developing adenocarcinoma of the stomach. Cancer Res 1995; 55:2111–2115.

18. Graham D. Evolution of concepts regarding *Helicobacter pylori*: from a cause of gastritis to a public health problem. Am J Gastroenterol 1994; 89:469–471.

19. Valle J, Kekki M, Sipponen P, Ihamaki T, Siurla M. Long-term course and consequences of *Helicobacter pylori* gastritis. Scand J Gastroenterol 1996; 31:546–550.

20. Beam E. *Helicobacter pylori* and peptic ulcer disease. Clin Rev 1995; 5:51–70.

21. Peterson W. *Helicobacter pylori* and peptic ulcer disease. N Eng J Med 1991; 324:1043–1048.

22. Babatvala N, Mayo K, Megraud F, Jennings R, Deeks J, Feldman R. The cohort effect and *Helicobacter pylori*. J Infect Dis 1993; 168:219–221.

23. Megraud F. Epidemiology of *Helicobacter pylori* infection: some fundamental questions. Eur J Gastroenterol Hepatol 1993; 5(suppl 2):S60–S63.

24. Thomas J, Gibson G, Darboe M, Dale A, Weaver L. Isolation of *Helicobacter pylori* from human feces. Lancet 1992; 340:1194–1195.

25. Drumm B, Perez-Perez G, Blaser M, Sherman P. Intrafamilial clustering of *Helicobacter pylori*. N Eng J Med 1990; 322:359–363.

26. Lewindon P, Lau D, Chan A, Tse P, Sullivan P. *Helicobacter pylori* in an institution for disabled children in Hong Kong. Dev Med Child Neurol 1997; 39:682–685.

27. Malaty H, Engstrand L, Pedersen N, Graham D. *Helicobacter pylori* infection: genetic and environmental influences. A study of twins. Ann Intern Med 1994; 120:982–986.

28. Malaty H, Graham D. Importance of childhood socioeconomic status on the current prevalence of *Helicobacter pylori* infection. Gut 1994; 35:742–745.

29. Mobley H, Hu L, Foxall P. *Helicobacter pylori* urease: properties and role in pathogenesis. Scan J Gastroenterol 1991; 187(suppl):39–46.

30. Ghiara P, Marchetti M, Blaser M, et al. Role of *Helicobacter pylori* virulence factors vacuolating cytotoxin, CagA, and urease in a mouse model of disease. Infect Immunol 1995; 63:4154–4160.

31. Malfertheiner P, Bode G. *Helicobacter pylori* and the pathogenesis of duodenal ulcer disease. Eur J Gastroenterol Hepatol 1993; 5(suppl 1):S1–S8.

32. Graham D, Lew GM, Klein P, et al. Effect of treatment of *Helicobacter pylori* infection on the long-term recurrence of gastric or duodenal ulcer. Ann Intern Med 1992; 116:705–708.

33. Laine L. Eradication of *Helicobacter pylori* reduces gastric and duodenal ulcer recurrence. Gastroenterology 1992; 103:1695–1703.

34. Rauws E, Tyygat G. Cure of duodenal ulcer associated with erradication of *Helicobacter pylori*. Lancet 1990; 335:1233–1235.

35. Eurogast S. An international association between *Helicobacter pylori* infection and gastric cancer. Lancet 1993; 341:1359–1362.

36. Forman D, Newell D, Fullerton F, et al. Association between infection with *Helicobacter pylori* and risk of gastric cancer: evidence from a prospective investigation. BMJ 1991; 302:1302–1305.

37. Parsonnet J. *Helicobacter pylori* as a risk factor for gastric cancer. Eur J Gastroenterol Hepatol 1993; 5(suppl 1):S103–S107.

38. Boot H, de Jong D, van Heerde P, Taal B. Role of *Helicobacter pylori* eradication in high-grade MALT lymphoma (letter; comment). Lancet 1995; 346:448–449.

39. Enno A, O'Rourke J, Howlett C, Jack M, Dixon M, Lee A. MALToma-like lesions in the murine gastric mucosa after long-term infection with *Helicobacter felis*. Am J Pathol 1997; 147:217–222.

40. Kelly S, Geraghty J, Neale G. *H. pylori,* gastric carcinoma, and MALT lymphoma. Lancet 1994; 343:418.

41. Montalban C, Manzanal A, Boixeda D, Redondo C, Bellas C. Treatment of low-grade gastric MALT lymphoma with *Helicobacter pylori* erradication. Lancet 1995; 345:798–799.

42. Sharp D. Worms, spirals, flukes as carcinogens (see comments). Lancet 1995; 345: 403–404.

43. Dunn B, Cohen H, Blaser C. *Helicobacter pylori.* Clin Microbiol Rev 1997; 10: 720–741.

44. Huang J, Hunt R. Review: eradication of Helicobacter. Problems and recommendations. J Gastroenterol Hepatol 1997; 12:590–598.

45. Rene W, Hulst V, Rauws E, et al. Prevention of ulcer recurrence after eradication of *Helicobacter pylori*: a prospective long-term follow-up study. Gastroenterology 1997; 113:1082–1086.

46. Graham D, Lew G, Evans D, Evans D, Klein P. Effect of triple therapy (antibiotics plus bismuth) on duodenal ulcer healing. Ann Intern Med 1991; 115:266–269.

47. Khalifa M. Familial achalasia, microcephaly, and mental retardation: case report and review of the literature. Clin Pediatr 1988; 27:509–512.

48. Wright C, Riddell R. Histology of the stomach and duodenum in Crohn's disease. Am J Surg Pathol 1998; 22:383–390.

49. Oberhuber G PA, Oesterreicher C, Novacek G et al. Focally Enchanced gastritis: A frequent type of gastritis in patients with Crohn's disease. Gastroenterology 1997; 112:698–706.

50. Ruuska T, Savilahti E, Maki M, Ormala T, Visakorpi J. Exclusive whole protein enteral diet versus prednisolone in the treatment of acute Crohn's disease in children. J Pediatr Gastroenterol Nutr 1994; 19:175–180.

51. Lenaerts C, Roy C, Vaillancourt M, Weber A, Morin C, Seidman E. High incidence of upper gastrointestinal tract involvement in children with Crohn's disease. Pediatrics 1989; 83:777–781.

52. Tally N, Shorter R, Phillips S, Zinsmeister A. Eosinophilic gastroenteritis: a clinicopathological study of patients with disease of the mucosa, muscle layer, and subserosal tissues. Gut 1990; 31:54–58.

53. Klein N, Hargrove R, Sleisenger M, Jeffries G. Eosinophilic gastroenteritis. Medicine 1970; 49:299–319.

54. Katz A, Goldman H, Grand R. Gastric mucosal biopsy in eosinophilic (allergic) gastroenteritis. Gastroenterology 1977; 73:705–709.

55. Hassall E, Dimmick J, Israel D. Parietal cell hyperplasia in children receiving omeprazole (abstr). Gastroenterology 1995; 108:A110.

56. Driman D, Wright C, Tougas G, Riddlell R. Omeprazole produces parietal cell hypertrophy and hyperplasia in humans. Dig Dis Sci 1996; 41:2039–2047.

57. Israel D, Hassall E, Dimmick J. Gastric polyps in children receiving omeprazole (abstr). Gastroenterology 1995; 108:A121.

58. Fitzgibbons PL JP. The effect of long-term acid suppression on gastric mucosal histology. Am J Clin Pathol 1998; 110:569–571.

59. Weinstein W, Lieberman D, Lewin K, Weber L, Berger M, Ippoliti A. Omeprazole-induced regression of Barrett's esophagus: a 2 year, randomized, controlled double blind trial (abstr). Gastroenterology 1996; 110:A294.

60. Soll A, Kurata J, McGuigan J. Ulcers, nonsteroidal antiinflammatory drugs, and related matters. Gastroenterology 1989; 96:561–568.

61. Lanza F. A guideline for the treatment and prevention of NSAID-induced ulcers. Am J Gastroenterol 1998; 93:2037–2046.

62. Mulberg A, Linz C, Bern E, Tucker L, Verhave M, Grand R. Identification of nonsteroidal anti-inflammatory drug–induced gastroduodenal injury in children with juvenile rheumatoid arthritis. J Pediatr 1993; 122:647–649.

63. Bellary SV IP, Lee FI. Upper gastrointestinal lesions in elderly patients presenting for endoscopy: relevance of NSAID usage. Am J Gastroenterol 1991; 86:961–964.

64. Larkai EN SJ, Lidsky MD, et al. Gastroduodenal mucosa and dyspeptic symptoms in arthritic patients during chronic nonsteroidal anti-inflammatory drug use. Am J Gastroenterol 1987; 22(11):1153–1158.

65. Gabriel SE, Jaakkimainen L. Bombardier C. Risk for serious intestinal complications related to use of nonsteroidal anti-inflammatory drugs: a meta-analysis. Ann Intern Med 1991; 115:787–796.

21

Celiac Disease

Isabel Polanco
Universidad Autónoma de Madrid and Hospital Infantil Universitario
"La Paz," Madrid, Spain

1 DEFINITION

Celiac disease (CD) is now recognized as an immunologically mediated enteropathy of the small intestine that is characterized by lifelong intolerance to gliadin and related prolamines from wheat and other cereals and occurs in genetically predisposed individuals. Symptoms result from structural damage to the mucosa of the small intestine, which causes malabsorption. Normal mucosal architecture is restored after a gluten-free diet is introduced, but villous atrophy reappears when gluten is reintroduced into the diet (gluten challenge). After years of gluten exclusion, relapse of intestinal lesions recurs with gluten challenge (1,2). It is the certainty of eventual relapse that differentiates CD from other childhood enteropathies and suggests that there is some additional property of the gluten molecules that affects enterocyte function or mucosal antigen presentation.

The concept that celiac disease is permanent has been questioned not only by the observation of long periods of unexplained clinical remission after gluten reintroduction (3) but also by reports of cases which, after having had a clear histological relapse while on a gluten-containing diet, subsequently showed partial or total recovery of the histological lesion (4).

The diagnosis of CD is made by three biopsies: one at presentation, one while the patient is on a gluten-free diet, and the third after a gluten challenge. Although pediatric gastroenterologists all agree on the need for an initial biopsy, there is debate about whether three biopsies are truly necessary (5,6).

2 EPIDEMIOLOGY

The true incidence of CD in susceptible populations may be dramatically higher than has previously been recognized and most cases may remain undiagnosed unless actively identified through mass serological screening (7). It is well known that CD affects females more than males (ratio 2:1).

CD occurs predominantly among individuals of European origin, with the highest incidence in the children and adults of Northern Europe and Scandinavia (from 1 in 300 to 1 in 1000). The west coast of Ireland has the highest reported incidence, with CD affecting over 1 in 300 of the entire population. Southern European populations also have a high incidence: Italy (1 in 1000), Spain (1 in 2000), the southwest of France (1 in 3500), and Portugal (1 in 4000) (8).

The incidence of CD has also been found to be elevated in North Africa (1 in 700) and in Israel (1 in 2000) (8). It is not rarely diagnosed in Latin America (Argentina, Uruguay, Chile, Cuba, etc.) (9). CD seems to be less frequent in the United States. The incidence of CD is less well known in Middle East, China, and India. A relationship between various factors (genetic background of the population, quality and quantity of gluten, the age at gluten introduction, and breast-feeding) and the diagnosis of CD has been described (8–10).

There is an increased risk of small bowel lymphoma in adults presenting with CD in midlife. Early presentation may therefore be advantageous, as a strict gluten-free diet will substantially reduce the risk.

3 GENETIC FACTORS

The earliest evidence that genetic factors are of significance in the susceptibility to CD consisted of isolated reports of multiple cases occurring within families. The hereditary basis for CD was also underlined by the finding of classical morphologic changes in the mucosa of the small intestine of 10% of asymptomatic family members. In addition, the high rate of concordance for the disorder among monozygotic twins (71%) emphasized the importance of genetic factors (11,12). Human leukocyte antigens (HLAs) appeared to be the main genetic factors in the susceptibility to CD. There is a strong association between CD and the major histocompatibility complex (MHC) type, with a particular class II allele (HLA-DQ) found in almost all patients. The first recognized genetic association was with class I tissue type, HLA-B8, which is inherited, and with linkage to the true class II susceptibility gene (13).

The MHC type determines the specificity of the peptide binding site on antigen-presenting cells. Class I molecules (e.g., HLA-B8) present antigen to CD8 T lymphocytes, whereas class II molecules (HLA-DP, -DR, or -DQ) present to CD4 T-helper cells. It is therefore important that the initial association with HLA-B8 was secondary, due to linkage disequilibrium with HLA-DQ2, which is found in over 90% of European patients. This implies that the intestinal CD4 cells, found within the mucosal lamina propria rather than the epithelial compartment, are of central importance in the disease.

The primary association of CD is the HLA-DQ dimer DQA1*0501/ DQB1*0201 the majority of patients and first-degree relatives (and up to 20% of normal controls in susceptible populations) may express this dimer on antigen-presenting cells. It is clear from the number of unaffected people that the possession of this haplotype is not enough in itself to cause gluten-induced changes, and the administration of extra gluten to HLA-identical siblings of celiac patients does not always result in pathological changes to the intestine (14). The HLA-DQ dimmer is also strongly linked to HLA-DR status. If children are of the HLA-DR3 tissue type, they will carry both the α and β DQ molecules on the same chromosome, whereas if they are HLA-DR5 and also HLA-DR7, they will carry one molecule on each chromosome (Fig. 1). The end result is the same, in that their antigen-presenting cells can together express these specific HLA-DQ mole-

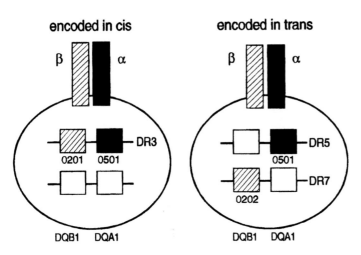

FIGURE 1   Patients with celiac disease who are DR3 or DR5/DR7 heterozygous may express the same HLA-DQ molecule, HLA-DQ(α1*0501,β1*02). The DQA1*0501 and DQB1*02 genes are located in *cis* (on the same chromosome) in DR3 individuals, whereas they are located in *trans* (on opposite chromosomes) in DR5/DR7 heterozygous individuals.

cules and thus present processed gluten peptides to the potentially reactive CD4 cells of the lamina propria.

The few CD patients who do not express the HLA-DQ (1*0501, 1*02) molecule are very often HLA-DR4, DQ8–positive. In this subset of patients, the primary susceptibility is most probably conferred by the HLA-DQ8 molecule (13,15).

4 PATHOLOGY

The proximal mucosa of the small intestine in patients with CD becomes abnormal on gluten ingestion and small bowel biopsy is essential to confirm the diagnosis. The abnormality is characterized by stunted or even absent villi associated with an increase in crypt length and cell numbers—the "flat mucosa." The flat gut lesion is characteristic but nonspecific of CD and a flattened jejunal biopsy may be seen in transient gluten intolerance, soy- and cow's-protein enteropathy, autoimmune enteropathy, acute viral enteritis, giardiasis, prolonged malnutrition, etc. In adults there are fewer causes of flattened jejunal mucosa; these include the Zollinger-Ellison syndrome, tropical sprue, giardiasis, oral contraceptives, and others.

On conventional histological examination (Fig. 2) there is an increased rate of crypt cell proliferation, and the volume of the mucosa lamina propria doubles. Surface epithelium is extensively affected; it is densely infiltrated with small

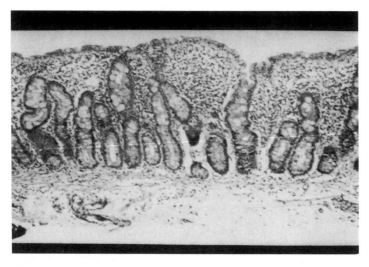

FIGURE 2 Histological section of a flat mucosa in untreated celiac disease.

lymphocytes, and enterocytes appear cuboidal or even flattened with scarcely discernible brush borders. The enterocyte cytoplasm is vacuolated and nuclei are sometimes pyknotic (16). The flat appearance of the mucosal surface in CD may, in fact, be caused by an increase in the volume of the intervillous tissues rather than an actual loss of villi. The enterocyte may be abnormal, showing a flattened or vacuolated appearance, with irregularities of the microvilli and mitochondria seen under the electron microscope.

There is an increased density of intraepithelial lymphocytes, which falls to normal values on a gluten-free diet but rises again after a gluten challenge. The T-cell receptors of these lymphocytes have an increased expression of the γ/σ heterodimer. This is fairly specific for celiac disease, but in infancy it may be found in other enteropathies (17). Table 1 provides a summary of the immunological features of CD.

TABLE 1 Immunologic Features of CD

	Normal small intestine	Celiac disease
Epithelial compartment		
Epithelial morphology	Tall columnar	Variable flattening or vacuolation
Cells per crypt	750	2600
Intraepithelial lympho- cytes per 100 epithe- lial cells	20–40	>40
CD8/CD4 cell ratio	9:1	7–9:1
% T cells	90	50–80
% T cells	10	20–50
Activation markers seen	No	No
Lamina propria		
Total volume	—	Doubled
Lymphocyte density	—	Unchanged
Lymphocyte numbers	—	Doubled
CD8/CD4 cell ratio	~1:1.5	~1:1.5
% T cells	<10	<10
Activation markers seen	No	Yes (CD4 cells)
Other inflammatory cell types in excess		Plasma cells (IgA > M > G) Mast cells Neutrophils

Source: Ref. 37.

All structural damage resolves on gluten withdrawal but recurs if gluten is reintroduced to the diet. Similar intestinal changes are frequently found in dermatitis herpetiformis (DH), an intensely itchy, chronic papulovesicular skin disorder caused by granular subepithelial IgA deposits in the upper dermis. Both the cutaneous and intestinal lesions regress with a gluten free-diet. DH is now considered as a specific skin manifestation of CD.

5 CLINICAL FEATURES

CD can present with a variety of clinical manifestations. A better knowledge of CD has permitted the identification not only of the classic forms of the disease, with its typical gastrointestinal symptoms, but also the identification of atypical forms, characterized by the presence of symptoms not referred to gastrointestinal pathology (Table 2).

In general, the first symptoms appear in the months following the introduction of gluten in the diet. The earlier that gluten is introduced, the shorter the interval between introduction and occurrence of the first symptoms. The first symptoms of CD, therefore, traditionally occur between 6 months and 2 years of age.

In a minority of children, diagnosis is not made until the age of 5 years. CD can therefore be diagnosed at any time up to adulthood (18) because symptoms have been either ignored or misinterpreted (e.g., short stature) or because the disease is truly asymptomatic.

5.1 Classic Presentation

There is considerable variation in the age of onset of symptoms in children with CD.

The characteristic features of the disease are most often encountered in infants 9 to 18 months of age. Within weeks or months of gluten introduction, the classical syndrome of chronic diarrhea, failure to thrive or weight loss, vomiting (especially before 9 months), and abdominal distention develops. The stools are softer, paler, looser, bulkier, more frequent, and more offensive than usual but seldom grossly greasy. Stools may be liquid, and dehydration may occur during exacerbation of the disease. Edema, hypocalcemia, anemia, and hematomas are characteristic of the celiac crisis. In contrast, stools are normal or even hard in up to 15% of cases. Anorexia is common and may precede digestive symptoms; it may be prominent and hence wrongly attributed to psychological troubles.

On physical examination, the child is severely impaired. He or she is pale, looks miserable, and is depressed or irritable (Fig. 3). There is a delay in psychomotor development. Weight is more affected than height. Subcutaneous fat disappears. Muscle wasting—affecting mostly the buttocks, thighs, and shoulders— contrast markedly with the prominent abdominal distention (Fig. 4).

TABLE 2 Clinical Presentation According to the Age of Onset
of Symptoms in CD

Symptoms	Signs
Classical presentation	
Chronic diarrhea	Abdominal distention
Anorexia	Buttock wasting
Abdominal distention	Malnutrition/growth failure
Weight loss	Pallor
Vomiting	Irritability
Irritability/lethargy	Psychomotor delay
	Hematomas
	Rickets
Presentation at older age	
Asymptomatic	Glossitis, aphtous ulcers
Absence of diarrhea	Short stature
Decreased appetite	Iron-deficiency anemia
Anorexia	Osteopenia
Growth failure	Bruising
Pubertal delay	Arthritis/arthralgia
Menstrual irregularities	Enamel hypoplasia
Abnormal (loose) stools	Cerebral calcifications
Arthritis/arthralgia	
Abdominal pain	
Constipation	
Presentation at adulthood	
Anxiety/depression	Glossitis, aphtous ulcers
Chronic diarrhea	Malnutrition
Anorexia	Spontaneous hemorrhage
Abdominal pain	Peripheral edema
Infertility	Isolated megaloblastic anemia
Paresthesias	Cramps/tetany
Nocturnal diuresis	Digital clubbing
Bone pain	Proximal myopathy
Cerebrospinal degeneration	Peripheral neuropathy
	Variety of rashes
	Hyposplenism

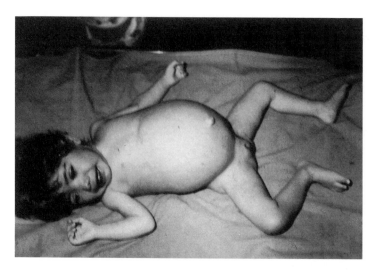

FIGURE 3 A girl with untreated celiac disease. She is pale and looks miserable and depressed.

5.2 Presentation at Older Age

Diagnosis of CD may be made in later childhood. Decreased appetite and abnormal stools are often revealed only on direct questioning. Constipation is more frequent at this stage than in infants. Dental enamel hypoplasia can be found in the permanent teeth, as well as cerebral calcifications, epilepsy, and other neurological disorders (18,19). In early school years, apparently isolated short stature is a frequent presentation. A mild degree of abdominal distention, microcytic anemia, or osteoporosis may lead the diagnosis.

CD has been implicated in more than 15% of cases of children with retarded growth. In these children, plasma growth hormone is low or normal, whereas the levels of insulin-like growth factor (IGF-1) activity are reduced (16,20) and can be returned to normal with the exclusion of gluten from the diet (20). On the other hand, the somatostatin concentration in the jejunal mucosa of untreated patients in an active phase of the disease was significantly elevated, as compared with controls and with those patients who had excluded gluten from their diets (21).

5.3 Asymptomatic and Atypical Presentations

CD may be asymptomatic and discovered only because of a systematic search through family studies or in children affected with conditions associated with

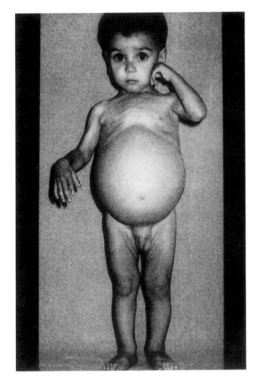

FIGURE 4   A 3-year-old boy with typical active celiac disease. Note his distended and prominent abdomen, muscle wasting, and severe malnutrition.

CD (Tables 3 and 4). Today there is a vast amount of literature describing new, unexpected extraintestinal symptoms or complications of CD. Atypical symptoms such as arthritis, arthralgia, or isolated megaloblastic anemia due to folic acid deficiency have been reported (18) as well as isolated symptomatology such as short stature, abdominal pain, muscular hypotony, edema, and bleeding without any other manifestations (Table 5).

5.4   Low-Grade Enteropathy in Celiac Disease

Recently, new concepts have emerged that have substantially changed our knowledge of CD and questioned its very definition. It is in fact now quite widely accepted that the term *celiac disease* should not be limited to patients with severe enteropathy, although subtotal villous atrophy is still considered by many to be the hallmark of the disease (22). In fact, the gluten-dependent enteropathy may also be quite mild; only epithelial infiltration may be present. With increasing

TABLE 3   Some Conditions Associated with CD

Dermatitis herpetiformis	Down's syndrome
Diabetes mellitus type I	Selective IgA deficiency
Autoimmune thyroiditis	Rheumatoid arthritis
Hypogammaglobulinemia	Vasculitis
Chronic active hepatitis	Primary biliary cirrhosis
Fibrosing alveolitis	Sjögren's syndrome
Crohn's disease	Ulcerative colitis
Systemic lupus erythematosus	Cow's-milk-protein enteropathy
Glomerulonephritis	

TABLE 4   Associated Disorders Found in 990 Children with CD at the Hospital Infantil Universitario "La Paz," Madrid

Dermatitis herpetiformis	34	Vitiligo	4
Isolated IgA deficiency	34	Down's syndrome	3
Diabetes mellitus type I	32	Cardiopathy	3
Asthma	6	Cystic fibrosis	1
Psoriasis	6	Fibrosing alveolitis	1
Chronic active hepatitis	6	Renal tubular acidosis	1
Epilepsy	6	Spinocerebellar degeneration	1
	Total = 138		

TABLE 5   Mode of Presentation in 990 Children with CD at the Hospital Infantil Universitario "La Paz," Madrid

Classic presentation: 574 cases (61,7%)
   Chronic diarrhea, abdominal distention, failure to thrive, anorexia, etc.
Atypical presentation: 356 cases (38,3%)

Short stature	74	Abdominal distention	36
Anemia	69	Bleeding	23
Constipation	68	Muscular hypotony	21
Abdominal pain	47	Edema	18

TABLE 6 Late-Relapser CD Patients: Clinical Data and Follow-Up

Patient	1	2	3	4	5
Sex	F	F	M	M	F
Year of birth	78	80	84	80	81
First gluten intake (months)	4	6	6	4	6
First symptoms (months)	15	18	17	24	18
Age of presentation (years months)	2,4	2,6	1,6	3,2	3,0
First biopsy specimen	SVA	SVA	SVA	SVA	SVA
HLA DR-DQ	3/7-DQ2	3/7-DQ2	3/7-DQ2	3/7-DQ2	3/7-DQ2
Duration of gluten-free diet (years, months)	3,8	3,6	4,6	2,10	3,0
Normal mucosa (years)	6	6	6	6	6
Duration of challenge (years)	14	12	8	12	11
Age at time of relapse (years)	?	?	?	?	?
Last normal biopsy	1998	1998	1998	1998	1998

severity of the histological picture, crypt hyperplasia will be seen. Sometimes the lesion is patchy.

The presence of immunohistochemical markers unique to CD, such as increased density of epithelial Y8+ T cells, may be of help in identifying gluten as the cause of these mild forms of enteropathy.

5.5 Latent Celiac Disease

It also has become widely accepted that CD patients may present with a severe or mild enteropathy at different times of life. There are, in fact, subjects who had a normal jejunal biopsy while on a regular diet while at some time in the past they had a flat jejunal biopsy that recovered on a gluten-free diet. For such subjects the definition of *latent* CD has been proposed (23,24). This definition can also be applied to ''late relapsers'' (3,25) (Table 6).

6 DIAGNOSIS

Based on the recommendations of the European Society for Paediatric Gastroenterology and Nutrition (ESPGAN), from 1970 the diagnosis of CD required three jejunal biopsies (1). The main diagnostic criteria were the following: 1) demonstration of abnormal jejunal mucosa at presentation on a gluten-containing diet, 2) a clear clinical and histological improvement on a gluten-free diet (GFD), and 3) deterioration of the jejunal mucosa after oral challenge with gluten.

ESPGAN revised the diagnostic criteria at its annual meeting in Budapest in 1989 (5). The ''revised criteria'' are summarized as follows:(1) demonstration of abnormal jejunal mucosa at presentation on a gluten-containing diet, (2) a clear-cut clinical improvement on a GFD, and (3) a control jejunal biopsy on a GFD is recommended if the patient was asymptomatic at the time of diagnosis and the clinical response to a GFD is equivocal.

6.1 The First and the Second Biopsies

The recognition of the many clinical forms of CD (classical, atypical, asymptomatic, latent) suggests that a clinical diagnosis of celiac disease may not be possible (25–27). The revised criteria for the diagnosis of CD (5) recommend a control jejunal biopsy after adherence to a GFD only in those cases when the patient was asymptomatic at the time of diagnosis and when the clinical response to a GFD was equivocal. In all the other patients a clear clinical remission on a strict GFD with disappearance of all symptoms should be the second and last step in the diagnosis.

Moreover, the main reason to repeat the small bowel biopsy in all cases of presumed CD after a course of treatment with a GFD is to make sure that the small bowel mucosal lesion has improved. Over recent years it has become clear that a person can exhibit a flat small bowel mucosa characteristic of CD without showing any symptoms or signs of malabsorption. This is the case in at least 10% of the relatives of CD patients, in a number of patients after gluten challenge, and in teenagers with CD who consume gluten (cheat on the diet).

The proportion of symptomatic patients with classical CD malabsorption has been estimated to be as low as 30 to 40% of all gluten-sensitive individuals, and it has been proposed that CD may generally be an asymptomatic condition. It is thus possible that a patient who is clinically well and who follows a GFD can still have small bowel lesions—for example, because she or he does not adhere faithfully to the diet. On the other hand, it is common clinical experience to follow classical celiac children who become and remain asymptomatic after some months on a GFD, although they "confess" to consuming gluten regularly. For this reason the diagnosis of CD, after or before adherence to a GFD, must rely not only on the presence or absence of clinical symptoms. Since it is well known that strict adherence to a GFD offers significantly better protection against malignancy to CD patients (28), control of the jejunal lesions should not be disregarded. In addition, if adherence to the GFD is strict and the small bowel histology is still abnormal, the presence of other gastrointestinal pathology remains a possibility. We believe that a second small bowel biopsy to determine the recovery of the intestinal lesions after GFD is mandatory in all cases of suspected CD.

6.2   The Value of Serological Markers

A noninvasive serological test for the screening of CD has long been sought, and some authors have pointed out that serological tests such as the determination of the serum titers of IgA antigliadin (AGA), antireticulin (ARA), antiendomysium (EmA), and antitisular transglutaminase (tTGA), alone or in combination, could replace the small bowel biopsy as a diagnostic test. However, the sensitivity and specificity of high titers of these serum antibodies vary widely from center to center (29).

Depending on the group of patients studied, sensitivities and specificities of IgA determination of 82 to 96% and 92 to 97%, respectively, have been reported. In clinical practice, however, results of the IgA/AGA tests are sometimes disappointing. Patients with IgA deficiency are missed, and elevated serum levels are found in gastrointestinal disorders other than CD, such as postinfection malabsorption, Crohn's disease, and food protein intolerance as well as in first-degree relatives of CD patients without intestinal alterations (30).

The value of serological markers is age-related. IgA AGA has been found to be the most useful marker in symptomatic children below 2 to 5 years of age and EmA in those older than 5 years and adults. Among our own patients, 10 children below age 2 at the onset of symptoms who had a flat mucosa and well-proven CD, with histological relapse after 6 to 12 months on a gluten challenge, had "falsely" negative EmA. Moreover, we have also observed "falsely" positive EmA in the following individuals: eight siblings of CD patients who had normal mucosa and five untreated CD children with severe villous atrophy, which reversed after withdrawal of gluten and had a normal mucosa after more than 8 years on a gluten-containing diet (Table 6). All of them were HLA-DR3-DQ2– positive and presented the heterodimers DQ 1∗0501 and DQ 1∗0201.

AGA determination alone is not enough, as 15 to 20% of CD patients remain AGA-negative (31) and false-positive AGA titers may frequently be observed in certain patient groups, as in Down's syndrome (32). AGA determination provides a sensitive parameter for monitoring the effectiveness of a GFD and for diagnosing CD in very young children. Serum IgA/EmA determination can be used to screen for CD in asymptomatic adolescents who do not adhere to a GFD and in whom the antigliadin antibody test has a false-negative rate of about 20%, although we have observed "falsely negative EmA" in eight well-proven celiac adolescents (classic ESPGAN criteria) with severe villous atrophy because of a lax diet.

6.3 The Gluten Challenge

According to the "revised criteria" of ESPGAN (5), gluten challenge followed by jejunal biopsy is recommended in the following circumstances: 1) If there is doubt about the initial diagnosis, 2) in communities with high incidence of other causes of enteropathy, 3) if the initial diagnosis is made under the age of 2 years, and 4) in adolescents intending to abandon the GFD.

However, the age of 2 years chosen in the "revised criteria" for not performing gluten challenge seems somewhat arbitrary (6). We agree that a flat jejunal biopsy specimen obtained from a white adult or older child in the western world is very indicative of CD, and gluten challenge followed by jejunal biopsy is not mandatory for the diagnosis of all cases of CD. A biopsy may be needed, however, in some cases irrespective to the age of onset of symptoms. Nevertheless, caution should be exercised in relaxing the diagnostic criteria until prospective studies about this subject performed in different centers are available. Individual circumstances should determine the precise approach to a particular patient.

Clinical practice shows that a gluten challenge under strict medical control is safe in most pediatric patients and has the well-known benefit of better compliance with a lifelong GFD due to both the doctor's and the patient's (and parents') knowledge that the diagnosis has been made as accurately as possible. In the last 31 years (1967–1998) we have diagnosed and followed 930 cases of well-established CD; we found no major complication in any of these after gluten challenge.

Finally, because a considerable number of patients show no clinical or functional alterations following gluten challenge even if they have already developed histological relapse (33), biopsy of the small intestine is the only acceptable method of evaluating the results of the gluten provocation. At present, measurement of EmA or tTGA antibodies in serum, which should be normal when the histological lesions recover, may be helpful to indicate the right moment to obtain the second and third biopsies after gluten challenge. The combination of the serological determinations seems to be an appropriate screening method for CD, but it is not diagnostic.

7 TREATMENT

A strict GFD with exclusion of gluten from wheat, rye, and barley is the universal approach to the management of CD and, in our opinion, must be recommended for life in both symptomatic and asymptomatic individuals (34,35).

Lifelong adherence to a strict GFD should be advised for all the children with CD in order to avoid the late complications of the disease (28,36). Adherence to a strict GFD is essential but not easy for CD patients, and a follow-up control of the asymptomatic CD patients by a gastroenterologist approximately once a year seems to be advisable. Celiac patients' associations help patients to adhere to a GFD and understand their disease better.

CD children adhering to a GFD, even when diagnosed late, reach their target height. Furthermore, it has been demonstrated that CD patients who adhere to a GFD are more likely to enjoy a normal life span.

The ingestion of very small amounts of gluten, even without the presence of clinical or serological responses, induces changes that are detectable morphometrically. The clinical response of patients with CD after starting a GFD is observed within days or weeks. The histological recovery, however, seems to take much longer and can be incomplete even after 2 years, especially in adults.

Although a GFD appears simple, in practice it represents a challenge to patients, dietitians, and physicians, since wheat products are added to many processed foods and are ubiquitous in the Occidental diet. This may be the reason why about 30% of adult patients do not adhere to a strict GFD and why about 25% of the patients who believe that they are following GFD are actually consuming gluten. It has been shown that most of these patients, although well and having normal biochemical parameters, show many abnormalities in their small intestinal biopsies. These facts should be discussed with such patients, and the physician should stress the importance of adhering to a gluten-free diet regardless of apparent gluten tolerance. Several helpful books distributed by the national celiac societies provide excellent dietary instructions and gluten-free recipes.

Adherence to ''gluten-free'' diets is difficult because sources of unintentional gluten intake are so numerous. These sources include contamination with wheat flour of foods that are "naturally" gluten-free, residual gluten in gluten-free wheat starch used for bread mixes, mislabeling of foods, and consumption of products that as yet have not been proven to be toxic to CD patients. Extensive lists of gluten-free foods are available. There is no guarantee of the completeness and validity of the lists, as all contributions (new entries, deletions, and changes) are voluntary. General awareness should be promoted to keep these lists updated. In the *Codex Alimentarius*, the definition of *gluten-free* is based on the nitrogen content of the gluten-containing cereal grains (0.05/100 g of these grains) on a dry-weight basis. It means the acceptance of roughly 100 mg of gliadin per 100 g of dry product derived from cereal grains. The problem is that this standard refers to the amount contained in a particular food item and not to the amount of food that can be taken by a person who is sensitive to it.

Patients with CD need careful support to provide them with up-to-date facts about a GFD. This may in part be given by the many celiac patient societies around the world. In addition, regular attendance at a celiac outpatient clinic, where a specially trained dietitian is available, is helpful. One of the well-known problems in the management of CD is poor dietary compliance among adolescents. Even those patients who claim to be compliant often have jejunal biopsy evidence of gluten ingestion and tend to be underweight.

There is much discussion about the use of wheat starch in manufactured gluten-free products. Although there is no evidence that the amount of gliadin contained in the gluten-free food made with wheat starch is a real danger to CD patients who eat it regularly, other authors suggest that it should be avoided.

Besides the GFD, CD patients may temporarily need a diet low in lactose. As constitutional hypolactasia is a common problem, it is frequently identified in patients having CD. These patients have fewer symptoms if they follow a GFD lactose–reduced diet supplemented with calcium (500 to 1000 mg daily).

Treatment with a GFD will lead to the restoration of normal hematological values in most patients. However, in the transitional period following initiation of the GFD, folic acid (5 to 10 mg daily) and iron are usually given. Vitamin B_{12} deficiency is relatively uncommon and is best treated with hydroxycobalamin 1 mg IM every 2 to 3 months.

The adherence to a GFD improves the absorption of vitamin D, but if osteomalacia is present, the administration of calciferol (1.25 mg or 50,000 U daily) may be necessary to achieve a cure.

In conclusion, the most serious potential complication from long-standing CD is malignancy. The risk of developing a small intestinal lymphoma is increased only in patients on a reduced gluten or normal diet. The role of a gluten-free diet in protecting against other malignancies has also been suggested.

A strict gluten-free diet has become the cornerstone of the management of CD patients and must be recommended for life in both symptomatic and asymptomatic individuals.

REFERENCES

1. Meuwisse GW. Diagnostic criteria in celiac disease. Acta Paediatr Scand 1970; 59: 461–463.
2. McNeish AS, Harms K, Rey J, Shmerling DH, Walker-Smith JA. Re-evaluation of diagnostic criteria for celiac disease. Arch Dis Child 1979; 54:783–786.
3. Polanco I, Larrauri J. Does transient gluten intolerance exist? In: Kumar PJ, Walker-Smith JA, eds. Celiac Disease: One Hundred Years. Middlesex, UK: Leeds University Press, 1990, pp 226–230.
4. Schmitz J, Arnaud-Battandier F, Jos J, Rey J. Long-term follow-up of childhood celiac disease: is there a natural recovery? Pediatr Res 1984; 18:1054.
5. Walker-Smith JA, Guandalini S, Schmitz J, Shmerling DH, Visakorpi JK. Revised criteria for the diagnosis of celiac disease: report of working group of ESPGAN. Arch Dis Child 1990; 65:909–911.
6. Polanco I, Mearin ML, Krasilnikoff PA. The diagnosis of celiac disease: one, two or three biopsies? Pediatrika 1996; 16:350–357.
7. Catassi C. Screening for celiac disease. In: Makki M, Collin P, Visakorpi JK, eds. Celiac Disease. Tampere, Finland: Celiac Disease Study Group, 1997, pp 23–33.
8. Greco L, Mäki M, Di Donato F, Visakorpi JK. Epidemiology of celiac disease in Europe and the Mediterranean area: a summary report on the multicentre study by the European Society of Pediatric Gastroenterology and Nutrition. In: Auricchio S, Visakorpi JK, eds. Common Food Intolerance: I. Epidemiology of Celiac Disease. Dynamic Nutrition Research Series, Vol 2. Basel: Karger, 1992, pp 25–44.
9. Polanco I, De Rosa S, Jasinski C. Celiac disease in Latin America. In: Auricchio S, Visakorpi JK, eds. Common Food Intolerance: I. Epidemiology of Celiac Disease. Dynamic Nutrition Research Series, Vol. 2. Basel: Karger, 1992, pp 10–29.
10. Polanco I, Vázquez C. The influence of breast feeding in celiac disease. Pediatr Res 1981; 75:1193.
11. Polanco I, Biemond I, van Leeuwen A, Schreuder I, Meera-Khan P, Guerrero J, d'Amaro J, Vázquez C, van Rood JJ, Peña AS. Gluten-sensitive enteropathy in Spain: genetic and environmental factors. In: McConnell RB, ed. The Genetics of Celiac Disease. Lancaster, UK: MTP Press, 1981, pp 211–234.
12. Mearin ML, Biemond I, Peña AS, Polanco I, Vázquez C, Schereuder G, de Vries R, van Rood JJ. HLA-DR phenotypes in Spanish celiac children: their contribution to the understanding of the genetics of the disease. Gut 1983; 24:532–537.
13. Sollid LM, Thorsby E. HLA susceptibility genes in celiac disease—genetic mapping and role in pathogenesis. Gastroenterology 1993; 105:910–922.
14. Polanco I, Mearin ML, Larrauri J, Biemond I, Wipkink-Bakker A, Peña AS. The effect of gluten suplementation in healthy siblings of children with celiac disease. Gastroenterology 1987; 92:678–681.
15. Spurkland A, Sollid LM, Polanco I, Vartdal F, Thorsby E. The CD associated HLA-DQ β heterodimer may be encoded by unusual haplotypes. Hum Immunol 1992; 5: 162–167.
16. Schmitz J. Celiac disease in childhood. In: Marsh MN, ed. Celiac Disease. Oxford, UK: Blackwell Scientific Publications, 1992, pp 17–48.
17. Kutlu T, Brousse N, Rambaud C, Le Deist F, Schmitz J, Cerf-Bensussan N. Numbers

of T cell receptor (TCR) + but not of TcR + intraepithelial lymphocytes correlate with the grade of villous atrophy in celiac patients on a long term normal diet. Gut 1993; 34:208–214.

18. Mäki M, Kallonen K, Lahdeaho ML, Visakorpi JK. Changing pattern of childhood celiac disease in Finland. Acta Paediatr Scand 1988; 77:408–412.

19. Gobbi G, Andermann F, Naccarato S, Banchini G, eds. Epilepsy and Other Neurological Disorders in Celiac Disease. London: John Libbey, 1997.

20. Hernández M, Argente J, Navarro A, Caballo N, Barrios V, Hervás F, Polanco I. Growth in malnutrition related to gastrointestinal diseases: celiac disease. Horm Res 1992; 38:79–84.

21. Arilla E, Hernández M, Polanco I, Roca B, Prieto JC, Vázquez C. Modification of somatostatin content and binding in jejunum from celiac children. J Pediatr Gastroenterol Nutr 1987; 6:228–233.

22. Ferguson A, Kingstone K, Gillett H. Is biopsy the sole diagnostic criterion? In: Makki M, Collin P, Visakorpi JK, eds. Celiac Disease. Tampere, Finland: Celiac Disease Study Group, 1997, pp 189–193.

23. Polanco I, Larrauri J, Prieto G, Guerrero J, Peña AS, Vázquez C. Severe villous atrophy appearing at different ages in two coeliac siblings with identical HLA haplotypes. Acta Paediatr Belg 1980; 33:276.

24. Mäki M. Holm H, Koskimies S, Visakorpi JK. Latent celiac disease. In: Mearin ML, Mulder CJJ, eds. Celiac disease. Dordrecht: Kluwer Academic Publishers, 1991, pp 153–156.

25. Polanco I. Continuing need for three biopsies in children. In: Makki M, Collin P, Visakorpi JK, eds. Celiac Disease. Tampere, Finland: Celiac Disease Study Group, 1997, pp 171–176.

26. Mulder Ch JJ, Mearin ML, Peña AS. Clinical and pathological spectrum of celiac disease (letter). Gut 1993; 34:740–741.

27. Polanco I, ed. Enfermedad celiaca. In: Actualidades en Gastroenterología y Hepatología. Vol 20. Barcelona: JR Prous, 1996.

28. Holmes GKT, Prior P, Lane MR, Pope D, Allen RN. Malignancy in celiac disease— effect of a gluten free diet. Gut 1989; 30:333–338.

29. Mulder CJJ, Rostami K, Marsh M. When is a celiac a celiac? Gut 1998; 42:594.

30. Ribes-Koninckx C, Giliams JP, Polanco I, Peña AS. IgA antigliadin antibodies in celiac disease and in inflammatory bowel disease. J Pediatr Gastroenterol Nutr 1984; 29:165–166.

31. Ascher H. Childhood Celiac Disease in Sweden: Changes in Epidemiology, Clinical Pattern and Diagnosis. Goteborg, Sweden: Göteborg University, 1996.

32. Von Blomberg BME, Mearin ML, Houwen RHJ, Peña AS. Serological assays for diagnosing celiac disease. Pediatrika 1996; 16:367–371.

33. Volta U, Molinaro N, Fusconi M, Cassani F, Bianchi FB. IgA antiendomysial antibody test: a step forward in celiac disease screening. Dig Dis Sci 1991; 36:752–756.

34. Pena AS. History of celiac disease: Dicke and the origin of the gluten-free diet. In: Mearin ML, Mulren CJJ, eds. Celiac Disease: 40 Years Gluten-Free. Dordrecht, The Netherlands: Kluwer Academic Publishers 1991, pp 3–7.

35. Polanco I, Prieto G, Molina M, Carrasco S, Lama R. Nutritional management of celiac disease. Pediatrika 1996; 16:386–389.
36. Holmes GKT. Long-term health risks for unrecognized celiac patients. Dyn Nutr Res 1992; 2:105–118.
37. Murch S, Walker-Smith J. Etiology and pathogenesis of childhood coeliac disease. Int Semin Paediatr Gastroenterol Nutr 1996; 5/2:11–15.

22

Chronic Abdominal Pain

Donna K. Zeiter and Jeffrey S. Hyams
University of Connecticut School of Medicine, Farmington, and
Connecticut Children's Medical Center, Hartford, Connecticut

1 INTRODUCTION

Recurrent abdominal pain (RAP) is a common complaint of pediatric patients. In a community-based study, 17 to 24% of both middle and high school students experienced abdominal pain that interfered with their activity (1). Because many children do not seem to have significant "organic" pathology, many physicians have thought of these children as having "psychosomatic" disease. The literature has suggested that 90 to 95% of children do not have organic causes of their pain; however, in one referral population, approximately 12% of children with abdominal pain had inflammation detected on upper endoscopy, 20% were found to have lactose malabsorption, and 4% were found to have inflammatory bowel disease (2).

The differential diagnosis of children with RAP is extensive and warrants a careful history, physical examination, and selective laboratory studies. Certain warning signs in both the history and physical examination can aid in directing further tests and many suggest the need for referral to subspecialists.

TABLE 1 Differential Diagnosis of Recurrent or Chronic Abdominal Pain in Infants and Children[a]

Gastrointestinal	Irritable bowel syndrome, constipation, carbohydrate intolerance, gastritis (*Helicobacter pylori*), intussusception, gastroesophageal reflux, inflammatory bowel disease, celiac disease, allergic gastroenteritis, Meckel's diverticulum
Hepatobiliary	Hepatitis, tumor, cholecystitis, choledochal cyst, gonococcal perihepatitis
Pancreatic	Pancreatitis, pancreatic pseudocyst
Infectious	Parasites (Giardiasis), familial Mediterranean fever
Anatomic	Malrotation, web, stricture, intestinal duplications, recurrent intestinal obstruction
Genitourinary	Urinary tract Infection, hydronephrosis, ureteropelvic junction obstruction, nephrolithiasis, ovarian cyst, ovarian torsion, pelvic inflammatory disease, dysmenorrhea, endometriosis, ectopic pregnancy
Metabolic/toxic	Diabetes mellitus, porphyria, lead poisoning, hyperparathyroidism, hyperlipidemia
Systemic	Angioneurotic edema, juvenile rheumatoid arthritis
Miscellaneous	Abdominal epilepsy, abdominal migraine

[a] Underlining indicates the more common causes.
Source: Ref. 4.

2 ETIOLOGY

The experience of abdominal pain combines somatic, visceral, and referred pain; therefore abdominal pain tends to be poorly localized and the quality difficult to describe (3). Although RAP is often secondary to gastrointestinal causes, physicians need to be aware of hepatobiliary, genitourinary, infectious, and metabolic diseases (Table 1) (4).

3 HISTORY

Where age-appropriate, the initial history should be obtained directly from the child. Attempt to obtain a complete description of the pain, unencumbered by medical terminology. The history should focus on the length of time the child has experienced pain, pain frequency, location and duration, association with meals, and nighttime awakening. Other associated symptoms—such as vomiting, diarrhea, and constipation—may help direct investigation. Also question the patient on systemic symptoms such as fever, joint pain, joint swelling, aphthous ulcerations, skin rashes, headache, pallor, diaphoresis, and dizziness.

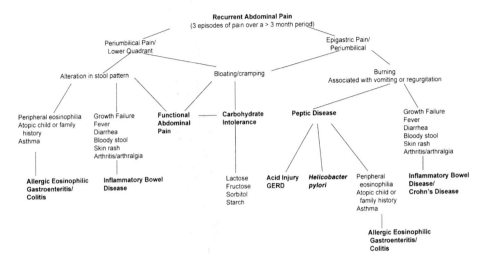

FIGURE 1 Key historical elements in evaluating gastrointestinal causes of recurrent abdominal pain. (From Ref. 4.)

Certain historical points may indicate the possibility of organic disease. These "red flags" include growth failure (weight or height), nighttime awakening, vomiting, blood in the stool or emesis, age less than 4 years, fever, arthritis/arthralgia, aphthous ulcer, skin rash, or family history of inflammatory bowel disease or peptic disease.

Figure 1 reviews a suggested approach to historical information and possible diagnoses in patients with RAP (4).

4 PHYSICAL EXAMINATION

The exam should begin with an accurate determination of weight, height, and vital signs. Give the child time to adjust to the physician by starting the physical examination away from the abdomen. Many younger children may be examined initially on the parent's lap. Evaluate the skin for rashes, turgor, and color. Joints are examined for swelling and redness, nail beds for color and clubbing. The abdominal examination should include visual assessment of the abdomen for distention and vascular anomalies, auscultation for bowel sounds and bruits, and percussion and palpation for liver span, spleen size, masses, and tenderness. Observation of the child's gait can reveal peritoneal signs. In female patients, a gynecological exam may be indicated. In the acute setting, the rectal exam is important in determining lateralization of tenderness as well as checking for mass effect and blood in the stool. In the patient with chronic abdominal pain, the rectal examination is often less informative; however, findings of fissures, tags, and fistulas on visualization of the anus may suggest underlying inflammatory bowel disease.

"Red flags" in the physical exam include fever, growth failure, arthritis, skin rashes (erythema nodosum/pyoderma gangrenosum), clubbing, organomegaly, peritoneal signs, masses, perianal disease, and blood in the stool.

5 DIAGNOSIS

5.1 Blood Tests

Initial evaluation of a patient with RAP should include a complete blood cell count, erythrocyte sedimentation rate, urinalysis, urine culture if indicated, and occult blood in the stool. In patients with vomiting or diarrhea, measurement of electrolytes may be indicated. Chemistries—including total protein, albumin, AST, ALT, alkaline phosphatase, and GGT—are useful in evaluating nutritional status and screening for liver disease if indicated by the history or physical exam. In patients with growth failure, abdominal pain and diarrhea, antigliadin IgA and IgG, and antiendomysial IgA can be used to screen for celiac disease (see Chap. 21).

In patients with dyspepsia, serology for *Helicobacter pylori* may be considered. Although still controversial, serological testing is difficult to interpret in children; it should not be used as the sole diagnostic test and cannot be used to monitor treatment (5). Also, multiple studies have failed to demonstrate a strong association between *H. pylori* and recurrent abdominal pain (5) (see Chap. 20).

In patients with RAP and no unusual components to the history and physical, nothing more than a screening complete blood count and erythrocyte sedimentation rate may be needed. However, if there is suspicion of other underlying disease, a number of radiographic and endoscopic tests are available (see Table 2) (6–8).

5.2 Radiography

In patients with chronic abdominal pain, an abdominal radiograph rarely contributes to the diagnosis. If the patient has persistent vomiting or peritoneal signs, an abdominal radiograph may demonstrate obstruction or perforation. A fecalith may be visible in 5 to 10% of children with acute abdominal pain (9). Constipation or obstipation may be demonstrated on plain film, helping to direct the type and extent of treatment.

TABLE 2 Pros and Cons of Diagnostic Testing

Test	When	Problems
Plain film	Suspected obstruction or perforation	Minimal radiation Low yield
Upper gastrointestinal (UGI) study	Excellent study for anatomy and intraluminal processes Not the study for gastroesophageal reflux	Radiation Preparation Expense
Lower gastrointestinal study	Used in patients with suspected obstruction Also useful in some patients with constipation to screen for Hirschsprung's disease	Radiation Perforation Preparation Uncomfortable
Ultrasound	Useful in evaluating multiple organs, including gallbladder, liver, spleen, pancreas, kidneys, appendix Also useful in evaluating abdominal masses (especially cystic structures)	Difficulty visualizing air-containing organs No bone penetration Ultrasonographer-dependent
CT	Excellent visualization of extraluminal abdominal structures	Radiation Sedation Intravenous contrast
MRI	Excellent visualization of extraluminal abdominal structures	Sedation (very sensitive to motion artifact)
Upper endoscopy	Useful to evaluate hematemesis, persistent vomiting, dysphagia, odynophagia, chronic diarrhea, evaluation of caustic ingestion, foreign body and evaluation of abnormality on UGI study	Risks include cardiac or respiratory depression Bleeding Perforation Infection Contraindicated in patients with suspected bowel perforation
Lower endoscopy	Useful in evaluating hematochezia, chronic diarrhea, inflammatory bowel disease, or familial polyposis syndromes	Risks are as indicated in upper endoscopy Contraindicated in patients with suspected bowel perforation

Source: Refs. 6–8.

5.3 Contrast Studies

Upper gastrointestinal (UGI) contrast studies are useful in delineating the anatomy of the esophagus, stomach, and duodenum. The initial swallow may be used to evaluate for abnormalities of the esophagus, including fistulas, vascular rings, webs, and hiatal hernias. Other anatomic anomalies—such as gastric outlet obstruction, duodenal web, and stricture and malrotation—are well visualized on UGI contrast studies. In the pediatric patient, UGI studies are not as sensitive as endoscopy in the evaluation of mucosal injury. UGI studies are also not the best test for gastroesophageal reflux. The small bowel and terminal ileum may also be visualized if the study is continued as a small bowel follow through.

Large bowel enema contrast studies are important in patients with evidence of obstruction of many causes, such as intussusception, volvulus, malrotation, meconium ileus, and Hirschsprung's disease (7). A number of contrast agents are used in the pediatric patient, including barium, water-soluble contrast, and air. In a patient with symptoms suggestive of intussusception (pain, vomiting, palpable mass, blood in the stool), an air-contrast barium enema may be both diagnostic and therapeutic. In patients with meconium ileus, use of a water-soluble contrast may also be therapeutic. The barium enema study are not considered the study of choice in demonstrating mucosal disease or polyps in the pediatric patient; however, colonoscopy and barium enema may complement each other.

5.4 Cross-Sectional Imaging

Abdominal sonography is a noninvasive test that provides excellent screening for diseases of the biliary tree, pancreas, or genitourinary tract (3). In patients of the appropriate age with pain and vomiting, ultrasonography can screen for intussusception, pyloric stenosis, and obstruction of the ureteropelvic junction. In patients with chronic recurrent abdominal pain, abdominal ultrasound appears to have limited yield. In one study, 81% of patients had a normal study and 19% had abnormalities detected, none of which contributed to the primary symptom of abdominal pain (6).

The use of computed tomography (CT) and magnetic resonance imaging (MRI) will depend on history, physical examination, and other laboratory findings. These tests are not used routinely in patients with chronic abdominal pain.

5.5 Endoscopy

Upper and lower endoscopy is useful in patients with suspected mucosal disease leading to abdominal pain. Upper endoscopy is indicated in those patients with hematemesis, persistent vomiting, dysphagia, odynophagia, chronic diarrhea, evaluation of caustic ingestion, foreign body, and evaluation of abnormality on UGI (3). In those patients with chronic recurrent abdominal pain who have not responded to medical therapy or who relapse once therapy is discontinued, endos-

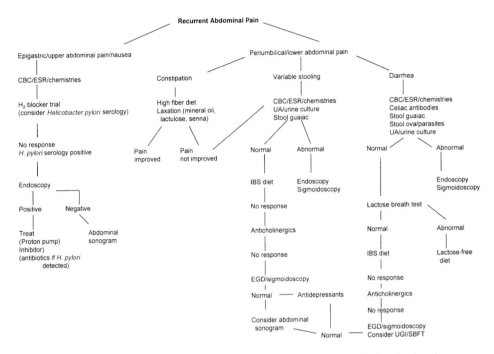

FIGURE 2 Suggested evaluation of patient with recurrent abdominal pain.

copy will identify the severity, extent, and composition (neutrophilic/eosino-philic) of any inflammation. Colonoscopy is indicated in those patients with hematochezia, chronic diarrhea, inflammatory bowel disease, or familial polyposis syndromes (3). In patients with chronic right-lower-quadrant abdominal pain, colonoscopy is the most sensitive way to evaluate for inflammation in the terminal ileum.

Figure 2 outlines a suggested approach to recurrent abdominal pain, including use of increasingly invasive testing.

6 RECURRENT ABDOMINAL PAIN AND THE FUNCTIONAL BOWEL DISORDERS

6.1 Introduction/Classification

Apley and Nash were the first investigators to review abdominal pain in 1000 English schoolchildren in 1958 (10). They defined RAP as three or more episodes of pain affecting activity over a 3-month period. Their conclusions were that "those with pains tend to be anxious, timid, fussy and overconscientious" (10).

With the availability of safe pediatric radiographic and endoscopic techniques, RAP can be divided into the "organic" diseases and "nonorganic" or functional disorders. The use of the term *functional* reflects our inability to identify altered tissue structure or function. Although many symptoms may overlap, symptom-based criteria are being used in an attempt to further define differences in patients with functional disorders to facilitate both research and treatment (11). In pediatrics, classification of functional bowel disorders is less well defined than in adults. However, three main categories are more commonly recognized: irritable bowel syndrome (IBS), functional dyspepsia, and functional abdominal pain.

Irritable bowel syndrome is defined by the use of the Manning (12) or Rome (13) criteria, which include abdominal pain relieved by stooling, alteration in stooling pattern ranging from diarrhea to constipation, feelings of incomplete evacuation, and abdominal distention. As in adults, IBS may be further subclassified as diarrhea-predominant, constipation-predominant, and variable (14).

Functional dyspepsia is the presence of pain, discomfort, nausea, bloating, and early satiety located in the upper abdomen. Ulcer-like dyspepsia has pain as the dominant complaint, while dysmotility-like dyspepsia has other upper abdominal symptoms as the primary complaint (14). In a recent prospective study, 49% of patients presenting for a pediatric gastroenterology evaluation for chronic abdominal pain had dyspepsia (15). Of these patients, 44% ultimately underwent endoscopy, with 62% having no identifiable inflammation on biopsy (15). Those with inflammation had esophagitis, gastritis, duodenitis, or *H. pylori* gastritis. No ulcers were detected (15). Suggested mechanisms of functional dyspepsia include dysmotility with delayed gastric emptying, delayed upper intestinal transit, or visceral hypersensitivity (14).

Functional abdominal pain is the term used to describe those patients who have abdominal pain but do not fulfill the criteria for IBS (14).

6.2 The Enteric Nervous System

The enteric nervous system (ENS) is a network of neurons whose cell bodies are located in the myenteric and submucosal plexuses of the bowel wall. These neurons serve to modulate many functions, including epithelial transport, secretion, sensation, and gastrointestinal motility (16,17). The ENS is inhibitory to the pacers of the smooth muscle composing the gastrointestinal tract. This function permits aboral waves of peristalsis (16). Sensory receptors relay information through the paravertebral ganglia via the vagus nerve and spinal cord, where information can be processes in the cortex, brainstem, limbic system, hypothalamus, and reticular formation (16). These, in turn, will activate reflexes, controlling the various motility patterns seen in the gastrointestinal tract.

Hypotheses as to the pathogenesis of functional bowel disorders focus on altered ENS responsiveness and how this may interact with external stimuli and higher cortical perception.

6.3 Mechanisms

Multiple mechanisms are most likely involved in the development of functional abdominal pain, including abnormal motility, enhanced visceral hypersensitivity, and psychosocial factors (18).

Although initially felt to be a primary cause of functional bowel disorders, altered motility does not seem to be as closely linked to symptoms as previously thought. Earlier studies demonstrated an increase in myoelectric activity with a pattern of three cycles per minute; however, more recent studies refute those findings (18). In some patients with constipation-predominant IBS, delayed transit has been demonstrated (19). Some patients with diarrhea-predominant IBS have decreased transit times (20). Most importantly, multiple studies have demonstrated that patients with IBS have increased, exaggerated motility in response to environmental stimuli such as stress, meals, and hormones (18).

Visceral hypersensitivity describes the phenomenon of increased sensitivity to distention and normal intestinal function as well as increased somatic referral of visceral pain, which is seen in patients with IBS (18). A number of studies using balloon distention of various parts of the colon have demonstrated that patients with IBS have lower thresholds for perceiving visceral pain on distention (without altered compliance), and the pain appears to have an altered referral pattern by comparison with normal controls (21–23). These patients also demonstrate a normal or increased tolerance of somatic pain (24).

Mechanisms for this visceral hypersensitivity include alteration in the modulation of the peripheral sensory neurons in the bowel wall and alteration in how this information in centrally synthesized. Mast cells and enterochromaffin cells located in the bowel wall appear to be innervated by the autonomic nervous system. When stimulated, these cells have the ability to secrete chemicals that may diffuse to afferent receptors, altering visceral sensation (25).

The central nervous system acts to integrate and modulate input from the periphery. There is evidence that the prefrontal and anterior cingulate cortices are involved in altered autonomic function, leading to perception of bowel distention (25). There is also evidence that stress leads to increased motility in the descending and sigmoid colon (25). It is difficult to determine whether stressful experiences or underlying psychiatric diagnoses lead to an altered central nervous system modulation and therefore to pain, or whether these maladaptive behaviors are in part related to an alteration in central processing associated with functional bowel disease.

Psychiatric profiles of patients with functional bowel disorders have been investigated. In a recent study reviewing data from the Medical Research Council National Survey of Health and Development, England, a cohort of children was followed for 20 years to evaluate the prognosis of those with abdominal pain (26). The incidence of pain compared favorably with that previously reported (between 17 and 20%). There was a significant association between abdominal pain in the children and illness in the parents, suggesting that parental anxiety may reinforce the child's anxiety about physical symptoms (26). Interestingly, the children were not maladjusted and did not have high scores on assessment for neuroses. However, childhood abdominal pain did have an association with increased likelihood of anxiety or depression in adulthood (26). Finally, children with abdominal pain did not have an increased likelihood of becoming adults with abdominal pain (26).

7   MANAGEMENT/TREATMENT

The management of patients with chronic abdominal pain is determined by the location and description of that pain. The majority of patients will ultimately be described as having functional abdominal pain/IBS. However, a subset of children will have epigastric/upper abdominal pain, bloating, or nausea—conditions known as dyspepsia. The discomfort may be related to meals or may be nocturnal and associated with poor feeding or vomiting. This upper abdominal pain may be caused by disorders ranging from gastroesophageal reflux, gastritis, esophagitis, and pancreatitis to functional dyspepsia. Ultimately, treatment will depend on the diagnosis.

Patients with dyspepsia and an otherwise normal physical and biochemical examination may initially be given therapeutic trials of antacids or H_2 blockers. Antacids are often a simple first-line therapy for patients with dyspepsia and are dosed at 0.5 mL/kg per dose after eating and before bed. Improvement in the epigastric pain, even transiently, may help support the presence of acid-peptic disease. If the patient fails to improve, a trial of H_2-receptor antagonists is both cost-effective and safe.

Patients who fail to respond to these maneuvers often require an endoscopy (see Chap. 32). Endoscopy is the most sensitive and specific means of identifying the presence and/or type of inflammation (allergic versus acid-peptic). *H. pylori* may also be identified on endoscopy. If the endoscopy is normal, the patient has functional dyspepsia. The potential mechanisms of functional dyspepsia are numerous and, in many ways, parallel those for other functional bowel disorders. Some patients have been found to have altered gastric myoelectric activity, gastric emptying, or antroduodenal motility (14). Additionally, patients may have an increased mucosal sensitivity to gastric acid (14).

Patients with functional dyspepsia may respond to antisecretory medications such as proton-pump inhibitors or cytoprotective agents such as sucralfate. Patients with dysmotility-like dyspepsia may respond to prokinetic medications such as metoclopramide or cisapride (14), although cisapride is no longer available in the United States.

In patients with IBS or functional abdominal pain, management and treatment are multifactorial, requiring input from the pediatrician, gastroenterologist, nutritionist and mental health professional. The ultimate goal of treatment is to relieve symptoms and to improve the patients' quality of life.

The physician should identify and address those fears that have led the parents to bring the child for evaluation. Depending on the severity of symptoms and the degree to which activity is impaired, directed noninvasive testing may help reassure the family. Education about functional bowel disorders should include a discussion of potential mechanisms and reassurance. It is important to validate the patient's experience of the pain as being real and not contrived while also pointing out how life events and stresses may play a part in the disease process.

Treatment often begins with dietary modification. Patients should avoid foods high in fat, alcohol, and caffeine. Foods with large amounts of poorly digestible carbohydrates (high-fructose corn syrup, sorbitol, stachyose, and raffinose) should be avoided, as these may lead to increased gas production, bowel distention, and pain. Lactose should not be discontinued routinely unless lactose intolerance is documented, as cow's-milk products often provide a large amount of calories. In patients with constipation-predominant IBS, diets high in fiber may help relieve discomfort and promote stooling, although the general and prolonged use of fiber in other forms of IBS remains controversial (18).

When these simple tactics fail to improve the patient's abdominal pain, anticholinergic medication is often the first line of therapy (27). Acetylcholine functions as a neurotransmitter at both the neuromuscular junction (nicotinic) and the ganglia of the autonomic nervous system and parasympathetic system (muscarinic). Because of this autonomic action, these medications affect the gastrointestinal tract by decreasing bowel tone and motility and decreasing secretion (27). The most common forms used include dicyclomine hydrochloride (Bentyl) and hyoscyamine sulfate (Levsin). A number of anticholinergic medications have been found to be more effective than placebo for controlling pain and improving quality of life and at this time are awaiting FDA approval (18).

In patients with refractory symptoms of IBS, antidepressants have been demonstrated to lead to improved pain control and global functioning via a number of potential mechanisms. Antidepressants have been shown to modify intestinal motility (28). Tricyclic antidepressants affect neurotransmission by blocking muscarinic receptors as well as serotonin and norepinephrine reuptake. This alteration in neurotransmitters may lead to the analgesic effect of antidepressants, which is independent of their psychotropic effects (29). In a retrospective review of 5 years of antidepressant use in patients with IBS, improvement was seen in 89% of patients, with remission of symptoms in 61% (30). In another controlled study comparing desipramine with placebo and atropine, 54% of patients reported improvement on desipramine, while 21% improved on atropine and 18% of the placebo group improved (31). Doses tend to be smaller than those used in major mental illness (18): 10 to 25 mg before bedtime.

In the ''biosychosocial'' approach to IBS, the affective state of the patient and his or her social and cultural environment play a vital role in the development and experience of disease. Psychological treatments have been demonstrated to improve patients' quality of life, and the issue of counseling as an adjunct to medical treatment and investigation should be raised early in the course of working with patients with IBS. A positive response seems to correlate with patients who relate the gastrointestinal symptoms to stress, are younger, and have lower levels of anxiety (18). There are currently no studies indicating whether one form of therapy is superior to another.

8   WHEN TO REFER

The initial assessment and management of most children with chronic abdominal pain should begin under the guidance of the primary care provider. If any of the red flags previously discussed appear in the history or physical, there should be a higher index for referral to a facility that can perform more invasive radiographic and endoscopic testing.

In patients with chronic abdominal pain, the surgeon is rarely the first line of referral. However, if patients develop evidence of obstruction (vomiting, abdominal distention), evidence of perforation (fever, peritoneal signs), or evidence of choledocholithiasis (jaundice, fever, right-upper-quadrant tenderness), they should first be stabilized in the emergency room and surgical consultation obtained.

In patients with functional bowel disorders as determined by history, physical, and limited laboratory evaluation, treatment with diet and anticholinergics can be initiated by the primary care physician. However, the use of antidepressants should be limited to the most refractory cases, and these children warrant evaluation by a pediatric gastroenterologist before beginning these medications.

In patients with dyspepsia, a trial of H_2 blockade may modify symptoms and may be managed through the primary care physician. If H_2 blockade does not lead to improvement, the input of a pediatric gastroenterologist with access to endoscopy may help to further clarify the source of the dyspepsia and aid in directing treatment.

Patients in whom there is a significant suspicion for lactose intolerance warrant a lactose breath test to document malabsorption before beginning the diet, which can be very restrictive (see Chap. 14).

Of course, in some cases families continue to be concerned about the possibility of an underlying illness despite directed testing, reassurance, and education. In these cases, the support of a subspecialty referral may be vital in helping direct the family toward the most effective treatments.

The pediatric patient with chronic abdominal pain can be the most challenging to evaluate and manage. These patients require careful histories and physical exams performed over multiple visits. Descriptions of the pain are often impossible to obtain from the child and reports are subject to the biases of the caregivers. Testing and referrals must be directed and individualized. Despite our poor understanding of the functional bowel diseases, the care of these patients provides an opportunity to treat the entire patient physically, socially, and psychologically.

REFERENCES

1. Hyams JS, Burke G, Davis PM, Rzepski B, Andrulonis PA. Abdominal pain and irritable bowel syndrome in adolescents: a community based study. J Pediatr 1996; 129(2):220–226.
2. Hyams JS, Treem WR, Justinich CJ, Davis P, Shoup M, Burke G. Characterization of symptoms in children with recurrent abdominal pain; resemblance to irritable bowel syndrome. J Pediatr Gastroenterol Nutr 1995; 20:209–214.
3. Antonson DL. Abdominal pain. Pediatr Endosc 1994; 4(1):1–21.
4. Zeiter D, Hyams JS. Abdominal pain in infants and children—what to watch for in the workup? Consultant Consult Primary Care 1997; 37:121–132.
5. Bujanover Y, Reif S, Yahav J. Helicobacter pylori and peptic disease in the pediatric patient. Pediatr Clin North Am 1996; 43(1):213–234.
6. Shannon A, Martin DJ, Feldman W. Ultrasonographic studies in the management of recurrent abdominal pain. Pediatrics 1990; 86:35.
7. Liu PCF, Stringer DA. Radiography: contrast studies. In: Walker WA, Durie PR, Hamilton JR, Walker-Smith JA, Watkins JB. Pediatric Gastrointestinal Disease: Pathophysiology, Diagnosis, Management, 2nd ed. Vol 2. Philadelphia: Mosby-Year Book, 1996; pp 1674–1712.
8. Shuckett BS, Babyn P, Stringer DA, Cohen MD. Cross-sectional imaging: sonography, computed tomography, magnetic resonance imaging. In: Walker WA, Durie PR, Hamilton JR, Walker-Smith JA, Watkins JB, eds. Pediatric Gastrointestinal Disease: Pathophysiology, Diagnosis, Management, 2nd ed. Vol 2. Philadelphia: Mosby-Year Book, 1996; pp 1713–1760.
9. Irish MS, Pearl RH, Caty MG, Glick PL. The approach to common abdominal diagnoses in infants and children. Pediatr Clin North Am 1998; 45(4):729–772.
10. Apley J, Naish N. Recurrent abdominal pain: a field survey of 1,000 school children. Arch Dis Child 1958; 33:165–170.
11. Drossman DA, Thompson WG, Talley NJ, Funch-Jensen P, Janssens J, Whitehead WE. Identification of sub-groups of functional gastrointestinal disorders. Gastroenterol Int 1990; 3(4):159–172.
12. Manning AP, Thompson WG, Heaton KW, Morris AF. Towards a positive diagnosis of irritable bowel. BMJ 1978; 2:653–654.
13. Thompson WG Dotevall G, Drossman DA, Heaton KW, Druis W. Irritable bowel syndrome: guidelines for the diagnosis. Gastroenterol Int 1989; 2:92–95.
14. Hyams JS, Hyman PE. Recurrent abdominal pain and the biopsychosocial model of medical practice. J Pediatr 1998; 133(4):473–478.
15. Hyams FS, Davis P, Sylvester FA, Zeiter DK, Justinich CJ, Lerer T. Dyspepsia in

children and adolescents: a prospective study. J Pediatr Gastroenterol Nutr 2000; 30:413–418.

16. Corazziari E. Neuro-enteric mechanisms of gastrointestinal motor function. J Pediatr Gastroenterol Nutr 1997; 25:S3–S4.

17. Guandalini S. Enteric nervous system: intestinal absorption and secretion. J Pediatr Gastroenterol Nutr 1997; 25:S5–S6.

18. Drossman DA, Whitehead WE, Camilleri M. Irritable bowel syndrome: a technical review for practice guideline development. Gastroenterology 1997; 122:2120–2137.

19. Cann PA, Read NW, Brown C, Hobson N, Holdsworth CG. Irritable bowel syndrome: relationship of disorders in the transit of a single solid meal to symptom patterns. Gut 1983; 24:405–411.

20. Vassallo MJ, Camilleri M, Phillips SF, Steadman CJ, Taley NJ, Hanson RB, Haddad AC. Colonic tone and motility in patients with irritable bowel syndrome. Mayo Clin Proc 1992; 67:725–731.

21. Accarino AM, Azpiroz F, Malagelada JR. Selective dysfunction of mechanosensitive intestinal afferents in irritable bowel syndrome. Gastroenterology 1995; 108:636–643.

22. Mertz H, Naliboff B, Munakata J, Niazi N, Mayer EA. Altered rectal perception is a biological marker of patients with irritable bowel syndrome. Gastroenterology 1995; 109:40–52.

23. Munakata J, Naliboff B, Harraf F, Kodner A, Lembo T, Chang L, Silverman DHS, Mayer EA. Repetitive sigmoid stimulation induces rectal hyperalgesia in patients with irritable bowel syndrome. Gastroenterology 1997; 112:55–63.

24. Cook IJ, Vaan Eeden A, Collins SM. Patients with irritable bowel syndrome have greater pain tolerance than normal subjects. Gastroenterology 1987; 93:727–733.

25. Schmulson MJ, Mayer EA. Evolving concepts in irritable bowel syndrome. Curr Opin Gastroenterol 1999; 15:16–21.

26. Hotopf M, Carr S, Mayou R, Wadsworth M, Wessely S. Why do children have chronic abdominal pain, and what happens to them when they grow up? Population based cohort study. BMJ 1998; 316:1196–1200.

27. Hardy SC, Walker A. Anticholinergic medications in pediatric gastrointestinal disease. Pediatr Rev 1994; 15(10):389–390.

28. Gorard DA, Libby GW, Farthing MJG. Effect of a tricyclic antidepressant on small intestinal motility in health and diarrhea-predominant irritable bowel syndrome. Dig Dis Sci 1995; 40:86–95.

29. Clouse RE. Antidepressants for functional gastrointestinal syndromes. Dig Dis Sci 1994; 39(11):2352–2363.

30. Clouse RE, Lustman PJ, Geisman RA, Alpers DH. Antidepressant therapy in 138 patients with irritable bowel syndrome: a five-year clinical experience. Aliment Pharmacol Ther 1994; 8:409–416.

31. Greenbaum DS, Mayle JE, Vanegeren LE, Jerome JA, Mayor JW, Greenbaum RB, Matson RW, Stein GE, Dean HA, Halvosen NA, Rosen LW. Effects of desipramine on irritable bowel syndrome compared with atropine and placebo. Dig Dis Sci 1987; 32:257–266.

23

Constipation and Encopresis

Vera Loening-Baucke
University of Iowa, Iowa City, Iowa

1 INTRODUCTION

Constipation and encopresis represent common problems in children. Constipation is a symptom not a disease. Many different disorders can cause the symptom of constipation. Constipation is most commonly due to functional reasons; in other words, it is not due to organic or anatomic causes or secondary to the intake of medication. We define encopresis as the involuntary loss of formed, semiformed, or liquid stool into the child's underwear in the presence of functional constipation after the child has reached the age of 4 years (1). Fecal incontinence is fecal soiling in the presence of an organic or anatomic lesion, such as myelomeningocele, some muscle diseases, or anorectal malformations.

The aims of this chapter are to describe the symptoms of functional constipation with or without encopresis in children 4 years of age or older, to present the differential diagnosis of constipation in this age group, to describe the evaluation and treatment of these children, and to report on treatment outcome.

2 ANATOMY AND PHYSIOLOGY

Very special control mechanisms are developed in the body to prevent loss of gas, stool, and urine. Unconscious regulation of bowel movements is a normal phenomenon after birth. Conscious regulation of bowel movements is achieved at an average age of 28 months. Fecal continence is the body's ability to recognize when the rectal ampulla fills; to discriminate whether the content is formed, liquid stool, or gas; and to retain the content until emptying it is socially convenient. The major structures responsible for continence and defecation are the external

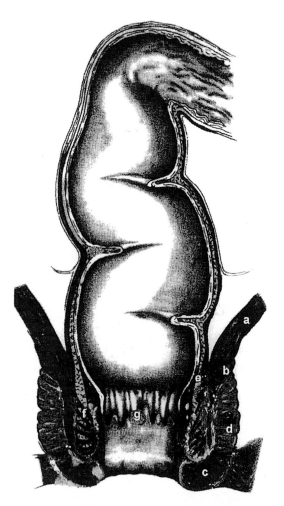

FIGURE 1 Anatomy of the anorectal area: (a) musculus levator ani; (b) m. sphincter ani externus, deep part; (c) m. sphincter ani externus, subcutaneous part; (d) m. sphincter ani externus, superficial part; (e) m. sphincter internus; (f) intersphincteric fascia; (g) linea dentata.

anal sphincter, the puborectalis muscle, the internal anal sphincter, and the rectum (Fig. 1). The factors responsible for maintaining fecal continence and that also facilitate defecation are the high-pressure zone in the anal canal, the anal and rectal sensory and reflex mechanisms, the viscoelastic properties of the rectum, and stool volume and consistency. Fecal material can be retained by contraction of the external sphincter and puborectalis muscle. Fecal material can be expelled by the combination of increased intra-abdominal pressure produced by closure of the glottis, fixation of the diaphragm, contractions of the abdominal muscles and rectal wall, and relaxation of the internal and external anal sphincters.

3 FUNCTIONAL CONSTIPATION

Some 96% of children pass stools from three times daily to once every other day, a pattern that persists until old age (2). Constipation is usually defined in terms of alterations in the frequency, size, consistency, or the ease in the passing of stool. Constipation in children can be defined by a stool frequency of less than 3 times per week, painful bowel movements, or stool retention with or without encopresis even when the stool frequency is ≥ 3 times per week.

Functional constipation may be thought of as a maladaptive response. In children, if defecation is painful, the pain-producing activity may be avoided by stool withholding. When the child decides not to have a bowel movement, he or she tightens the external anal sphincter and muscles of the pelvic floor. The rectum adjusts to the contents and the urge to defecate gradually passes. The repetition of this process creates a vicious cycle, as successively greater amounts of stool are built up in the rectum with longer exposure to its drying action. Children may ignore the call to stool, which results in fecal retention leading to suppression of the rectal sensation. In some, pain and fear prevent the relaxation of the pelvic floor muscles during defecation.

Encopresis exists when the retained stool—whether formed, soft, or semi-liquid—leaks to the outside around the accumulated firm stool mass. When stool retention remains untreated for a prolonged period of time, the rectal wall stretches and a megarectum develops. The intervals between bowel movements become increasingly longer and the rectum becomes so large that the stored stool can be felt as an abdominal mass that reaches up to the umbilicus, or sometimes even above. In some cases, stool distends the whole colon (megacolon). Some children may not have stool palpable through the abdominal wall, either because they have recently passed a large bowel movement or because they have soft fecal loading of their megarectum, which may not be recognized by an inexperienced examiner.

Prevalence rates for constipation between 18 to 28% have been reported from Brazil and 34% from Great Britain (3). Most often constipation is short-lived and of little consequence; however, chronic constipation most often follows an inadequately managed acute problem. Some 5% of the otherwise healthy 4- to 11-year-old schoolchildren in Great Britain have been reported to have chronic constipation which lasts for >6 months (3).

No single mechanism is responsible for chronic functional constipation. Constitutional and inherited factors, such as intrinsic slow motility, contribute to constipation. Constipation can cause painful bowel movements and fear of defecation that leads to voluntary withholding of stool. There seems to be two age peaks for the worsening of constipation. The first peak is during toilet training while the second occurs when a child begins to attend school, when toilet use is regulated to special times and toilets may not be clean and private. Another cause for constipation has been intolerance of cow's-milk protein (4). We found this to be a rare cause of constipation in children.

4 ENCOPRESIS

In the United States, only 25 to 30% of children are reliably toilet trained by 2 years of age and 80% by 3 years. Because of the relatively wide range in age for achieving bowel control among normal children, the definition of encopresis is applied only to children who are at least 4 years of age (1). Encopresis is the involuntary passage of formed, semiformed, or liquid stool into the child's underwear and is a complication of long-standing constipation. Although the fecal soiling is involuntary, it can be prevented for short periods of time if the child concentrates carefully on closing the external anal sphincter. Encopresis is reported to affect 2.8% of 4-year-old children, 1.5% of 7- to 8-year-old children, and 1.6% of 10- to 11-year-old children. The male-to-female ratio for encopresis ranges from 2.5:1 to 6:1.

The clinical features of constipation with fecal retention are listed in Table 1. Some children will have intermittent soiling. A period free of soiling may occur after a huge bowel movement, which may obstruct the toilet, and soiling will resume only after several days of stool retention. Usually, the consistency of stool found in the underwear is loose or clay-like. Sometimes the core of the impaction breaks off and a firm stool is found in the underwear. Occasionally, a full bowel movement is passed into the underwear. Many children display retentive posturing. Instead of using the bathroom and sitting down for defecation and relaxing the pelvic floor at times when an urge to defecate is felt, the retentive child will contract the pelvic floor and gluteal muscles often in standing position in an attempt to avoid defecation.

Children with encopresis often deny the presence of stool in their underwear and even the accompanying foul and penetrant odor. Many children hide their soiled underwear, and most have a nonchalant attitude regarding the enco-

TABLE 1 Clinical Features of Constipation with Fecal Retention

Difficulties with defecation begin early in life (in 49% of children prior to 1
    year of age)
Passage of very large stools
Obstruction of the toilet by the stools
Symptoms due to the increasing accumulation of stool
  Retentive posturing
  Encopresis
  Abdominal pain and irritability, anal or rectal pain
  Anorexia
  Urinary symptoms
    Daytime urinary incontinence
    Nighttime urinary incontinence
    Urinary tract infection
Unusual behaviors in an effort to cope with the encopresis
  Nonchalant attitude regarding the encopresis
  Hiding of soiled underwear
  Lack of awareness of an encopretic episode
Dramatic disappearance of most symptoms following the passage of a
    huge stool

presis. Parents usually find this situation very frustrating, and soiling becomes a major issue of contention between the parent and the child.

4.1 Complications of Constipation

Encopresis is the most obvious complication of constipation, but other complications are frequently seen (Table 2). Chronic abdominal or anal and rectal pain is reported by approximately one-half of the children. Fifty-two percent of our chronically constipated and encopretic children suffered from abdominal pain. Severe attacks of abdominal pain can occur either daily, just before a bowel movement, or for several days prior to a large bowel movement. Many children suffer from vague, chronic abdominal pain while some patients with large stool masses throughout the entire colon may not experience any abdominal pain. Other primary complications of constipation are urinary symptoms such as daytime and/or nighttime urinary incontinence and urinary tract infections. Daytime urinary incontinence was present in 29% of chronically constipated and encopretic children, bed wetting in 34%, and one or more urinary tract infections in 33% of girls and 3% of boys (5). Other urinary problems—such as vesicoureteral

TABLE 2 Complications of Chronic Constipation

Encopresis
Pain
  Abdominal pain
  Anal or rectal pain
Anorexia
Urinary complications
  Daytime urinary incontinence
  Nighttime urinary incontinence
  Urinary tract infection
  Vesicoureteral reflux
  Urinary retention
  Megacystis
  Ureteral obstruction
Rarely, life-threatening events such as shock or toxic megacolon
Social exclusion by siblings, parents, peers, and teachers

reflux, urinary retention, megacystis, and ureteral obstruction—were seen less frequently.

Life-threatening events such as severe shock and toxic megacolon are fortunately rare but have been observed by both the author and others.

The social stigma that goes along with increased flatulence and the odor of encopresis can be devastating to the child's self-esteem and acceptance by siblings, parents, peers, and teachers.

5 INVESTIGATIONS

5.1 Clinical Investigation

The history (Table 3) should include information regarding the general health of the child and the presenting signs and symptoms. A careful history must elicit the intervals, amount, diameter, and consistency of bowel movements deposited into the toilet and of stools deposited into the underwear at the present time. The amount, intervals, diameter, and consistency of bowel movements are important because some children may have daily bowel movements but evacuate incompletely, as evidenced by periodic passage of very large amounts of stool of hard to loose consistency, or the presence of a fecal abdominal mass. Do the stools clog the toilet? Is stool withholding present? What was the age at onset of constipation and/or soiling? Was there a problem with the timing of passage of meconium? The character of the stools is reviewed from birth for

TABLE 3 Encopresis and Soiling

History	Physical examination

Complete, with special attention to:
  Stooling habits
    Character of stools in toilet
    Character of stools in underwear
    Stool-withholding maneuvers
  Age of onset of constipation/soiling
  Abdominal pain
  Urinary symptoms:
    Day wetting
    Bed-wetting
    Urinary tract infections
  Dietary habits
	Complete, with special attention to:
	  Abdominal examination
	  Anal inspection
	  Rectal digital examination
	  Neurologic examination, including testing of perianal sensation

consistency, caliber, volume, and frequency. Is abdominal pain present? Are urinary incontinence or urinary tract infection present? What are the dietary habits? At what age was cow's milk introduced into the diet, and did that cause any problems?

The physical examination (Table 3) should be thorough in order to rule out an underlying disorder. Weight and height should be plotted. The remainder of the general examination should focus on features of systemic disease. An abdominal fecal mass can be palpated in approximately half of these children. Sometimes the mass extends throughout the entire colon, but more commonly the mass is felt suprapubically and midline, sometimes filling the left or the right lower quadrant. In many cases, inspection of the perineum shows fecal material but may also show evidence of streptococcal disease or fissures. The position of the anus and its size must be assessed. Often the rectum is packed with stool, which may be of hard consistency; more commonly, the outside of the fecal impaction will feel like clay with a rock-hard core. Sometimes the retained stool can be soft or even loose. In some children who recently had a large bowel movement, rectal fecal retention may not be felt. A low anal pressure during digital rectal examination suggests either fecal retention with inhibition of anal resting pressure, a disease involving the external or internal anal sphincter, or both. In cooperative children, the neurological examination should include perineal sensation testing using a cotton swab. Loss of perianal skin sensation can be associated with various neurological diseases of the spinal cord.

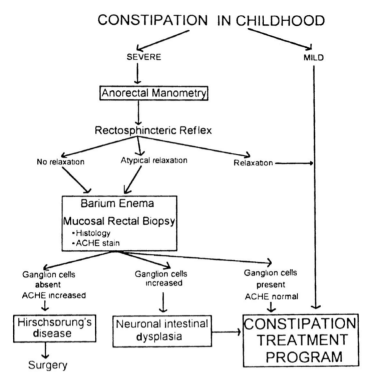

FIGURE 2   Algorithm for the application of diagnostic tests in constipated children. ACHE, acetylcholinesterase stain. (From Ref. 6.)

5.2   Laboratory Investigation

Most children with functional constipation with or without encopresis require no or minimal laboratory workup (Fig. 2). A careful history and physical examination helps differentiate between the various entities described in Table 4 and allows the physician to make a decision regarding requirements for blood studies (deficiency or excess of thyroid or adrenal hormones, electrolyte imbalances, calcium levels, and endomysial antibodies to rule out celiac disease), urine culture, x-ray studies, anorectal manometric studies, or rectal biopsy. Special investigations are indicated in the presence of any symptoms suggestive of Hirschsprung's disease and when anorectal malformation or postoperative state are complicating factors. These children may need to be investigated by radiological studies, anorectal manometry, and/or rectal biopsy.

    Radiological studies are usually not indicated in uncomplicated constipa-

TABLE 4   Causes of Constipation with or Without Fecal Soiling

Functional constipation in >90%
Neurogenic constipation
   Hirschsprung's disease
   Disorders of the spinal cord, such as myelomeningocele, tumor
   Cerebral palsy, hypotonia
Constipation secondary to anal lesions
   Anal fissures
   Anterior location of the anus
   Anal stenosis and anal atresia
Chronic intestinal pseudo-obstruction
Constipation secondary to endocrine and metabolic disorders
   Hypothyroidism
   Renal acidosis
   Diabetes insipidus
   Hypercalcemia
Constipation secondary to neuromuscular disorders
   Myotonic dystrophy
   Muscular dystrophy
Constipation induced by drugs
   Methylphenidate
   Phenytoin
   Imipramine hydrochloride
   Phenothiazine
   Antacids
   Codeine-containing medication

tion. A plain abdominal film can be very useful in assessing the presence or absence of retained stool, its extent, and whether or not the lower spine is normal. A plain radiograph of the abdomen is particularly useful in an encopretic child with absence of a fecal mass on abdominal and rectal examination, in children who vehemently refuse the rectal examination, or in children who are markedly obese. When there is overflow soiling, failure to appreciate the degree of fecal retention in these children can lead to erroneous treatments that further delay effective defecation or lead to misdirected psychotherapy.

    A barium enema is unnecessary in uncomplicated cases of constipation (Figs. 3A and 3B); however, an *unprepped* barium enema is helpful in the assessment of Hirschsprung's disease (Figs. 3C and 3D), in which a transition zone between aganglionic and ganglionic bowel may be observed. This test is useful in other neuronal disorders in which extensive bowel dilatation may be seen and

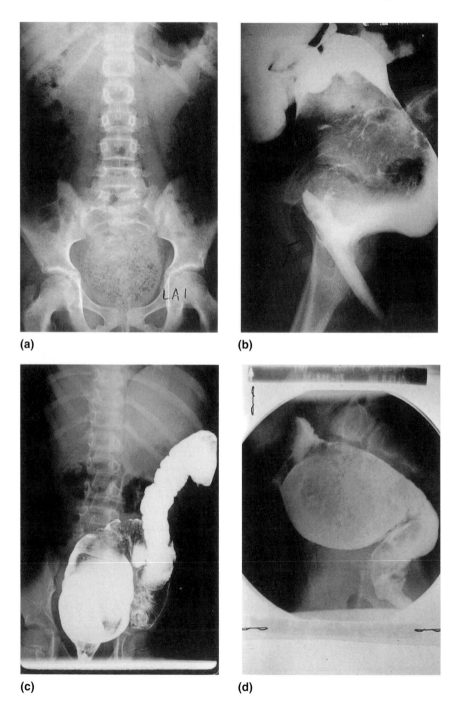

(a)

(b)

(c)

(d)

in the evaluation of the postsurgical patient operated for anal atresia or Hirsch-sprung's disease. Determination of total gastrointestinal transit time (time needed for an ingested substance to appear in stool) provides an objective measure of the severity of constipation in children but does not influence the initial decision of how to treat the constipation.

Anorectal manometry or, if not available, a barium enema is the first step to be taken in patients in whom the history reveals early onset of constipation, severe constipation, absence of fecal soiling, or small-diameter stools or when the physical examination reveals failure to thrive, an empty or small rectal am-pulla with impacted stools in the proximal colon, or when there is persistence of constipation despite adherence to the bowel management program. The main clinical role of anorectal manometry is in the evaluation of children with severe constipation, in whom Hirschsprung's disease must be excluded.

At the University of Iowa, anorectal manometry is most often performed with a commercially available probe containing three microtransducers spaced 5 cm apart and a latex balloon at the tip, which is connected to a transducer (Fig. 4). One transducer lies in the rectum and another one in the anal canal; the latex balloon lies in the rectum, 5 cm above the rectal pressure transducer. The rectosphincteric reflex, also called the anorectal inhibitory reflex, is present in healthy children (Fig. 5A) and in children with functional constipation and enco-presis (Fig. 5B). In a constipated child with a dilated rectum, larger volumes for balloon distention may be necessary to elicit the reflex. The rectosphincteric re-flex is absent in Hirschsprung's disease (Fig. 5C). The rectosphincteric reflex is absent because of the absence of ganglion cells that would transmit this disten-tion reflex. The rectosphincteric reflex has been reported to be absent, atypical, or normal in patients with neuronal intestinal dysplasia. Barium enema and rec-tal biopsy must be performed in all patients with absent or atypical rectosphinc-teric reflex.

FIGURE 3 (a) Anteroposterior abdominal x-ray from a 10-year old girl with functional constipation and encopresis. A large fecal bolus can be seen in the rectum just above the symphysis. (b) The lateral view of a barium enema in the same child reveals the large fecal bolus in the rectum and dilatation of the rectum down to the anal canal. The catheter in the rectum lies along the anterior wall and the levator sling is prominent, suggesting an anterior loca-tion of the anus. (c) Anteroposterior view of a barium enema in a 9-year-old boy with Hirschsprung's disease. The dilated rectum is seen high above the symphysis. A small aganglionic rectum is seen below the distended rectum. This is better seen in the lateral view of the barium enema (d), where the dilated part is the ganglionated rectum above the transition zone; below is the small-diameter aganglionic bowel.

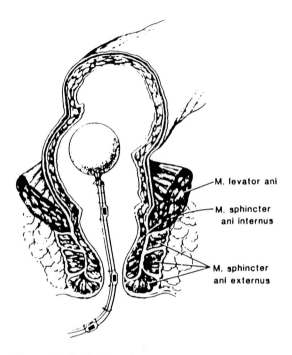

M. levator ani

M. sphincter
ani internus

M. sphincter
ani externus

FIGURE 4   Technique for recording anal and rectal pressures. A commercially available probe containing three microtransducers spaced 5 cm apart and a latex balloon connected to a transducer, is used. One transducer lies in the rectum and another one in the anal canal. The base of the rectal distention balloon lies 5 cm above the rectal pressure transducer in the rectum.

Histological and histochemical information is obtained through the rectal biopsy. The presence or absence of ganglion cells can be evaluated from the superficial suction rectal biopsy. False-negative results are possible, particularly in patients with short-segment Hirschsprung's disease. Absence of ganglion cells with increased staining of nerve trunks with acetylcholinesterase stain are diagnostic for Hirschsprung's disease. Full-thickness biopsies performed by a surgeon are necessary for the evaluation of other abnormalities of both the myenteric and submucosal plexuses, such as in hypoganglionosis or hyperganglionosis.

We have performed numerous manometric studies in children with functional constipation and encopresis and have documented many abnormalities, including increased threshold to rectal distention and decreased rectal contractility as compared to controls (7). In follow-up, after 3 years of therapy, many children will show continued abnormalities of anorectal function, leaving them

A: CONTROL CHILD

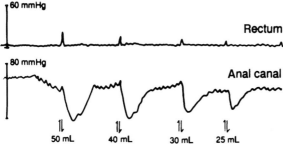

B: CHRONIC CONSTIPATION AND ENCOPRESIS

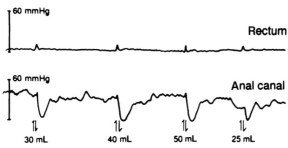

C: HIRSCHSPRUNG'S DISEASE

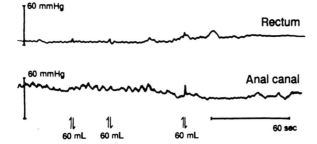

FIGURE 5 (A) This recording is from a healthy 10-year-old boy. The arrows indicate distention of a rectal balloon with air for 1 sec, which results in a decrease in anal pressure, called the rectosphincteric or anorectal inhibitory reflex. (B) Recordings in children with idiopathic constipation with and without encopresis are similar. The relaxation of the internal anal sphincter with rectal distention of similar volumes may not be as deep. (C) Here distention of a rectal balloon with air for 1 sec produces no decrease in anal pressure. The absent rectosphincteric reflex in this 12-year-old boy with severe constipation and intermittent soiling is due to Hirschsprung's disease.

at risk for recurrent problems. Another abnormality is the contraction of the external anal sphincter and pelvic floor muscles instead of relaxation during defecation attempts. This abnormality is called *abnormal defecation pattern* or *abnormal defecation dynamics*. It is found in many constipated children who respond poorly to conventional treatment (7).

6 TREATMENT OF CHRONIC CONSTIPATION WITH ENCOPRESIS

Most children with chronic constipation with or without encopresis will benefit from a precise, well-organized therapeutic plan. Treatment includes various forms of behavioral therapy and psychological approaches and is designed to clear fecal retention, prevent future retention, and promote regular bowel habits. The treatment of constipation with or without encopresis is comprehensive and has four phases: 1) education; 2) removal of the fecal retention; 3) prevention of reaccumulation of stools through reconditioning to normal bowel habits and laxative use, and 4) withdrawal of treatment.

6.1 Education

We point out that constipation began long before the encopresis was first noted. We stress that the stooling problem is not caused by a disturbance in the psychological behavior of the child and is not the parents' fault. Soiling occurs involuntarily and usually without the awareness of the child, although the child may be able to prevent soiling for short periods if he or she concentrates carefully on closing the external anal sphincter. The child and parent are told that many children are troubled with this condition and that we understand the condition and its treatment. We explain normal defecation to the child and parents. We discuss realistic expectations for response to therapy. We stress that months to years of treatment will be necessary. In most cases, a detailed plan eliminates the parents' and the child's frustration and improves compliance for the prolonged treatment necessary. Some of the parents do not possess the skills necessary to effectively manage their child's behavior, specifically in relation to following a demanding regimen. These parents need to be identified so that the educational efforts can be optimized. In addition, a caring relationship is established. Success of treatment depends on the ability of the physician to draw the child and his parents into a therapeutic relationship.

6.2 Removal of Fecal Retention

For removal of the fecal retention, a hypertonic phosphate enema (135 mL) can be used. In most children, one to two enemas result in good bowel cleanout.

Severe vomiting with hypernatremia, hyperphosphatemia, hypocalcemia, hypo-kalemia, dehydration, seizures, coma, and death have been reported in few children <5 years of age after a single hypertonic phosphate enema. Therefore, in children who have never received a hypertonic phosphate enema before, the first time enema should be given in the clinic or doctor's office. Normal (isotonic) saline enemas may be used but are often not effective. Cleansing soap-suds enemas should be avoided because they can result in bowel necrosis, perforation, and death. Tap-water enemas should be avoided as well, as they can cause water intoxication by dilution of serum electrolytes, leading to seizures or even death. Children with megarectum or megacolon who do not respond to phosphate enemas can be disimpacted with a hyperosmolar milk of molasses enema (1:1 milk and molasses) with the infusion stopped when the child indicates discomfort (200 to 600 mL). The milk of molasses enema may have to be repeated. If disimpaction is not achieved with enemas, the child is admitted to the hospital for oral lavage with polyethylene glycol-electrolyte solution. The lavage solution is given orally or by nasogastric tube until clear fluid is excreted through the anus. Large volumes are necessary for bowel cleanout; the average is 12 L given over 23 hr at a rate of 14 to 40 mL/kg/hr. It is recommended to give 5 to 10 mg metoclopramide by mouth 15 min prior to the lavage solution to reduce nausea and vomiting. For a child who vehemently fears enemas, the fecal mass can be softened and liquefied with large quantities of oral mineral oil or osmotic agents, with the administration continued until the fecal mass is passed. Fecal soiling, abdominal pain, and cramping may increase during the administration of oral solutions to remove fecal retention.

6.3 Prevention of Reaccumulation of Stools

The child must be reconditioned to normal bowel habits by regular toilet use. The child is encouraged to sit on the toilet for up to 5 min three to four times a day following meals. The gastrocolic reflex, which goes into effect shortly after a meal, should be used to his or her advantage. Both child and parents must be instructed to keep a daily record of bowel movements, fecal soiling, urinary incontinence, and medication use. This helps to monitor compliance and to make appropriate adjustments in the treatment program by parents and/or physician. If necessary, positive reinforcement is given for effort and later for success by using star charts, little presents, television viewing, or computer game time as rewards.

    The role of dietary fiber in the treatment of chronic functional constipation is controversial. Additional fiber has no value when colorectal tone is diminished in the child who has functional fecal retention. Later, when the tone is restored, additional fiber is of great value to improve defecation. Recommended are several

TABLE 5 Suggested Dosages of Commonly Used Laxatives

	Age	Dose
Milk of magnesia	>6 months	1–3 mL/kg body weight per day, divided in one or two doses
Mineral oil	>6 months	1–5 mL/kg body weight per day, divided in one or two doses
Lactulose or sorbitol	>6 months	1–3 mL/kg body weight per day, divided in one or two doses
Senna (Senokot) syrup	1–5 years	5 mL with breakfast, maximum 5 mL twice daily
	5–15 years	10 mL with breakfast, maximum 10 mL twice daily

servings daily from a variety of fiber-rich foods such as whole-grain breads and cereals, fruits, vegetables, and legumes. Dietary fiber increases water retention and provides substrate for bacterial growth.

In most constipated patients, daily defecation is maintained by the daily administration of laxatives beginning in the evening of the clinic visit. Laxatives should be used according to body weight and severity of the constipation. Suggested dosages of commonly used laxatives are given in Table 5. The choice of medication for functional constipation does not seem as important as the children's and parents' compliance with the treatment regimen. There is no set dosage for any laxative. There is only a starting dosage that must be adjusted to induce one to two bowel movements per day that are loose enough to ensure complete daily emptying of the lower bowel and to prevent soiling and abdominal pain. Once an adequate dosage is established, it is continued for approximately 3 months to help the distended bowel regain some of its function. Usually, regular bowel habits are established by that time. Then, the dosage may be reduced in small decrements while maintaining a daily bowel movement without soiling. Laxatives must be continued for several months sometimes years at the right dose to induce daily soft stools.

The mechanism of action of milk of magnesia is the relative nonabsorption of magnesium and the resultant increase in luminal osmolality. For severe constipation with rock-hard stools, the starting dosage of milk of magnesia is 2 to 3 mL/kg body weight per day, given with the evening meal. For children who have fecal retention of mostly soft-formed stools, usually 1 mL/kg body weight daily is adequate.

Mineral oil is converted into hydroxy fatty acids, which induce fluid and electrolyte accumulation. Dosages range from 1 to 5 mL/kg body weight per day. Long-term use of mineral oil has been reported to be safe. A major concern about long-term mineral oil use had been its action as a lipid solvent, which could interfere with absorption of the fat-soluble vitamins. This concern has been dismissed by a study showing negligible reduction of plasma levels of vitamins A and E after 4 months of mineral oil use. Mineral oil should never be force-fed or given to patients with dysphagia or vomiting because of the danger of aspiration pneumonia. Anal seepage of the mineral oil, often causing an orange stain, is an undesirable side effect, especially in children who go to school.

Lactulose and sorbitol are nonabsorbable carbohydrates, which are hydrolyzed to short chain fatty acids by the colonic flora. They cause increased water content of the stool by their osmotic effects and that of their metabolites. Both are cheap and easily taken when mixed in soft drinks.

Senna has an effect on intestinal motility as well as on fluid and electrolyte transport and will stimulate defecation. We use senna when liquid stools produced by osmotic laxatives are retained, when the child refuses milk of magnesia, mineral oil, or sorbitol; and in children with fecal incontinence and constipation due to organic or anatomic causes. Other centers use senna more frequently for functional constipation.

6.4 Psychological Treatment

Adherence to the treatment program will improve the constipation and encopresis in all children. The presence of coexisting behavioral problems is often associated with poor treatment outcome. If the coexisting behavior problem is secondary to chronic constipation and encopresis, it improves with treatment. Children who do not improve should be referred to a psychologist for further evaluation, because continued problems can be due to noncompliance or control issues by the child and/or the parent. Psychological intervention, family counseling, and occasional hospitalization to get a treatment program started have helped some of these unfortunate children.

6.5 Follow-Up Visits and Weaning from Medication

Since the management of chronic constipation and encopresis requires considerable patience and effort on the part of the child and parents, it is important to provide necessary support and encouragement through frequent office visits. Parents are encouraged to call the doctor's office. Progress should initially be assessed monthly and later less frequently by reviewing the stool records and repeating the abdominal and rectal examination to make sure that the problem is adequately managed. If necessary, dosage adjustments are made and the child and parents are encouraged to continue with the regimen. After regular bowel habits are established, the frequency of toilet sitting is reduced and the medication dosage is gradually decreased to a dosage that maintains one bowel movement

TABLE 6   Frequent Therapy Mistakes by Physicians and Parents

Mistakes by physicians:
  Not removing the fecal retention
  Removing the fecal retention but failing to prescribe stool softeners or
    laxatives
  Giving too low a dose
  Not controlling the adequacy and success of therapy with a rectal
    examination
  Stopping the laxative too soon
  Not providing continuing support and follow-up
Mistakes by parents:
  Not insisting that the child uses the toilet at regular times for defecation
    trials
  Not giving the medication daily
  Discontinuing the laxatives as soon as the encopresis has disappeared

daily and prevents encopresis. Fiber intake is encouraged at that time. After 6 months, a further reduction or discontinuation of the medication is attempted. However, treatment must resume if constipation recurs.

6.6   What Can Go Wrong with the Treatment?

Physicians as well as parents make frequent mistakes (Table 6). Mistakes by physicians are treatment with stool softeners and laxatives without prior removal of the fecal retention, giving too low a dose, not controlling the adequacy and success of therapy with a rectal examination, stopping the laxative too soon, and not providing education, anticipatory guidance, continuing support, and regular follow-up. Mistakes by the parents include not insisting that the child uses the toilet at regular times for defecation trials, not giving the medication daily, or worse, discontinuing the laxatives as soon as the encopresis has disappeared.

7   OUTCOME

With this bowel management program, almost every patient will experience dramatic improvement in constipation and soiling. Complete recovery, defined as at least three bowel movements per week with no fecal soiling while off laxatives, is less frequently seen. A 1-year follow-up study of 97 patients ≥5 years of age treated at the Encopresis Clinic at the University of Iowa showed that 43% of patients had recovered (7). A 1-year follow-up study from Australia showed that 51% of patients receiving laxatives and behavior modification had recovered, but only 36% did so if they had received behavior modification alone (8). The duration of laxative treatment in more than 300 patients in Great Britain showed that 22% of patients required regular laxative use for <6 months, 44% for <12 months, and 56% for >12 months (9).

What is the long-term outcome? In our 4-year follow-up study of 215 children ≥5 years of age with functional constipation and encopresis treated with our bowel management program, we found that 65% had recovered. A 5-year follow-up study from Italy revealed that 48% had recovered (10). The recovery rates for patients younger than 4 years old were similar.

8   NEWER TREATMENT APPROACHES

The laxative and behavioral approach had been described in 1963. Since then only a few new treatment approaches, biofeedback, cisapride, and elimination of cow's-milk protein have been suggested and explored. Cisapride is now off the market because of safety concerns.

8.1   Biofeedback Treatment

A problem occurring in 25 to 53% of constipated patients is abnormal defecation dynamics—an abnormal contraction of the external anal sphincter and pelvic floor muscles during defecation (7). The external anal sphincter and pelvic floor consist of striated muscles that are under voluntary control. These muscles are amenable to biofeedback treatment and the children can be taught to relax these muscles during defecation.

Several uncontrolled biofeedback studies had suggested that children with abnormal defecation dynamics were significantly less likely to recover after 1 year of conventional laxative treatment than children with normal defecation dynamics. For biofeedback treatment, the child is shown the differences between his own manometric tracing from the anal canal and rectum and/or electromyographic (EMG) tracing from the external anal sphincter and the tracings from a normal individual. The child then attempts to produce relaxations or tracings similar to the normal external anal sphincter relaxations he or she was shown. Constant verbal reinforcement, visual reinforcement (recording), and/or sound reinforcement (the EMG recording stylus produced less noise) are given when correct responses are made.

In a randomized study, we evaluated the effect of biofeedback treatment on the clinical outcome 7 and 12 months later. At 7 months, 5% of conventionally treated and 55% of conventional plus biofeedback–treated patients had recovered ($p < 0.01$). At 12 months, 16% of conventionally treated and 50% of conventional plus biofeedback–treated patients had recovered ($p < 0.05$) (11). Six years later, there was no difference in outcome between children with abnormal defecation dynamics who had received biofeedback treatment or not. Since then, three more randomized biofeedback studies have been published, none of them showed a significant benefit of biofeedback (11).

8.2 Withdrawal of Cow's Milk

Intolerance to cow's-milk protein occurs in 0.3 to 7.5% of otherwise normal infants, with 82% exhibiting their first symptoms within 4 months of life, and 89% by 1 year of age. Intolerance to cow's-milk protein is a transient disorder; 28% of children were tolerant to cow's milk challenge by the age of 2 years, 56% by 4 years, and 78% by 6 years (12). Intolerance to cow's-milk protein most often causes vomiting and diarrhea but can also cause allergic rhinitis, asthma, eczema, and constipation. In a study of 206 infants with intolerance to cow's-milk protein, 6% had constipation that was unresponsive to varied additions of carbohydrates, juices, fruits, and malt, anal dilatation and laxatives. In them, normal stooling occurred after complete withdrawal of cow's milk from the diet (13). Recently, Iacono et al (4) compared cow's milk with soy milk in a double-blind, crossover study in 65 constipated children who were refractory to previous treatment with laxatives. These children were 11 to 72 months of age. Of these children, 75% had anal fissures and perianal erythema or edema and 68% recovered from constipation while receiving soy milk. In them, constipation recurred in 1 to 3 days after challenge with cow's milk. Children with a response to soy milk had a higher frequency of coexisting rhinitis, dermatitis, bronchospasm, anal fissures, erythema, and edema than those without a response. Shah et al. (14) reported from London that 55% of 20 constipated children who were refractory to conventional therapy responded to cow's-milk withdrawal. A closer look at the data indicates that 79% of the 14 children with atopy were cured, while none of the 6 children without such history responded to cow's-milk withdrawal. Therefore, an elimination trial of cow's milk should be tried in all constipated children unresponsive to increase in dietary fiber and laxative treatment and in particular in those with a history or signs of atopy.

9 CONSTIPATION WITH OR WITHOUT FECAL INCONTINENCE

Constipation in the presence of an organic disease or an anatomic abnormality can also be accompanied by loss of liquid or solid matter or gas. Rare organic conditions for constipation should be considered and ruled out. Usually this can be accomplished with a history, physical examination, and, if necessary, anorectal manometry, barium enema, and rectal biopsy. The list of causes for diseases causing constipation is long and given in Table 4, but more than 90% of children with constipation have functional constipation as the cause. Constipation can be due to drugs, neurological causes such as spinal disorders (myelomeningocele, spinal tumor, spinal trauma or spinal infection), Hirschsprung's disease, cerebral palsy, generalized hypotonia, or mental retardation. Constipation is often seen in children after repair of anal atresia. Intractable constipation is seen in children with chronic intestinal pseudo-obstruction. Other causes are endocrine, metabolic, and neuromuscular disorders.

9.1 Myelomeningocele

Myelomeningocele is a congenital neural tube defect that occurs in approximately 1 in 1000 births. As a result of aggressive medical and surgical treatment, 90% of the children survive. Fecal incontinence occurs in most of the children with myelomeningocele. Patients with low lesions suffer from severe constipation with overflow fecal incontinence. Patients with high lesions suffer from fecal incontinence.

Varying degrees of nerve impairment exist in these patients, the most common being loss of anal and/or rectal sensation. Many are unable to differentiate sensations produced by gas from those produced by liquid or solid feces. The second most common impairment is loss of external anal sphincter and levator ani function. A bolus of feces cannot be retained when rectal contractions and reflex relaxation of the internal anal sphincter occur because the external anal sphincter cannot be squeezed voluntarily.

9.2 Hirschsprung's Disease

Hirschsprung's disease (congenital aganglionic megacolon) is rare but must be considered in the differential diagnosis of a child of any age with severe constipation. The incidence is about 1 in 5000 births. Boys are four times more likely to be affected than girls.

Hirschsprung's disease usually presents in the newborn period with constipation, abdominal distention, vomiting, diarrhea, or bloody diarrhea. The severity of the disease ranges from complete obstruction that is relieved only by surgery to a mere transient meconium retention; some cases are even less severe. In infants and toddlers, Hirschsprung's disease presents with constipation and stools of small diameter (ribbon-like stools). Rectal examination reveals the rectum to be empty of stool and small in diameter. Although many children with Hirschsprung's disease fail to thrive, not all are sickly, underweight, and anemic.

The chief complaint of older children, adolescents, and adults with Hirschsprung's disease is severe constipation. It is sometimes difficult to differentiate older patients with Hirschsprung's disease from patients with functional megacolon by history or even physical examination. Patients with either disease present with infrequent bowel movements and abdominal distention. Table 7 lists the differences in presentation between children with functional constipation and those with Hirschsprung's disease who were at least 5 years of age at diagnosis.

The absence of the rectosphincteric reflex during anorectal manometry (Fig. 5C), a transition zone in the unprepped barium enema study with the narrowed aganglionic segment distally and a dilated segment proximally (Fig. 3D), and the absence of ganglion cells in the submucosal and myenteric plexuses in the rectal biopsy differentiate between patients with Hirschsprung's disease and those with functional megacolon. The extent of bowel involved with aganglionosis varies and is best demonstrated with a barium enema. In the study by Klein, the rectum with or without the sigmoid was involved in 58% of patients, a longer segment was involved in 26%, and the total colon; sometimes, in addition, the small bowel was involved in 12% (16). The treatment of Hirschsprung's disease is the surgical resection of the segment of bowel that lacks ganglion cells (see Chap. 33).

Constipation and fecal incontinence are common problems postoperatively in patients with Hirschsprung's disease.

TABLE 7 Functional Constipation Versus Hirschsprung's Disease in Children over 5 Years of Age

	Functional constipation[a] $n = 215$	Hirschsprung's disease[b] $n = 15$
Stool size	Large in 98%	Small to large
Failure to thrive	3%	Uncommon
Constipation from birth	10%	53%
Constipation prior to age 1 year	49%	67%
Stool withholding	71%	rare
Abdominal pain	51%	87%
Abdominal fecal mass	42%	93%
Fecal retention in the rectum	96%	27%
Size of rectal ampulla	Large in 80% Normal in 20%	Small to large
Fecal soiling	90%	33%

[a] Unpublished data from the University of Iowa
[b] *Source*: Ref. 15.

9.3 Anorectal Malformations

The reported overall incidence of anorectal anomalies varies from 1 in 3000 to 1 in 15,000 live births. Anorectal malformations are classified into low translevator, intermediate, and high (supralevator) types and most are recognized at birth.

The concept of an anterior location of the anus, the mildest form of an anorectal malformation, has been proposed as a cause of constipation. Anterior location of the anus is more common in females and is associated with a posterior shelf that interferes with evacuation (see Fig. 3B). The surgical repositioning of the anus into a more posterior location supposedly corrects the presence of the posterior shelf and facilitates the passage of stool. The concept of an anteriorly placed anus and a posterior rectal shelf causing constipation does not stand the test of an objective critical analysis. Many girls have an anterior location of the anus without constipation and few patients benefit from anoplasty.

The presence of a rectal opening located anterior to the center of the anal sphincters, called *perineal fistula*, is sometimes recognized only later in life. The anal orifice is not surrounded by sphincter muscles; they are located in the normal position. Patients suffer from constipation and fecal incontinence. These patients benefit from surgical positioning of the anal opening into the center of the sphincter muscles.

Anal stenosis and secondary megacolon are seen in many children following surgical correction of imperforate anus. Symptoms are passage of small-diameter stools and a tight anal canal felt during the rectal examination. Treatment consists of anal dilatation and sometimes anoplasty.

The anatomic development of the anal sphincters and rectum determines the degree of fecal incontinence in patients who have undergone surgery for anal atresia. Incontinence is associated with abnormal function of the rectum or the anal sphincters. Patients with low anal atresia often have fecal incontinence due to constipation and will have good continence as soon as the constipation is adequately treated. Patients with the high type anal atresia are often incontinent of stool as children but may experience some improvement during the teenage years.

9.4 Cerebral Palsy and Hypotonia

Many children with cerebral palsy, generalized hypotonia, or mental retardation, particularly those who are neurologically impaired, experience constipation. In tube-fed children, the absence of dietary fiber may cause constipation. In other children, poor defecatory efforts are due to decreased skeletal muscle tone and weak coordination. Abnormalities in the central nervous system as well as sensory and motor abnormalities due to affected enteric neurons may be responsible for constipation.

9.5   Pseudo-obstruction

Intractable constipation is seen in children with chronic intestinal pseudo-obstruction, a rare but devastating disease that occurs in both sexes. Chronic intestinal pseudo-obstruction can be either localized or disseminated and results in motor dysfunction at various levels of the gastrointestinal tract, involving the esophagus, stomach, duodenum, small bowel, and large bowel. Patients with large bowel involvement commonly present with severe constipation with megacolon. The term *chronic intestinal pseudoobstruction* covers a variety of different disorders. In some cases, a specific myopathy is the problem; in others a degeneration of the ganglia or the nerves occurs; and in some cases, no specific histological alteration has been detected. The disorder is familial in some cases. Onset often occurs in childhood. In many patients, symptoms are recurrent and mainly include constipation, diarrhea, and gaseous abdominal distention. The urinary tract can be involved too.

A cause of intestinal pseudo-obstruction can be neuronal intestinal dysplasia. Neuronal intestinal dysplasia can mimic Hirschsprung's disease in the neonatal period, with symptoms of intestinal spasticity, diarrhea, bloody stools, enterocolitis, and stool retention. The abnormalities on the rectal biopsy are hyperplasia of the submucosal and myenteric plexuses, although not every ganglion is involved; a moderate increase in acetylcholinesterase activity; and mucosal inflammation (17). Clinical improvement will occur with time in localized disease, and sometimes bowel resection is necessary. Neuronal intestinal dysplasia type B presents with chronic constipation and megacolon in children 6 months to 6 years of age. In the newborn period, it presents sometimes with a meconium plug. The biopsy shows numerous ganglia in the submucosal and myenteric plexuses consisting of giant and small ganglion cells and a moderate increase in acetylcholinesterase activity (17). Although a considerable megacolon develops, the clinical course is often benign.

9.6   Other Causes

Children with myotonic dystrophy or muscular dystrophy may have fecal incontinence, constipation, abdominal cramping, or abdominal distention. Some of these children may have a fecal impaction. Most patients have low anal resting and squeeze pressures.

Pellet stools are seen in hypothyroidism and metabolic disorders associated with water depletion, such as renal acidosis, diabetes insipidus, or hypercalcemia.

Drugs such as anticonvulsants (phenytoin), psychotherapeutic agents (methylphenidate, imipramine hydrochloride, phenothiazine), and codeine-containing cough syrups can cause constipation.

10   TREATMENT OF CONSTIPATION WITH OR WITHOUT INCONTINENCE

An appropriate treatment plan is developed using the symptoms and results of the rectal examination and, if necessary, the results of the anorectal manometric evaluation or rectal biopsy. Treatment options include medical therapy with senna, suppositories, glycerin, phosphate, or large-volume saline enemas, frequent manual removal of feces, behavior modification, biofeedback training, or a combination of these.

Treatment with osmotic laxatives in patients with weak anal sphincters and fecal impaction is rarely successful. The constipation is relieved but fecal incontinence increases. Increasing dietary fiber; producing regular daily bowel movements with daily administration of senna; or emptying the rectum regularly with suppositories, enemas, or digital maneuvers can improve the incontinence in most of these children. For those who continue with severe fecal incontinence despite optimal medical management, a novel technique was introduced by Malone et al. in 1990 (18). They reported the formation of a continent appendicocecostomy through which the cecum could be intermittently catheterized and an antegrade enema administered. In this way the colon could be regularly cleaned, usually every 2 days, rendering the child soiling-free. As antegrade enema, half a phosphate enema (64 mL) diluted in an equal volume of saline and then washed through with 100 to 200 mL of saline or polyethylene glycol electrolyte solution can be used. Antegrade enema administration has helped most of our 25 patients with persistent constipation and/or fecal incontinence due to myelomeningocele, post–anal atresia and Hirschsprung's disease. The procedure has been modified, with some surgeons implanting a button gastrostomy or a trap-door device into the cecum or the terminal ileum.

11   SUMMARY

Functional constipation and encopresis are common in childhood. Other causes of constipation are ruled out by history and physical examination and, if necessary, by anorectal manometry, barium enema, and rectal biopsy. Successful treatment of constipation and encopresis requires a combination of parent and patient education, medical therapy, nutritional intervention, behavioral intervention, and long-term compliance with the treatment regimen. The conventional treatment approach, which consists of behavior modification and laxatives, improves the constipation and encopresis in all patients who comply with the treatment program. Recovery rates are approximately 50% after 1 year. Biofeedback treatment is not better than conventional treatment. In some children, if cow's-milk protein intolerance is suspected of being the problem, a period of dietary elimination should be tried. Intolerance of cow's-milk protein is a rare cause of constipation.

Every physician should be able to develop an appropriate treatment program for most of his or her patients with constipation, encopresis, or fecal incontinence. Only a few patients—young patients with severe constipation starting at birth, older patients who do not respond to treatment, patients with a history and physical findings compatible with Hirschsprung's disease, and patients who have been operated for Hirschsprung's disease or anorectal malformation—need to be referred for further diagnosis and management.

REFERENCES

1. Diagnostic and Statistical Manual of Mental Disorders, 4th ed (DSM-IV). Washington, DC: American Psychiatric Association, 1987.
2. Weaver LT. Bowel habit from birth to old age. J Pediatr Gastroenterol Nutr 1988; 7:637–639.
3. Yong D, Beattie RM. Normal bowel habit and prevalence of constipation in primary school children. Amb Child Health 1998; 4:277–282.
4. Iacono G, Cavataio F, Montalto G, Florena A, Tumminello M, Soresi M, Notarbartolo A, Carroccio A. Intolerance of cow's milk and chronic constipation in children. N Engl J Med 1998; 339:1100–1104.
5. Loening-Baucke V. Urinary incontinence and urinary tract infection and their resolution with treatment of chronic constipation of childhood. Pediatrics 1997; 100:228–232.
6. Loening-Baucke V. Chronic constipation in children. Gastroenterology 1993; 105: 1557–1564.
7. Loening-Baucke V. Factors determining outcome in children with chronic constipation and faecal soiling. Gut 1989; 30:999–1006.
8. Nolan TM, Debelle G, Oberklaid F, Coffey C. Randomised trial of laxatives in treatment of childhood encopresis. Lancet 1991; 338:523–527.
9. Clayden GS. Management of chronic constipation. Arch Dis Child 1992; 67:340–344.
10. Staiano A, Andreotti MR, Greco L, Basile P, Auricchio S. Long-term follow-up of children with chronic constipation. Dig Dis Sci 1994; 39:561–564.
11. Loening-Baucke V. Biofeedback training in children with functional constipation. Dig Dis Sci 1996; 41:65–71.
12. Bishop JM, Hill DJ, Hosking CS. Natural history of cow milk allergy: clinical outcome. J Pediatr 1990; 116:862–867.
13. Clein NW. Cow's milk allergy in infants. Pediatr Clin North Am 1954; 4:949–962.
14. Shah N, Lindley K, Milla P. Cow's milk and chronic constipation in children. N Engl J Med 1999; 340:891–892.
15. Barnes PR, Lennard-Jones JE, Hawley PR, Todd IP. Hirschsprung's disease and idiopathic megacolon in adults and adolescents. Gut 1986; 27:534–541.

16. Klein MD, Philippart AI. Hirschsprung's disease: three decades' experience at a single institution. J Pediatr Surg 1993; 28:1291–1294.
17. Fadda B, Maier WA, Meier-Ruge W, Schaerli A, Daum R. Neuronal intestinal dysplasia: a critical 10-year analysis of clinical and bioptic results. Z Kinderchir 1983; 38:305–311.
18. Malone PS, Ransley PG, Kiely EM. Preliminary report: the antegrade continence enema. Lancet 1990; 336:1217–1218.

24

Motility Disorders

Carlo Di Lorenzo
University of Pittsburgh and Children's Hospital of Pittsburgh,
Pittsburgh, Pennsylvania

1 INTRODUCTION

It may be argued that the main job of the bowel is to ''move'' its contents from one end to the other. Digestion and absorption may take place only in the presence of highly coordinated contractions allowing mixing, propulsion, and expulsion of luminal contents. Such motor activity is controlled by the intrinsic activity of the enteric nervous system under the modulating action of the autonomic nervous system and the gastrointestinal hormones. The importance of motility disorders as a major cause of gastrointestinal problems has become increasingly recognized over the past few years. Advances in diagnostic methodology have provided new insights into the ontogeny, physiology, and pathology of gastrointestinal motility. Most information on normal and abnormal gastrointestinal motility in children has been acquired using water-perfused catheters positioned in the esophagus, stomach, duodenum, and colon (Fig. 1). The motility of the gastric fundus, pylorus, and ileum still requires further studies to be fully elucidated. Developments in the field of pharmacological treatment of motility disorders have resulted in a new class of drugs, the prokinetic agents. It is estimated that approximately 50% of children visiting a pediatric gastroenterologist have symptoms at least in part

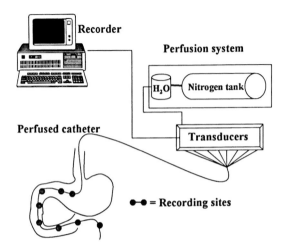

FIGURE 1 Schematic representation of gastrointestinal manometry.

related to abnormal motility. General practitioners are commonly asked to evaluate infants and children with gastroesophageal reflux, constipation, or irritable bowel syndrome, and an understanding of the role of motility in the pathophysiology of these conditions may lead to more effective diagnosis and treatment. Table 1 lists some of the conditions in which motility abnormalities have been demonstrated. This chapter is divided into sections discussing disorders related to the abnormal motor function of the different areas of the gastrointestinal tract.

TABLE 1 Conditions Involving Abnormalities in Motility

Gastroesophageal reflux
Achalasia
Diffuse esophageal spasm
Rumination syndrome
Gastroparesis
Toddler's diarrhea
Recurrent abdominal pain
Nonulcer dyspepsia
Irritable bowel syndrome
Intestinal pseudo-obstruction
Other neuromuscular diseases (diabetes, scleroderma, neuronal intestinal
  dysplasia)

2   ESOPHAGEAL MOTILITY DISORDERS

The esophagus is a hollow conduit with sphincters at each end whose main goal is to stay empty in spite of numerous intrusions from above or below. Functionally, the esophagus may be divided into three areas: the upper esophageal sphincter (UES), the esophageal body, and the lower esophageal sphincter (LES). The UES is a striated muscle that is tonically closed due to continuous neural excitation. It opens during swallowing, contracts during inspiration, and protects the airway from gastric content during episodes of gastroesophageal reflux (GER). The esophageal body has striated muscle in the upper third, mixed striated and smooth muscle in the middle third, and only smooth muscle in the lower third. This is important to remember because there are motility disorders that affect only the striated or the smooth muscle, causing dysfunction of the upper or the lower part of the esophagus, respectively. Swallowing initiates the primary peristalsis, a contraction that clears the esophagus from pharyngeal contents. Secondary peristalsis eliminates gastric content during episodes of GER. The LES is a high-pressure area between the esophagus and the stomach; this constitutes the main barrier against GER. The LES relaxes 1 to 2 sec after swallowing and remains open for 6 to 8 sec. An impaired LES function, characterized either by a low-pressure sphincter or a sphincter with an excessive frequency of relaxations, leads to GER, a condition covered elsewhere in this book (see Chap. 19).

2.1   Disorders of the Upper Esophageal Sphincter

The most common disorder of the UES is *cricopharyngeal achalasia*, involving the failure of the UES to open completely or to open in synchrony with pharyngeal contractions. Symptoms suggestive of cricopharyngeal achalasia include choking, tracheal aspirations with repetitive coughing episodes, nasopharyngeal regurgitation, drooling, and poor eating (1). Often, patients are more symptomatic on swallowing liquids as opposed to solids, a differentiating characteristic from patients with a fixed, lumen-occluding lesion. Dysfunctions of the UES are often accompanied by other evidence of neurological or muscular disease, such as cerebral palsy, familial dysautonomia, Silver-Russell syndrome, 5p⁻ (cri-du-chat) syndrome, muscular dystrophy, and minimal-change myopathy (2). Arnold-Chiari malformations have also been associated with dysphagia and UES dysfunction in young children, and brainstem magnetic resonance imaging should be performed in children with cricopharyngeal achalasia to seek such malformation. Surgical decompression of Arnold-Chiari malformation leads to complete clinical and manometric resolution (3). The diagnostic assessment of a child with suspected UES dysfunction begins with a complete examination of mouth, neck, and cranial nerves. Videofluoroscopy and nasopharyngeal endoscopy are the most accurate diagnostic means to assess UES function. A modified barium swallow with different consistency boluses ("cookie swallow") allows a careful assessment of the pharyngeal and esophageal portion of the swallowing process. Cricopharyngeal achalasia is demonstrated radiologically as a horizontal "bar" during swallowing, often accompanied by aspiration of radiopaque material (Fig. 2). Esophageal manometry provides information complementary to the radiological study (4). Conservative treatment of UES dysfunction may be indicated in young infants, because spontaneous improvement may occur. Dietary modifications include elimination of foods and liquids that are easily aspirated. Foods with thicker consistency are usually better tolerated because of their adherence to the pharyngeal wall. Drinking of thickened liquids through a straw may also be helpful in controlling the volume of ingested liquids. In older children, resolution of symptoms has been achieved with either bougienage, surgical and laser myotomy, and injection of botulinum toxin (5). Difficulty in swallowing due to decreased pressure of pharyngeal contractions may be one of the presenting symptoms of botulism. Nitrazepam has been associated with delayed cricopharyneal relaxation, causing drooling and aspiration (6).

2.2 Disorders of the Esophageal Body and the Lower Esophageal Sphincter

Primary esophageal motility disorders include mostly conditions affecting the esophageal smooth muscle, such as GER, achalasia, and diffuse esophageal spasm. There are also systemic diseases that cause abnormal esophageal motility, such as scleroderma or other connective tissue diseases. Table 2 summarizes the manometric features of the most common esophageal motility disorders.

Achalasia is the most common primary esophageal motor disorder and is characterized by 1) increased or normal LES pressure, 2) absent or incomplete LES relaxation in response to a swallow, 3) loss of esophageal peristalsis, and 4) elevated intraesophageal pressure (1). When there are nonperistaltic, spasmlike contractions, the disease is classified as *vigorous achalasia*. Achalasia is thought to result from postganglionic denervation of the esophageal smooth muscle. More recently, it has been reported that vasoactive intestinal polypeptide and nitric oxide are absent in the gastroesophageal junction of patients with achalasia (7). Mean age at the time of diagnosis in children is 8.8 years. Achalasia should be suspected in children presenting with progressive dysphagia, recurrent emesis, weight loss, chest pain, and aspiration pneumonia. It starts as an obstruction at the level of the gastroesophageal junction with subsequent dilatation of the lower esophagus due to absence of esophageal peristalsis. A plain chest x-ray showing a widened mediastinum, esophageal air-fluid level, or absence of gastric air may suggest the diagnosis. A conclusive diagnosis of achalasia is made by barium swallow or esophageal manometry. The characteristic x-ray appearance is a dilated distal esophagus with tapering at the LES, giving the distal esophagus a "bird's beak deformity" (Fig. 3). The esophageal manometry reveals absence of

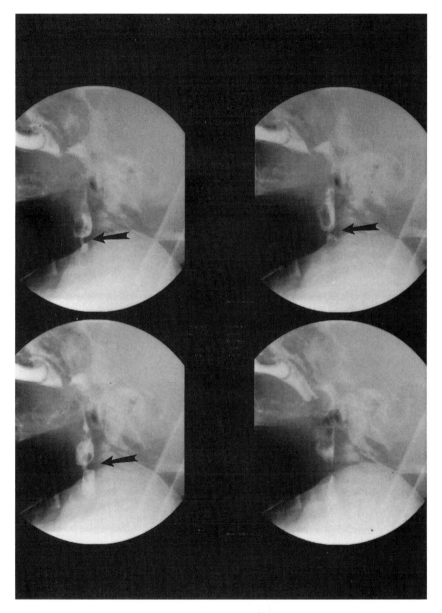

FIGURE 2 Modified barium swallow demonstrating a persistent "bar" (arrows) during swallowing in a 3 month-old child with cricopharyngeal achalasia.

TABLE 2 Manometric Characteristics of Esophageal Motility Disorders

Disorder	LES	Esophageal body	UES and upper esophagus
Achalasia	Normal or high pressure Incomplete or absent relaxation	Aperistaltic or simultaneous contractions	Normal
Esophageal spasm	Normal or high basal pressure Complete relaxation	High amplitude, prolonged, propagated or simultaneous contractions	Normal
Scleroderma or other connective tissue diseases	Hypotensive or absent Complete relaxation	Absent or decreased amplitude	Normal
GER	Normal or hyotensive Complete relaxation Excessive frequency of relaxations	Decreased amplitude and failed peristalsis in presence of esophagitis	Normal

Key: LES, lower esophageal sphincter; UES, upper esophageal sphincter; GER, gastro-esophageal reflux.

peristalsis, which is the hallmark of the disease, and incomplete LES relaxation. Therapy is based on relief of the functional LES obstruction. In patients who have suffered extreme weight loss, it is also important to provide nutritional rehabilitation. Pharmacotherapy with nitrates and calcium channel blockers decreases the LES pressure and facilitates esophageal emptying. However, the benefit is short-lasting and there are significant long-term side effects. The major role of pharmacotherapy is to provide relief of symptoms until more definitive interventions can be performed (8). Intrasphincteric injection with botulinum toxin, a potent inhibitor of acetylcholine release from nerve terminals, has been found to provide short-term (3 to 9 months) benefit in treating children with achalasia and may be used in patients who are poor surgical candidates. The two most successful modalities for a definitive cure are pneumatic dilatation and esophageal myotomy. The pneumatic dilatation is accomplished using inflatable balloons that forcefully stretch the LES. The most common surgical procedure used for acha-

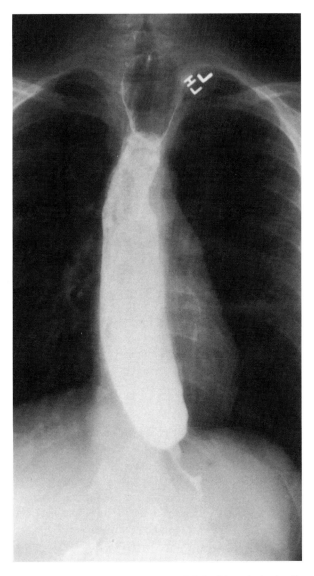

FIGURE 3 Barium swallow in a child with achalasia. Note the esophageal dilation, with air-fluid level in the upper esophagus and "breaking" in the lower esophagus.

lasia is the Heller myotomy. Compared to pneumatic dilatation, myotomy seems to have better long-term results (9). New laparoscopic and thoracoscopic approaches are reducing the morbidity associated with this procedure. Postsurgical complications include GER and persistence of obstructive symptoms.

Abnormal esophageal peristalsis can cause dysphagia for both solids and liquids and chest pain. A spastic disorder of the esophagus should be suspected only when cardiopulmonary causes of chest pain have been excluded and an endoscopy has ruled out esophagitis. Children presenting only with chest pain and no evidence of cardiopulmonary disease may be given first a therapeutic trial with a proton-pump inhibitor, since a large group of patients will respond to acid suppression. When symptoms persist, it may be time to determine whether a spastic disorder of the esophagus is present. Unlike the situation in patients with achalasia, in those with diffuse esophageal spasm the esophagus retains its ability to propagate primary peristaltic contractions most of the time. Radiographically, there may be the appearance of a "corkscrew" esophagus. Manometry reveals contractions of greater than normal amplitude and prolonged duration, with approximately 30% occurring simultaneously at different levels of the esophagus. At times, there are multipeaked, repetitive contractions following a single swallow. Treatment involves the use of smooth muscle relaxants. In contrast, children with esophagitis often have low-amplitude contractions leading to ineffective peristalsis and clearance of refluxed material. The prevalence of impaired motility increases with the most severe form of esophagitis. Abnormal esophageal motility may have a pathogenic role in GER disease by prolonging the contact time between the esophageal mucosa and the gastric refluxate. Finally, children with an esophageal atresia repair often continue to have dysphagia, vomiting, and chronic respiratory symptoms. Motility studies of these children demonstrate markedly abnormal motility in the distal esophagus with absent peristalsis and low or absent LES pressure. The etiology of the esophageal motor dysfunction in these children remains unclear. Guidelines for the use of esophageal manometry in children have recently been published by the North American Society for Pediatric Gastroenterology and Nutrition. They emphasize that esophageal manometry is generally not useful in the diagnosis or medical treatment of GER disease (10).

3 GASTRIC MOTILITY DISORDERS

Functionally, the stomach may be divided into two regions: proximal (the fundus and the top third of the body) and distal stomach (the bottom two-thirds of the body, the antrum and the pylorus). The proximal stomach expands when food is ingested and functions as a reservoir. It then slowly contracts and moves its content to the distal stomach. The distal stomach breaks down solid food, emptying it into the duodenum with phasic, powerful, coordinated contractions. Only particles with a diameter smaller than 1 to 2 mm go through the pylorus.

3.1 Delayed Gastric Emptying

Disorders in gastric motility cause disruption of the normal storage, trituration, and emptying of food. Delayed gastric emptying in the absence of a mechanical obstruction is known as gastroparesis. Symptoms of gastroparesis include postprandial fullness, anorexia, early satiety, bloating, emesis several hours after the meal, halitosis, and epigastric pain. Delayed gastric emptying in children has a variety of mechanical and nonmechanical causes (Table 3). Postviral gastroparesis is an entity recently described in children and accounts for many acquired forms of delayed gastric emptying (11). It follows a short viral illness, often a gastroenteritis, and is associated with postprandial antral hypomotility. In most cases the symptoms resolve spontaneously within 6 to 24 months. Abnormal gastric motility may be associated with disordered esophageal and/or small bowel motility and be part of a generalized motility disorder known as pseudo-obstruction.

The evaluation of a child with a suspected gastric motility disorder begins with the identification of the clinical conditions that are likely to interfere with gastric emptying. It is important to rule out mechanical causes of obstruction, such as peptic ulcer disease, which may cause pylorospasm and deformity of the gastric outlet. In infants, hypertrophic pyloric stenosis must be ruled out by either ultrasonography or radiographic study. A suggested plan of assessment is summarized in Figure 4.

In adults the most accurate and sensitive measure of gastric emptying is the emptying scan. Radionuclide markers are incorporated into either the liquid or the solid component of a meal and a gamma camera measures the amount of radioactivity emptied over time. Being minimally invasive, quantitative, and physiological (ordinary meals are used), radionuclide testing has gained wide acceptance in pediatrics as well. In infants, the meal used is usually milk or formula. Ideally, the composition and volume of milk should be standardized according to body size. In practice, many children are on modified feeding regimens, and standardization is particularly difficult. Eggs labeled with ^{99m}Tc sulfur colloid are used to evaluate the gastric emptying of solids in older children. The results are expressed as percentage of radioactivity remaining in the stomach after one (liquid meals) or 3 hr (solid meals) or as time to emptying half of the meal ($t_{1/2}$). Scintigraphic studies in younger or uncooperative children are complicated by the requirement for the subjects to lie motionless for extended periods, a challenging requirement for many infants. The proper interpretation of emptying scan should be performed only in laboratory with standardized technique and established control population values.

Barium studies of the upper gastrointestinal tract are nonphysiological (ingestion of barium makes many children nauseated), insensitive, and nonquantitative and will demonstrate delays in gastric emptying only in severe cases. Thus,

TABLE 3   Causes of Delayed Gastric Emptying

Mechanical obstruction
  Hypertrophic pyloric stenosis
  Peptic ulcer
  Status post–gastric surgery
  Bezoar
Drugs
  Anticholinergics
  Opiates
  Tricyclic antidepressants
  Phenothiazines
  Somatostatin
  Adrenergic agonists
  Aluminum antacids
  Calcium channel blockers
  GABA
  L-dopa
Neuromuscular
  Diabetes
  Connective tissue diseases
  Muscular dystrophy
  Intestinal pseudo-obstruction (myopathic and neuropathic)
  Vagotomy
  Familial dysautonomia
Infectious
  Rotavirus
  Epstein-Barr virus
  Cytomegalovirus
  Herpes zoster
  Norwalk agent
Metabolic
  Hyperglycemia
  Hypothyroidism
  Hypokalemia
  Hypocalcemia
Psychiatric disorders
  Depression
  Anorexia nervosa
End-stage renal disease
Idiopathic

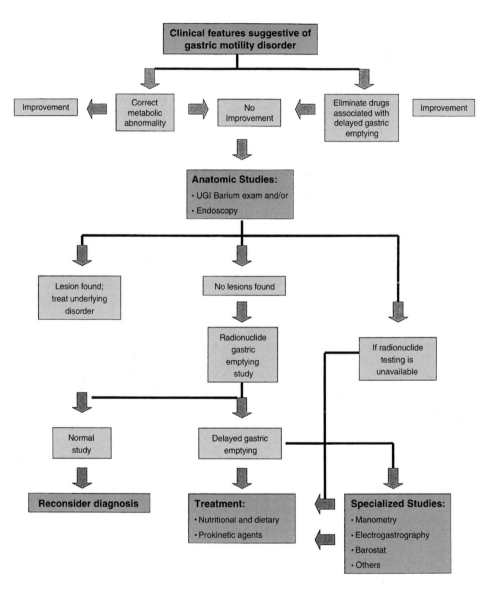

FIGURE 4   Assessment of the child with suspected gastric motility disorder. (Reproduced and modified with permission from Moore JG. Gastroparesis: pathogenesis and evaluation. In: Champion MC, Orr WC, eds. Evolving Concepts in Gastrointestinal Motility. Cambridge, MA: Blackwell Science, 1996, pp 87–107.)

radiological contrast studies should not be relied upon for a diagnosis of a gastric motility disorder. Real-time ultrasonography may be used to estimate gastric volume and gastric motor activity. The ultrasound probe is placed over the epigastrium of a supine patient. The gastric emptying time is assessed by measuring the width of the gastric antrum at selected levels before and after the test meal (12). It is a test that is very operator-dependent and has not yet gained wide acceptance.

Specialized studies used to assess the gastric motor function include manometry, electrogastrography, and the electronic barostat. Such tests are available only in selected referral centers and in some cases are still considered as investigational. *Manometry* measures the strength and the coordination of antral contractions during fasting and after ingestion of a meal. It may also be used to evaluate the potential for prokinetic drugs such as erythromycin to provide a therapeutic benefit. In postviral gastroparesis, manometry demonstrates absence of antral contractions in the postprandial period. Children with rumination, a behavioral disorder characterized by effortless regurgitation of partially digested food, display characteristic pressure changes after ingestion of a meal, allowing differentiation from children with intrinsic motility disorders. *Electrogastrography* (EGG) records gastric myoelectric activity from the abdominal surface with electrodes placed on the skin. It has been used in children of all ages, including preterm infants. Abnormalities of gastric electric rhythm are found in many children with delayed gastric emptying. The restoration of normal gastric rhythm has been associated with symptomatic improvement (13). The use of EGG as a diagnostic technique in children still requires standardization of electrode placement, duration of the test, study analysis, and interpretation. The *barostat* is a device that measures pressures and isobaric volume changes in a balloon, which may be placed in different parts of the gastrointestinal tract. It has been used to measure changes in tone in the gastric fundus and to evaluate gastric visceral sensitivity. The barostat has also been used to evaluate gastric wall compliance and gastric receptive relaxation in newborn infants (14).

Children with gastroparesis may benefit from dietary changes. A "mechanical soft diet" is encouraged, avoiding solid foods with large amount of indigestible residue, such as raw fruits and vegetables, skins, seeds, tough meats. Fatty meals delay gastric emptying and should also be avoided. Liquids empty more rapidly than solids and the use of high-calorie blenderized formulas is recommended. Drugs that improve gastric emptying include cisapride, erythromycin, metoclopramide, and domperidone (not available in the United States). Whenever possible, drugs should be administered in liquid formulations to facilitate their delivery to the small bowel, where they can be absorbed. Enteral nutrition through a nasoduodenal or gastroduodenal feeding catheter may be necessary in children not responding to dietary and pharmaceutical intervention who are not able to maintain their weight.

3.2 Rapid Gastric Emptying

Rapid gastric emptying is found at times in children who have undergone gastric surgery (vagotomy, pyloroplasty, fundoplication), leading to a constellation of symptoms known as *dumping syndrome*. The rapid gastric emptying of meals rich in carbohydrates in the proximal bowel causes sudden distention of the duodenum and draws fluids into the bowel, producing abdominal pain, fullness, nausea, and weakness (*early* dumping). Late symptoms occur 60 to 150 min after the ingestion of the meal and include palpitation, sweating, hunger, diaphoresis, and syncope (*late* dumping). These symptoms are believed to result from a rebound hypoglycemia induced by the supraphysiological release of insulin in the early postprandial period. Diagnosis is based on typical symptoms, documentation of the changes in glycemic values, and the result of the gastric emptying scintiscan. Treatment involves dietary modifications, with a diet high in protein and fat and low in carbohydrates, restricted fluid intake, and use of uncooked starches. Octreotide, a long-acting somatostatin analogue, has been used to delay gastric emptying in some children with dumping syndrome.

4 INTESTINAL MOTILITY DISORDERS

Once the triturated food leaves the stomach, the process of digestion and absorption begins. The proximal jejunum has many propagating contractions that spread the intestinal content, exposing it to a large area of mucosa and facilitating digestion. In contrast, the distal jejunum and the ileum have tonic, segmenting contractions and retain food longer in order to maximize absorption of nutrients. Finally, the distal ileum generates high-amplitude, rapidly propagating contractions that expel the food through the ileocecal valve into the colon. This highly coordinated sequence of intestinal contractions is under complex myogenic, neural, and hormonal control. The patterns of gastrointestinal motor activity differ during fasting and after the ingestion of food. In the fasted state, the stomach, small intestine, and gallbladder participate in a cycle of motor quiescence and activity. This cycle is known as *migrating motor complex* (MMC) and consists of three distinctive phases that occur in sequence and slowly migrate along the length of the small bowel. Phase 1 is characterized by motor quiescence and is followed by a period of apparently random contractions of variable amplitude, called phase 2. Phase 3 is a 5- to 10-min period with a distinctive pattern of intense, uninterrupted, propagating contractions occurring at a frequency of 3 per min in the stomach, 11 to 12 per min in the duodenum, and 7 to 9 per min in the distal ileum. Each cycle lasts 100 to 200 min, and the cycle length is shorter in younger children. The onset and migration of MMCs in the small bowel is generated and maintained by the intrinsic nervous system of the gut and is independent of extrinsic nerves. Feeding abolishes the cyclic pattern and replaces it with a postprandial pattern, characterized by random, phasic contractions (similar to phase 2 activity) that may last several hours, after which the fasting pattern resumes if no food is ingested. The ability to switch to a fed motility pattern is regulated by extrinsic nerves and is lost in patients with vagotomy or bowel denervation.

Abnormalities in small bowel motility have been identified in many functional gastrointestinal disorders. It has been suggested that abnormal small bowel motility may play a pathogenic role in some children with severe abdominal pain or nonulcer dyspepsia (15,16). Abnormal propagation of contractions may cause ineffective propulsion of the luminal content, causing uncomfortable segmental distention of the small bowel. High-pressure or prolonged tonic contractions may stimulate bowel wall proprioreceptors and be perceived as painful. It is believed that some children with recurrent abdominal pain may have an exaggerated motor response to a heterogeneous group of physical or psychosocial stimuli. However, it remains unclear whether the abnormalities in motility have any etiological role in causing symptoms or are merely epiphenomena found in an organ, the intestine, capable of only a limited repertoire of motor responses. In performing motility testing, there is often a poor temporal correlation between motility abnormalities and symptoms. Some children have symptoms when manometry is normal while others have abnormal contractions but no symptoms. Only a minority of children and adults with nonulcer dyspepsia have a significant delay in gastric emptying or small bowel transit. Because manometric studies rarely provide direct insight into the pathogenesis of functional bowel disorders, they should not be performed to confirm or rule out a diagnosis of nonulcer dyspepsia or irritable bowel syndrome. Recently, criteria for the clinical diagnosis of childhood functional bowel disorders have been published with the purpose of decreasing the amount of diagnostic testing often performed in these children (17).

Abnormal motility has also been described in toddler's diarrhea, an entity described as a persistent, unexplained diarrhea typically occurring in children between 1 and 4 years of age. Children with toddler's diarrhea have intermittently loose stools, occurring up to 6 to 8 times a day and often containing undigested material but without blood or pus. Despite the abnormal stools, children with this condition may be thriving and the diarrhea rarely lasts beyond the age of 5 years. It has been suggested that children with toddler's diarrhea have an inadequate postprandial motor response, with MMCs that continue to cycle even after feeding, causing a more rapid small bowel transit time (18). A high-fat diet, which activates the ''ileal break'' and delays intestinal transit, is often used in children with toddler's diarrhea to decrease the volume and frequency of bowel movements.

4.1 Chronic Intestinal Pseudo-obstruction

The most severe form of intestinal dysmotility is chronic intestinal pseudo-obstruction (CIP), which refers to a heterogeneous group of disorders with similar clinical features (19). A pediatric working group has defined pediatric chronic intestinal pseudo-obstruction as "a rare, severe, disabling disorder characterized by repetitive episodes or continuous symptoms and signs of bowel obstruction, including radiographic documentation of dilated bowel with air-fluid levels, in the absence of a fixed, lumen-occluding lesion" (20). Based on this definition, CIP should be diagnosed only when a mechanical obstruction has been ruled out. In reality, there are many other severe forms of motility disorders involving the small bowel that do not necessarily present with dilated loops of bowel. These are often referred to as "mild forms" of CIP. The most common symptoms in children with CIP are vomiting, nausea, abdominal distention, constipation, decreased oral intake, and weight loss. Stasis may lead to bacterial overgrowth, with the subsequent development of diarrhea, flatulence, steatorrhea, and worsening abdominal distention. About one-third of CIP infants have associated neuromuscular disease of the urinary bladder (hollow visceral myopathy or hollow visceral neuropathy). These infants may be at high risk for recurrent urinary tract infections. Table 4 summarizes symptoms suggestive of CIP in chldren. Pseudo-obstruction may represent the intestinal manifestation of a systemic diseases, such as scleroderma or diabetes, or may reflect a primary disorder of the intestinal neuromuscular system. More than 90% of childhood forms of CIP are primary and approximately 50% are congenital. One-third of infants born with CIP die in the first year of life, succumbing to the acute and chronic complications of total parenteral nutrition (TPN). A poor outcome (death or TPN dependence) is more common in children with malrotation, short-bowel syndrome, urinary tract involvement, and myopathic histology (21).

There is no single test diagnostic of CIP. The most important step in the diagnosis of CIP is to have a high index of suspicion and consider this diagnosis early in order to avoid repeated laparotomies searching for bowel obstructions. Abdominal radiographs reveal dilated loops of small bowel except in patients who are not being fed and have venting enterostomies. Contrast radiology should be performed using water-soluble material to avoid the formation of barium concretions. Contrast studies show dilated loops of bowel with very slow transit

TABLE 4 Symptoms and Signs Suggestive of Intestinal Pseudo-obstruction

---

Coexistence of upper and lower gastrointestinal symptoms (vomiting, abdominal distention, constipation)
Weight loss
No symptom-free intervals
Symptoms since birth
Other organ involvement (urinary system, autonomic nervous system)
No evidence of bowel obstruction on radiologic studies

---

through a featureless intestine. Esophageal motility is often normal in children with CIP, and a normal esophageal manometry does not rule out CIP. The measurement of gastroduodenojejunal motility is very important in the evaluation of the child with CIP. Small bowel motility is always abnormal in children with CIP involving the upper gastrointestinal tract (22). Other diagnoses, including factitious disorders or behavioral problems in the child or the family, should be considered when the manometry study is normal. In children with myopathy, manometry reveals hypomotility, with infrequent low amplitude contractions. In subjects with neuropathy, there are normal amplitude and uncoordinated contractions. Often MMCs are absent and are replaced by prolonged clusters of nonpropagating contractions. Antroduodenal manometry may also provide important prognostic information, determine the areas of the gastrointestinal tract involved in the disease, and assess the potential for a drug to provide therapeutic benefit. In children, absence of MMCs is often associated with requirement for partial or total parenteral nutrition and a poor response to cisapride (23).

4.1.1 Therapy

Treatment of childhood CIP is challenging and requires a team effort with the participation of nutritionists, pain management specialists, surgeons, occupational therapists, urologists, and mental health personnel. Dehydration and electrolyte abnormalities should be corrected. Systemic diseases causing CIP need to be treated or ruled out. Because malnutrition is a frequent consequence of CIP at all ages, it is essential to identify and address nutritional deficiencies appropriately. Nutritional sufficiency is critical for the child's normal growth and development as well as for maximizing bowel function. Subjects with motility disorders tolerate low-fat, homogenized, or liquid meals better than regular meals. When any type of oral intake fails, gastrostomy and jejunostomy feedings should be tried before considering the use of parenteral nutrition. Bacterial overgrowth contributes to the abnormal transit in CIP by increasing gas production and distending the intestinal lumen. Mucosal inflammation may further decrease motility and absorption. Antibiotic treatment of bacterial overgrowth often improves small bowel symptoms.

The most severe forms of CIP rarely improve substantially with the use of prokinetic drugs. Cisapride increases small bowel motility and may be beneficial to some children with mild forms of CIP. Other children may be helped by the use of erythromycin, a motilin agonist, which improves gastric motility, and octreotide, a long-acting somatostatin analogue, which acts mainly on the small bowel (24). Less favorable in children with CIP has been the experience with metoclopramide, domperidone, leuprolide, and misoprostol.

Surgery should be limited to the placement of venting enterostomies. Gastrostomies are often placed to decrease the frequency of vomiting and decompress the dilated stomach and proximal bowel. Gastrointestinal motility may improve as the dilated areas resume a more normal diameter. Jejunal feeding tubes may be placed through the gastrostomy to simultaneously decompress the stomach and provide enteral nutrition. Ileostomies are particularly beneficial in children with colonic involvement. It is important to maximize enteral feedings even when parenteral nutrition is used so as to delay the onset of TPN-related hepatobiliary disorders (cholestasis, gallstones, and cirrhosis). The ability of the bowel to tolerate enteral feedings must be reassessed at regular intervals because of the possibility, in CIP, of alternating periods of more and less severe symptoms.

5 COLONIC MOTILITY DISORDERS

The colon is more than just a storage organ. It mixes and reabsorbs approximately 90% of the ileal effluent, ferments and utilizes unabsorbed carbohydrates, and expels dietary fiber, bacteria, and other undigested solids. The consistency and volume of the stool depends on the interaction among the ability of the mucosa to absorb luminal fluids, the physical characteristics of the stool, and the colonic transit time. Food reaches the cecum within 3 to 4 hr of ingestion; it may then take several more hours to reach the rectum. Transit is especially slow in the right side of the colon. Characteristics of normal and abnormal colonic motility have recently been clarified in children with the use of water-perfused catheters placed endoscopically with the tip in the cecum (26). There are two types of normal motor activity: (1) low-amplitude tonic and phasic contractions, mixing luminal contents, and (2) high-amplitude propagated contractions (HAPCs), propelling stools from the right side of the colon to the rectum. The HAPCs are the manometric equivalent of the ''mass movements'' classically described in the radiology literature. Colonic motility increases after a meal (the ''gastrocolonic response'') and upon awakening. Infants and young children have a particularly striking motility response to the ingestion of food, producing clusters of HAPCs after eating, often associated with the evacuations of stool. The number of HAPCs decreases with age and normal adults have 2 to 4 HAPCs per day. Once the HAPCs carry the stool to the distal colon, the rectal wall is distended and there is a reflex contraction of the rectum and relaxation of the internal anal sphincter, pushing fecal material into the anal canal. The sensitive lining of the anoderm perceives the stool and a decision is made whether to expel it or to postpone defecation by contracting the external anal sphincter and the puborectalis muscle. If defecation is delayed, a Valsalva maneuver is then needed to push the stool into the anal canal again and produce a bowel movement. The basic regulatory control mechanisms controlling defecation are present in the newborn, with only the conscious decision of contracting and relaxing the skeletal muscles (external anal sphincter, puborectalis, and abdominal muscles) developing at the time of toilet training. Any disruption of this sequence of motor events may lead to constipation. The most common cause of constipation in pediatrics is a conscious decision made by the child to delay defecation after experiencing an unpleasant evacuation (see Chap. 23). In children with this form of functional (or behavioral) constipation, the motility of the colon is normal. The only abnormal motor activity in a chronically constipated child is found in the rectum, which may become so dilated that it may not be able to generate enough pressure to propel the stool into the anal canal.

In children, neuromuscular colonic diseases are nearly always primary and in most cases present during the first year of life. Abnormalities in the colonic nervous system range from aganglionosis to hyperaganglionosis. Aganglionosis is the hallmark of Hirschsprung's disease, which is found in less than 1% of children presenting for the first time with constipation. For a more detailed discussion of Hirschsprung's disease, refer to the chapter on constipation. Other colonic neuromuscular diseases are even less common than Hirschsprung's disease. Intestinal neuronal dysplasia (IND) is a condition that has recently received much attention. It is characterized by hyperplasia of the myenteric and submucosal plexuses and an abnormal distribution of neural elements. It has been suggested that the incidence of this condition is higher than previously thought and that it can be associated with Hirschsprung's disease, proximal to the aganglionic segment. The causal relation between histological findings of IND and clinical symptoms has been questioned. It has also been postulated that the pathological abnormalities may be secondary to the chronic stasis of stool and stretching of the bowel. The pathological diagnosis of every neuromuscular colonic disease different from Hirschsprung's disease is challenging due to the lack of age and location control specimens. A recent multicenter study concluded that there is still a high interobserver variation with regard to the different morphological features and final diagnosis of IND (26). In view of the lack of uniform criteria for the diagnosis of colonic neuromuscular diseases, other diagnostic studies need to be performed in the child who is refractory to conventional treatment for constipation and does not have Hirschsprung's disease. Such studies may be considered especially in the child who does not fit the typical presentation of functional constipation (Table 5).

Ingestion of radiopaque markers has been used to differentiate generalized colonic disease from functional constipation. Healthy children excrete swallowed markers within 48 hr. In children who withhold stools, the markers are retained in the rectum for several days. In colonic motility disorders, the markers accumulate in the areas with abnormal motor function. When a generalized colonic motility disorder is suspected, full-thickness biopsies or colonic manometry studies can differentiate between neuropathy and myopathy and identify the diseased segments. In the absence of generalized colonic dilatation, children whose contractions do not increase following a meal and/or do not produce HAPCs are believed to have a colon neuropathy. Children with no colonic contractions or persistently low-amplitude contractions are more likely to have a myopathy.

TABLE 5 "Red Flags" for a Colonic Neuromuscular Disease in a Constipated Child

Onset during the first 6 months of life
Lack of response to conventional behavioral and medical treatment
No fecal soiling
No stool-withholding behavior
Upper gastrointestinal symptoms
Failure to thrive
Empty rectum

6 RECENT ADVANCES

In the past few years there has been a tremendous amount of interest in the study of motility disorders, leading to exciting new information regarding their pathophysiology, diagnosis and treatment. Much attention has been centered on the role that the interstitial cells of Cajal (ICC) and nitric oxide (NO) play in coordinating motility and sphincter function. The ICC are considered the pacemaker cells of the gut because their network generates the slow waves of depolarization of the gut smooth musculature, allowing the cells to contract. The tyrosine-kinase receptor c-*kit* has been found to be a specific marker for ICC, and it binds to the cytokine stem cell factor (SCF). Mice with a defective c-*kit*/SCF system do not develop ICC, have a disorganized motility pattern, and are not able to tolerate enteral feedings. Recent studies indicate that the distribution of ICC is abnormal in both hypertrophic pyloric stenosis and Hirschsprung's disease, suggesting that both conditions may share a common pathophysiological defect (27). Other motility disorders, including pseudo-obstruction, may be related to abnormalities in ICC.

Nitric oxide is a molecule generated from L-arginine by catalysis of NO synthase enzymes. It has a very short half-life and cannot be stored. Nitric oxide has now been recognized as the primary neurotransmitter of nonadrenergic-noncholinergic nerves, which mediate the majority of inhibitory responses in the gastrointestinal tract. It seems to have an important role in co-ordinating esophageal peristalsis, LES relaxation, gastric accommodation, sphincter of Oddi opening, and internal anal sphincter relaxation. The absence or the overexpression of NO leads to abnormal motility. Inhibitors of NO synthase accelerate intestinal and colonic motility, decrease number of LES relaxations, increase gastric and gallbladder emptying, and attenuate perception of visceral nociceptive stimuli. Deficiency of NO is found in achalasia, pyloric stenosis, and Hirschsprung's disease (28). It is conceivable that the use of NO and NO inhibitors will be possible in the future for the treatment of gastrointestinal motility and functional bowel disorders. Currently, nonspecific activation or inhibition of this ubiquitous molecule may cause undesired neurological, cardiovascular, and immunological side effects, making its use as a therapeutic agent problematic.

Progress has also been made in understanding the genetics of some forms of motility disorders. Several genetic markers for familial and sporadic forms of Hirschsprung's disease have been identified. It has become clear that Hirschsprung's disease is a multigenic disorder with incomplete penetrance and variable expressivity. Mutations in the chromosome 10 mapped RET proto-oncogene have been associated with long-segment aganglionosis and are found in multiple endocrine neoplasia (MEN) 2A, MEN 2B, papillary thyroid carcinoma, and familial medullary thyroid carcinomas. Endothelin-B receptor genes and endothelin-3 genes have been recogized as susceptibility genes for the shorter forms of Hirschsprung's disease and are found in type 2 Waardenburg syndrome. Other gene abnormalities have been identified in smaller subgroups of patients. All the genetic defects identified so far account for about 50% of all forms of Hirschsprung's disease. These genetic abnormalities are thought to cause impaired neuronal crest migration and differentiation (29). They may constitute a model for study of the development of more generalized forms of motility disorders. Identification of these and other genetic markers may permit prenatal diagnosis of motor disorders in the future.

Finally, exciting advances have been made in the treatment of some of the most severe forms of motility disorders. It is now possible to implant gastric and intestinal pacemakers aimed at coordinating motility. Small bowel transplantation has emerged as a definitive cure for patients with the most severe forms of chronic pseudo-obstruction. All patients on TPN with frequent septic episodes, limited intravenous access for nutritional support, and established or impending liver failure should be considered transplant candidates. Different centers have transplanted patients with pseudo-obstruction by using isolated small bowels or multiviscera including stomach, small bowel, colon, liver and pancreas. The 3-year patient and graft survival has been 65%, similar to that of other types of small bowel transplant (30).

REFERENCES

1. Del Rosario F, Di Lorenzo C. Achalasia and other motor disorders. In: Willie R, Hyams JS, eds. Pediatric Gastrointestinal Disease: Pathophysiology, Diagnosis, Management, 2nd ed. Philadelphia, Saunders, 1999, pp 189–197.
2. Staiano AM, Cucchiara S, De Vizia B, Andreotti MR, Auricchio S. Disorders of upper esophageal sphincter motility in children. J Pediatr Gastroenterol Nutr 1987; 6:892–898.
3. Putnam PE, Orenstein SR, Pang D, Pollack IF, Proujansky R, Kocoshis SA. Cricopharyngeal dysfunction associated with Chiari malformation. Pediatrics 1992; 89: 871–876.

4. Kahrilas PJ. Esophageal motility disorders: pathogenesis, diagnosis, treatment. In: Champion MC, Orr WC, eds. Evolving Concepts in Gastrointestinal Motility. Cambridge, MA: Blackwell Science, 1996, pp 15–45.
5. Del Rosario JF, Orenstein SR. Common pediatric esophageal disorders. Gastroenterologist 1998; 6:104–121.
6. Wyllie E, Wyllie R, Cruse RP, Rothner AD, Erenberg. The mechanisms of nitrazepam-induced drooling and aspiration. N Engl J Med 1986; 314:35–38.
7. Mearin F, Mourelle M, Guarner F, Salas A, Riveros-Moreno V, Moncada S, Malagelada J. Patients with achalasia lack nitric oxide synthase in the gastroesophageal junction. Eur J Clin Invest 1993; 23:724–728.
8. Maksimak M, Perlmutter DH, Winter HS. The use of nifedipine in the treatment of achalasia in children. J Pediatr Gastroenterol Nutr 1986; 5:883–886.
9. Okike N, Payne WS, Neufeld DM, Bernatz PE, Pairolero PC, Sanderson DR. Esophagomyotomy versus forceful dilatation for achalasia of the esophagus: results in 899 patients, Ann Thorac Surg 1979; 28:119–125.
10. Gilger MA, Boyle JT, Sondheimer JM, Colletti RB. Indication for pediatric esophageal manometry. J Pediatr Gastroenterol Nutr 1997; 24:616–618.
11. Sigurdsson L, Flores A, Putnam PE, Hyman PE, Di Lorenzo C. Postviral gastroparesis: presentation, treatment and outcome. J Pediatr 1997; 131:751–753.
12. LiVoti G, Tulone V, Bruno R, Cataliotti F, Iacono G, Cavataio F, Balsamo V. Ultrasonography and gastric emptying: evaluation in infants with gastroesophageal reflux. J Pediatr Gastroenterol Nutr 1992; 14:397–399.
13. Cucchiara S, Minella R, Riezzo G, Vallone G, Vallone P, Castellone F, Auricchio S. Reversal of gastric electrical dysrhythmias by cisapride in children with nonulcer dyspepsia. Dig Dis Sci 1992; 37:1136–1140.
14. Di Lorenzo C, Mertz H, Rehm D, Mayer EA, Hyman PE. Gastric sensory response in newborn infants. Gastroenterology 1994; 106:A488.
15. Pineiro-Carrero VM, Andres JM, Davis RH, Mathias JR. Abnormal gastroduodenal motility in children and adolescents with recurrent functional abdominal pain. J Pediatr 1988; 113:820–825.
16. Di Lorenzo C, Hyman PE, Flores AF, Kashyap P, Tomomasa T, Lo S, Snape WJ Jr. Antiduodenal manometry in children and adults with severe nonulcer dyspepsia: do they have the same disease? Scand J Gastroenterol 1994; 29:799–804.
17. Rasquin-Weber A, Hyman PE, Cucchiara S, Fleisher DR, Hyams JS, Milla PJ, Staiano A. Childhood functional gastrointestinal disorders. Gut 1999; 45(2):1160–1168.
18. Fenton TR, Harries JT, Milla PJ. Disordered small bowel motility: a rational basis for toddler's diarrhea. Gut 1983; 24:897–903.
19. Di Lorenzo C. Pseudo-obstruction: current approaches. Gastroenterology 1999; 116:980–987.
20. Rudolph CD, Hyman PE, Altschuler SM, Christensen J, Colletti RB, Cucchiara S, Di Lorenzo C, Flores AF, Hillemeier AC, McCallum RW, Vanderhoof JA. Diagnosis and treatment of chronic intestinal pseudo-obstruction syndrome in children: report of a consensus workshop. J Pediatr Gastroenterol Nutr 1997; 24:102–111.
21. Heneyke S, Smith VV, Spitz L, Milla PJ. Chronic intestinal pseudo-obstruction: treatment and long term follow up of 44 patients. Arch Dis Child 1999; 81:21–27.
22. Hyman PE. Chronic intestinal pseudo-obstruction. In: Hyman PE, Di Lorenzo C

eds. Pediatric Gastrointestinal Motility Disorders. New York: Academy Professional Information Services, 1994, pp 115–128.

23. Di Lorenzo C, Flores AF, Buie T, Hyman PE. Intestinal motility and jejunal feedings in children with chronic intestinal pseudo-obstruction. Gastroenterology 1995; 108: 1379–1385.

24. Di Lorenzo C, Lucanto C, Flores AF, Idries S, Hyman PE. Effect of sequential erythromycin and octreotide on antroduodenal manometry. J Pediatr Gastroenterol Nutr 1999; 29:293–296.

25. Di Lorenzo C, Flores AF, Reddy SN, Hyman PE. Colonic manometry differentiates causes of intractable constipation in children. J Pediatr 1992; 120:690–695.

26. Koletzko S, Jesch I, Faus-Kebler T, Briner J, Meier-Ruge W, Muntefering H, Coerdt W, Wessel L, Keller KM, Nutzenadel W, Schmittenbecher P, Holschneider A, Sacher P. Rectal biopsy for diagnosis of intestinal neuronal dysplasia in children: a prospective multicenter study on interobserver variation and clinical outcome. Gut 1999; 44:853–861.

27. Vanderwinden JM, Liu H, De Laet MH, Vanderhaegen JJ. Study of interstitial cells of Cajal in infantile hypertrophic pyloric stenosis. Gastroenterology 1996; 111:279–288.

28. Vanderwinden JM, De Laet MH, Schiffmann SN, Mailleus P, Lowenstein CJ, Snyder SH, Vanderhaegen JJ. Nitric oxide synthase distribution in the enteric nervous system of Hirschsprung's disease. Gastroenterology 1993; 105:969–973.

29. Klein MD, Burd RS. Hirschsprung's disease. In: Willie R, Hyams JS, eds. Pediatric Gastrointestinal Disease: Pathophysiology, Diagnosis, Management, 2nd ed. Philadelphia: Saunders, 1999, pp 489–498.

30. Sigurdsson L, Reyes J, Kocoshis SA, Mazariegos G, Abu-Elmagd KM, Bueno J, Di Lorenzo C. Intestinal transplantation in children with chronic intestinal pseudo-obstruction. Gut 1999; 45:570–574.

25

Food Allergy

Uzma Shah and W. A. Walker
Harvard Medical School and MassGeneral Hospital and Children's
Hospital, Boston, Massachusetts

1 INTRODUCTION

Food allergy as an adverse reaction to food was originally described by Hippocrates (460–370 B.C.) and Lucretius (95–55 B.C.). Since then extensive studies have been done to find effective methods of diagnosis, particularly so as to eliminate unnecessarily restrictive diets, which in themselves could lead to malnutrition and failure to thrive. More importantly, food allergies may be very severe and can result in fatal complications.

   The purpose of this chapter is to provide a brief review of the pathogenesis, clinical manifestations, diagnosis, and management of food allergies in children.

2 DEFINITIONS

For the purpose of simplification, a number of definitions have been used to describe food reactions. An adverse reaction is a clinically abnormal reaction after the ingestion of a food or additive (1). Such reactions may be secondary to food hypersensitivity or food intolerance. An allergic reaction to food is a specialized form of food intolerance due to an aberrant immune response, while food intolerance is a non-immune-mediated event in response to ingested foods that may include toxins such as aflatoxins and staphylococcal toxins (2). The majority of adverse food reactions, however, are due to food intolerance (2).

It is only recently that attempts have been made to use uniform definitions and diagnoses for food allergies. Confusion in terminology as well as variations in the diagnosis and reporting of symptoms have also made prevalence determination in a population very difficult (3,4). The incidence of food allergies in children has been estimated to be between 0.3 and 7.5% (5–8), while in adults the incidence is 0.3 to 2 percent. Burkes et al. and Sampson et al. (9–13) have also demonstrated an increase in food allergy in atopic children.

3   PATHOPHYSIOLOGY

While almost any food can be allergenic, the most frequently implicated foods include fish, cow's milk, soy, peanuts, nuts, and wheat (14–16). Being heat- and enzyme-resistant, the majority of these allergens are water soluble glycoproteins with molecular weights of 10,000 to 60,000 Da.

The mucosal immune system forms an effective barrier to the transport of intact macromolecules across the intestinal epithelium, and both immune and nonimmune mediated factors play a role in providing mucosal defense. Microbial flora in the intestinal lumen prevent the growth of pathogens (17), while surface glycoprotein, intestinal peristalsis, and enzymatic activity provide further protection (19). Some transfer of intact protein does occur through the enterocyte, via tight junctions, and through the M cell (20,21). Immune mechanisms involve the gut-associated lymphoid tissue or GALT, which comprises the reticuloendothelial system of the liver, Peyer's patches, mesenteric lymph nodes, and intraepithelial lymphocytes (22,23). Activation of lymphocytes results in the proliferation of T and B cells and then migration to the lymphatics to reach the systemic circulation. In the mucosa, B cells further differentiate into antibody-producing cells (24–28). On subsequent reexposure to antigen, IgA is produced in the lamina propria. A secretory component is attached to the IgA and aids in the transport of IgA across the epithelium and also prevents adherence of microbes to the mucosa. It also prevents proteolytic digestion of the IgA molecule in the intestinal lumen (19,29) (Fig. 1).

Under normal circumstances, food antigen exposure leads to the development of oral tolerance, with the activation of CD8+ suppressor T lymphocytes and suppression of systemic IgG and IgM production. Failure in the development of oral tolerance leads to food hypersensitivity reactions (30–32).

Although, according to Coombs and Gell, there are four major types of immunological allergic reactions, the most frequent type is an IgE-mediated hypersensitivity response (19,22). In genetically susceptible individuals, antigen exposure leads to the production of antigen-specific IgE, which plays a central role

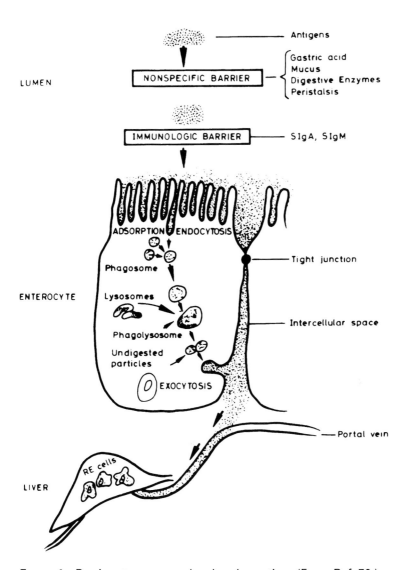

FIGURE 1   Barriers to macromolecular absorption. (From Ref. 70.)

in the inflammatory response and the release of inflammatory mediators such as cytokines, prostaglandins, leukotrienes, serotonin, histamine, etc. In type 2 reactions, complement activation and cytolysis follow antigen–antibody interactions. In type 3 allergic responses, antigen–antibody complexes are formed that damage the mucosa. In type 4 reactions, a delayed-type of hypersensitivity response occurs, with the involvement of sensitized T cells. Allergic reactions to food may be further categorized as immediate or delayed.

4   CLINICAL MANIFESTATIONS

Gastrointestinal symptoms are among the most frequent clinical manifestations and occur in 50% of patients. Symptoms may occur hours or even days after exposure to the food antigen and may vary from mild to severe.

4.1   Allergic Gastroenteropathy

Characterized by eosinophilic infiltration of the mucosa, this entity occurs in three forms, with variable involvement of the intestine. The type most frequently seen is the mucosal variety, where eosinophilic infiltration is limited to the mucosa. Other types include the transmural and serosal types. Mucosal disease presents with nausea, vomiting, abdominal pain, and diarrhea; it may be associated with occult blood loss and iron deficiency anemia as well as failure to thrive. Transmural disease may manifest itself with obstructive symptoms, while serosal disease may present with ascites and abdominal pain (33).

4.2   Food-Induced Enterocolitis

Occurring mainly in infants less than 3 months of age, this condition is most frequently due to an allergenic antigen in cow's-milk protein and soy. Clinical presentations include vomiting, regurgitation, diarrhea, malabsorption, and failure to thrive. Stools may contain eosinophils and neutrophils; there may be associated steatorrhea and occult blood loss.

4.3   Food-Induced Colitis

Also occurring in infants in the first few months of life, this entity comprises allergies mostly to soy and milk protein. Disease is limited to the colon. Colonic biopsies show ulceration, edema, and eosinophillic infiltration that resolves with the removal of the offending antigen from the diet (21,34).

4.4   Celiac Disease

Also known as gluten-sensitive enteropathy, celiac disease occurs more frequently in certain populations across the globe, such as in the Irish, and may be associated with the HLA markers DR4 and DQW2 (see Chap. 21). Allergy exists to the gliadin fraction of gluten derived from wheat and the disease manifests itself in children as failure to thrive, abdominal pain, malabsorption, short stature, iron deficiency anemia, rickets, and irritability. Characteristic features include abdominal distention and muscle wasting (35,36).

4.5 Infantile Colic

Allergy to milk has also been implicated in infantile colic. Lothe et al. found that colic occurred in 24 of 27 infants allergic to milk, with resolution of symptoms after removal of milk from the diet (37). Jakobsson et al. also showed that milk in the maternal diet may produce symptoms in breast-fed babies, with improvement in symptoms after elimination of cow's milk from the maternal diet (38).

Extragastrointestinal manifestations of food allergies are numerous and involve several systems. Cutaneous manifestations include eczema and urticaria. Rhinitis, asthma, and anaphylaxis may occur. Food allergies are also thought to play a role in the etiology of diabetes mellitus, nephrotic syndrome, and arthritis.

4.6 Allergic Esophagitis

Some patients with chronic symptoms of gastroesophageal reflux despite medical therapy may have allergic esophagitis. The histological appearance of esophageal eosinophils has been correlated with esophagitis and gastroesophageal reflux in children. Esophageal eosinophilia that persists despite antireflux therapy may suggest allergic esophagitis. In a study by Liacouras et al. (39) of 1809 patients, 20 had persistent symptoms and esophageal eosinophilia. Histological examination revealed 34.2 ± 9.6 eosinophils per high power field in the patients with primary eosinophilic esophagitis who did not respond to antireflux therapy, in contrast to 2.26 ± 1.16 eosinophils per high power field in those who did respond to antireflux therapy. All the study patients responded rapidly to steroid treatment. A food elimination and challenge test was recommended when physicians or parents chose not to use steroids. Walsh et al. also identified a group of pediatric patients characterized by an allergic history, lack of response to antireflux therapy, normal pH probe study results, and a large number of eosinophils in esophageal biopsy specimens that represent examples of allergic esophagitis (40).

5 DIAGNOSIS

A good history and physical examination are critical in making a diagnosis of food allergy (Table 1). It is extremely important to elucidate, by using food recall, which food ingredient may be causing the problem. Important information to be obtained includes the timing of the allergic response after exposure to the food

TABLE 1   Diagnosis of Food Allergy

History and physical examination
Food diary
Elimination diet
RAST, ELISA testing
Skin testing
Food challenges
Endoscopy and intestinal biopsy

Key: RAST, radioallergosorbent test;
ELISA, enzyme-linked immunosorbent
assay.

antigen, the duration and nature of the allergic response, and the treatment required. The presence of nongastrointestinal manifestations in the respiratory system, such as asthma, or cutaneous disease, such as eczema, should be ascertained. A family history of allergies may be helpful in making the diagnosis. Physical examination focuses on searching for signs of allergy, such as eczema, urticaria, or wheezing.

5.1   Skin Tests

Skin testing with dilute concentrations of food extracts has been done with a pinprick technique to diagnose food allergies. The test detects specific IgE antibody for the applied antigen and can detect at least 80% of the IgE-mediated responses, but it is inconclusive for non-IgE-mediated reactions. While results are usually available within 10 to 20 min (31,41), positive and negative controls are also required along with the food allergen. Positive controls with histamine and negative controls with saline are frequently used. A wheal of 3 mm or greater in size is considered positive (22,42). There is a risk of anaphylaxis with the use of skin tests; hence such testing should be done only in a controlled environment. A positive skin test implies that the patient's symptoms may be related to the food allergen tested; however, the positive predictive value of the test is less than 50% (22). The predictive value of the test depends on factors such as the age of the patient and the allergen tested, with greater positivity for antigens such as wheat (75%) and eggs (50%) and in children below 1 year of age (33,43). A negative skin test has a greater than 95% negative predictive value (15,22,44,45). However, skin tests after a severe reaction may be temporarily negative due to anergy (46).

5.2   Laboratory Investigations

Serum testing for antigen-specific IgE can be done using a test called the radioallergosorbent test or RAST. It can be used for testing against various food antigens at the same time and is not only convenient but can be particularly useful in patients with skin rashes, etc. However, disadvantages include a limited number of antigens available for testing and the high cost of the test (47).

The enzyme-linked immunosorbent assay (ELISA) detects antigen-specific IgE and has similar limitations as the RAST. The ELISA does not expose the laboratory personnel to radiation, as the RAST does. However, markedly elevated IgE levels can interfere with the ELISA and the RAST and give falsely elevated results.

Peripheral eosinophilia, eosinophils in the nasal mucus and stool, and elevated serum IgE levels suggest IgE-mediated disease. Sicherer et al. studied cow's milk–specific IgE levels in children less than 3 years of age in comparison with children greater than 9 years of age with persistent milk allergy. The children with persistent symptoms of milk allergy had significantly greater levels of whole milk–and casein-specific IgE (48). In another study by Majamaa et al. the diagnostic accuracy of various tests such as serum IgE levels, skin testing, and patch testing was determined. Of the 143 infants with cow's-milk allergy that were tested, oral milk challenge was positive in 50%. Of these patients 26% had elevated IgE levels. In contrast, only 14% of these patients had positive skin tests and 44% had positive results with the patch test (49). Further testing, such as endoscopic biopsies are restricted to cases where a definitive diagnosis is required. Tests such as intestinal mast-cell histamine release and the detection of circulating immune complexes are of academic interest alone.

5.3 Elimination Diets and Food Challenges

Elimination diets involve the elimination of the offending food from the diet for a 2 to 4-week period. When no particular food is suspected, elimination of common food allergens is tried. However, care must be taken not to impose unnecessarily restrictive diets, which in themselves would lead to inadequate nutrition and failure to thrive. Elemental diets such as Vivonex and Neocate and formulas such Nutramigen and Pregestimil provide non- or hypoallergenic blends that can be used in these restrictive diets. Continuation of symptoms suggests that etiologies other than food allergy may be responsible for the symptoms and alternate diagnoses need to be sought.

Food challenges are performed to confirm food allergy. It is extremely important that all food challenges be performed under strict medical supervision, as such testing may be potentially life-threatening if an anaphylactic reaction occurs in response to the food antigen. A history of such a reaction is a contraindication to food challenges. Testing may include an open method, where both the patient and the physician are aware of the food antigen; a single-blinded method, where only the physician is aware; and a double-blinded approach, where both physician and patient are unaware of the nature of the food antigen (18). The latter is used as a "gold standard" for food allergy testing, as it can be used where symptoms are vague and ill-defined (7,50).

Food challenges require a 2-week period of removal of the offending antigen from the diet prior to testing. The food antigen is administered in small doses and increased incrementally over a period of time until symptoms occur (13,46,51). A positive challenge indicates that the food may be responsible for the symptoms produced but does not indicate the immune mechanism involved.

6 MANAGEMENT

Treatment of food allergies involves elimination of the allergenic food from the diet (Fig. 2). Most children are allergic to only one food (52). It is important to make sure that a nutritionist is involved in designing the diet with the necessary eliminations to ensure an appropriate caloric intake and growth. Parents are instructed on reading food labels to look for those hidden ingredients that may be problematic for the food-allergic child.

Most infants with allergy to cow's milk will also be allergic to soy protein (44). Casein hydrolysates such as Nutramigen and Pregestimil and free amino acid diets such as Vivonex and Neocate have been used successfully in children with allergy to milk and soy protein (45,54,55).

Anaphylactic reactions are treated with epinephrine, and it is critical that patients with histories of such reactions carry epinephrine with them at all times. An identification bracelet with the allergies listed is helpful.

Mast-cell stabilizers such as sodium cromoglycate and ketotifen have limited use in the treatment of food allergy. Similarly steroids have no use in the treatment of food allergies except in eosinophilic gastroenteropathy (7,55).

The delayed introduction of solid foods and exclusive breast-feeding in the first 6 months of life may prevent the development of food allergies (20,56,57). Breast milk carries various immune protective factors, including IgA, that may play a role in early immune protection in the infant's gastrointestinal tract (8). Patients with a strong family history of atopic disease may benefit from the elimination of allergenic foods from the maternal diet as well, as small amounts of intact protein pass into breast milk (58). Controversy exists, however, on the implementation of strict maternal diets in an attempt to prevent the development of food allergies in the infant (59,60).

The intestinal microflora is an important constituent of the gut mucosal barrier (61,62). In its absence, macromolecular transport across the intestinal epithelium may increase. Isolauri et al. suggest that specific strains of intestinal microflora may be protective against allergic sensitization. Oral bacteriotherapy with probiotics such as *Lactobacillus GG* has been shown to alleviate the intestinal inflammation in patients with food allergy (63,64). It has been previously shown that *Lactobacillus GG* promotes antigen-specific immune responses, particularly in the IgA class (63,64). Antigen uptake at Peyer's patches may be

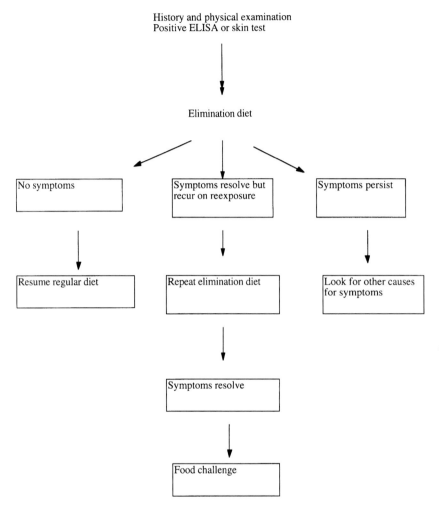

FIGURE 2   Algorithm for approach to a patient with suspected food allergy.

reduced and may potentiate the production of IFN-γ by T cells that in turn inhibit the detrimental effects of TNF-α at the intestinal epithelium (65,66).

7   SUMMARY

Most children outgrow their food allergy within a few years. In a retrospective review by Sicherer et al. of the patients followed for milk allergy for a median period of 25 months, loss of sensitivity to cow's milk occurred in 6 of 10 patients and loss of sensitivity to soy protein in 2 of the 8 patients studied (67). However, allergy to peanuts, fish, and eggs tends to persist longer (68,69). While a good history and physical examination are very important in the diagnosis of food allergy, it would be wise to refrain from strict elimination diets except where absolutely warranted. Further research is still needed on the appropriate timing and degree of food allergen avoidance in early infancy that may help in preventing food allergy.

REFERENCES

1. American Academy of Allergy and Immunology/National Institute of Allergy and Infectious Disease. NIH Publication No 84-2422. Adverse Reactions to Food. Bethesda MD: National Institute of Health, 1984, pp 1–6.
2. Nichaman MZ, Mcpherson RS. Estimating prevalence of adverse reactions to foods: principles and constraints. J Allergy Clin Immunol 1986; 78:148–154.
3. Opper FH, Burakoff R. Food allergy and intolerance. Gastroenterologist 1993; 1: 211–220.
4. Rossiter MA. Food Intolerance: a general pediatrician's view. J R Soc Med 1985; 78:17–20.
5. Marks DR, Marks LM: Food allergy: manifestations, evaluation and management. Postgrad Med 1993; 93:191–201.
6. Buckley RH, Metcalfe D. Food allergy. JAMA 1982; 248:2627–1631.
7. Metcalfe DD. Food hypersensitivity. J Allergy Clin Immunol 1984; 73:749–762.
8. Walker EC. Food allergy. Am Fam Physician 1988; 38:207–212.
9. Zeiger RS, Heller S, Mellon MH, et al. Effect of combined maternal and infant food-allergen avoidance on development of atopy in early infancy: a randomized study. J Allergy Clin Immunol 1989; 84:72–89.
10. Bock SA. Prospective appraisal of complaints of adverse reactions to foods in children during the first 3 years of life. Pediatrics 1987; 79:683–688.
11. Altman DR, Chiaramonte LT. Public perception of food allergy. J Allergy Clin Immunol 1996; 97:1247–51.
12. Host A, Halken S. A prospective study of cow milk allergy in Danish infants during the first three years of life. Allergy 1990; 45:587–596.
13. Hoffman KM, Sampson HA. Evaluation and management of patients with adverse food reactions. In Bierman CW, Pearlman DS, Shapiro CG et al., eds. Allergy, Asthma and Immunology from Infancy to Adulthood. Philadelphia: Saunders, 1996, pp 665–686.
14. Sampson HA. Food allergies, Oski F, DeAngelis CD, Feigin RD, eds. Principles and Practice of Pediatrics. Philadelphia: Lippincott, 1994, pp 227–232.
15. Bock SA, Atkins FM. Patterns of food hypersensitivity during sixteen years of double blind, placebo-controlled food challenges. J Pediatr 1990; 117:561–567.
16. Kemp AS. Food allergy in children. Aust Fam Physician 1993; 22:1959–1963.
17. Donaldson RM. Normal bacterial population of the intestine and their relation to intestinal function. N Engl J Med 1964; 270:994–1001.
18. Atkins FM, Metcalfe DD. The diagnosis and treatment of food allergy. Annu Rev Nutr 1984; 4:233–255.

19. Pang KY, Walker WA, Bloch KJ. Intestinal uptake of macromolecules: differences in distribution and degradation of protein antigen in control and immunised rats. Gut 1981; 22:1018–1024.

20. Duggan C, Walker WA. Protein intolerance, in Oski FA, DeAngelis CD, Feigin RD, eds. Principles and Practice of Pediatrics. Philadelphia: Lippincott, 1994, pp 1887–1890.

21. Stern M. Allergic enteropathy. In: Walker WA, Durie PR, Hamilton JR, et al., eds. Pediatric Gastrointestinal Disease. St Louis: Mosby 1996, pp 677–692.

22. Burks AW, Sampson H. Food allergies in children. Curr Probl Pediatr 1993; 23: 230–252.

23. Patrick MK, Gall DG. Protein intolerance and immunocyte and enterocyte interaction. Pediatr Clin North Am 1988; 35:17–34.

24. Walker WA, Isselbacher KJ. Uptake and transport of macromolecules by the intestine: possible role in clinical disorders. Gastroenterology 1974; 67:531–550.

25. Triger DR, Cynamon MH, Wright R. Studies on hepatic uptake of antigen: 1. Comparison of inferior vena cava and portal vein routes of immunisation. Immunology 1973; 25:941–950.

26. McDermott MR, Bienenstock J. Evidence for a common mucosal immunological system: 1. Migration of immunoblasts into intestinal, respiratory and genital tissue. J Immunol 1979; 122:1892–1897.

27. Lessof MH. Food allergy and intolerance, in Lachmann PJ, Peters K, Rosen FS, eds. Clinical Aspects of Immunology. Boston: Blackwell, 1993, pp 1067–1080.

28. Sampson HA. The immunopathogenic role of food hypersensitivity in atopic dermatitis. Acta Derm Venerol 1992; 176:S34–S37.

29. Sampson HA, Fomon SJ. Antigen antibody interactions and adverse reactions to food, in Fomon SJ, ed. Nutrition of Normal Infants. St Louis: Mosby 1993, pp 395–408.

30. Seidman E. Food allergic disorders of the gastrointestinal tract, in Roy CC, Silverman A, Allagille D, eds. Pediatric Clinical Gastroenterology. St Louis: Mosby 1995, pp 374–384.

31. Sampson A, Metcalfe DD. Food allergies. JAMA 1992; 268:2840–2844.

32. Sampson HA. The immunopathogenic role of food hypersensitivity in atopic dermatitis. Acta Derm Venereol 1992; 176:S34–S37.

33. Bock SA, Sampson HA. Food allergy in infancy. Pediatr Clin North Am 1994; 41: 1047–1067.

34. Proujansky R, Winter HS, Walker WA. Gastrointestinal syndromes associated with food sensitivity. In: Barness LA, ed. Advances in Pediatrics. Vol 35. St Louis: Mosby, 1988, pp 219–238.

35. Wright R, Roberston D. Immunologically mediated damage, local and distant. In: Brostoff J, Challacombe SJ, eds. Food Allergy and Intolerance. London: Ballière Tindall, 1987, pp 237–247.

36. Kelly CP, Feighery CF, Gallagher RB et al. Diagnosis and treatment of gluten sensitive enteropathy. Adv Intern Med 1990; 35:341–364.

37. Lothe L, Lindberg T. Cows milk protein causes infantile colic in breast fed infants: a double blind cross over study. Pediatrics 1989; 83:262–266.

38. Jakobbson I, Lindberg T. Cow's milk protein causes infantile colic in breast fed infants: a double blind cross over study. Pediatrics 1983; 71:268–271.

39. Liacouras CA, Wenner WJ, Brown K, et al. Primary eosinophilic esophagitis in children: successful treatment with oral corticosteroids. J Pediatr Gastroenterol Nutr 1998; 26:380–385.

40. Walsh SV, Antonioli DA, Goldman H, et al. Allergic esophagitis in children: a clinicopathological entity. Am J Surg Pathol 1999; 23(4):390–396.

41. Sampson HA, McCaskill CC. Food hypersensitivity and atopic dermatitis: evaluation of 113 patients. J Pediatr 1985; 107:669–675.

42. Lemanske RF Jr, Taylor SL. Standardized extracts, foods. Clin Rev Allergy 1987; 5:23–36.

43. Sampson HA, Albergo R. Comparison of results of skin tests. RAST and double blind placebo controlled food challenges in children with atopic dermatitis. J Allergy Clin Immunol 1984; 74:26–33.

44. Committee on Nutrition, American Academy of Pediatrics. Food hypersensitivity. In: Barness LA, ed. Pediatric Nutrition Handbook, Elk Grove Village, IL. American Academy of Pediatrics 1993, pp 274–285.

45. Bousvaros A, Walker WA. Food allergy. In Steihm ER, ed. Immunologic Disorders in Infants and Children. Philadelphia: Saunders 1996, pp 707–741.

46. Watson WTA. Food allergies in children: diagnostic strategies. Clin Rev Allergy Immunol 1995; 13:347–359.

47. Sicherer SH. Sampson HA. Cow's milk protein specific IgE concentrations in 2 age groups of milk allergic children and children achieving tolerance. Clin Exp Allergy 1999; 29(4):507–512.

48. Majamaa H, Moisio P, Holm K, et al. Cow's milk allergy. Diagnostic accuracy of skin prick and patch test and specific IgE. Allergy 1999; 54(4):346–351.

49. Bock SA. Food sensitivity: a critical review and practical approach. Am J Dis Child 1980; 134:973–982.

50. Butkus SN, Mahan LK. Food allergies: immunological reactions to food. J Am Diet Assoc 1986; 86:601–608.

51. Terho EO, Savolainin J. Diagnosis of food hypersensitivity. Eur J Clin Nutr 1996; 50:1–5.

52. Metcalfe DD. Allergic reactions to food. In: Frank MM, Austen KF, Claman HN, et al, eds. Samter's Immunological Diseases. Boston: Little Brown, 1995, pp 1357–1360.

53. Crespo JF, Pascual C, Burks AW, et al. Frequency of food allergy in a pediatric population from Spain. Pediatr Allergy Immunol 1995; 6:39–43.

54. Sampson HA, James JM, Bernhisel-Broadbent J. Safety of an amino acid derived infant formula in children allergic to cow's milk. Pediatrics 1992; 90:463–465.

55. Sampson HA, Buckley RH, Metcalfe DD. Food allergy. JAMA 1987; 258:2886–2890.

56. Stern M. Gastrointestinal allergy. In: Walker WA, Durie PR, Hamilton JR, eds. Pediatric Gastrointestinal Disease. St Louis: Mosby, 1991, pp 557–574.

57. Zeiger RS. Prevention of food allergy in infancy. Ann Allergy 1990; 65:430–441.

58. Dannaeus A. Food allergy in infancy and children. Ann Allergy 1987; 59:124–126.

59. Chandra RK, Puri S, Suraiya C, et al. Influence of maternal food antigen avoidance

during pregnancy and lactation on incidence of atopic eczema in infants. Clin Allergy 1986; 16:563–571.

60. Falth-Magnusson K, Kjellman NIM. Development of atopic disease in babies whose mothers were receiving exclusion diet during pregnancy. J Allergy Clin Immunol 1987; 80:868–875.

61. Fuller R. Probiotics in human medicine. Gut 1991; 32:439–442.

62. Wells CL, Maddaus MA, Jechorek RP, Simmons RL. Role of intestinal anaerobic bacteria in colonization resistance. Eur J Microbiol Infect Dis 1988; 7:107–113.

63. Isolauri E, Majamaa H, Arvola T, Rantala I, et al. Lactobacilli casein strain GG reverses increased intestinal permeability induced by cows milk in suckling rats. Gastroenterology 1993; 105:1643–1650.

64. Majamaa H, Isolauri E, Saxelin M, et al. Lactic acid bacteria in the treatment of acute rotavirus gastroenteritis. J Pediatr Gastroenterol Nutr 1995; 20:222–228.

65. Halpern GM, Vruwink KG, Van de Water G, et al. Influence of long term yogurt consumption in young adults. Int J Immunother 1991; 7:205–210.

66. Hernandez-Pando R, Rook GAW. The role of TNF-alpha in T cell mediated inflammation depends on the Th1/Th2 cytokine balance. Immunology 1994; 82:591–595.

67. Sicherer SH, Eigenmann PA, Sampson HA. Clinical features of food protein induced enterocolitis syndrome. J Pediatr 1998; 133(2):214–219.

68. Sampson HA, Scanlon SM. Natural history of food hypersensitivity in children with atopic dermatitis. J Pediatr 1989; 115:23–27.

69. Tariq SM, Stevens M, Mathew S, et al. Cohort study of peanut and tree nut sensitization by age 4 years. BMJ 1996; 313:514–517.

70. Sanderson IR, Walker WA. Uptake and transport of macromolecules by the intestine: possible role in clinical disorders (an update). Gastroenterology 1993; 104:630.

26

Gastrointestinal Bleeding

William R. Treem
Duke University Medical Center and Duke Children's Hospital,
Durham, North Carolina

1 INTRODUCTION

Gastrointestinal bleeding is among the most frightening events that can confront a parent or child. Faced with the myriad of potential causes and locations for bleeding and the anxiety of the parent and child, the pediatrician may feel challenged by what appears to be a complex problem of differential diagnosis and treatment. By following some simple guidelines, one can adopt a rational, expeditious, cost-effective approach, which will narrow the differential diagnosis and focus the evaluation on a few diagnostic tests. This chapter reviews the differential diagnosis and assessment of the infant and child with gastrointestinal bleeding.

2 GUIDELINES FOR ASSESSMENT AND FORMULATION OF A DIFFERENTIAL DIAGNOSIS

Table 1 lists the ''ten commandments'' for the assessment of gastrointestinal bleeding. All of these can be accomplished with a careful history and physical examination and with a minimum of procedures and tests in the office, emergency room, or hospital setting. The likely diagnosis will dictate whether the patient can be managed in the primary care setting or—if further diagnostic radiographic

TABLE 1 "Ten Commandments" for the
Assessment of Gastrointestinal Bleeding

Assess hemodynamic stability
Remember, common things are common
Factor in the age of the patient
Note the color of the emesis or stool
Use the nasogastric tube
Beware of pseudobloods
Assess for a change in bowel habit
Examine for signs of obstruction or perforation
Always examine the anus and rectum
Avoid using barium x-rays in favor of endoscopy

---

or endoscopic studies are required—should be referred to a pediatric gastroenter-ologist or surgeon.

2.1 Assess Hemodynamic Stability

The first and most important step in the evaluation of the child with gastrointesti-nal bleeding is the determination of hemodynamic stability. Even before the vital signs are taken, signs of poor perfusion must be sought, including pallor, livedo reticularis, coolness of the extremities, slow capillary refill (greater than 2 sec), weakness, and lethargy. When interpreting the vital signs, it is important to re-member that a young child's main early compensatory mechanism for dealing with impending shock is an increase in heart rate. Tachycardia and a narrowed pulse pressure are earlier signs of shock than hypotension. Determining whether the patient has orthostatic signs of increased heart rate or falling blood pressure is an important part of the assessment.

Any signs and symptoms of hemodynamic instability should prompt ag-gressive intervention to establish one or more large-bore intravenous lines; pro-vide supplemental oxygen; send for baseline laboratory assessment of hemoglo-bin, platelet count, clotting factors, electrolytes, liver enzymes, and renal function; request cross-matched blood from the blood bank; and infuse a large bolus of saline quickly in order to maintain perfusion. The value of the initial hematocrit may not be as accurate as the child's vital signs, color, and perfusion in determining the severity of blood loss and the need for volume replacement. It is important to remember that equilibrium of the hematocrit after acute blood loss may take 24 hr or more, so the hematocrit may appear falsely high in the face of impending shock. Also, most children have excellent cardiac, pulmonary, and renal function and can adapt to substantial blood loss without a noticeable alteration in cardiopulmonary function provided that the blood has been lost slowly. A child with a very low hematocrit and little or no signs of shock has likely lost blood via the gastrointestinal tract over a prolonged period of time. In this situation, overzealous, rapid replacement with blood may result in fluid overload, pulmonary edema, and congestive heart failure. A prolonged prothrombin time suggests severe liver disease, biliary obstruction, or chronic malabsorption of fat and fat-soluble vitamins and indicates the need for parenteral vitamin K or clotting factors to help stop the bleeding and prepare the patient for further invasive diagnostic tests. A platelet transfusion should be given if there is active bleeding and the platelet count is less than 50,000/mm^3 or if a diagnostic endoscopy with biopsies or a therapeutic procedure is planned.

2.2 Common Things Are Common

Tables 2 to 4 list both common and uncommon causes of upper and lower intestinal bleeding divided by age, site, and presenting symptom. It is important to remember that certain problems are common in each group. For example, the infant presenting with streaks of red blood in otherwise normal stool most likely

TABLE 2 Common Causes of Upper Gastrointestinal Bleeding

Symptom	Infant (0–2 years)	Child (2–12 years)	Adolescent (>12 years)
Hematemesis (bright red blood)	Gastritis	Gastritis	Gastritis
	Gastric ulcer	Peptic ulcer	Peptic ulcer
		Mallory-Weiss tear	Mallory-Weiss tear
		Esophageal varices	Esophageal varices
Hematemesis (coffee ground)	Gastritis	Esophagitis	Esophagitis
	Nasogastric tube trauma	"Prolapse gastrophy"	"Prolapse gastropathy"
	Swallowed maternal blood	Gastritis (viral, NSAIDs)	Viral, NSAIDs
		Helicobacter pylori	*Helicobacter pylori*
		Peptic ulcer	Peptic ulcer
Melena	Gastritis	Gastritis	Gastritis
	Duodenal ulcer	Duodenal ulcer	Duodenal ulcer
		Esophageal varices	Esophageal varices

TABLE 3 Common Causes of Lower Gastrointestinal Bleeding

Symptom	Infant (0–2)	Child (2–12)	Adolescent (>12)
Painless melena	Meckel's diverticulum		
Melena with pain, obstruction, perforation	Necrotizing enterocolitis, intussusception		
Hematochezia with diarrhea, crampy pain	Infectious colitis, Hirschsprung's enterocolitis	Infectious colitis, ulcerative colitis, Crohn's disease, HUS, HSP	Infectious colitis, ulcerative colitis, Crohn's disease, HUS, HSP
Painless hematochezia without diarrhea	Anal fissure, eosinophilic colitis, lymphonodular hyperplasia	Anal fissure, juvenile polyp, lymphonodular hyperplasia	Anal fissure, ulcerative proctitis, perianal Crohn's disease

Key: HUS, hemolytic uremic syndrome; HSP, Henoch-Schönlein purpura.

has an anal fissure or eosinophilic colitis secondary to cow's-milk or soy protein intolerance and is much less likely to have a colonic hemangioma or rectal ectopic gastric mucosa. Similarly, the infant vomiting bright red blood in the newborn nursery is likely suffering from a gastric ulcer, gastritis, or esophagitis secondary to stress rather than bleeding from a gastric or duodenal duplication. A child with retching and vomiting of gastric contents which initially is food, then is bile stained, and then tinged with brown flecks likely has minor mucosal bleeding engendered by the recurrent prolapse of fundic gastric mucosa through the gastroesophageal junction (prolapse gastropathy) (1). Much less frequently, severe retching and/or coughing results in significant esophageal bleeding from a Mallory-Weiss tear of the mucosa at the gastroesophageal junction. Although there are exceptions, esophageal variceal bleeding usually does not occur before 2 years of age, even in children with cirrhotic lesions from early infancy such as biliary atresia or early extrahepatic causes of portal hypertension, such as cavernous transformation of the portal vein.

Painless rectal bleeding in a toddler is much more likely to be from a juvenile inflammatory polyp than from an arteriovenous malformation or a Meckel's diverticulum. Blaming rectal bleeding on hemorrhoids in children under the age of 10 years is usually a mistake, since hemorrhoids are very rare in young children

TABLE 4 Uncommon Causes of Gastrointestinal Bleeding
by Site

Esophagus
    Infectious esophagitis (*Candida*, herpes, cytomegalovirus)
    Esophageal pill ulcer
    Caustic ingestion
    Foreign body
    Mucositis (chemotherapy)
Stomach
    Infectious gastritis (cytomegalovirus)
    Gastric duplication cyst
    Dieulafoy's diease
    Gastric hemangiomas
    Hereditary hemorrhagic telangiectasia
    Portal gastropathy
    Gastric varices
    Leiomyoma (myosarcoma)
Duodenum
    Hemobilia
    Duodenal hematoma
    Duplication cyst
    Graft-versus-host disease
    Dieulafoy's disease
Small intestine
    Graft-versus-host disease
    Crohn's disease with ileal ulcer
    Intussusception with lead point
    Lymphoma
    Vascular malformation
    Polyposis syndrome (Peutz-Jegher)
    Ileal duplication
Colon
    Arteriovenous malformation
    Hemangiomas
    Amebiasis
    Viral colitis (cytomegalovirus, adenovirus)
    Familial adenomatous polyposis
Anorectum
    Hemorrhoids
    Sexual abuse
    Rectal prolapse
    Solitary rectal ulcer
    Rectal varices

even in the presence of constipation; if present, they may point to portal hypertension (2). Bloody mucous diarrhea in a young child is usually an infectious diarrhea caused by a bacterial pathogen such as *Salmonella*, *Shigella*, *Campylobacter jejuni*, *Yersinia Enterocolitica*, or *Clostridium difficile*. The practice of performing a barium enema on any young child presenting to the emergency room with bloody, mucous stools in order to rule out intussusception should be discouraged, since this is a rare cause of blood in the stool, and does not present with diarrhea. Also, the presence of barium will obscure efforts to arrive at the proper diagnosis.

2.3 Factor in the Age of the Patient

Figure 1 shows the likely age at presentation of the common etiologies of gastrointestinal bleeding in children. In the newborn, upper gastrointestinal bleeding is often secondary to gastritis or gastric and duodenal ulceration. In sick premature neonates, this phenomenon is attributed to the "stress" of premature birth accompanied by respiratory disease, infection, and ischemic bowel disease. However, it has also been reported in seemingly normal full-term infants in the first 48 hr of life (3). Certain lesions such as allergic or eosinophilic colitis, intussusception, and Meckel's diverticulum are almost always seen only during the first 2 years

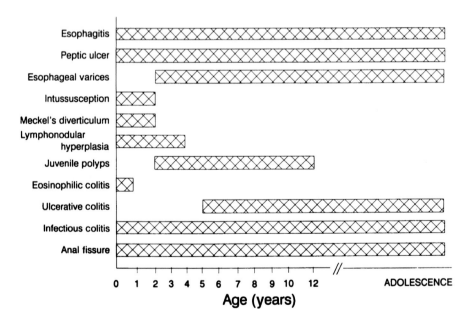

FIGURE 1 Common etiologies of gastrointestinal bleeding in children: likely age at presentation. (From Ref. 50.)

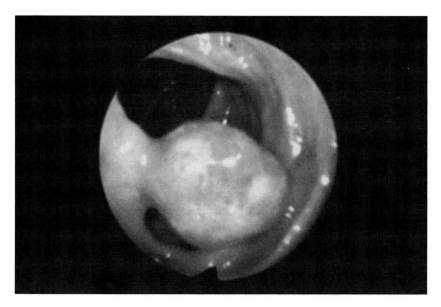

FIGURE 2 Endoscopic photograph of a juvenile inflammatory polyp in the sigmoid colon of a 4-year-old with painless hematochezia. (From Ref. 50.)

of life. In contrast, it is unusual to see gastrointestinal bleeding from esophageal varices, juvenile polyps, or inflammatory bowel disease before the age of 2 years. Bloody diarrhea may signify the presence of infectious colitis in virtually all pediatric age groups. However, eosinophilic colitis, necrotizing enterocolitis, and enterocolitis secondary to Hirschsprung's disease are more likely in infants in the first few months of life; whereas ulcerative colitis, Crohns disease, Henoch-Schönlein purpura, and hemolytic-uremic syndrome (often caused by infection with *Escherichia coli* 0157-H7) are much more likely to be responsible in older children and adolescents. A child under the age of 4 presenting with bright red boood per rectum after a viral illness and with multiple submucosal nodules in the colon is likely to have lymphonodular hyperplasia; this is a benign, self-limited illness that has occasionally been associated with immunodeficiency and food allergies. Children with familial polyposis syndromes rarely develop multiple colonic polyps and lower gastrointestinal bleeding before the age 7 to 10 years.

2.4 Note the Color of the Emesis or Stool

Hematemesis with red blood and ''coffee grounds'' (denatured hemoglobin) or a bloody nasogastric aspirate confirms bleeding from the upper gastrointestinal tract. Those lesions that bleed more briskly, including esophageal or gastric varices and large gastric or duodenal ulcers, will result in frankly bloody emesis. Forceful vomiting or retching can lead to bleeding from a mucosal laceration at the gastroesophageal junction, (a Mallory-Weiss tear). In contrast, more indolent bleeding from peptic esophagitis, postviral gastritis, and gastritis induced by non-steroidal anti-inflammatory drugs (NSAIDs) will manifest itself as coffee-ground emesis. Chronically indwelling nasogastric tubes or gastrostomy tubes and skin-level devices may provoke gastric mucosal erosions and slow oozing with coffee-grounds emesis.

Bright red blood per rectum (hematochezia) with otherwise normal stools or spots of red blood on the toilet tissue or in the toilet imply bleeding from anal, rectal, or left-sided colonic lesions such as anal fissures, a juvenile polyp (Fig. 2), or a limited proctitis secondary to cow's milk–protein allergy or ulcerative proctitis. Allergic protocolitis usually affects infants fed formula based on cow's-milk protein in the first 3 months of life; aside from mucous and blood streaks in their stool, these infants are usually completely well. This disorder can also affect breast milk–fed infants, since small amounts of cow's-milk proteins are found in human breast milk if the mother is consuming them in her diet (4). Affected infants typically recover within 2 weeks if their feeding is changed to a protein-hydrolysate formula or the mother eliminates cow's milk from her diet (see Chap. 25).

In contrast, bright red blood mixed with mucus and loose stools suggests left-sided or diffuse colitis caused by infectious, pseudomembranous, or ulcer-ative colitis. Common pathogens causing infectious colitis in immunocompetent and immunocompromised children are listed in Table 5. Copious amounts of red blood or even darker clots mixed with stool (melena) are more characteristic of the bleeding from a colonic arteriovenous malformation or Meckel's diverticu-lum. "Currant-jelly stools" are potentially indicative of ischemic bowel lesions

TABLE 5 Causes of Infectious Colitis with Bleeding in Immunocompetent and Immunocompromised Children

Immunocompetent[a]	Immunocompromised
Salmonella	Cytomegalovirus
Campylobacter jejuni	Adenovirus
Shigella	Herpes simplex
Yersinia enterocolitica	Candida
Clostridium difficile	
E. coli 0157-H7	
Aeromonas hydrophilia	
Entamoeba histolytica	

[a] Can affect immunocompromised patients as well.

such as those seen with an intussusception. Bleeding duodenal lesions or even esophageal varices may present with melena if the bleeding is brisk enough, but they more often manifest themselves as either dark, tarry stools or hematemesis.

2.5 Use the Nasogastric Tube

One of the simplest ways to differentiate upper tract bleeding from lower tract bleeding is to pass a nasogastric tube and lavage with room-temperature saline. In the absence of frank hematemesis, it is often difficult to determine the location of the bleeding, especially if the presentation is with black tarry stools or melena. A positive nasogastric aspirate directs the search for a source of bleeding to the upper gastrointestinal tract. A negative aspirate does not completely rule out the possibility of duodenal bleeding or hemobilia (bleeding into the biliary tract) but suggests that the bleeding originates beyond the ligament of Treitz in the small intestine or the colon. Direct aspiration from a preexisting gastrostomy tube is not a reliable procedure because of the anterior location of this tube and the likely posterior location of the blood pooling in the gastric fundus.

The nasogastric tube can also act as a gauge of the severity of continued upper gastrointestinal bleeding. Gastric lavage with room-temperature saline should be continued until the return is clear. Most patients can be effectively lavaged with a nasogastric sump tube—12 Fr in small children and 14 to 16 Fr in older children. The recommended volume of each infusion depends on age: 30 to 50 mL for infants and 100 to 200 mL for older children. Room-temperature rather than iced saline should be used because the latter can contribute to hypothermia, especially in small infants, and can inhibit clotting capability (5).

2.6 Beware of Pseudobloods

Table 6 lists potential pitfalls in the diagnosis of gastrointestinal bleeding in children. Consideration of the possibility that the child does not have true gastrointestinal bleeding is particularly important when he or she looks well and the physical examination is normal. Factitious hematochezia (red or purple tinge to the stool) can be seen with certain artificial food colorings used in drinks, Jell-O, breakfast cereals, and syrups for liquid medications. Tomato skins, peach skins, and even beets can look like bits of blood in the stool in a child with diarrhea and a rapid transit time. Dark gray or black stools can be caused by the ingestion of iron preparations. Pepto-Bismol, purple grapes and grape juice, spinach, licorice, blueberries, and dirt. Blood exogenous to the gastrointestinal tract is a common cause of pseudogastrointestinal bleeding. Swallowed maternal blood in a breast-fed infant or nasopharyngeal blood in an infant or other child with epistaxis, a nasogastric tube, or a recent tonsillectomy or adenoidectomy may mimic true gastrointestinal hemorrhage. The Kleinhauer and Apt-Downey tests are used to differentiate maternal blood from infant blood in the stomach contents of breast-fed infants

TABLE 6 Potential Pitfalls in the Diagnosis of Gastrointestinal Bleeding in Children

Extraintestinal blood	Pseudobloods	Black stools	False positive	False negative
Maternal blood[a]	Red syrup (medications)	Iron	Red meat	Vitamin C
Epistaxis	Red dyes (foods)	Pepto-Bismol	Tomatoes	Old stool
Nasogastric tube trauma	Red Jell-O	Grape juice	Cherries	
Facial, oropharyngeal trauma	Fruit punch	Purple grapes	Turnips	
	Peach, tomato skins	Spinach		
	Beets	Chocolate		
		Blueberries		
		Licorice		
		Dirt		

[a] Swallowed at time of birth, or from cracked nipples in a breast-fed baby.

with presumed upper gastrointestinal tract bleeding by discriminating between fetal and maternal hemoglobin on the basis of resistance to changes in pH. In a form of Munchausen syndrome by proxy, the stool or emesis may be contaminated with blood other than the child's. A determination of the blood type or the finding of nucleated red blood cells in the bloody sample (usually not seen with human blood) can raise suspicion of this possibility.

Most commonly used tests to verify blood in the stool are based on leuko-dyes (guaiac, orthotolidine), which use the peroxidase-like reactivity found in hemoglobin to induce an oxidative reaction with the reagent; producing a blue color. Ingestion of red meats with animal blood (even when well cooked), and certain plants with peroxidase activity—such as horseradish, turnips, tomatoes, and fresh red cherries—will lead to false-positive test rsults. Consumption of vitamin C, even in the amounts found in standard multivitamin preparations, and storage of the specimen longer than 4 days may produce false-negative test results. More sensitive and specific tests of blood in the stool are available and are based on a fluorometric assay of porphyrin (HemoQuant) or on the use of antihemoglobin antibodies (6,7).

2.7 Assess for a Change in the Bowel Habit

Painless bleeding presenting with no change in bowel habit must be distinguished from that occurring in the setting of diarrhea, abdominal pain, tenesmus, or constipation. Hematochezia accompanying a history of hard, infrequent, or large stools passed with straining almost always signals the presence of an anal fissure or some other perianal or anal lesion. Red blood here is often found on the side of the stool or on the paper when the child wipes the anus. Children with perianal streptococcal infections may withhold stool and become constipated because of fear of painful bowel movements, which cause bleeding when passed. Perianal fissures and fistulas with secondary infection and abscess formation may be the most overt symptom of Crohn's disease or chronic granulomatous disease and can lead to stool withholding, hard stools, and minor loss of bright red blood per rectum. Chronic rectal prolapse secondary to straining from constipation or cystic fibrosis will occasionally be associated with some ischemia of the prolapsed rectal mucosa and hematochezia. Rarely, children with constipation and a history of fecal impaction may have a solitary rectal ulcer thought to be secondary to internal prolapse of the posterior rectal wall mucosa (8).

Blood and mucus mixed with diarrheal stool usually signals a more diffuse mucosal colonic inflammatory lesion, including infectious colitis, ulcerative colitis, or Crohn's disease involving the colon. Occasionally, ulcerative colitis limited to the rectum (ulcerative proctitis) can present without diarrhea or even with constipation because of the limited mucosal involvement and the pain urgency experienced with defecation, leading to stool withholding. However, most children with ulcerative colitis have more extensive involvement of their colon at first presentation and present with crampy abdominal pain, tenesmus, diarrhea, and then progressively mucous, bloody stools. Most children and adolescents with infection caused by *E. coli* 0157-H7 will have a 5 to 7 day prodrome of bloody diarrhea secondary to an intestinal vasculitis before they show any signs of oliguria, hematuria, hypertension, hyperkalemia, and renal failure (9).

Although brisk bleeding into the intestinal lumen acts as a cathartic, the bleeding secondary to esophageal varices, Meckel's diverticulum, or arteriovenous malformations is not usually preceded by diarrhea and is most often painless and sudden, with no previous change in the bowel habit. Another common cause of painless rectal bleeding with no history of diarrhea or constipation is juvenile polyps. These inflammatory pedunculated polyps (Fig. 2) are usually found on the left side of the colon, are often solitary, and rarely have adenomatous changes. In contrast to the major bleeding and hemodynamic compromise often seen in children with Meckel's diverticulum and arteriovenous malformations, most children with juvenile polyps have frequent episodes of minor loss of bright red blood per rectum with no change in vital signs and no anemia.

2.8   Examine for Signs of Obstruction or Perforation

Blood in the emesis or stool is always frightening to the child and parents; however, its presence most often does not signal a life-threatening or serious problem. A careful abdominal and rectal examination can help separate those few patients with signs of a surgical abdomen, suggesting a perforated viscus or bowel obstruction, accompanying the gastrointestinal bleeding. Bloody emesis or stool in the setting of a distended abdomen may indicate a perforated ulcer, midgut volvulus (secondary to malrotation), or a perforated viscus secondary to Crohn's disease in an older child or necrotizing enterocolitis (NEC) in an infant. Although intestinal involvement in NEC may be extensive, it is most often found in the ileum and right colon. Rarely, infants with pyloric stenosis can develop prepyloric stasis ulcers and present with hematemesis.

Bloody diarrhea in an infant with a distended abdomen should raise questions of Hirschsprung's disease with enterocolitis. Diffuse inflammatory colitis resulting in transmural inflammation, ischemia, ileus, or even perforation can be seen in older children with the bowel vasculitis of Henoch-Schönlein purpura, severe pseudomembranous colitis, or even ulcerative colitis with toxic megacolon. In the last case, the patient with ulcerative colitis will suddenly convert from having multiple bloody, mucousy stools to having few or no stools. Increased abdominal distention, decreased bowel sounds, and increasing diffuse abdominal pain and peritoneal signs signal the onset of gross colonic dilatation. Relatively minor bleeding into the lumen may be accompanied by massive bleeding into the bowel wall in children with Henoch-Schönlein purpura and in those suffering blunt abdominal trauma. The resulting bowel wall hematoma causes intense abdominal pain and, if large enough, relative intestinal obstruction. Because the third portion of the duodenum crosses the spine and can be pinned against the bony prominence, this is a common place for hematomas caused by blunt abdominal trauma. Abdominal trauma may also fracture intrahepatic blood vessels or damage the gallbladder, leading to bleeding into the intrahepatic and extrahepatic bile ducts. Some blood may flow into the small intestine, but a much larger amount may collect in the gallbladder, giving rise to a condition known as *hemobilia* (10). When the relatively small amount of blood in the emesis or stool does not correlate with the drop in hematocrit and the degree of hemodynamic compromise, a search for hidden reservoirs of gastrointestinal blood loss—such as bowel wall hematomas, hemobilia, or blood filled congenital gastric or duodenal duplication cysts—should be undertaken.

If there are signs of bowel obstruction and a palpable abdominal sausage-shaped mass, intussusception is the likely cause of hematochezia. Although obstruction, a sausage-shaped mass, and currant-jelly stools are classic presenting symptoms of intussusception, these findings are often missing. In the most recent large series, only 21% of 583 patients presented with the classic triad of colicky abdominal pain, vomiting, and the passage of bloody, mucous stool (11). Blood in the stool was present in only 37% of patients and only 15% of patients had detectable bleeding if symptoms of colicky abdominal pain were present for less than 12 hr. Infants and toddlers with an intussusception may be well, then briefly irritable or inconsolable, and then lapse into a stuporous state before passing a bloody stool. Most cases occur between 2 months and 2 years of age, although intussusception does occur in older children, where it is associated with a ''lead point'' and can present recurrently. Such precipitating lesions include Meckel's diverticulum, duplication cysts, polyps, hemangiomas, or neoplasms, particularly lymphomas. Intussusception is a recognized complication of Henoch-Schönlein purpura, cystic fibrosis, and Peutz-Jeghers syndrome.

2.9 Always Examine the Anus and Rectum

Failure to examine the anal area and the rectum will result in missing obvious causes of lower gastrointestinal bleeding and the administration of unnecessary tests. Disorders in this area usually result in the passage of bright red blood on the side of the stool or on the toilet paper or the toilet water may be stained red (hematochezia). Anal fissures are common in infants and children and are most often secondary to trauma from the passage of hard, large stools. Such fissures are superficial, often painful, and usually located in the midline (12 and 6 o'clock). In contrast, fissures due to Crohn's disease are often deeper, eccentric to the midline, most often painless, and accompanied by skin tags and fistulous tracts. Other causes of perianal disease—including fissures, fistulas, and abscesses—are chronic granulomatous disease and immunodeficiency syndromes. Hemorrhoids are unusual in young children and may signal the presence of portal hypertension. Rectal prolapse can be associated with mucosal injury and hematochezia; occasionally, a rectal polyp on a long stalk may protrude through the anus, mimicking a rectal prolapse. Most solitary juvenile inflammatory polyps are located in the left colon, and some can be palpated in the rectal canal with a careful digital rectal examination.

2.10 Avoid Using Barium X-rays in Favor of Direct Endoscopic Examination

In the era of pediatric endoscopy, there is little indication for the use of barium x-rays in the evaluation of gastrointestinal bleeding in children, especially after plain films of the abdomen have excluded bowel obstruction or perforation. Previous studies comparing barium radiography and upper endoscopy in infants and children have shown that the bleeding site is identified in only 18% of cases with barium examination but in 90 to 100% of cases with endoscopy in children with esophagitis and gastritis, and in 55 and 94% of cases, respectively, in children with ulcers (12). Similarly, a barium enema has no role in the initial evaluation of a patient with hematochezia or melena and only delays diagnosis by preventing the collection of adequate stool specimens for culture and delaying colonoscopic mucosal examination. The exception to this rule is a case in which intussusception is likely, and in this setting many radiologists favor the use of air rather than barium enemas to diagnose and reduce intussusception.

3 HISTORY AND PHYSICAL EXAMINATION

From the previous discussion, it is clear that a careful history and physical examination will narrow the diagnostic possibilities and suggest a diagnosis. In addition to the considerations outlined above, the physician should consider the family history, past and present medical history, medication history, and accompanying mucocutaneous and other physical findings in the evaluation of the cause of gastrointestinal bleeding.

3.1 Family and Past Medical History

A family history of peptic ulcer disease and/or *Helicobacter pylori* infection should be sought. *H. pylori* is associated with more than 90% of cases of recurrent duodenal ulcer and primary gastritis. *H. pylori*–associated ulcers are relatively uncommon in children as compared with adults. More commonly, children present with nodular antral gastritis as a mucosal manifestation of *H. pylori* infection

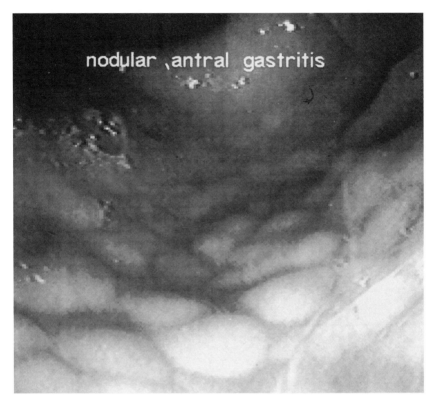

FIGURE 3 Submucosal nodules characteristic of nodular antral gastritis secondary to *H. pylori* in a 15-year-old with hematemesis.

(13) (Fig. 3). These "nodules" are characterized histologically by prominent lymphoid aggregates. Epidemiological evidence points to human to human spread of *H. pylori* in family units (14). Chronic upper gastrointestinal bleeding leading to guaiac-positive stools and profound iron deficiency anemia in patients with vague epigastric pain and minimal gastrointestinal symptoms has been reported in children with antral gastritis secondary to *H. pylori* (15). Rarely, adolescents with *H. pylori* present with hematemesis and acute serious upper gastrointestinal bleeding as a result of erosive gastritis and gastric ulcer.

A family history of inflammatory bowel disease (Crohn's disease and ulcerative colitis) in a parent or other first-degree relative considerably raises the risk in the related child. Some polyposis syndromes, such as familial adenomatous polyposis, are transmitted via autosomal dominant inheritance; a family history of polyposis, lower gastrointestinal bleeding, and early colon cancer is almost always apparent.

The past and proximate medical history may also offer important clues to the etiology of the bleeding. Certain underlying congenital malformations and systemic diseases are associated with conditions that give rise to gastrointestinal bleeding. Children with mental/motor retardation and cerebral palsy are commonly affected by severe chronic gastroesophageal reflux and chronic constipation. Since these patients are unable to give a history, symptoms of dyspepsia, heartburn, abdominal pain, and rectal pain may not be recognized prior to the onset of esophageal or anorectal bleeding. A malfunctioning ventriculoperitoneal shunt with chronically increased intracranial pressure and the subsequent development of peptic ulcer disease is a rare cause of hemorrhage in this population. Other underlying diseases associated with chronic gastroesophageal reflux include cystic, fibrosis, Down's syndrome, previous repair of esophageal atresia, progressive systemic sclerosis, and familial dysautonomia.

A history of recurrent infections, thrush, and chronic diarrhea suggests the possibility of an immunodeficiency state. *Candida albicans*, herpes simplex, and cytomegalovirus can infect the esophagus in children with acquired and congenital immunodeficiency states and cause ulceration and mucosal blood loss, usually presenting with symptoms of dysphagia, odynophagia, chest pain, and occasionally fever and vomiting. Both common variable immunodeficiency and selective IgA deficiency are associated with lymphonodular hyperplasia, which is a cause of painless lower intestinal bleeding in young children usually under the age of 4 years (16). The mechanism of bleeding is thought to be thinning of the surface epithelium over the enlarged hyperplastic submucosal lymphatic tissue, with eventual ulceration and bleeding (Fig. 4). Nodules of lymphoid tissue are found throughout the gastrointestianl tract, but they are most prominent in the rectum and sigmoid colon in children with hematochezia.

A history of travel to areas endemic for traveler's diarrhea and parasitic infestation in a patient with bloody diarrhea or even melena should prompt stool and serum investigations for enteroinvasive *E. coli*, amebiasis, ascariasis, strongyloidiasis, and hookworm. Pathogens that cause watery diarrhea such as *Giardia* and *Cryptosporidium* do not cause colitis or invasive enteritis and are not associated with gastrointestinal blood loss. In patients with bloody diarrhea, a dietary history may reveal recent exposure to potentially contaminated foods such as chicken, unpasturized milk, and undercooked hamburger, implicated in outbreaks of *Salmonella, Yersinia enterocolitica*, and hemolytic uremic syndrome secondary to *E. coli* 0157-H7 (17). Children in the pediatric intensive care unit, particularly those with increased intracranial pressure (brain tumor, hydrocephalus, encephalitis, trauma), acute renal failure, fulminant hepatic failure, sepsis, coagulopathy, severe burns, and severe congenital heart disease are particularly at risk for severe gastrointestinal bleeding.

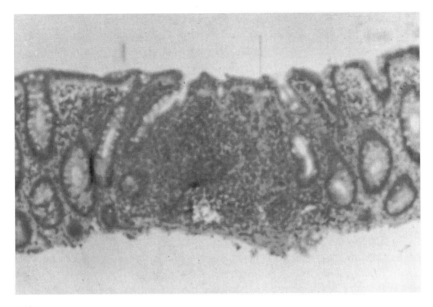

FIGURE 4   Biopsy of the left colon in a 3-year-old with mucous, blood-streaked stool and lymphonodular hyperplasia. Submucosal lymphoid nodule is erupting through the mucosal epithelium.

3.2   Medication History

Multiple medications are associated with esophageal, gastric, and even intestinal inflammation and ulceration. In the neonatal intensive care nursery, indomethacin to close a patent ductus arteriosus, tolazoline to reduce pulmonary vascular hypertension, and dexamethasone to stimulate lung maturity have all been associated with severe upper gastrointestinal hemorrhage from hemorrhagic gastritis or gastric ulcer. Chronic ingestion of aspirin or other NSAIDs (ibuprofen, naproxen, ketoralac) in patients with collagen vascular disease, juvenile rheumatoid arthritis, or other conditions can incite bleeding in the upper gastrointestinal tract. Children with severe asthma treated with theophylline and prednisone have an increased risk of gastritis and gastric ulcer (18). Adolescents taking tetracycline antibiotics for acne and other conditions have developed esophageal ulcers and bleeding (19). Children receiving anticonvulsant therapy with phenobarbital and phenytoin may develop gastrointestinal hemorrhage secondary to a profound coagulopathy correctable with vitamin K administration. However, gastrointestinal bleeding is an uncommon manifestation of coagulopathy unless there is also a mucosal lesion (e.g., esophagitis, gastritis, ulcer). Many chemotherapeutic agents—including methotrexate, doxorubicin, cytosine arabinoside, actinomycin

D, 5-fluorouracil, and bleomycin—cause a form of mucosal injury known as mucositis. Radiation potentiates this injury, which causes diffuse mucosal ulceration of the oropharynx, esophagitis, stomach, and, to a lesser extent, small and large intestine.

Clostridium difficile toxin–induced colitis is suspected if the patient has been exposed to antibiotics within 1 month of presentation. Almost every antibiotic has been implicated as a potential inciting agent. *C. difficile* may also be epidemic in neonatal intensive care nurseries and even in day care centers where only an index case may have been exposed to antibiotics, with other cases being colonized and infected to human-to-human spread (20).

3.3 Mucocutaneous and Other Associated Physical Findings

Table 7 lists systemic diseases and syndromes associated with significant gastrointestinal bleeding along with cutaneous and other physical stigmata, which are clues to the diagnosis. Vascular malformations of the intestinal tract, although rare, are an important cause of blood loss in neonates and young children. In about half the cases, cutaneous hemangiomas suggest the presence of gastrointestinal mucosal hemangiomas (Fig. 5). Cutaneous hemangiomas with hemihypertrophy suggest the inherited condition Klippel-Trenaunay syndrome (21). Bluish, soft, compressible skin nodules—especially noticeable on the soles of the feet and the palms of the hands—are pathognomonic of blue-rubber-bleb nevus syndromes, where dozens of similar submucosal or even transmural venous malformations stud the stomach, small intestine, and colon (22) (Fig. 6). Cutaneous telangiectasis and recurrent epistaxis are found in hereditary hemorrhagic telangiectasia (Osler-Weber-Rendu syndrome), where gastrointestinal bleeding may be the presenting symptom in the second decade of life (23). Girls with Turner's syndrome, with webbed necks and short stature, can suffer profound gastrointestinal blood loss from venous malformations or diffuse hemangiomas (24). Children with congenital aortic valve disorders may have secondary vascular ectatic lesions (angiodysplasia) throughout the gastrointestinal tract.

Most gastrointestinal polyps in children are benign juvenile inflammatory polyps that present with painless hematochezia and are not associated with other physical stigmata. However, multiple polyposis syndromes do present in childhood with acute and chronic bleeding, including familial adenomatous polyposis and familial juvenile polyposis coli. Other colonic (and intestinal or gastric) polyposis syndromes in childhood are often recognizable by distinctive physical findings. Pigmentation of the lips, buccal mucosa, face, and palmar and plantar surfaces suggests the diagnosis of Peutz-Jegher syndrome. Gardner's syndrome, caused by the same genetic mutation responsible for familial adenomatous polyp-

TABLE 7 Systemic Diseases and
Syndromes Associated with
Gastrointestinal Bleeding

Multiple telangiectasias
  Hereditary hemorrhagic telangiectasia
  Aortic valve disorders
Venous malformations
  Turner's syndrome
  Blue-rubber-bleb nevus syndrome
Hemangiomas
  Klippel-Trenaunay syndrome
  Diffuse neonatal hemangiomas
Fragile vascular walls
  Ehlers-Danlos syndrome
  Pseudoxanthoma elasticum
Inflammatory bowel disease
  Glycogen storage disease 1B
  Behcet's disease
  Hermansky-Pudlak syndrome
Lymphonodular hyperplasia
  IgA deficiency
  Common variable immunodeficiency
Polyposis
  Familial adenomatous polyposis
  Garner's syndrome
  Juvenile polyposis coli
  Peutz-Jegher syndrome
  Cronkhite-Canada syndrome
  Turcot's syndrome
Ulcers
  Systemic mastrocytosis
  Zollinger-Ellison syndrome

---

osis, is characterized by retinal lesions and epidermoid cysts, fibromas, and osteomas of the skull, mandible, and other bones (25). Other polyposis syndromes include Cronkhite-Canada syndrome, associated with alopecia, onychodystrophy, and hyperpigmentation; and Turcot's syndrome, associated with café au lait spots and brain tumors. Benign leiomyomas and even malignant leiomyosarcomas are an unusual but well-recognized cause of severe colonic and gastroduodenal bleeding in children.

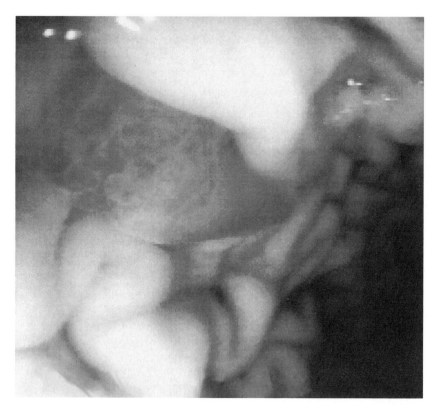

FIGURE 5 Gastric hemangioma in a 6-year-old with multiple skin hemangiomas and chronic iron-deficiency anemia.

Disorders associated with white cell defects and cyclic neutropenia can give rise to lesions mimicking those of Crohn's disease and result in gastrointestinal bleeding. These include glycogen storage disease type 1b, with visceromegaly and hypoglycemia, and Hermansky-Pudlak syndrome, associated with albinism (26,27). Perirectal lesions, antropyloric granulomatous inflammation, and ileocolonic lesions mimicking Crohn's disease can also be part of the spectrum of chronic granulomatous disease. Connective tissue disorders, especially Ehlers-Danlos syndrome type IV (ecchymotic) and pseudoxanthoma elasticum, are associated with intestinal bleeding as a consequence of fragile vascular epithelium (28). Both spontaneous colonic perforation and hemorrhage have been reported in Ehlers-Danlos syndrome. Blood in the stool in patients with epidermolysis bullosa can result from esophageal and rectal strictures, anal fissures, and friable perianal skin (29). Endoscopy is relatively contraindicated in these diseases,

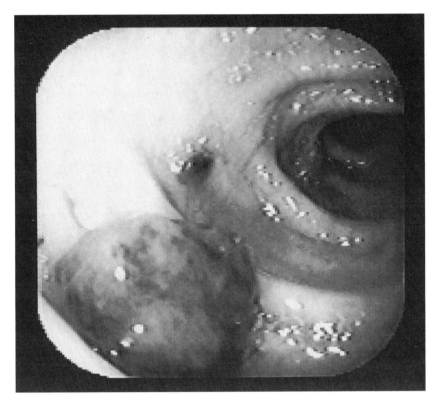

FIGURE 6 Right colonic vascular malformations in a 10-year-old with blue-rubber-bleb nevus syndrome with black tarry stool.

where these procedures may damage and tear fragile bullae and mucosal vessels and lead to increased bleeding.

The finding of splenomegaly or hepatosplenomegaly points to portal hypertension and varices secondary to cirrhosis or portal vein thrombosis as the cause of gastrointestinal hemorrhage (Fig. 7). Other stigmata of chronic liver disease—such as jaundice, clubbing, spider angiomas, caput medusae, and ascites—support the suspicion that varices or portal gastrophy are the cause of bleeding. However, their absence does not preclude the presence of cirrhosis or portal hypertension. With massive bleeding, the congested spleen may shrink dramatically, only to reappear after resuscitation with fluid and blood products. Hemorrhoids and occasionally rectal varicosities may occur in some children with portal hypertension and cause significant bleeding.

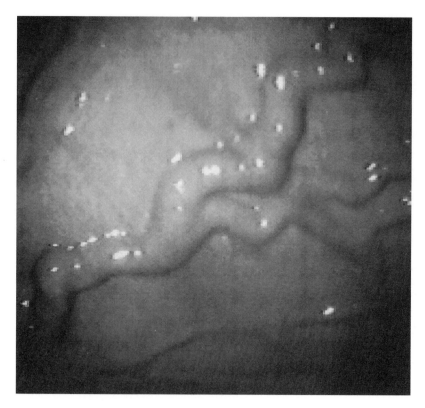

FIGURE 7 Gastric varices in an adolescent with cavernous transformation of the portal vein and portal hypertension.

4 LABORATORY EXAMINATION

Several basic laboratory tests are useful adjuncts to diagnose the source of gastrointestinal (GI) bleeding. The complete blood count (CBC) is probably the most useful, not only to assess the severity of the bleeding by measurement of the hemoglobin and hematocrit but also to help distinguish those lesions that cause acute bleeding from those giving rise to chronic blood loss. Evidence of iron deficiency anemia (hypochromic, microcytie–appearing red blood cells and a low mean corpuscular volume (MCV)) suggests chronic blood loss; which in a patient with melena would favor a duodenal ulcer over esophageal varices or a Meckel's diverticulum as the cause of the bleeding. In a patient with bloody diarrhea, evidence of iron deficiency would suggest a chronic inflammatory bowel disease (Crohn's disease or ulcerative colitis) rather than an acute infectious colitis or vasculitis. A low white blood cell (WBC) count and platelet count would be expected in a patient with portal hypertension, esophageal varices, an enlarged spleen, and hypersplenism. This constellation of findings is sometimes seen in children with chronic liver disease progressing to cirrhosis, including those with biliary atresia, cystic fibrosis, alpha-1-antitrypsin deficiency, parenteral nutrition–induced cholestatic liver disease, autoimmune chronic active hepatitis, and Wilson's disease. Portal hypertension in children can also be the rsult of portal venous obstruction (cavernous transformation of a portal vein) and hepatic venous obstruction (Budd-Chiari syndrome). In these patients, an evaluation for leukemia or other malignancy may delay the ivestigation for severe underlying chronic liver disease and other caues of portal hypertension.

Most infectious colitides and ulcerative colitis result in thrombocytosis as part of the acute-phase response to infection and inflammation. However, thrombocytopenia in the setting of bloody diarrhea should prompt consideration of hemolytic uremic syndrome, where the consumption of platelets and the appearance of schistocytes and fragments of red blood cells seen on the blood smear may be one of the earliest signs of vasculitis and intravascular hemolysis. In the infant or child with hematochezia, the presence of peripheral eosinophilia in the WBC differential suggests the possibility of eosinophilic colitis secondary to food protein allergy (most often due to cow's-milk protein). Stool Gram's stains with multiple polymorphonuclear leukocytes suggest infectious or inflammatory colitis, whereas the presence of eosinophils or Charcot-Leyden granules in the stool supports the diagnosis of eosinophilic (allergic) colitis.

An elevated blood urea nitrogen (BUN) commonly accompanies severe gastrointestinal bleeding due to bacterial metabolism of blood proteins to ammonia and conversion to urea. Hypovolemia and secondary renal hypoperfusion can also contribute to azotemia. An elevated blood BUN/creatine ratio has been used to segregate upper from lower GI bleeding in children without renal disease. In one study, all BUN/creatinine ratios greater than 30 corresponded to patients with documented upper GI bleeding sources (30). However, the majority of children with upper GI bleeding in this study had ratios less than 30, as did all children with lower GI bleeding. A low serum total protein and albumin suggest a chronic inflammatory small bowel or colonic lesion resulting in protein-losing enteropathy, such as Crohn's disease or even ulcerative colitis. Elevated aminotransferases, bilirubin, and alkaline phosphatase or gamma glutamyl transpeptidase should raise questions not only about the possibility of intrinsic liver disease but also about hemobilia secondary to trauma, a tumor (rhabdomyosarcoma), or a vascular malformation.

5 INDICATIONS AND SEQUENCE FOR DIAGNOSTIC TESTS

The guidelines discussed above should enable the physician to narrow the elevation to a few suspected entities causing bleeding in the upper or lower GI tract.

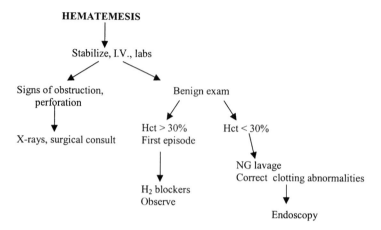

FIGURE 8 Algorithm for the approach to the child with hematemesis.

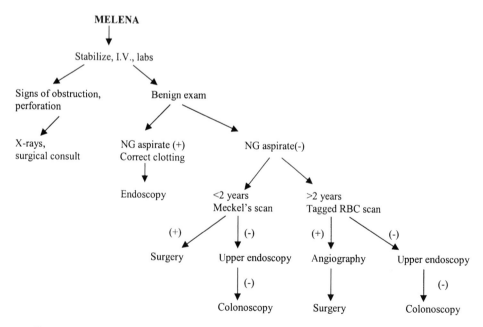

FIGURE 9 Algorithm for the approach to the child with melena.

The algorithms shown in Figures 8 and 9 suggest a sequence of diagnostic tests for the evaluation of hematemesis and melene. Use of these algorithms will be influenced and modified by the patient's age, signs of hypoperfusion or shock, physical findings suggesting obstruction or perforation, and a history of changes in the bowel habit.

5.1 Diagnostic Upper Gastrointestinal Endoscopy

GI-endoscopy has become the mainstay of the evaluation of both the infant and child with upper-GI bleeding (see Chap. 32). For the patient with hematemesis or melena and a positive nasogastric lavage, upper endoscopy is the procedure of choice. In any neonate or child with abdominal distention, abdominal pain, or peritoneal signs, a flat-plate and upright or left lateral decubitus film of the abdomen should be done first to exclude bowel obstruction, free intra-abdominal air, or pneumatosis intestinalis. In spite of the diagnostic accuracy of upper-GI endoscopy, not every child with upper tract bleeding must undergo this procedure. For the child whose history is compatible with acute self-limited bleeding (viral gastritis, drug-induced gastritis), who is hemodynamically stable, and who has a hematocrit of greater than 30%, conservative therapy with fluids, antacids, and H_2-receptor antagonists is appropriate. If the bleeding persists, there are recurrent episodes of upper tract bleeding, or the first acute episode results in hemodynamic instability and significant anemia, upper-GI endoscopy should be performed as soon as possible after stabilization and resuscitation.

5.2 Adjunctive Medical Therapy for Serious Upper-Tract Hemorrhage

It is always preferable to defer upper-GI endoscopy until after the bleeding has stopped, the patient has received fluid and blood-product resuscitation, and the stomach has been lavaged. This will maximize the safety and efficacy of both diagnostic and therapeutic endoscopy. Occasionally, bleeding is torrential, and aggressive diagnostic and therapeutic measures must proceed in an unstable patient. Medical therapy for significant upper-tract bleeding can help control the hemorrhage and stabilize the patient for endoscopy. Table 8 summarizes available nonendoscopic methods for the control of upper-GI bleeding. Octreotide, a synthetic somatostatin analogue, has all but replaced vasopressin as adjunctive medical therapy to control variceal bleeding in children (31). In any child with the possibility of significant bleeding from esophageal or gastric varices, a bolus of 1 μg/kg (up to a maximum of 100 μg) of intravenous octreotide should be given, followed immediately by a continuous infusion of octreotide starting at a rate of 1 μg/kg/hr. This can be increased by 1 μg/kg/hr every 6 hr up to 4 μg/kg/hr. Intravenous octreotide has also been used successfully to slow bleeding from nonvariceal unidentified sources in the small intestine and from diffuse small

TABLE 8 Pharmacologic Therapy for Acute Gastrointestinal Bleeding

Therapy	Dose
Vasoconstriction	
Octreotide (somatostatin analog)	(IV) 1 μg/kg bolus (max 100 μg), followed by 1 μg/kg/hr continuous
Vasopressin	(IV) 0.1 U/min/1.73 m² continuous (increase up to 0.4 U/min/1.73 m²)
Acid blockade	
Ranitide	(IV) 4 mg/kg/day continuous or divided q 6 h
Famotidine	(IV) 0.4–0.8 mg/kg/dose q 8 h
Omeprazole	(PO) 1–2 mg/kg/day divided q 12 h (maximum 40 mg q 12 h)
Cytoprotection	
Sucralfate	(PO) 100 mg/kg/day divided q 6 h (max 1 g q 6 h)
Misoprostol (prostaglandin analog)	(PO) 100–200 μg/dose tid (adult dose)

intestinal lesions secondary to severe graft-versus-host disease in recipients of bone marrow transplants. Rarely, it will be necessary to treat with intravenous vasopressin. Current recommendations are to begin infusing the drug at a rate of 0.1 U/min/1.73 m² and increase the dose by 0.05 U/min hourly up to a maximum of 0.4 U/min/1.73 m². In children less than 5 years of age, we do not ordinarily exceed 0.2 U/min. Children seem more resistant than adults to the major complications of myocardial ischemia, arrhythmias, hypertension, and peripheral ischemia, and they usually tolerate the invariable hyponatremia and fluid retention well.

When a child is actively bleeding from esophageal or gastric varices, a Mallory-Weiss tear, Dieulaboy's lesion, or some other esophageal or gastric fundal lesion, it may be necessary to stop the bleeding with tamponade in order to buy time for stabilization, pharmacological intervention, and preparation for therapeutic endoscopy or surgery. Temporary control of bleeding can be obtained with a Sengstaken-Blakemore, Linton, or Minnesota tube. After sedating and intubating the patient, this tube is usually passed via the oral route because of its size. The gastric balloon is inflated to a volume between 60 and 200 mL and pulled up toward the gastroesophageal junction, effectively tamponading the bleeding site. Traction is maintained on the tube and a second nasoesophageal tube is passed in order to aspirate accumulating saliva and blood from any ongoing esophageal hemorrhage. If esophageal bleeding continues in spite of traction on the gastric balloon, the esophageal balloon is inflated to a maximum of 40 mmHg. The length of the esophageal balloon may be excessive and occlude the pharynx in infants and small children. We have successfully used a radial balloon catheter (15 to 18 mm in diameter, 3 to 8 cm in length) to tamponade esophageal bleeding from varices or esophageal ulcers in infants.

H_2-receptor antagonists do not appear to affect fatality rates, rebleeding, or the need for surgery in adults with acute hemorrhage from a peptic ulcer. However, there are now several recent studies supporting the use of H_2-receptor antagonists to prevent bleeding in children in the intensive care unit who are at increased risk of gastrointestinal bleeding (32–34). The proper intravenous doses of cimetidine, ranitidine, and famotidine in critically ill children are summarized in Table 8. Two cytoprotective agents, sucralfate and misoprostol, can be used to treat indolent upper-GI bleeding from gastric erosions and hemorrhagic gastritis. Misoprostol, a prostaglandin analogue, is used primarily to counteract the ulcerogenic effects of NSAIDs in children with juvenile rheumatoid arthritis and other rheumatic diseases. Sucralfate is composed of sucrose and aluminum sulfate salts and binds to denuded gastric mucosal surfaces, protecting them from continued injury by pepsin, bile salts, and other mucosal irritants (35). Problems associated with chronic use of sucralfate include aluminum toxicity in patients undergoing dialysis, binding of other orally administered drugs, and the potential to form bezoars in the stomach.

5.3 Therapeutic Upper-Tract Endoscopy

There are a number of effective techniques available to pediatric endoscopists to stop significant upper-GI bleeding. Different techniques are more suitable for specific lesions. Nonvariceal gastric erosions and ulcers can often be controlled with circumferential injections of 0.25 to 0.5 mL of 1:10,000 epinephrine via a sclerotherapy needle introduced down the biopsy channel of the endoscope. Once the bleeding has slowed, epinephrine directed into a bleeding vessel can be injected, or a thermocoagulation device can be aplied to the bleeding site. Both the bipolar electrocoagulation device (BICAP) and the heater probe rely on the generation of heat to coagulate the surrounding tissue. These devices will only fit through the biopsy channel of a larger endoscope (at least 9.8 mm in external diameter). Tamponade is achieved with firm diet pressure directly on the vessel, and then two to four pulses of 30 J are delivered to coagulate the lesion. The argon plasma coagulator (APC) relies on the delivery of energy by an ionized stream of argon gas delivered via a catheter inserted through the scope (36). The advantage of this method is that it does not require direct contact with the bleeding site; it does not require direct en face application of the probe to the lesion; and the depth of burn (dessication) is at most 3 mm into the tissue. This device is best suited for diffuse superficial lesions such as multiple hemangiomas, erosions, or telangiectasis (Fig. 10).

The injection of sclerosing agents directly into esophageal varices via a catheter inserted into the biopsy channel of the upper endoscope has proven successful in children, with obliteration of esophageal varices being achieved in 75 to 92% of pediatric patients after multiple sessions (37). The techniques of sclerotherapy used in children are similar to those employed in adults, with some differences in the size of the sclerotherapy needles and the volume of injection. Most often, a 25-gauge sclerotherapy needle is used, and no more than 2.0 mL of sclerosant per injection. The maximum cumulative dose of the sclerosing agent is 0.8 mL/kg body weight per session, not to exceed 20 mL. Sclerosants favored are similar to those used in adults, with the majority of series in children reporting

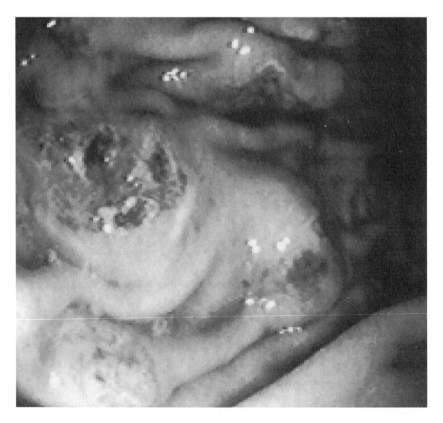

FIGURE 10 Gastric hemangiomas after treatment with the argon plasma coagulator (APC).

the use of sodium tetradecyl sulfate or sodium morrhuate. The most common significant complications of injection sclerotherapy are esophageal ulceration and stricture, which occur in approximately 25 and 15%, respectively, of all children treated. Endoscopic variceal ligation (banding) has been successfully carried out in children and is rapidly replacing injection sclerotherapy because of the reduced potential for stricture formation (38). Because of the increased external diameter of the endoscope when it is fitted with the band-applicator tip, this procedure almost always requires endotracheal intubation to protect the integrity of the airway, and also general anesthesia. The development of multiple ligation devices has allowed the application of up to six bands per session without having to remove and reload the device.

5.4 Diagnostic Colonoscopy and Enteroscopy

Colonoscopy is the first procedure to consider in children with bright red blood per rectum. It is also indicated in children with melena after an upper tract lesion has been ruled out by a negative nasogastric asirate and/or upper endoscopy. Contraindications to colonoscopy include 1) the presence of fulminant colitis or toxic megacolon; 2) signs of perforation or peritonitis; 3) pneumatosis intestinalis on an abdominal radiograph; and 4) signs suggesting intussusception. Relative contraindications include bleeding disorders or impaired platelet function, recent bowel surgery, profound neutropenia, and signs of partial or complete bowel obstruction. Colonoscopy is not necessary for many children with the acute onset of bloody diarrhea, in whom infections, including pseudomembranous colitis induced by *C. difficile* toxin, should first be ruled out with the appropriate stool specimens and cultures. The presence of an anal fissure or other anal lesion to account for hematochezia should also preclude colonoscopy unless the location and characteristics of the anal fissures suggest perianal Crohn's disease (39). The presence of the classic rash of Henoch-Schönlein purpura or the characteristic hematological and urinary sediment findings of hemolytic uremic syndrome would obviate the need for colonoscopy to diagnose bowel vasculitis. A limited proctosigmoidoscopy may be all that is needed to make a diagnosis of ulcerative colitis or pseudomembranous colitis in a very sick patient. Often, this limited procedure can be accomplished without sedation or with minimal intravenous conscious sedation. This is an advantage for patients with fulminant colitis in whom narcotic sedation may precipitate a profound ileus and/or toxic megacolon.

A mistake that is often made is to decrease the bowel preparation regimen or avoid it for a child with significant lower-GI bleeding. Although blood can act as a cathartic and precipitate diarrhea in children, omission of a bowel preparation before colonoscopy will often obscure the localization of the bleeding site. In the interest of shortening the time before colonoscopy in a bleeding child and with the protection of intravenous fluid administration, nasogastric and orally administered polyethylene glycol solutions are often the best method of obtaining adequate bowel preparation. This method also avoids the potential for severe hyperphosphatemia or hypermagnesemia when phosphate enemas or oral phosphate and magnesium solutions are administered to children with diffusely inflamed colons and small intestines. Approximately 80 mL/kg of the polyethylene glycol solutions are usually needed, up to a maximum of 4 L. These are administered at a rate of approximately 10 mL/min for younger children and 20 to 25 mL/min for older children (40).

The recent introduction of long enteroscopes has allowed endoscopic investigation of the small bowel to localize sites of occult bleeding between the ligament of Treitz and the ileocecal valve. With the exception of bleeding from a Meckel's diverticulum, bleeding caused by focal small bowel lesions is rare in children. Isolated penetrating ileal ulcers and ileal ulcers in conjunction with Chrohn's disease have been reported to cause significant bleeding in children. Vascular malformations can affect the small intestine as part of a number of the syndromes listed in Table 7. Graft-versus-host disease may severely affect the small bowel, with a relative sparing of the colon and stomach; rejection after small intestinal transplantation may be relatively focal, sparing the duodenum and proximal jejunum and more severely affecting the distal jejunum and ileum.

5.5 Therapeutic Colonoscopy

Colonoscopy can be used to control lower-GI bleeding from polyps, hemangiomas and other vascular malformations, and large ulcers secondary to inflammatory or infectious causes. Juvenile polyps are a major cause of hematochezia in children between the ages of 2 and 12 years, with a peak incidence between 4 and 7 years of age (41). Most patients present with streaks of red blood without diarrhea or pain and a few with prolapse of the polyp through the anus. Approximately 75% of the polyps are in the rectum and sigmoid colon; however, polyps can appear anywhere in the colon. They range in size from 0.1 to 3.0 cm and are usually pedunculated on a moderate to long stalk (Fig. 2). The surface is often hemorrhagic. Some children present with passage of a moderate amount of blood and clots after autoamputation of the polyp, leaving a bleeding stalk. Most children have more than one polyp at the time of presentation, with some having more than 10. Most polyps in children as so-called juvenile retention polyps composed primarily of fibrous stroma permeated by acute and chronic inflammatory cells with cystically dilated glands scattered throughout the stroma. These polyps rarely have adenomatous changes, but recent series stress the need for careful pathological examination of juvenile polyps because of an increased incidence of potential malignant change in children with multiple polyps and polyps on the right side of the colon (42).

Polypectomy using a diathermy snare inserted via the colonoscope is safe and effective in children. General anesthesia is required only in very young children or those patients with widespread polyps requiring multiple polypectomies and a prolonged procedure. In contrast to older reports, a recent series of colonoscopic polypectomies in children reported no major complications of perforation, sepsis, or significant hemorrhage (43). Occasionally, delayed bleeding from a residual stalk will occur and can be treated successfully with epinephrine or use of the argon plasma coagulator. The colon, especially the right side, is thinner-walled and the energy delivered by any thermal or laser device must be reduced in order to avoid perforation. Approximately 20% of children undergoing polypectomy will have later bleeding from recurrent juvenile polyps.

5.6 Nuclear Medicine and Interventional Vascular Radiological Techniques

Abdominal scintigraphy with technetium 99m pertechnetate, which rapidly binds to the gastric mucosa, has been most useful in making the diagnosis of Meckel's diverticulum in children. Because the vast majority of Meckel's diverticula that cause bleeding contain ectopic gastric mucosa, this test has an 85 to 90% sensitivity, which may be enhanced by the use of priming agents such as pentagastrin or H_2-receptor antagonists (44). The diverticulum is visualized as a well-demarcated focus of high-intensity activity located anywhere in the abdomen but most often within 100 cm of the ileocecal valve in the right lower quadrant. Active bleeding at the site may enhance detection but is not necessary for visualization of the lesion. Larger accumulations of radionuclide can result from ectopic gastric mucosa in lesions other than Meckel's diverticula—including enteric duplications; gastric heterotopia in the duodenum, jejunum, or ileum; or gastric metaplasia in Barrett's esophagus. False-positive results occur with ureteral obstruction, arteriovenous malformations, hemangiomas, or an inflammatory mass such as that seen in Crohn's disease (45). In patients with Crohn's disease, the uptake is most often poorly demarcated and is not simultaneous with uptake seen in the stomach, as it is in those with a Meckel's diverticulum.

Tagged red blood cell scans may be useful in detecting intermittent bleeding in the gastrointestinal tract of at least 500 mL/day (46). In this test, approximately 50 mL of the patient's RBCs are removed and labeled with technetium 99m and then reinjected into the patient, who is being monitored by a gamma counter. Images are taken every 5 min for the first hour to detect extravasation of the tagged RBCs into the intestinal lumen. Additional images are taken at regular intervals for up to 24 hr in order to detect an accumulation of labeled cells at a focal area of the intestine. Confusion about the exact site of bleeding is inherent in the test because of intestinal peristalsis, which propels extravasated blood distally. Angiography and/or endoscopy is needed to confirm the precise location of the bleeding site.

With improved techniques and experience, angiography is being used more often in children to localize sources of gastrointestinal bleeding and to administer therapy to stop the bleeding (47). Ongoing hemorrhage at a rate of 0.5 mL/min or greater is needed for angiography to identify the bleeding source accurately. Once the patient is hemodynamically stable and has established adequate urine output, the angiographer can insert a femoral artery catheter and systematically evaluate branches of the celiac axis and superior and inferior mesenteric arteries. Arterial injection of contrast material is followed by rapid-sequence exposures to include the arterial and venous phases of the injection. Rapid sequence filming allows visualization not only of extravasation of dye into the lumen, indicating active bleeding, but also a mucosal blush, representing a vascular lesion (hemangioma), or local early venous filling, indicative of an arteriovenous malformation. Once the bleeding lesion is identified, the catheter can be left in position for selective infusion of vasopressin or for embolization using Gelfoam or coils. The presence of bleeding can also be used for accurate identification of the site of bleeding during surgery, when methylene blue can be injected through the catheter with the abdomen open and the bowel exposed. Angiography in children carries a higher complication rate than in adults approaching 4% in children below 5 years of age (48). The main complication is femoral artery spasm.

Recently, the transjugular intrahepatic portosystemic shunt (TIPS) procedure has been carried out in children with recurrent upper-GI bleeding secondary to esophageal and/or gastric varices (49). This is particularly useful in children with cirrhotic liver lesions who are awaiting liver transplantation. In this technique, a catheter is adanced down the internal jugular vein into the inferior vena cava and out the right hepatic vein. A needle is then advanced through the wall of the hepatic vein and across the liver parenchyma to enter a branch of the right portal venous system. A stent is deployed between the two vessels, constructing an intrahepatc portosystemic shunt and thus decompressing the high-pressure portal venous system and decreasing blood flow through the varices.

6   WHAT CAN GO WRONG

The most common mistakes made by referring pediatricians in patients with GI bleeding are (1) inadequate examination of the perianal and anorectal area; (2) inadequate history, to exclude ''pseudobloods''; (3) overuse of barium and other radiological techniques; (4) lack of use of the nasogastric tube to localize the bleeding to the upper gastrointestinal tract and assess its severity; (5) failure to divide lower-GI bleeding into lesions that cause painless rectal bleeding with no change in bowel habits from those associated with tenesmus, crampy pain, and mucous, bloody diarrhea; and (6) failure to appreciate the significance of the

CBC as an indication of acute versus chronic bleeding, allergic gastroenteropathy, or chronic liver disease with portal hypertension and hypersplenism. By following the ten commandments for the assessment of GI bleeding in children outlined above, the primary practitioner should be able to avoid these pitfalls and arrive at a diagnosis quickly and efficiently. Reasons for referral to a tertiary care center include a first GI bleeding episode with hemodynamic compromise; repetitive episodes of minor bleeding; bleeding with other indications of a chronic underlying GI condition, such as Crohn's disease or ulcerative colitis; the need for therapeutic endoscopy to control present or future bleeding; the presence of bleeding with signs of obstruction or perforation; and the presence of persistent iron deficiency anemia with no known bleeding source.

REFERENCES

1. Laine L, Weinstein WM. Subepithelial hemorrhages and erosions of human stomach. Dig Dis Sci 1988; 33:490–503.
2. Heaton ND, Davenport M, Howard ER. Symptomatic hemorrhoids and anorectal varices in children with portal hypertention. J Pediatr Surg 1992; 27:833–835.
3. Goyal A, Treem WR, Hyams JS. Severe upper gastrointestinal bleeding in healthy full-term neonates. Am J Gastroenterol 1994; 189:613–616.
4. Lake AM, Whitington PE, Hamilton SR. Dietary protein-induced colitis in breast fed infants. J Pediatr 1982; 101:906–911.
5. Ponsky JL, Hoffman M, Swayngim DS: Saline irrigation in gastric hemorrhage: effect of temperature. J Surg Res 1980; 28:204–206.
6. Ahlquist DA, McGill DB, Schwartz S. Fecal blood levels in health and disease: a study using HemoQuant. N Engl J Med 1985; 312:1422–1425.
7. Frommer JJ, Kupparis A, Brown MK. Improved screening for colorectal cancer by immunological detection of occult blood. BMJ 1988; 296:1092–1095.
8. Niv Y, Bat L. Solitary rectal ulcer syndrome—clinical, endoscopic, and histologic spectrum. Am J Gastroenterol 1986; 48:486–491.
9. Robson WLM, Leung AKC, Kaplan BS. Hemolytic-uremic syndrome. Curr Probl Pediatr 1993: 23:16–33.
10. Czerniak A, Thompson JN, Hemingway AP. Hemobilia: a disease in evolution. Arch Surg 1988; 123:718–721.
11. Bruce J, Huh YS, Cooney DR. Intussusception: evolution of current management. J Pediatr Gastroenterol Nutr 1987; 6:663–669.
12. Ament ME, Berquist, Vargas J. Fiberoptic upper endoscopy in infants and children. Pediatr Clin North Am 1988; 35:141–151.
13. Bujanover Y, Konikoff F, Barataz M. Nodular gastritis and *Helicobacter pylori*. J Pediatr Gastroenterol Nutr 1990; 11:41–44.
14. Peterson WL. *Helicobacter pylori* and peptic ulcer disease N Engl J Med 1991; 324: 1043–1048.
15. Drumm B, Sherman P, Cutz E, Karmali M. Association of *Campylobacter pylori*

on the gastric mucosa with antral gastritis in children. N Engl J Med 1987; 316: 1557–1561.

16. Ament ME, Ochs HD, David SD. Structure and function of the gastrointestinal tract in primary immunodeficiency syndrome: a study of 39 patients. Medicine 1973; 52: 227–239.

17. Boyce TG, Swerdlow DL, Griffin PM. *Escherichia coli* 0157:H7 and the hemolytic-uremic syndrome. N Engl J Med 1995; 333:364–368.

18. Drumm B, Rhoads JM, Stringer DA. Peptic ulcer disease in children: etiology, clinical findings and clinical course. Pediatrics 1988; 82:410–416.

19. Kato S, Kobayaski M, Sato H. Doxycycline-induced hemorrhagic esophagitis: a pediatric case. J Pediatr Gastroenterol Nutr 1988; 7:762–764.

20. Bartlett J. Clostridium difficile: history of its role as an enteric pathogen and the current state of knowledge about the organism. Clin Infect Dis 1994; 18:5265–5272.

21. Schmitt B, Posselt HG, Waag KL. Severe hemorrhage from intestinal hemangiomatosis in Klippel-Trenauney syndrome: pitfalls in diagnosis and management. J Pediatr Gastroenterol Nutr 1986; 5:155–159.

22. Wong SH, Lau WY. Blue rubber-bleb nevus syndrome. Dis Colon Rectum 1982; 25:371–375.

23. Perry WH. Clinical spectrum of hereditary hemorrhagic telangiectasis (Osler-Weber-Rendu disease). Am J Med 1987; 82:989–997.

24. Burge DM, Middleton AW, Kamath R, Fasher BJ. Intestinal haemorrhage in Turner's syndrome. Arch Dis Child 1981; 56:557–569.

25. Foulkes WD. A tale of four syndromes: familial adenomatous polyposis, Gardner syndrome, attenuated APC, and Turcot syndrome. Q J Med 1995; 88:853–863.

26. Roe TF, Thomas DW, Gilsanz V. Inflammatory bowel disease in glycogen storage disease type 1b. J Pediatr 1986; 109:55–59.

27. Garay SM, Gardella JE, Fazzini EP, Goldring RM. Hermansky-Pudlak syndrome: pulmonary manifestations of a ceroid storage disorder. Am J Med 1979; 66:737–747.

28. Nardone DA, Reuler JB, Girard DE. Gastrointestinal complications of Ehler-Danlos syndrome. N Engl J Med 1979; 300:863–866.

29. Ergun GE, Lin AN, Dannenberg AJ, Carter DM. Gastrointestinal manifestations of epidermolysis bullosa, a study of 101 patients. Medicine (Baltimore) 1992; 71:121–127.

30. Felber S, Rosenthal P, Henton D. The BUN/creatinine ratio in localizing gastrointestinal bleeding in pediatric patients. J Pediatr Gastroenterol Nutr 1988; 7:685–689.

31. Lamberts SWJ, van der Lely AJ, de Herder WW, Hofland LJ. Octreotide. N Engl J Med 1996; 334:246–254.

32. Treem WR, Davis PM, Hyams JS. Suppression of gastric acid and secretion by intravenous administration of famotidine in children. J Pediatr 1991; 118:812–815.

33. Blumer JL, Rothstein FC, Kaplan BS, Pharmacokinetic determination of ranitidine pharmacodynamics in pediatric ulcer disease. J Pediatr 1985; 107:301–306.

34. Lloyd CW, Margin WJ, Taylor BD, Hauser AR. Pharmacokinetics and pharmacodynamics of cimetidine and metabolites in critically ill children. J Pediatr 1985; 107: 295–300.

35. McCarthy DM. Sucralfate. N Engl J Med 1991; 325:1017–1025.

36. Grund KE, Farin G. New principles and applications of high-frequency surgery, including argon plasma coagulation. Gastrointest Endosc 1997; 47:15–23.
37. Hassall E, Berquist WE, Ament ME, et al. Sclerotherapy for extrahepatic portal hypertension in childhood. J Pediatr 1989; 116:69–73.
38. Fox VL, Carr-Locke DL, Connors PJ, Leichtner AM. Endoscopic ligation of esophageal varices in children. J Pediatr Gastroenterol Nutr 1995; 20:202–208.
39. Markowitz J, Grancher K, Rosa J. Highly destructive perianal disease in children with Crohn's disease. J Pediatr Gastroenterol Nutr 1995; 21:149–153.
40. Wyllie R, Kay M. Esophagogastroduodenoscopy, colonoscopy and related techniques. In: Wyllie R, Hyams J, eds. Pediatric Gastrointestinal Disease: Pathophysiology, Diagnosis, and Management. Philadelphia: Saunders, 1993, pp 967–998.
41. Cynamon HA, Milov DE, Andres JM. Diagnosis and management of colonic polyps in children. J Pediatr 1989; 114:593–598.
42. Hoffenberg EJ, Sauaia A, Maltzman T, Knoll K, Ahnen DJ. Symptomatic colonic polyps in childhood: not so benign. J Pediatr Gastroenterol Nutr 1999; 28:175–181.
43. Mestre JR. The changing pattern of juvenile polyps. Am J Gastroenterol 1986; 81: 312–317.
44. Treves S, Grand RJ, Eraklis AJ. Pentagastrin stimulation of Technetium-99m uptake by ectopic gastric mucosa in a Meckel's diverticulum. Radiology 1978; 128:711–719.
45. Rodgers BM, Youssef S. "False positive" scan for Meckel diverticulum. J Pediatr 1975; 87:239–240.
46. Driscoll DM. The role of radionuclide imaging in the diagnosis of gastrointestinal bleeding in children. Radiography 1986; 52:237–243.
47. Afshani E, Berger PE. Gastrointestinal tract angiography in infants and children. J Pediatr Gastroenterol Nutr 1986; 5:173–186.
48. Jacobson B, Curtin H, Rubenson A. Complications of angiography in children and means of prevention. Acta Radiol [Diagn] (Stockh) 1980; 21:257–261.
49. Heyman M, LaBerge JM. Role of transjugular intrahepatic portosystemic shunt in the treatment of portal hypertension in pediatric patients. J Pediatr Gastroenterol Nutr 1999; 29:240–249.
50. Treem WR. Gastrointestinal bleeding in children. Gastrointest Clin North Am 1994; 4:75–97.
51. Treem WR. Gastrointestinal hemorrhage in children. Pract Gastroenterol 1997; 21: 21–38.

27

Inflammatory Bowel Disease

George Marx and Ernest G. Seidman
University of Montreal and Ste. Justine Hospital, Montreal,
Quebec, Canada

1 INTRODUCTION AND DEFINITIONS

The term *inflammatory bowel disease* (IBD) is generally used to refer to either ulcerative colitis (UC) or Crohn's disease (CD). Recognition of these conditions in the pediatric age group is very important, since the incidence of IBD peaks in the second decade of life (1,2). Despite significant advances in our understanding of intestinal immunology, the etiology of these chronic, spontaneously relapsing disorders remains unknown. They are generally grouped together in view of their many shared epidemiological, pathogenic, histological, and clinical characteristics (1). In most instances, these conditions can be readily differentiated on the basis of clinical, endoscopic, radiological, histological, and serologic data (1,3,4). However, an "indeterminate colitis" subgroup exists, representing about 10% of all cases of chronic colitis, with features insufficiently characterized to be classified as either CD or CU (1,3). This chapter summarizes the state of the art in the diagnosis and management of pediatric IBD—a major challenge to the health care team.

The chronic inflammation of UC remains confined to the mucosal lining of the colon in a continuous manner (Figs. 1a and 2a). The disease begins in the rectum and proceeds proximally to a varying but homogeneous extent in all cases

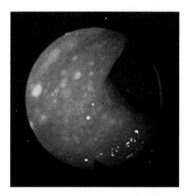

FIGURE 1a Colonoscopic image of ulcerative colitis. The disease affects the colon in a continuous manner.

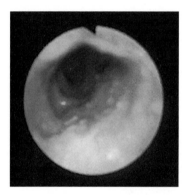

FIGURE 1b Colonoscopic image of Crohn's disease (CD). The asymmetric, inhomogenous and segmental bowel involvement characterizes CD, as one of the major criteria differentiating it from ulcerative colitis.

unless treatment (systemic or topical) is administered (1). Histologically, acute (neutrophils, eosinophils) and chronic (lymphocytes, plasma cells, monocytes, macrophages) inflammatory cell infiltrates of mucosa are seen, as well as crypt abscesses, distortion of the mucosal glands, and goblet cell depletion. Except in rare cases with toxic megacolon, the inflammation does not extend into the submucosa, muscularis propria, or serosa.

In contrast to UC, CD is a transmural disease that may involve any segment of the gastrointestinal tract, from the mouth to the anus. The asymmetrical, inhomogeneous, and segmental bowel involvement characterizes CD as one of the

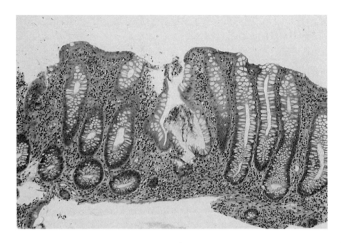

FIGURE 2a   Histologic image of ulcerative colitis. Histologically, acute (neutrophils, eosinophils) and chronic (lymphocytes, plasma cells, monocytes, macrophages) inflammatory cell infiltrates of mucosa are seen, as well as crypt abscesses, distortion of the mucosal glands, and goblet cell depletion. Except in rare cases with toxic megacolon, the inflammation does not extend into the submucosa, muscularis propria, or serosa.

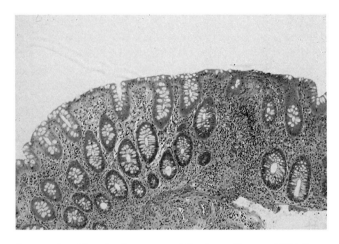

FIGURE 2b   Histologic image of Crohn's disease (CD). In contrast to ulcerative colitis, CD is a transmural disease. Histologically, affected areas primarily demonstrate chronic inflammatory cell infiltrates. Whereas noncaseating granuloma formation is diagnostic for CD, this is seen only in a minority of cases, usually early in the course of the disease.

major criteria differentiating it from UC (Figs. 1b and 2b). In children, the most
frequently involved area is the terminal ileum (75% of cases in our experience).
More than 50% of our pediatric CD patients have colonic involvement, usually
of the cecum and proximal ascending colon. Disease restricted to the large bowel
is encountered in about 10 to 15% of cases (1). Histologically, affected areas
primarily demonstrate chronic inflammatory cell infiltrates. Whereas noncaseating granuloma formation is diagnostic for CD, this is seen in only a minority of
cases, usually early in the course of the disease. Regions of diseased bowel are
separated by uninvolved segments of normal intestine, resulting in the typical
"skip lesions."

It is essential to exclude any potential infectious gastrointestinal disorder
that can mimic IBD in terms of the symptoms and signs as well as endoscopic,
histological, and even radiological findings. Potential microbial pathogens include *Salmonella, Shigella, Campylobacter, Yersinia enterocolitica, Aeromonas
hydrophilia, Entamoeba histolytica, Mycobacterium tuberculosis, Giardia, Di-
entamoeba fragilis, Clostridium difficile,* and *Histoplasma* (1).

2   EPIDEMIOLOGY AND PATHOGENESIS

Despite intensive research efforts, the etiology of IBD remains unknown. As in
adults, environmental, genetic, and immunological factors have been implicated
(Fig. 3). Recent population studies confirmed that the incidence of CD has increased in the United States from 1 to 6.9 cases per 100,000 person-years, comparing 1940 and 1993 irrespective of gender (5). However, the incidence was
found to have stabilized between 1973 and 1991. In view of the very low mortality associated with CD, the overall prevalence increased by 46%, from 60 to 133
per 100,000 inhabitants between 1980 and 1991. Another important finding was
a significant decrease in the median age at diagnosis, from about 44 years in
1940 to just below 30 in 1993. This impressive difference reflects the increasing
number of new cases of CD in the pediatric age group. Indeed, prior to 1954,
pediatric cases were rarely diagnosed, whereas 17% of the cases in 1990 were
under the age of 20 (5). The incidence of CD in Scotland, as an area representative
of Europe, was 3 to 5 cases per 100,000 inhabitants (2). The age-specific incidence for CD in individuals 15 to 19 years of age was 16 to 20 per 100,000, and
2 to 5 per 100,000 for those below age 15.

The situation for UC is somewhat different. A greater variation of incidence
has been described in the various studies published prior to 1998, likely due to
the difficulties of ascertainment of mild and asymptomatic disease. Generally
speaking, it seems that the incidence of UC has changed little over the last decade
(2,6). It has been estimated that the incidence of UC between the ages of 10 and
19 years is 23 cases per 100,000 age-specific population (2,5).

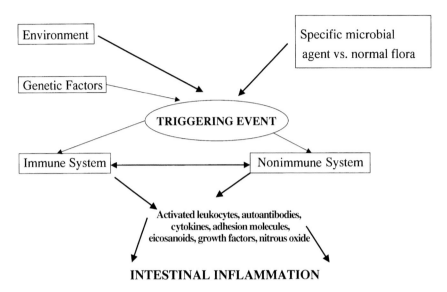

FIGURE 3 Multifactorial pathogenesis of inflammatory bowel disease.

Several epidemiological factors concerning susceptibility to IBD are summarized in Table 1. There is a relatively high prevalence of both UC and CD in the economically developed countries of northern and western Europe, the United States, and Canada. The incidence is higher in Canada and the northern United States compared to the southern states. In several countries, the prevalence in Ashkenazi Jews is two to four times higher than in the population as a whole (7). In Montreal, a striking number of new cases of CD have recently been seen in children born to parents who emigrated from countries where IBD is much rarer (South and Central America, the Caribbean, North Africa, Spain and Portugal, and the Middle East). A recent study showed that IBD in African-American children is more prevalent than previously believed, ranging from 7 to 12 per 100,000 (8). The crude incidence rate for all children with CD was 8.8 per 100,000 over the same period. Similarly, the incidence of UC in African-American children varied from 5 to 6.9 per 100,000, with a crude childhood incidence of 5.3 per 100,000 (8). This important study points out that the generally accepted assumption of a predisposition for IBD among Caucasians no longer holds.

2.1 Breast-Feeding and Early Weaning

Although there is some evidence to suggest that a lack of breast-feeding or early weaning may be a risk factor, other studies have not confirmed these findings (9).

TABLE 1 Putative Environmental and Etiopathogenic Factors Involved in the Development of Inflammatory Bowel Disease

Environmental factors	Lack of breast-feeding (early weaning)
	Perinatal infections
	History of cow's milk allergy (UC)
	Northern industrialized countries
	"Sanitized" childhood environment
	Smoking (protective for UC)
	Western diet
	Oral contraceptive use (CD)
Intestinal permeability	First-degree family members of patients with CD have increased intestinal permeability
Genetic factors	Increased familial aggregation (CD > UC)
	High concordance rate in monozygotic twins
	Association with other genetically determined diseases
Putative infectious agents	*Mycobacterium paratuberculosis*
	Listeria monocytogenes
	Paramyxovirus
Immunologic mechanisms	Excessive proinflammatory cytokines
	Relative deficiency of anti-inflammatory cytokines
	Th1 lymphocytes activated in CD
	Th2 lymphocytes activated in UC
Nonimmune cell	Intestinal epithelial cells, mesenchymal cells, enteric nervous system, endothelial cells

Key: UC, ulcerative colitis; CD, Crohn's disease.

2.2 Smoking

Smoking appears to have a protective role in UC, and cessation of smoking has been linked to relapses (10). On the other hand, smoking as well as the use of oral contraceptives are independent risk factors for clinical, surgical, and endoscopic recurrence in CD and have an adverse effect on postoperative disease activity (11). Both of the latter risk factors can be modified and are of potential relevance among adolescents.

2.3 Dietary Factors

A plausible link between diet and IBD would appear to be self-evident, since IBD affects the very site of nutrient absorption. However, studies linking excessive sugar and deficient fruit and vegetable fiber intake have not been substantiated (12). The relative efficacy of elemental diets in inducing remission in CD but not UC is suggestive of a role for dietary factors in the inflammatory process (12–16).

In addition to eliminating dietary antigens, elemental diets alter the composition and quantity of dietary fatty acids (12,13). Dietary polyunsaturated fatty acids of the omega-6 family (linoleic acid) are incorporated into cell membranes as arachidonic acid. This then serves as the substrate for the production of eicosanoids released by activated immune cells via the lipoxygenase and cyclo-oxygenase (COX 1 and 2) pathways. On the other hand, diets low in omega-6 fatty acids reduce the release of these proinflammatory mediators, such as leukotriene B4 (LTB$_4$). Dietary marine oils are omega-3 fatty acids that can also be incorporated into leukocyte membranes. They compete with arachidonic acid metabolites, thereby decreasing LTB$_4$ production (13,14). Our "western diet" has shifted partly from excessive consumption of saturated fats to a high consumption of omega-6 fatty acids. The latter are present in oils derived from most vegetables, other than olives. In parts of the world where marine oils (omega-3) or olive oil (omega-9) are consumed abundantly, the incidence of IBD is much lower (1). These observations have led to trials using marine oil supplements in preventing relapses in CD, as detailed below.

2.4   Intestinal Permeability

Increased intestinal permeability has been long been implicated in the pathogenesis of CD (1,17). It has been observed that some asymptomatic first-degree relatives of patients with CD have an increasing intestinal permeability (18). However, other studies have not confirmed these findings. Although this could represent a predisposing factor leading to inflammation, the heightened permeability is likely secondary to the inflammation (17,19,20).

2.5   Familial and Genetic Factors

There is now very strong evidence that genetic factors play a role in susceptibility to inflammatory bowel disease (21,22). In fact, the single most important risk factor for IBD is a positive family history (1). There is a high prevalence and disease concordance for IBD (particularly for CD) in monozygotic twins. The prevalence is also higher in first-degree relatives as compared with spouses. The variable frequency of disease observed in different ethnic groups also supports disease susceptibility genes. Ashkenazi Jews have a higher incidence of CD than non-Jews in their community (23). Familial aggregation is commonly observed, with a 5 to 20% likelihood of contracting IBD among first-degree relatives. Siblings of a patient with CD are 17 to 35 times more likely to develop the disease than the general population (24,25). A familial trend is also observed in the clinical characteristics of CD, including disease localization, age of onset, and disease type (fistulizing, stenosing, etc.) (24–26). The available data indicate that an intrinsic genetic factor underlies the susceptibility to IBD and determines its specific type. Nevertheless, the data are inconsistent with a simple Mendelian autosomal recessive mode of inheritance and suggest a complex, oligogenetically inherited disease with variable penetrance.

The association of IBD with other diseases of known genetic predisposition also supports its importance in the pathogenesis of IBD. Examples relevant to a pediatric population include the Hermansky-Pudlak syndrome, Turner syndrome, cystic fibrosis, and ankylosing spondylitis. All these diseases are linked to genes of the major histocompatibility complex (MHC). Some are associated with certain class II antigens. For example, ankylosing spondylitis in combination with CD is associated with human lymphocyte antigen HLA-B 27 and HLA-Bw60 (27). Other disorders that have been linked to genes of the MHC are associated with IBD, including psoriasis, atopy, celiac disease, type 1 diabetes, multiple sclerosis, autoimmune hemolytic anemia, autoimmune hepatitis, and primary sclerosing cholangitis.

A concept that further supports the relevance of genes to predisposition of IBD is that of genetic anticipation, defined as a progressively earlier disease onset in successive generations (26). It must be noted, however, that there is a disparity between the rapid increase of CD during the last few decades and any plausible changes in the genetic makeup of stable populations during the same period of time. Yet unknown environmental factors are clearly critical to develop IBD through an interaction of multiple predisposing but not sanctioning genes (17,19,20).

2.6 Infectious Agents

Many microbial pathogens have been purported to cause IBD, particularly CD. *Mycobacterium paratuberculosis*, paramyxoviruses such as measles, and *Listeria monocytogenes* are currently the agents that are most often implicated (17). The isolation of mycobacterial species in tissue from CD patients has led to therapeutic trials using antimycobacterial drugs in IBD (28). However, the lack of an immune response to these organisms, as well as their detection in control specimens, has cast doubt on their role.

Wakefield and coworkers have provided provocative evidence to suggest that a persistent measles viral infection induces focal granulomatous vasculitis, leading to CD (29). Paramyxovirus-like structures were visualized in the vascular endothelium by electron microscopy, and measles antigen and DNA were localized to granulomas and endothelial cells. Further supportive evidence was provided by epidemiological studies showing that the likelilhood of CD in the pediatric age group was observed to be very high in individuals born to a mother who had a measles infection during pregnancy (17). However, other investigators, using PCR, immunohistochemical techniques, or serological studies, have not confirmed the findings in favor of the measles infection theory (17,30,31).

More recently, Wakefield et al. also implicated a relationship between the measles-mumps-rubella (MMR) vaccine, bowel inflammation, and autism (32). In a group of 12 children, an association was found between pervasive developmental disorders and ileal-lymphoid-nodular hyperplasia and/or a mild, nonspecific colitis. In 8 of these patients, the parents described the onset of the child's behavioral problems following the MMR vaccine. However a 14-year prospective Finish study (31) showed no correlation between MMR vaccination, IBD, and pervasive developmental disorder. Further study in this area is under way.

2.7 Immunological Aspects

The prevailing view is that the pathogenesis of IBD involves dysregulation of the mucosal immune response to factors present within the gut lumen (17,19,20). Antigenic stimuli of microbial or dietary origin are continuously stimulating the gut-associated lymphoid tissue (GALT). Normally, secreted immunoglobulins, proteolytic enzymes, the mucous gel layer, and epithelial tight junctions efficiently exclude these luminal factors. Mucosal inflammation in response to pathogens normally occurs in a controlled fashion, with the host's GALT immunoregulatory mechanisms capable of down-regulating the inflammatory response. As a result, in the normal host, intestinal inflammation is self-limited. In IBD patients however, the mucosal immune system, once activated by an infection, appears to be incapable of down-regulating itself spontaneously (19,20). The normal unresponsiveness or tolerance to normal luminal antigens is abrogated in IBD, presumably as a result of genetic factors. An imbalance in the production of proinflammatory and down-regulatory cytokines ensues, resulting in altered intestinal epithelial cell proliferation, apoptosis, and changes in immune and absorptive functions (17,19,20). Inflamed intestinal tissue in IBD contains increased levels of proinflammatory cytokines such as interleukin (IL)-1, IL-6, IL-8, IL-12, IL-15 and TNF-α. On the other hand, the production of down-regulating cytokines (such as IL-4, IL-10, and transforming growth factor beta TGF-β) is diminished. The overproduced proinflammatory cytokines have multiple local effects, including the recruitment of other inflammatory cells through the increased expression of vascular adhesion molecules, excessive eicosanoid production, eosinophil degranulation, induction of nitric oxide synthase in macrophages and neurotrophils, and increased collage production (17,19,20,33). Il-1 and IL-6, potent stimuli for the hepatic production of acute-phase proteins, are capable of inducing other extraintestinal manifestations of IBD, such as fever. Reactive oxygen metabolites produced by neutrophils participating in the local inflammatory response are po-

tent cytotoxins, inducing cell injury or apoptosis (33,34). Products of inflammatory cells—such as histamine, prostaglandins, and leukotrienes—induce chloride
secretion by epithelial cells, contributing to diarrhea (35).

2.8 Nonimmune Cells

Although activated immune cells are the principal mediators of tissue damage
in IBD, the other cells populating the mucosa are involved. Intestinal epithelial
cells, mesenchymal cells, and nerve, neuroendocrine, and endothelial cells all are
implicated in the pathogenesis of IBD. Their interactions with immune cells in a
variety of complex events are likely of critical yet poorly understood importance.

2.9 Psychological Factors

It was long fashionable to implicate psychosocial stress as playing a key role in
the pathogenesis of IBD. However, no causal relationship has ever been demonstrated. Carefully conducted studies have not indicated that stressful life events
or depressed mood precipitates exacerbations (36). Nevertheless, psychosocial
factors are critically important to the child with IBD, affecting response to therapy
and quality of life.

3 CLINICAL MANIFESTATIONS

3.1 Crohn's Disease

The signs and symptoms of CD depend upon the bowel segment(s) involved.
Virtually any gastrointestinal symptom may be encountered at diagnosis (Table
2). Extraintestinal manifestations (Table 3) are observed in 25 to 35% of patients
and may be the sole initial manifestation in some cases (37,38). Typically, the
child presents with a history of recurrent episodes of cramping or colicky abdominal pain, often aggravated by eating. In some, the pain may increase prior to
defecation, which then might bring some relief. Loose, frequent stools are often
noted. Urgency to defecate and nocturnal diarrhea are generally present when
the colon is involved. Although bloody and mucus-containing bowel movements
are more typical of UC, they may be present in patients with Crohn's colitis as
well. Massive lower intestinal hemorrhage is a rare but potentially life-threatening manifestation of CD.

　　　Commonly, appetite progressively decreases during the initial stages or
during acute exacerbations of the disease, leading to anorexia. Nausea and vomiting can accompany the anorectic state but may indicate a severe colitis or an
intestinal obstruction. These symptoms are also commonly observed in patients
with proximal GI involvement (39). Extraintestinal manifestations—which may
include aphtous stomatitis or cheilitis, arthralgias or arthritis, fever, erythema

TABLE 2 Intestinal Manifestations and Extent of Involvement in Pediatric Crohn's Disease and Ulcerative Colitis

Intestinal symptoms	Crohn's disease	Ulcerative colitis
Rectal bleeding	+	+++
Diarrhea	+	+++
Abdominal pain	+++	+
Anorexia	+++	+
Vomiting	++	+
Intestinal involvement	Focal, transmural disease, granulomas	Homogeneous, superficial mucosal inflammation
Proximal mid–small bowel	+	−
Distal ileum	+++	+
Colon	++	+++
Rectum	++	+++
Anus	+++	−

TABLE 3 Extraintestinal Manifestations of Crohn's Disease and Ulcerative Colitis

Extraintestinal manifestations	Crohn's disease	Ulcerative colitis
Fever	+++	++
Perianal lesions	+++	−
Growth failure	+++	+
Aphtous mouth ulcers	+++	+
Arthritis	++	++
Erythema nodosum	+	+
Clubbing	++	+
Ankylosing spondylitis	+	+
Pyoderma gangrenosum	+	+
Episcleritis, uveitis	+	+
Primary sclerosing cholangitis	+	+
Hepatic steatosis	+	+
Pericarditis	−	+
Thromboembolic disease	+	+
Pancreatitis	+	+
Amyloidosis	Rare	Rare

nodosum, pyoderma gangrenosum, conjunctivitis or uveitis—may predominate over the intestinal symptoms. Those most often associated with CD are fever, aphtous mouth ulcers, and perianal lesions. Joint complaints and perianal lesions such as fissures, fistulas, or abscesses are generally seen more frequently in patients with colonic involvement (1). Low-grade fever is a typical finding in 70% of children, usually in the late afternoon and evenings. Fever of unknown origin in the pediatric age group should include CD in the differential diagnosis.

The potential complications of growth impairment and pubertal delay are unique to the pediatric CD population. The majority of patients are below the third percentile in weight and height when first diagnosed (12,14,40). The causes of malnutrition in children with IBD are summarized in Table 4. The impaired growth, leading to short stature, and the accompanying delayed maturation of secondary sexual characteristics are, for many adolescent IBD patients, more troubling and debilitating than the underlying disease.

3.2 Ulcerative Colitis

The most consistent symptoms of UC are frequent stools mixed with blood and mucus, accompanied by lower abdominal cramping (Table 2). The severity of symptoms usually correlates with the extent and degree of disease involvement. Nocturnal diarrhea is a sign of more extensive colonic involvement. Urgency with incontinence is encountered in about 25% of cases. The presence of tenes-

TABLE 4 Potential Causes of Undernutrition, Growth Failure, and Delayed Puberty in Patients with Inflammatory Bowel Disease

Causative factor	Explanation
Decreased nutrient intake	Disease-induced
	Iatrogenic
Malabsorption	Diminished absorptive surface
	Bacterial overgrowth
	Bile salt deficiency
Increased gut losses	Protein-losing gastroenteropathy
	Bleeding
	Electrolytes, minerals, trace metals
Drug-nutrient interactions	Corticosteroids (calcium, protein)
	Sulfasalazine (folate)
	Cholestyramine (fat, vitamins)
Increased requirements	Sepsis, fever
	Increased cell turnover
	Replace losses: catch-up growth

mus reflects rectal involvement. Postprandial diarrhea is also common, perhaps due to the gastrocolonic reflex. The abdominal pain is usually not as severe as in CD, is often colicky, and typically most intense prior to defecation. In some cases it is worse after the ingestion of food and, as in CD, may be relieved by defecation. Anorexia and nausea are often present in the acute stage of moderate to severe disease. Diminished intake due to lack of appetite accounts for weight loss. Exudative loss of protein through the inflamed bowel is the major cause of hypoalbuminemia. As in CD, the extraintestinal manifestations (Table 3) may precede the intestinal symptoms (37,38). Episodes of arthralgias and arthritis often coincide with colonic symptoms and constitute the most common extraintestinal finding in children with UC (1,37). Low-grade fever, peaking in the evening, may be noted. Weight loss may be present but is generally not as severe as in CD. Growth impairment, much less common than in CD, is seen in about 10% of cases. Erythema multiforme or erythema nodosum is encountered in only about 2% of cases. Pyoderma gangrenosum is a rare but potentially severe manifestation in children with UC. Aphthous stomatitis is seldom seen in children with UC versus those with CD. Ankylosing spondylitis has been reported in IBD in association with HLA-B27. Ocular manifestations such as uveitis occur infrequently in pediatric cases and are almost never seen early after diagnosis. Patients should be screened for liver enzyme abnormalities prior to instituting IBD therapy. Autoimmune hepatitis and primary sclerosing cholangitis, seen in about 3% of children with IBD, are more common in UC than in CD. The typical changes in the latter are concentric fibrosis around the bile ducts that progress to their obliteration. Either of these hepatic complications can lead to cirrhosis and are important to screen for. UC is also considered a risk factor for thromboembolic complications, as in CD.

4   DIAGNOSTIC METHODS

In the majority of cases, a thorough history and physical examination are highly suggestive of IBD. Laboratory measures, radiological and endoscopic studies, as well as histological analysis of the mucosal pathology are primarily utilized to confirm the diagnosis and to verify the extent and distribution of the disease (Fig. 4). As in adults, the symptoms of IBD in pediatric patients depend largely on the site and extent of the mucosal inflammation. However, the diagnosis of IBD is more often missed or delayed in children because of the greater frequency of nonspecific symptoms at presentation. Furthermore, school-aged children often (20%) consult a physican because of functional abdominal pain, which may lead to unnecessary and costly investigations. There has thus been much interest in the validation of noninvasive screening tests for IBD, much like those developed for celiac disease (41).

TABLE 5   Differential Diagnosis of Crohn's Disease and Ulcerative Colitis

Differential diagnosis	Crohn's disease	Ulcerative colitis
Infectious		
Appendicitis	++	+
Mesenteric adenitis	++	−
Enteritis (*Yersinia enterocolitica, Escherichia coli;* *Campylobacter jejuni, Salmonella, Shigella, Enta-moeba histolytica, Giardia lamblia, Mycobacterium tuberculosis*)	++	+
Pseudomembraneous or antibiotic-associated colitis	++	+++
Vascular disorders		
Hemolytic uremic syndrome, Henoch-Schöenlein pur-pura, Behçet's disease, polyarteritis nodosum, sys-temic lupus erythematosis, ischemic bowel dis-ease, dermatomyositis	+	+++
Immunodeficiency disorders	+	+
Iatrogenic		
Radiation, chemotherapy (typhlitis), graft-vs.-host dis-ease	+	+
Obstetrical and gynecological		
Ectopic pregnancy, ovarian cysts, tumors, endometri-osis	+	+
Allergic		
Eosinophilic gastroenteritis	+	+
Neuromuscular		
Hirschsprung's disease, pseudo-obstruction syn-dromes	+	++
Others		
Intussusception, Meckel's diverticulum, tumors	+	++

4.1   Laboratory Evaluation

At the time of first presentation, screening tests should include stool examinations for enteric pathogens. The detection of *Clostridium difficile* toxin is particularly relevant in the pediatric age group, as antibiotic-associated or pseudomembranous colitis is a much underdiagnosed condition. In the absence of frank hematochezia, fecal search for occult blood and leukocytes can be helpful. A complete blood count and erythrocyte sedimentation rate (ESR) are very helpful. Although not specific for IBD, patients usually have a microcytic, hypochromic anemia, an elevated platelet count, and a high ESR. Routine biochemical analysis often re-veals a low serum albumin, primarily due to the exudative enteropathy. Serum electrolytes may show low potassium if diarrhea is profuse. The blood urea nitro-

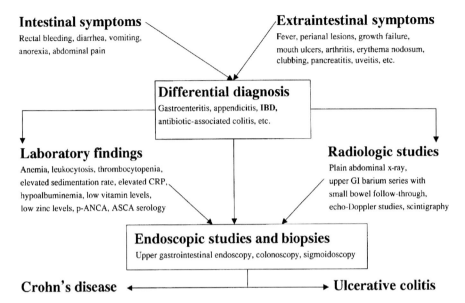

FIGURE 4   Diagnostic algorithm for inflammatory bowel disease.

gen (BUN) may be elevated if the patient is dehydrated. More often, however, it is low due to inadequate protein intake relative to losses in the catabolic state. Thrombocytosis, hypoalbuminemia, and high serum levels of the acute-phase protein orosomucoid correlate well with histological inflammation in patients with IBD (42). Markers of the acute-phase response such as C-reactive protein, orosomucoid, and the ESR are more likely to be elevated in patients with CD than those with UC (43).

Anemia, most frequently secondary to iron deficiency, may also be attributed to folic acid and/or vitamin B_{12} deficiency, malnutrition, and, rarely, autoimmune hemolysis. Increased levels of proinflammatory cytokines—such as IL-1, TNF-α, and interferon-gamma—can diminish erythropoiesis by inhibiting erythropoietin production and impairing iron metabolism (44). In malnourished patients, measurement of calcium, phosphorus, magnesium, zinc, and vitamin A, D and E status is important as part of the evaluation of micronutrient status (12,16).

As noted above, novel serological assays have recently been tested for their ability to differentiate between IBD and non-IBD in pediatric patients and, furthermore, to distinguish between UC and CD (4,41,44). The results clearly established that perinuclear antineutrophil cytoplasmic antibodies (pANCA) and anti–*Saccharomyces cerevesiae* antibodies (ASCA) were highly specific for UC and CD, respectively. ASCA react to oligomannosidic epitopes of the dietary organism commonly referred to as brewers' or bakers' yeast. It is unclear why increased

ASCA titers are specific for CD, as they are absent in other disorders with excessive small bowel permeability, such as untreated celiac disease (4). Furthermore, these tests had high positive predictive value (both more than 95%) in discriminating between IBD and non-IBD patients. The combination of ANCA screen by enzyme-linked immunosorbent assay (ELISA), followed by immunofluorescence with the additional confirmatory step for perinuclear staining (pANCA) using DNAse treatment of neutrophils with bound antibodies, increased the disease specificity of the assay in UC from 70 to 92% (4). The combined use of both pANCA and ASCA assays gave an overall agreement of 68% with the final diagnosis on the basis of clinical, endoscopic, radiographic and histopathologic criteria. Moreover, double positive testing (IgA and IgG) for ASCA was 100% specific for CD (4). A small proportion of CD patients are pANCA-positive, usually those with a ''UC-like'' distal colitis (4). Although the differentiation between CD and UC with the above assays was therefore imperfect, they are very useful when the patient is ASCA-positive and pANCA-negative (44). The high negative predictive value of ASCA makes it particularly attractive as a screening method in patients with nonspecific symptoms and a normal physical exam (45). It remains unclear whether pANCA and ASCA are useful in monitoring disease activity.

Radiologic assessment of skeletal bone age is indicated in children with unexplained short stature to determine whether delayed maturation is present. Recent studies have confirmed that children with IBD are at risk for osteopenia as compared with normal children (46,47). Bone mineral density (BMD) was measured by dual-energy x-ray absorptiometry. Trabecular rather than cortical bone was predominantly involved, as seen in the lumbar spine and femoral neck. Low BMD was more prevalent in children with CD versus those with UC, especially females. In order not to overestimate osteoporosis due to growth failure with delayed bone maturation in IBD, BMD values in pediatric patients with CD should take into consideration bone age delay. Interpretation of BMD on the basis of bone or height age, rather than chronological age, resulted in a diminution of the overall frequency of abnormally low BMD from 44% to 26 to 30% (46). The latter prevalence correlates with the results of studies in adult patients. BMD evaluation, correated for bone or height age, should be part of the management of IBD in children, particularly in CD, or in patients who have received corticosteroids.

4.2   Imaging Studies of the GI Tract

In a patient with symptoms or signs highly suggestive of IBD, radiological investigations should include a complete upper gastrointestinal series with small bowel follow-through (48). Colonoscopy has superseded barium studies as the preferred method of assessment of the colon due to its greater sensitivity. Moreover, it provides the opportunity to provide tissue for histological evaluation. Barium enemas still have a certain advantage in the preoperative evaluation, particularly when assessing for fistulas and stenoses.

Early radiological findings in CD of the small bowel include mucosal wall thickening with superficial aphthous ulcerations. As the disease progresses, focal as well as linear mucosal ulcerations are seen as well as pseudopolyp formation with a cobblestone appearance. Later on, the fibrotic process often leads to dilatation of bowel loops proximal to stenotic zones ("string sign") with rigid walls and diffuse narrowing, usually affecting the terminal ileum. When the colon is involved, there is loss of haustrations, ulcerations, extensive edema and, finally, shortening of the ("lead pipe") colon. Duodenal and jejunal disease is characterized roentgenographically by presence of edema, stenotic segments, and strictures with dilatation of proximal loops.

In the child with severe colitis, plain films of the abdomen and a limited rectosigmoidoscopy should be done rather than a barium enema. Contrast studies are absolutely contraindicated in the presence of colonic dilatation. There have been reports of toxic megacolon occuring within 48 h of a barium enema. In cases with severe colitis, thickening of the colonic wall is usually readily apparent on the plain abdominal film, and "thumbprinting" may be seen. Toxic megacolin is characterized by colonic dilatation (more than 8 cm), and small bowel distention (49). Early changes on barium studies in UC are nonspecific. Usually, as in CD, there is a loss of haustration and signs of mucosal inflammation prior to the development of superficial ulcerations.

Computed tomography is helpful in searching for abscesses, evaluating phlegmons, and revealing relationships between adjacent organs and loops of bowel, especially regarding fistulization to the bladder and vagina. Magnetic resonance imaging is valuable in assessing perineal abscess and fistula formation.

Our recent studies (45,50) suggest that Doppler ultrasonographic assessment of the abdomen is very useful as a diagnostic tool to screen for IBD in patients without frank signs of disease. This noninvasive technique can also assist as a preliminary assessment of the extent and distribution of disease. As well, vessel density estimation by Doppler sonography correlates with CD activity and may be useful in following the course of the disease, as well as response to therapy (45,50). In cases of partial bowel obstruction, radioisotopic leukocyte scans can be helpful in distinguishing between inflammatory narrowing of bowel loops and fixed fibrotic strictures. In the former situation, medical therapy may be beneficial, whereas the latter cases will require resection or strictureplasty.

4.3 Endoscopic Assessment

Endoscopy and mucosal biopsies have become indispensable tools in the diagnosis and monitoring of intestinal disorders. In general, colonoscopy should be performed in lieu of a barium enema. If the patient is severely ill, flexible rectosigmoidoscopy without insufflation of air can be employed judiciously. Although the endoscopic appearances of CD and UC are occasionally similar, certain features of CD are distinctive (Fig. 1). Rectal sparing is an exception in untreated UC but not uncommon in patients with CD. Patchy lesions or aphtous ulcers interspersed with normal-appearing mucosa are typical of CD involving the colon (Fig. 1a). Multiple deep, fissuring ulcers may be present, resulting in islands of normal mucosa and pseudopolyp formation. The ileocecal valve may appear granular and edematous, and the terminal ileum is often markedly nodular, scattered with linear ulcers. Upper gastrointestinal endoscopy is helpful in cases with upper GI symptoms (39). In patients with proximal CD, multiple foci of erythema, mucosal erosions, thickened folds, and a nodular mucosa are most often seen. Occasionally, a cobblestone pattern with longitudinal ulcers may be observed.

In UC, the changes are diffuse and homogeneous, spreading proximately from the rectum (Fig. 1b). In untreated cases, the latter is involved uniformly and most severely. The mucosa is granular without its normal glistening appearance as well as erythematous, and the normal vascular pattern is obscured by edema. In more severe cases, the mucosa is excessively friable, with bleeding spontaneously or on contact. Detailed histological examination of multiple mucosal biopsies obtained endoscopically is indispensable to making a definitive diagnosis of UC or Crohn's colitis (Fig. 2). Biopsies should always be taken in normal-appearing as well as involved mucosa, since microscopic inflammation and/ or granulomas may be present. When possible, inspection and biopsies of the terminal ileum should be attempted.

4.4 Differential Diagnosis

If the inflammatory process involves both the small and the large intestine, there is no doubt that one is dealing with CD. An exception to this rule is UC with "backwash ileitis." When the colon alone is involved, one has to rely on biopsy findings or on the presence of skip lesions, which are not compatible with UC.

Enteric infections, appendicitis, ovarian pathology, neoplasia, and intussusception as well as mesenteric adenitis may all present with lower abdominal pain. The differential diagnosis of chronic pain includes the irritable bowel syndrome, food intolerance, celiac disease, recurrent functional abdominal pain, peptic disease, and urinary tract pathology. Table 5 summarizes the disorders that should be taken into consideration in the differential diagnosis.

4.5 Assessment of Disease Severity

A variety of laboratory indices have been developed to assess the severity of disease activity (51). Endoscopic evaluation has been shown to correlate very poorly with symptoms, as bowel inflammation with ulcerations may persist despite induction of clinical remission with corticosteroids. Elevated levels of acute-phase reactants such as ESR, C-reactive protein (CRP), and serum orosomucoid are sensitive, albeit non-specific markers of disease activity (51). Elevations in the platelet count and reduced serum albumin levels are also frequently used. More recently, IL-6 levels were reported to discriminate between inflammatory and fibrostenosing disease (52). Stool markers of protein loss such as fecal alpha-1 antitrypsin generally have inadequate sensitivity (53). Stool cytokine measurement (IL-1β, IL-1RA, and TNF-α) was also recently shown to be useful for monitoring disease activity (54).

Intestinal permeability, measuring 5-h urinary excretion ratio of lactulose/ L-rhamnose was significantly increased in patients with active CD and extensive UC (55). However, no correlation was found between this permeability marker and the pediatric CD activity index. In our experience (53), the pediatric adaptation of the National Cooperative Crohn's Disease Study Group Crohn's Disease Activity Index serves as a useful clinical evalutaion (Table 6). In this PCDAI, the child's "infirm days" serve as an estimate of quality of life. For each day the child was unable to attend school or to participate fully in extracurricular activities, 5 points were added, to a maximum of 35 points per week. Chronic malnutrition and growth failure are not taken into consideration in this PCDAI and must be assessed separately. As noted above, Doppler ultrasound of the abdomen is useful as an accurate, objective and non-invasive measure of CD activity (45,40).

5   MANAGEMENT

The major goals in managing IBD are to induce and maintain remission of disease activity. This is essential to ensure normal growth and development in young patients. The yet obscure etiology and pathogenesis of IBD—along with its highly variable severity, extent, and clinical course—render it difficult to achieve an optimal therapy for all cases. Ideally, therapy should also minimize toxicity and side effects. Medical therapy for IBD has advanced remarkably in recent years (56). Therapeutic alternatives include 5-aminosalicylic acid (5-ASA) formulations, corticosteroids including budesonide, immunomodulatory drugs such as azathioprine, 6-mercaptopurine and thalidomide, metronidazole and other antibiotics, immunosuppresants such as methotrexate and cyclosporine, and newer biological therapies such as monoclonal antibodies TNF-α in addition to nutritional therapy, and surgery (Figs. 5 and 6). Although surgery is very useful for selected cases of complicated CD (strictures, fistulas, and abscesses), it is not curative as in the case of UC.

5.1   Aminosalicylate Compounds

The therapeutic efficacy of aminosalicylates was first suggested by studies using sulfasalazine (SASP) for arthritis in patients with concurrent IBD. The active

TABLE 6   Modified Pediatric Crohn's Disease Activity Index

Modified pediatric CDAI		Calculation
Total number of diarrheal stools for each of previous 7 days		X2
Abdominal pain for each of previous 7 days		X5
None	= 0	
Mild	= 1	
Moderate	= 2	
Severe	= 3	
General well-being for each of previous 7 days		X7
Well	= 0	
Below par	= 1	
Poor	= 2	
Very poor	= 3	
Terrible	= 4	
Extraintestinal complications over the past week		X20
Arthritis and arthralgias	= 1	
Skin or mouth lesions	= 1	
Iritis or uveitis	= 1	
Anorectal lesion	= 1	
Other fistulas	= 1	
Fever over 38°C	= 1	
Infirm days (school attendance/extracurricular activities)		X number of
No = 0, Yes = 5		days per week
Abdominal mass		X10
None	= 0	
Fullness	= 2	
Definite	= 5	
Hematocrit (normal lower limit for age-actual hct.)		X6
Body weight deficit		
1–(actual body weight/ideal weight for height) × 100		

Interpretation: Mild-to-moderate disease, <150; moderate relapse, 150–300; moderate–severe relapse, 300–450; severely ill, > 450.
Source: Adapted from Ref. 53.

moiety was subsequently found to be 5-aminosalicylate (5-ASA). Better-tolerated 5-ASA formulations were developed based on their release characteristics. Aminosalicylates are recommended as first-line treatment for both UC and CD in presentations. These include SASP, mesalamine, balsalazide, and olsalazine. Treatment is generally given orally at a dose of 50 to 75 mg/kg/day to a maximum of 4.8 g administered in three divided doses. Intolerance reactions (headache; gastrointestinal distress, especially nausea; hypersensitivity reactions, such as skin eruptions and hemolytic anemias) are less often encountered with 5-ASA

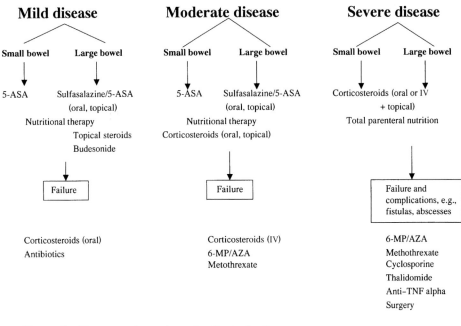

FIGURE 5   Therapeutic options for Crohn's disease.

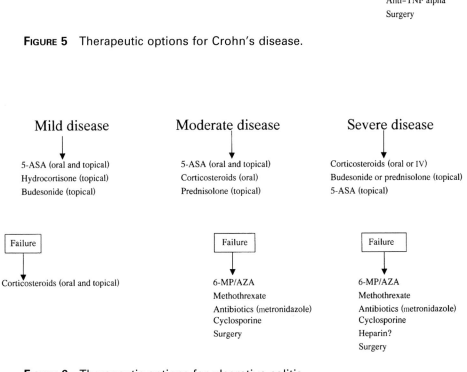

FIGURE 6   Therapeutic options for ulcerative colitis.

than SASP. Other rare complications include hepatotoxicity, granulocytopenia, thrombocytopenia, pancreatitis, and eosinophilic pneumonia (57).

UC is a superficial mucosal disease and is therefore well suited to treatment with topical agents effective at the mucosal level. Thus, in addition to oral therapy, 5-ASA can be administered alone or in combination with topical enemas or suppositories (corticosteroids or mesalamine) in order to control left-sided colitis or proctitis. It is important to achieve high concentration of 5-ASA at the site of disease. SASP and olsalazine are unique in that they are released only in the colon and are available in forms other than tablets, as a suspension or as a powder, respectively. They are therefore suitable for treating young children unable to swallow pills. However, both of these formulations have more frequent side effects than other 5-ASA formulations. Olsalazine has been observed to be less effective in controlling colitis than SASP. 5-ASA is combined with steroids or cyclosporin for more severe cases of UC. The choice of 5-ASA for CD depends on the distribution of the disease. SASP and mesalamine have been shown to be of benefit with ileal and colonic disease but have not been helpful for proximal disease. SASP and 5-ASA are also useful in maintaining remission in cases of colitis, whether due to UC or CD.

5.2   Corticosteroids

Systemic corticosteroids have long been the main treatment for moderate to severe active IBD. Oral prednisone induces remission in 65 to 75% of patients within 4 weeks of initiation. Generally, 1 mg/kg per day of prednisone is given, to a maximum of 40 mg/day (57). The dose is sometimes increased to 2 mg/kg/day (maximum 60 mg/day) in cases failing to improve within 2 weeks. In more severe cases, parenteral corticosteroid therapy is recommended. Progressive reduction of the dose is usually initiated within 1 month, with the aim of completely discontinuing steroid therapy after a few months. Maintenance therapy with SASP or 5-ASA is generally employed during the steroid weaning process. Nevertheless, almost half of the children with IBD are unable to come off steroid treatment without a flare of their disease. Such steroid-dependent patients are best managed with immunomodulatory therapy, as discussed below.

Steroid use is associated with numerous side effects, which are intolerable for many patients. These include acne, facial puffiness (moon face), hirsutism, striae, cataracts, aseptic necrosis of the femoral head, hypertension, depression, growth impairment, myopathy, and osteopenia with compression fractures (Table 7). Side effects can be reduced to a certain extent by adopting alternate-day dosing of prednisone and avoiding a nocturnal dose. Steroids have not been shown to be of benefit as maintenance therapy. It has been noted that alternate-day, low-dose prednisone may reduce symptomatic flares without inhibiting linear growth (58). However, confirmation from randomized controlled trials is lacking. Budesonide, a well-absorbed and rapidlly catabolized corticosteroid, has the advan-

TABLE 7 Major Side Effects of Drugs Commonly Used in Inflammatory Bowel Disease

Drugs	Side effects
Aminosalicylates Sulfasalazine 5-ASA/mesalamine/olsalazine Topical 5-ASA (enema, suppository)	Headaches, nausea, hypersensitivity reactions with skin involvement, hepatotoxicity, pancreatitis, granulocytopenia, thrombocytopenia Side effects of topical applications seldom encountered
Corticosteroids Prednisone Topical hydrocortisone (enema) Budesonide	Acne, moon facies, striae, growth impairment, hypertension, aseptic necrosis or bone fractures, depression or other mood alterations, sleep disorder, osteopenia, myopathy Budesonide has less systemic side effects
Antimetabolite therapy 6-Mercaptopurine Azathioprine Methotrexate	Pancreatitis, hepatitis, leukopenia Teratogenicity (methotrexate)
Immunosuppressive therapy Cyclosporine Tacrolimus	Nephrotoxicity, headaches, paresthesias, hirsutism, oral thrush Diabetes
Biological therapy Antitumor necrosis factor alpha	Serum sickness–like reactions Lupus-like syndrome Lymphomas?
Antibiotics Metronidazole	Long-term use: peripheral neuropathy

tage of causing fewer glucocorticoid-related systemic side effects. An ileal release preparation has been observed to induce remission in 50 to 69% of patients with active CD (59).

5.3 Immunosuppressive Drugs

5.3.1 Antimetabolite Immunomodulatory Therapy

6-Mercaptopurine (6-MP) and its prodrug azathioprine (AZA) have both cytotoxic and immunomodulatory properties. The incorporation of their active 6-thioguanine nucleotide (6-TG) metabolites into the DNA and RNA of hematopoietic cells reduces the proliferation of T and B lymphocytes and impairs their effector function. The main benefits of 6-MP and AZA in the treatment of IBD is their ability to maintain remission and as steroid-sparing agents (60). Due to their slow onset of action (2 to 6 months), these agents are not considered appropriate immediate therapeutic options for patients presenting with severe active disease. Although the majority of studies have been carried out in CD, similar benefits of 6-MP/AZA use have been demonstrated among UC patients (61). A recent retrospective study by Kirschner examined the safety AZA and 6-MP in pediatric IBD (62). These drugs are well tolerated in most children and adolescents. Only 8 to 10% of patients had acute toxicity that required cessation of therapy, usually due to acute pancreatitis or leukopenia. The identification of mutations of the gene that catabolizes 6-MP, thiopurine methyltransferase (TPMT), can reduce the risk of bone marrow toxicity by identifying highly susceptible patients prior to initiating therapy (63). Patients with heterozygous TPMT mutations can be safely and effectively treated with lower doses of AZA or 6-MP (63). Monitoring 6-TG and 6-MMP metabolite levels allows physicians to individualize and hence optimize therapy using these drugs. The vast majority of the patients thus treated achieve prolonged remission off corticosteroids successfully (63). These medications are being utilized with increasing frequency in pediatric IBD. Their proven beneficial effects include steroid-dependent and resistant cases as well as fistulizing disease. A recent randomized, placebo-controlled trial demonstrated that the early prophylactic use of 6-MP (1.5 mg/kg/day) significantly decreased the relapse rate and steroid requirements in newly diagnosed pediatric CD (64). Methotrexate is considered to be an antimetabolite due to its antagonistic effect on folic acid metabolism. A study examined the results of low-dose, weekly subcutaneous methotrexate (15 mg/m^2 weekly SC) in pediatric patients that had failed therapy with 6-MP (65). Among the 14 cases, 9 showed symptomatic improvement after 4 weeks of therapy. Until the long term risks and benefits of methotrexate are fully known, this therapy should be considered for children with CD who fail to respond to conventional therapy, including those with significant complications from 6-MP/AZA.

5.3.2 T Lymphocyte Immunosuppressive Therapy

Cyclosporin A (CsA) is a fungal product that was discovered to inhibit T-cell responses. Its immunomodulatory effects are achieved by blocking lymphocyte cytokine production, particularly IL-2. This reduces further activation and proliferation of T-helper cells. The efficacy of intravenous CsA among patients with severe UC has been demonstrated (56,60,66). Although immediate surgery can be avoided, the benefits must be weighted against the risk of severe complications, including life-threatening opportunistic infections. In addition, most patients relapse upon CsA withdrawal. Further studies are needed to determine the long-term outcome of using CsA as a bridge to 6-MP or AZA. In CD, intravenous CsA (4 mg/kg/day) has also been shown to be effective for closure of fistulas. As noted for severe UC, it is primarily used as a bridge to therapy with a longer-acting immunomodulatory therapy, usually with 6-MP/AZA or methotrexate. CsA may also be effective when given orally if trough CsA levels between 250 and 400 ng/mL are achieved. Side effects of CsA treatment include reversible nephrotoxicity, headaches, paresthesias, and infections (Table 7). Until further studies with longer follow-up are conducted, the use of CsA should be restricted to those IBD patients with severe, steroid-resistant disease who require a drug with a rapid therapeutic onset. Other biological therapies, such as anti-TNF antibodies, have largely replaced the use of CsA for CD. Another immunomodulator, tacrolimus or FK 506, is considered to be even more potent than CsA. Scant data from trials with this drug in IBD have been carried out, although case reports suggest a beneficial effect in fistulizing CD.

5.4 Biological Therapies

The new ''biological'' therapies have emanated from studies carried out in transgenic or gene-knockout models of IBD in mice. These novel agents are engineered to specifically target integral steps in the cascade that contributes to mucosal inflammation, either by blocking proinflammatory cytokines or by administering anti-inflammatory cytokines. Infliximab is a human/mouse chimeric anti-TNF-α neutralizing antibody that is the only biological treatment currently approved by the U.S. Food and Drug Administration and the Health Protection Branch of Health Canada. Studies have demonstrated that this antibody is rapidly and relatively highly effective for inducing remission in active, therapy-refractory inflammatory CD. The clinical benefits of a single infusion of 5 mg/kg are generally observed within 2 weeks and last for 4 to 8 weeks in about two-thirds of cases (67). This treatment is also effective in closing fistulas, particularly in the perineum (68). Experience in the pediatric age group is limited but shows similar trends. Although this approach is relatively safe, infusion reactions have been described. The formation of anti-infliximab antibodies has been reported to give rise to hypersensitivity reactions upon readministration. Given the uncertainty of long-term sequelae, particularly the risk for lymphomas, this modality of therapy in children is likely to be restricted to the most severe cases. Other new treatments that inhibit TNF-α are being investigated, including CDP571, a humanized monoclonal anti-TNF antibody, and Etarnercept, a recombinant TNF-receptor fusion protein (69).

IL-10, a product of T-helper type 2 cells, is an endogenous anti-inflammatory cytokine that down-regulates the production of proinflammatory cytokines such as TNF-α and IL-1β. Administration of recombinant human IL-10 has shown some clinical efficacy in treatment of active CD when given intravenously (70). Although not yet approved, further clinical trials are currently underway using this therapy, as well as with IL-11. Antisense nucleotides are short segments of DNA that bind to specific corresponding mRNA, leading to their degradation and interfering with transcription. Studies are currently underway to examine the efficacy of antisense oligonucleotides to adhesion molecules (71) or to transcription factor such as NFαB.

5.5   Antibiotics

Antibiotic therapy, especially metronidazole with or without ciprofloxacin, has been employed for some time for perianal disease or for closing fistulas (56,72). Intra-abdominal abscess developing as a result of fistulization is generally treated with broad-spectrum antibiotics directed against stool flora and commonly includes ampicillin, gentamicin, clindamycin, or metronidazole. Metronidazole has been shown to be effective in treating colonic CD but not for small-intestinal disease. However, the long-term use of metronidazole has been associated with peripheral neuropathy (Table 7).

5.6   Nutritional Therapy

The potential role of nutritional therapy in children with IBD is generally accepted, especially for CD as primary therapy to induce remission or as adjunctive therapy to maintain remission and enhance growth (73,74). Although several randomized controlled trials have suggested that elemental and semielemental diets are as effective as steroids, meta-analysis has shown a statistical advantage for corticosteroids (75). Nevertheless, nutrition is still a logical choice as primary therapy for active CD in selected cases. Patients who tend to respond best are those with newly diagnosed CD involving the terminal ileum with or without the cecum (76). Patients with long-standing disease or extensive colitis appear to respond less favorably. Although steroids usually induce remission, their use, unlike that of nutritional therapy, is associated with loss of mineral bone density and impaired linear growth (77). Another situation favoring diet as primary therapy involves adolescents who refuse to accept a course of corticosteroids due to concerns for cosmetic or other adverse effects (76).

   Major drawbacks to the use of nutritional therapy include its relatively high cost, unpleasant taste, and the monotony of exclusive defined formula diets. The availability of flavor packets has improved the acceptance and oral tolerance of elemental and semielemental formulas and has allowed complete elimination of tube feedings in 60% of our patients. Whatever the choice of formula, the major point is to avoid parenteral nutrition unless the enteral route has failed or is containdicated. Defined formulas are as effective as parenteral nutrition and certainly safer and less costly.

   A multicenter study examined the potential benefits of exclusive enteral nutrition using a semielemental diet on a cyclical basis, 1 out of every 4 months, with low-dose alternate-day prednisone (0.30 mg/kg every other day) for 16 months (78). The group that received intermittent semielemental diet had significantly fewer relapses and markedly improved growth velocity, compared with the group treated with prednisone. In addition to improving symptoms, elemental diets reduce excessive intestinal permeability, reverse the protein-loosing enteropathy, and decrease intestinal and systemic markers of inflammation (79).

The mechanisms of action of nutritional therapy remain unknown. Several theories have been postulated: removal of dietary antigens; reduction of proinflammatory nutrients such as omega-6 fatty acids and nucleotides; altered eicosanoid production, bowel gut hormones, and flora; as well as diminished pancreatic, hepatobiliary, and intestinal secretions (74). Novel formulas including cytokines such as TGF-β or antioxidants are currently under investiation, with promising results.

5.7 Surgery

Unlike UC, CD is not a surgically curable condition. Surgical interventions are thus usually reserved for complication of CD (Table 8). Intractability of symptoms has been reported to imply a poor prognosis postoperatively, with clinical relapse within 1 year in 50% of cases (80). In contrast, patients undergoing surgery for ileal strictures or local abscesses have a 50% recurrence rate after only 5 years. An exploratory surgery may be done in the initial stage of the disease if the patient presents with severe abdominal pain mimicking an acute appendicitis. Indications for elective surgery include intractability of disease, repeated bouts of partial bowel obstruction, or an abscess that fails to respond to conservative measures. Enteroenteric fistulas are usually left alone. Enterovesical fistulas are not absolute indications of operative treatment, although most patients will require surgery eventually. Perianal disease also calls for a conservative approach.

TABLE 8 Primary Surgical Indications in Pediatric Inflammatory Bowel Disease

Crohn's disease	Ulcerative colitis
Failure of medical therapy	Prolonged steroid dependence, intolerance to immunosuppressive agents
Hemorrhage	Hemorrhage
Fulminant colitis with or without toxic megacolon	Fulminant colitis with or without toxic megacolon
Perforation	Perforation
Obstruction of upper and/or lower GI tract	Chronic active, unremitting disease
Fistulas: enteroenteral, enterocutaneous, enterovesical, enterovaginal	
Intractable perirectal disease	
Growth failure	Growth failure
High-grade dysplasia, carcinoma	High-grade dysplasia, carcinoma

Abscesses should be drained and fistulas laid flat or treated with setons when possible. Although surgical resection has not been shown to influence the natural history of CD, successful removal of inflamed bowel can lead to dramatic growth acceleration and attainment of normal adult height. The mechanism of catch-up growth after surgery remains unclear. Many patients may advance through puberty during the postoperative year. Right hemicolectomy, limited small-bowel resection, strictureplasty, and subtotal colectomy with ileostomy are all options, depending on individual circumstances (81).

The greatest distinction of Crohn's colitis and UC is undoubtedly the fact that surgical removal of the entire colon and rectum is curative for UC. The major factors leading to surgery (82) are intractable disease (64%), refractory growth failure (14%), toxic megacolon (6%), hemorrhage (4%), perforation (3%), and cancer prophylaxis (2%). Despite the relative success of CsA and other immunosuppressive agents, it should be recalled that colectomy can be a lifesaving procedure in a child with fulminant colitis or toxic megacolon.

The increased risk of developing colon cancer with onset of UC during childhood is well established. Proctocolectomy in one or two stages has been the most commonly practiced and accepted operation. If rectal involvement is mild, some surgeons prefer to carry out a colectomy and ileoanal anastomosis in one stage. Meticulous supervision of the conserved rectum is mandatory, since it may be a site for cancer development. Successful ileoanal-endorectal anastomosis after total colectomy and a mucosal proctectomy is often acehived. The rectal mucosa is stripped from its muscular wall and the ileal mucosa is sutured on. The creation of a neorectum with an ileal pouch affords decreased stool frequency. This is now the treatment of choice in the pediatric population. An important factor regarding continence is the level at which the ileoanal anastomosis is performed (83).

6 PROGNOSIS

Unlike CD, for which no satisfactory maintentance therapy has been found, the long-term use of sulfasalazine or 5-ASA has significant protective value against disease exacerbations in children with UC. Eventually, surgical intervention can cure UC.

For most children with CD, the disease course is generally one of periodic exacerbations and remissions. Only a minority of patients (5%) have a prolonged remission after initial presentation. Another 5% have perpetual inflammation with severe symptoms that require continual aggressive medical therapy and multiple surgical procedures. Although the causes of most exacerbations remain unclear, intercurrent viral illness seems to be a common precipitating factor. For those patients with long-standing Crohn's disease of the colon, the risk of malignancy is increased, as observed in UC (84).

7 CONCLUSIONS

Advances in our understanding of the underlying pathogenesis of autoimmune disorders have led to major therapeutic inroads using novel approaches. The relatively few new treatment approaches that have been the subject of clinical investigation in adult IBD patients point to the need for properly conducted studies in pediatric IBD. Although nutritional therapy, corticosteroids, and the aminosalicylates have been joined by the increasing use of immunosuppressive drugs (azathioprine, 6-MP, methotrexate, cyclosporine), none of these treatment strategies is ideal for children. Whatever the strategy employed to induce a remission, its completeness and duration through puberty are important factors in achieving optimal growth. A principal aim in the management in pediatric IBD should be to reduce the relapse rate while assuring adequate nutrition and linear growth.

REFERENCES

1. Seidman E. Inflammatory bowel disease. In: Pediatric Clinical Gastroenterology, 4th ed. Roy C, Silverman A, Alagille D, eds. St-Louis: Mosby; 1995; pp 417–493.
2. Logan RFA. Inflammatory bowel disease incidence: up, down or unchanged. Gut 1998; 42:309–311.
3. Chong SKF, Blackshaw AJ, Boyle S, Williams CB, Walker-Smith JA. Histologic diagnosis of chronic inflammatory bowel disease in childhood. Gut 1985; 26:55–59.
4. Ruemmele FM, Targan SR, Levy G, Dubinsky M, Braun J, Seidman EG. Diagnostic accuracy of serological assays in pediatric inflammatory bowel disease. Gastroenterology 1998; 115:822–829.
5. Loftus EV Jr., Silverstein MD, Sandborn WJ, Tremaine WJ, Harmsen WS, Zinsmeister AR. Crohn's disease in Olmsted County, Minnesota, 1940–1993: Incidence, prevalence, and survival. Gastroenterology 1998; 114:1161–1168.
6. Ferguson A. Assessment and management of ulcerative colitis in children. Eur J Gastroenterol Hepatol 1997; 9:858–863.
7. Sonnenberg A, McCarty DJ, Jacobsen SJ: Geographic variation of inflammatory bowel disease within the United States. Gastroenterology 1991; 100:143.
8. Ogunbi SO, Ransom JA, Sullivan K, Schoen BT, Gold BD. Inflammatory bowel disease in African-American children living in Georgia. Pediatrics 1998; 138:103–107.
9. Koletzko S, Sherman P, Corey M, et al: Role of infant feeding practices in development of Crohn's disease in childhood. Br Med J 1989, 298:1617–1618.
10. Thomas GAO, Rhodes J, Green JT: Inflammatory bowel disease and smoking—a review. Am J Gastroenterol 1998, 93:144–149.
11. Timmer A, Sutherland LR, Martin F, and the Canadian Mesalamine for Remission of Crohn's Disease Study Group: Oral contraceptive use and smoking are risk factors for relapse in Crohn's disease. Gastroenterology 1998, 114:1143–1150.
12. Seidman EG, Nutritional management of inflammatory bowel disease. Gastroenterol Clin North Am 1989;18:129–155.

13. Ruemmele F, Roy CC, Levy E, Seidman EG. The role of nutrition in treating pediatric Crohn's disease in the new millennium. J Pediatr 2000; 136:285–291.

14. Seidman EG: Nutritional therapy for Crohn's disease: lessons from the Ste.-Justine Hospital experience. Inflamm Bowel Dis 1997; 3:49–53.

15. Beattie RM, Bentsen BS, Macdonald TT. Childhood Crohn's disease and the efficacy of enteral diets. Nutrition 1998; 14:345–350.

16. Seidman EG, LeLeiko N, Ament M, et al. Nutritional issues in pediatric inflammatory bowel disease. J Pediatr Gastroenterol Nutr 1991;12:424–438.

17. Cohen, MB, Seidman E, Winter H, Colletti R, Kirschner B, Balistreri W, Grand R. Controversies in pediatric inflammatory bowel disease. Inflamm Bowel Dis 1998; 4:203–227.

18. Hollander D, Vadheim C, Brettholz E, Pettersen GM, Delahunty T. Rotter JI. Increased intestinal permeability and inflammation in Crohn's disease. Ann Intern Med 1986; 105:883–885.

19. Dionne S, Ruemmele FM, Seidman EG. Immune pathogensis of IBD, in Inflammatory Bowel Disease. Bistrian BR, Walker-Smith JA, eds. Nestlé Nutrition Workshop Series, Clinical & Performance Programme. Vol 2. Philadelphia: Lippincott-Raven; 1999: 41–57.

20. Fiocchi C. Inflammatory bowel disease: etiology and pathogenesis. Gastroenterology 1998; 115:182–205.

21. Satsangi J, Jewell DP, Bell JI. The genetics of inflammatory bowel disease. Gut 1997; 40:572–574.

22. Brant SR, Yifan F, Fields CT, et al. American families with Crohn's disease have strong evidence for linkage to chromosome 16 but not chromosome 12. Gastroenterology 1998; 115:1056–1061.

23. Roth M-P, Petersen GM, McElree C, Vadheim CM et al. Familial empiric risk estimates of inflammatory bowel disease in Ashkenazi Jews. Gastroenterology 1989; 97:900–904.

24. Mayberry JF, Rhodes J, Newcombe RG: Familial prevalence of inflammatory bowel disease in relatives of patients with Crohn's disease. Br Med J 1980; 280:84.

25. Monson U, Bernell O, Johansson C, et al. Prevalence of inflammatory bowel disease among relatives of patients with Crohn's disease. Scand J Gastroenterol 1991; 26: 302–306.

26. Grandbastien B, Peeters M, Franchimont D, Gower-Rousseau C, et al. Anticipation in familial Crohn's disease. Gut 1998; 42:170–174.

27. Purmann J, Zeidler H, Bertrams J, et al. HLA antigens in ankylosing spondylitis associated with Crohn's disease. Increased frequency of the HLA phenotype B27-B44. J Rheumatology 1988; 15:1658–1661.

28. Graham DY, Markesich DC, Yoshimura HH, Mycobacteria and inflammatory bowel disease. Results of culture. Gastroenterology 1987; 92:436–442.

29. Wakefield AJ, Pittilo RM, Sim R, et al. Evidence of persistent measles virus infection in Crohn's disease. J Med Virol 1993; 39:345–353.

30. Smith MS, Khan K, Bradley NJ, et al. IgG antibodies to measles virus in children with inflammatory bowel disease. Gastroenterology 1994; 107:576–589.

31. Peltola H, Patja A, Leinikki P, Valle M, Davidkin I, Paunio M. No evidence for

measles, mumps, and rubella vaccine-associated inflammatory bowel disease or autism in a 14-year prospective study. Lancet 1998; 351:1327–1328.

32. Wakefield AJ, Murch SH, Anthony A. Ileal-lymphoid-nodular hyperplasia, nonspecific colitis, and pervasive development disorder in children. Lancet 1998; 351:637–640.

33. Yamada T, Grisham MB. Pathogenesis of tissue injury: role of reactive metabolites of oxygen and nitrogen. In Targan SR, Shanahan F., eds: Inflammatory Bowel Disease from Bench to Bedside. Baltimore: William & Wilkins: 1994:133–150.

34. Levy E, Rizwan Y, Thibault L, Lepage G, Brunet S, Bouthillier L, Seidman EG. Altered lipid profile, lipoprotein composition and oxidant and antioxidant status in pediatric Crohn's disease. Am J Clin Nutr 2000; 71:807–815.

35. Murch MW, Chang EB. Diarrhea in Inflammatory Bowel Disease. In Targan SR, Shanahan F, eds: Inflammatory Bowel Disease From Bench to Bedside. Baltimore: William & Wilkins; 1994: 239–254.

36. North CS, Alpers DH, Helzer JE, et al. Do life events or depression exacerbate inflammatory bowel disease? Ann Intern Med 1991; 114:381–386.

37. Hyams JS. Extraintestinal manifestations of inflammatory bowel disease in children. J Pediatr Gastroenterol Nutr 1994; 19:7–21.

38. Levine JB, Lukawski-Trubish D. Extraintestinal considerations in inflammatory bowel disease. Gastroenterol Clin North Am 1995; 24:633–646.

39. Lenaerts C, Roy CC, Vaillancourt M, Weber AM, Morin CL, Seidman E. High incidence of upper GI tract involvement in children with Crohn's disease. Pediatrics 1989; 83:777–781.

40. Saha MT, Ruuska T, Laippala T, Lenko L. Growth of prepubertal children with inflammatory bowel disease. J Pediatr Gastroenterol Nutr 1998; 26:310–314.

41. Hoffenberg E, Fidanza S, Sauaia A: Serologic testing for inflammatory bowel disease. J Pediatr 1999, 134:447–452.

42. Holmquist L, Ahren C, Fällström SP. Relationship between results of laboratory tests and inflammatory activity assessed by colonoscopy in children and adolescents with ulcerative colitis and Crohn's disease. J Pediatr Gastroenterology Nutr 1989; 9:187.

43. Means RT Jr., Krantz SB. Progress in understanding the pathogenesis of the anemia of chronic disease. Blood 1992; 80:1639.

44. Seidman E. Are serological tests for IBD useful to clinicians? Inflamm Bowel Dis 1999; 5:237.

45. Seidman EG, Dubinsky M, Patriquin H, Marx G, Theoret Y: Recent developments in the diagnosis and management of paediatric inflammatory bowel disease. In: Trends in Inflammatory Bowel Disease Therapy 1999. Williams CN et al., eds. Dordrecht, The Netherlands: Kluwer; 2000: 87–95.

46. Herzog D, Bishop N. Gloreiux F, Seidman EG. Interpretation of bone mineral density values in pediatric Crohn's disease. Inflamm Bowel Dis 1998; 4:261–267.

47. Gokhale R, Favus MJ, Karrison T, Sutton M, Rich B, Kirschner BS. Bone mineral density assessment in children with inflammatory bowel disease. Gastroenterology 1998; 114:902–911.

48. Lichtenstein JE. Radiologic pathologic correlation of inflammatory bowel disease. Radiol Clin North Am 1987; 25:3–24.

49. Sheth SG, LaMont JT. Toxic megacolon. Lancet 1998; 351:509–513.
50. Spalinger JH, Patriquin H, Miron M-C, Dubois J, Herzog D, Seidman EG. Doppler sonography in pediatric Crohn's disease: vessel density in the diseased bowel reflects disease activity. Radiology 2000; 217:787–791.
51. Dubinskty MC, Seidman EG, Diagnostic markers of inflammatory bowel disease. Curr Opin Gastroenterol 2000; 16:337–342.
52. Reinisch W, Gasche C, Tillinger W, et al. Clinical relevance of serum interleukin-6 in Crohn's disease: single point measurements, therapy monitoring, and prediction of clinical relapse. Am J Gastroenterol 1999, 94:2156–2164.
53. Herzog D, Delvin E, Seidman EG. Fecal a1-antitrypsin: a marker of intestinal versus systemic inflammation in pediatric Crohn's disease? Inflamm Bowel Dis 1996; 2: 236–243.
54. Saidi T, Mitsuyama K, Toyonaga A, et al. Detection of pro- and anti-inflammatory cytokines in stools of patients with inflammatory bowel disease. Scand J Gastroenterol 1998; 33:616–622.
55. Miki K, Moore DJ, Butler RN, et al. The sugar permeability test reflects disease activity in children and adolescents with inflammatory bowel disease. J Pediatr 1998; 133:750–754.
56. Stein R, Hanauer S. Medical therapy for inflammatory bowel disease. Inflamm Bowel Dis 1999; 28:297–321.
57. Walker-Smith JA. Therapy of Crohn's disease in childhood. Baillière's Clin Gastroenterol 1997; 11:593–610.
58. Del Rosario F, Orenstein SR, Neigut DA, Giarusso V, Wolfson N, Kocoshis SA. Retrospective analysis of alternate-day prednisone as maintenance therapy for Crohns disease. Clin Pediatr 1998; 37:413–419.
59. Rutgeerts P, Lofberg R, Malchow H, et al. A comparison of budesonide with prednisolone for active Crohn's disease. N Engl J Med 1994; 331:842.
60. Sandborn WJ. A review of immune modifier therapy for inflammatory bowel disease: azathioprine, 6-mercaptopurine, cyclosporine and methotrexate. Am J Gastroenterol 1996; 91:423–433.
61. Pearson DC, May GR, Fick GH, Sutherland LR. Azathioprine and 6-mercaptopurine in Crohn's disease. A meta-analysis. Ann Intern Med 1995; 123:132–142.
62. Kirschner B. Safety of azathioprine and 6-mercaptopurine in pediatric patients with inflammatory bowel disease. Gastroenterology 1998; 115:813–821.
63. Dubinsky MD, Lamothe S, Yang HY, Targan SR, Sinnett D, Theoret Y, Seidman EG. Pharmacogenomics and metabolite measurement for 6-mercaptopurine therapy in inflammatory bowel disease. Gastroenterology 2000; 118:705–713.
64. Markowitz J, Grancher BS, Kohn N, et al. A multicenter trial of 6-mercaptopurine and prednisone therapy in newly diagnosed children with Crohn's disease. Gastroenterology 2000; 119:895–992.
65. Mack DR, Young R, Kaufmann SS, Ramey L, Vanderhoof JA. Methotrexate in patients with Crohn's disease after 6-mercaptopurine. Pediatrics 1998; 132:830–835.
66. Cohen RD, Stein R, Hanauer SB. Intravenous cyclosporin in ulcerative colitis: a five year experience. Am J Gastroenterol 1999; 94:1587–1592.
67. Targan SR, Hanauer SB, van Deventer SJ, et al. A short term study of chimeric

monoclonal antibody cA2 to tumor necrosis factor alpha for Crohn's disease. N Engl J Med 1997;337:1029–1035.

68. Present DH, Rutgeerts P, Targan S, et al. Infliximab for the treatment of fistulas in patients with Crohn's disease. N Engl J Med 1999; 340:1398–1405.

69. Sandborn W, Hanauer S. Antitumor necrosis factor therapy for inflammatory bowel disease: a review of agents, pharmacology, clinical results and safety. Inflamm Bowel Dis 1999; 5:119–133.

70. Van Deventer SJ, Elson CO, Fedorak RN. Multiple doses of intravneous IL-10 in steroid-refractory Crohn's disease. Gastroenterology 1997; 113:383–389.

71. Yacyshyn BR, Bowen-Yacyshyn MB, Jewell L, et al. A placebo-controlled trial of ICAM-1 antisense oligonucleotide in the treatment of Crohn's disease. Gastroenterology 1998; 114:1133–1142.

72. Bernstein LH, Frank MS, Brandt LJ, et al. Healing of perianal Crohn's disease with metronidazole. Gastroenterology 1980; 79:357–365.

73. O'Sullivan MA, O'Morain CA. Nutritional therapy in Crohn's disease. Inflamm Bowel Dis 1998; 4:45–53.

74. Ruemmele F, Roy CC, Levy E, Seidman EG. The role of nutrition in treating pediatric Crohn's disease in the new millennium. J Pediatr 2000; 136:285–291.

75. Griffith AM, Ohlsson A, Sherman PM, Sutherland LR. Meta-analysis of enteral nutrition as a primary treatment of active Crohn's disease. Gastroenterology 1995; 108: 1056.

76. Seidman EG. Nutritional therapy for Crohn's disease: lessons from the Ste-Justine Hospital experience. Inflamm Bowel Dis 1997; 3:49.

77. Markowitz J, Grancher K, Rosa J, et al. Growth failure in pediatric inflammatory bowel disease. J Pediatr Gastroenterology Nutr 1994; 16:373.

78. Seidman EG, Jones A, Issenman R, Griffith A. Relapse prevention/growth enhancement in pediatric Crohn's disease: Multicenter randomized controlled trial of intermittent enteral nutrition versus alternate day prednisone. J Pediatr Gastronenterol Nutr 1996; 23:344.

79. Teahon K, Smethurst P, Person M, et al. The effect of elemental diet on permeability and inflammation in Crohn's disease. Gastroenterology 1991; 101:84.

80. Griffith AM, Wesson DE, Shanding B, et al. factors influencing postoperative recurrent of Crohn's disease in childhood. Gut 1991; 32:491–495.

81. Davies G, Evans CM, Shand WS, Walker-Smith JA. Surgery for Crohn's disease in childhood: influence of site and disease and operative procedure on outcome. Br J Surg 1990; 77:891–894.

82. Telander RL. Surgical management of inflammatory bowel disease in children: In Telander R (ed): Problems in General Surgery: Surgical Treatment of Inflammatory Bowel Disease. Philadelphia: Lippincott; 1993.

83. Martin LW, LeCoultre C, Schubert WK. Total colectomy and mucosal proctectomy with preservation of continence. Ann Surg 1977; 186:477–480.

84. Gillen CD, Walmsley RS, Prior P, et al. Ulcerative colitis and Crohn's disease: a comparison of the colorectal cancer risk in extensive colitis. Gut 1993; 34:778.

28

Chronic Diarrhea

John Angus Walker-Smith
University of London, London, England

1 DEFINITIONS

Diarrhea may be defined as the frequent passage of loose stools or, more accurately, as the passage of an increased volume of stool water, stool volume of >200 mL/m^2 of surface area per day indicates the presence of diarrhea. Alternatively, stool weight of >150 to 200 mg/m^2 of surface area per day of watery stool is another definition of diarrhea.

In clinical practice for children, such precise measurements cannot be achieved. Therefore, diarrhea in infancy and early childhood may be defined as an increase in stool frequency associated with a change in the nature of the stool—that is, a change to loose or watery stools. It must be remembered that the normal breast-fed infant may pass frequent loose stools. Yet when a breast-fed infant gets diarrhea, there is a departure from the normal stool pattern, with increase of volume and frequency.

1.1 Chronic Diarrhea

Chronic diarrhea may be defined as diarrhea of more than 2 weeks duration. Chronic diarrhea may be associated with malabsorption of one or more essential nutrients. This usually occurs when there is significant small intestinal mucosal damage or pancreatic exocrine insufficiency. When such malabsorption is severe and persistent, malnutrition may result, with important secondary complications. These include secondary immunocompetence and further impairment of the gastrointestinal function, such as failure of pancreatic secretion.

There are many reasons why chronic diarrhea may be associated with a nutritional deficiency. These include inadequate intake due to anorexia, defective digestion and absorption of digested food with excessive calorie losses in the stools, and finally the less well understood factors related to increased metabolic demands.

When malnutrition is associated with chronic diarrhea, this is most frequently due to disease of the small intestinal mucosa, the major organ of absorption in the body. Delayed growth or failure to thrive may result in infants, especially when chronic diarrhea is accompanied by inadequate nutrient supply of dietary protein, carbohydrate, or fat. The intake of specific nutrients such as zinc may also be of critical importance. The proportion of energy required for growth is highest at birth and falls thereafter. Malnutrition has its greatest effect on growth during the first 3 years of life, as infants have less nutritional reserves. In developed communities, malnutrition due to chronic diarrhea in childhood is now a declining problem, but it remains a major problem in developing communities.

1.2 Pathophysiology

Whether it is acute or chronic, there are two basic mechanisms for diarrhea: secretory and osmotic. Both may occur simultaneously in individual disease entities—e.g., in celiac disease and chronic inflammatory bowel disease.

1.3 Secretory Diarrhea

Secretory diarrhea results from a disturbance in the balance between absorption, which occurs primarily via the villous epithelial cells, and secretion, which occurs primarily via the crypt cells. Absorption of fluid secondary to sodium transport is accompanied by electrogenic and neutral sodium pumps. These pumps are inhibited by second messengers (cylic AMP, cyclic GMP, and calcium), which may be produced by bacterial enterotoxins such as cholera toxin, neurohumoral substances such as vasoactive intestinal peptide (VIP), and inflammatory cell products such as prostaglandins. Active secretion of chloride may also increase with many of the secondary messengers. Other causes of secretory diarrhea include inborn defects of electrolyte transport and congenital defects of bile salt absorption.

1.4 Osmotic Diarrhea

Osmotic diarrhea is caused by the ingestion of solutes that cannot be digested or absorbed (e.g., the indigestible disaccharide lactulose) or by diseases that interfere with absorption of solutes (e.g., lactose intolerance due to lactase deficiency). Carbohydrate malabsorption is the commonest cause of osmotic diarrhea. It may result from a primary deficiency of disaccharidase enzymes or of transport mechanisms such as the glucose-galactose system. However, it is most often the result of a secondary deficiency of disaccharidases as a sequel to small intestinal mucosal disease. In these circumstances the nonabsorbed sugar may be fermented by colonic microflora to produce lactic and other acids, further increasing the osmotic load and irritating the colon. Fat malabsorption is another cause. It may result from pancreatic insufficiency and bile salt depletion in addition to reduced surface area as a consequence of small intestinal enteropathy. Protein-losing enteropathy may occur in states of altered gut permeability, as when there is inflammatory bowel disease or in situations when there is obstruction to lymphatic blood vessels (e.g., lymphangiectasia), and this also contribute to osmotic diarrhea.

2 CAUSES

From a practical clinical perspective, chronic diarrhea in childhood may be classified under the following broad headings (although these categories may overlap, they provide a useful background knowledge for planned investigations):

2.1 Important Causes

Infections—postenteritis syndrome (persistent diarrhea)
Carbohydrate intolerance—primary and secondary
Food-sensitive small intestinal enteropathies—permanent and temporary
Motility disorders—toddler's diarrhea or chronic nonspecific diarrhea
Chronic inflammatory bowel disease—Crohn's disease and ulcerative colitis
Autoimmune enteropathy
Intractable diarrhea syndromes of infancy—e.g., tufting enteropathy and microvillus atrophy
Pancreatic disease—cystic fibrosis and Swachmann's syndrome
Bile salt deficiency—congenital and acquired
Inborn errors of metabolism—primary absorptive defects
Hormonal disorders—Venner-Morrison syndrome (pancreatic cholera)
Surgical causes—massive small intestinal resection and postoperative blind loop syndrome

3 INVESTIGATIONS

3.1 Stool Examination

Observation of the child's stool will show whether it is watery or blood or mucus is present. Watery diarrhea, when chronic, suggests carbohydrate malabsorption,

TABLE 1   Features of Osmotic
and Secretory Diarrhea

	Osmotic	Secretory
Fasting	Stops	Continues
Fecal osmolality	400	280
Na^+	30	100
K^+	30	40
$(Na^+ + K^+) \times 2$	120	280
Solute gap	280	0

while blood and mucus suggest inflammatory bowel disease. Microscopy may be useful to identify leukocytes, suggesting inflammation. It is very important to collect watery stools for the presence of reducing substances and measuring stool pH (1). As modern diapers are very good absorbers of water, it is essential that the stool be collected properly either by placing a urine container over the anus or by doing a rectal examination and catching the stool. The stool should be tested for reducing substances. From a practical standpoint, 1% or more is regarded as abnormal and suggests carbohydrate malabsorption, especially when the stool is acid.

In certain circumstances, such as the severe intractable diarrhea of infancy, the measurement of stool electrolytes may be helpful diagnostically. Table 1 indicates the difference in composition of electrolytes between osmotic and secretory diarrhea.

Fecal elastase is now recognized as a valuable test for the diagnosis of pancreatic disease (2). Fecal alpha-1-antitrypsin is a useful measure for protein-losing enteropathy (3). In the developing world, fecal leukocytes, fecal occult blood and fecal lactoferrin have been used in the workup of patients to identify those children who may have infectious diarrhea and so require microbiological investigation, so that antibiotic therapy may be instituted promptly. A recent met-analysis (4) suggests that fecal lactoferrin is the most accurate test. It has not been evaluated in chronic inflammatory bowel disease.

3.2   Microbiological Studies

Most gastrointestinal infections have cleared up by 2 weeks, but in some cases (e.g., shigellosis), they can become chronic, so stools should be cultured for bacterial pathogens and examined for cysts, ova, and parasites, including *Giardia lamblia*. Stools should be examined for the presence of viruses by electron microscopy or by enzyme-linked immunosorbent assay (ELISA) when there is evidence of immunodeficiency, as in these circumstances chronic viral excretion may occur.

3.3 Hormonal Studies

Circulating hormone and urine levels give important diagnostic information for rare tumors, such as VIPoma, causing hormonal disease (Verner-Morrison syndrome).

3.4 Sweat Test

Cystic fibrosis must be excluded by the performance of a sweat test to detect elevated sweat sodium.

3.5 Hydrogen Breath Tests

Hydrogen in the breath is the result of the breakdown within the intestine of substrates that have been eaten. Normally, after eating, no hydrogen appears in breath for 1 to 3 hr—i.e., until the ingested substrate reaches the bacteria of the colon. An earlier peak occurs if there is abnormal bacterial growth within the small intestinal lumen. Higher-than-normal levels are found when malabsorbed carbohydrates reach the colon.

These tests, therefore, can give information concerning intestinal transit and bacterial overgrowth as well as the absorption of sugar. They are most useful for older children with chronic diarrhea. They are not as useful for children with acute diarrhea or for diagnosis in infants, where estimation of stool reducing substances is more useful, because hydrogen production may be affected in acute diarrhea. Beyond infancy, however, stool reducing substances are not useful because of the efficacy of colonic salvage. Then a lactose hydrogen breath test is useful, especially for the diagnosis of late-onset lactose intolerance (5).

3.6 Hematological Studies

An elevated erythrocyte sedimentation rate (ESR) and C-reactive protein (CRP) level in a child with chronic diarrhea suggests the possibility of chronic inflammatory bowel disease (6). A low ferritin is a valuable indicator of iron deficiency, a frequent accompaniment of celiac disease and inflammatory bowel disease. A full blood count will also provide evidence of anemia, which may occur in such children. Serum and red cell folate are important investigations, but folate deficiency is now uncommon in children. However, when folic acid deficiency occurs, it suggests celiac disease. A high platelet count suggests chronic inflammatory bowel disease.

3.7 Immunological Studies

Immune deficiency may predispose to chronic diarrhea—e.g., IgA deficiency. Therefore serum immunoglobulins, serum IgG subsets, and T-cell subsets are all useful investigations. IgA antiendomysial antibody is very useful for the diagnosis of celiac disease with a high specificity (7). Although there can be false-positive values in infancy (8), IgA deficiency must always be excluded.

3.8 Radiology and Imaging

Barium studies may be very useful in making the diagnosis of Crohn's disease when there is involvement of the terminal ileum or sometimes more extensive small bowel involvement (see Chap. 27). The technique of acceleration and compression is a valuable aid to diagnosis (9,10). Computed tomography (CT) scans may occasionally give diagnostically useful information.

3.9 Small Intestinal Biopsy

This may be performed endoscopically or with the pediatric Crosby capsule (11). Small intestinal biopsy is a vital diagnostic technique for chronic diarrhea in children. Celiac disease still cannot be diagnosed in any other way (12). Children should not be diagnosed as having celiac disease and given a gluten-free diet without a biopsy first. There is a wide range of disorders where the small intestinal mucosa is abnormal (i.e., enteropathy) and they are listed in Table 2.

3.10 Ileocolonoscopy

This technique combined with multiple mucosal biopsies is essential for the diagnosis of both Crohn's disease and ulcerative colitis in childhood (13).

TABLE 2 Causes of Small Intestinal Enteropathy

Age less than 2 years
  Postenteritis enteropathy: infective enteropathy
  Postenteritis enteropathy: food-sensitive enteropathy
  Cow's milk–sensitive enteropathy
  Celiac disease
  Transient gluten intolerance
  Autoimmune enteropathy
  Syndrome of intractable diarrhea
Age more than 2 years
  Celiac disease
  Autoimmune enteropathy
  Crohn's disease

3.11   Postenteritis Enteropathy: Infective Enteropathy

3.11.1   Initial Infection

Postenteritis enteropathy may result from persistent infection that continues to cause damage to the small intestinal mucosa. This is a declining problem in developed countries but is still very important in developing countries (14). The best example is provided by infection with classical enteropathogenic strains of *Escherichia coli* (EPEC). These can produce chronic diarrhea and damage the small intestinal mucosa (Fig. 1). This may occur as "traveler's diarrhea with a vengeance" (15). This concerns children known to be well in the land of their birth (e.g., United Kingdom or United States) but who develop severe diarrhea when taken to their ancestral homeland (e.g., the Indian subcontinent or Mexico), where they may be exposed to new pathogens in a contaminated environment. Small intestinal biopsy in these children shows an enteropathy with clear evidence of infection—for example, on histological section, bacteria may be identified on the surface of the mucosa, adhering to the enterocytes (Fig. 1). In the developing world *E. coli* infection may be the most important cause of postenteritis syndrome.

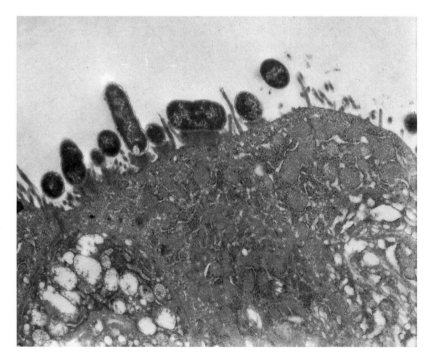

FIGURE 1   Enteropathogenic *E. coli* adhering to surface of enterocyte (electron micrograph).

Cryptosporidiosis is an important cause of this syndrome. It can occur as a primary infection in immunocompetent individuals (16) as well as in those who are immunodeficient, such as AIDS patients.

Persistent small intestinal mucosal inflammation occurs in immunodeficiency, both congenital and acquired syndromes (e.g., AIDS), where, for example, rotavirus as well as *Cryptosporidium* may persist with an enteropathy. Chronic rotavirus infection is always associated with disturbed immune function.

The postenteritis syndrome of infancy and early childhood is distinct from postinfective malabsorption or tropical sprue in adults. Indeed, folate deficiency is not a feature of the postenteritis syndrome in infancy and early childhood, although tropical sprue may occur in older children (17).

3.11.2 Secondary Infection

An enteropathy in a child with the postenteritis syndrome may also be caused by a secondary or acquired infection. For example, Phillips has found astrovirus and adenovirus in the mucosa of children having a biopsy for postenteritis syndrome who presumably have had intercurrent illnesses, accounting for the virus in the abnormal mucosa (14). However the overall clinical picture appears as one continuing illness, and it is only by testing for infective agents in the stools, etc., that intercurrent events will be recognized.

3.12 Postenteritis Enteropathy: Food-Sensitive Enteropathy

There is evidence that some children with a postenteritis enteropathy have a food-sensitive enteropathy (18), most often cow's milk–sensitive enteropathy (i.e., an enteropathy that which responds to elimination of cow's milk (Fig. 2) (see Chap. 25). This is an important cause of chronic diarrhea and failure to thrive in infancy. Again, however, it is becoming less common in western communities, probably both related to declining frequency of gastroenteritis and the development of less sensitizing cow's-milk formulas (19). Small intestinal biopsy remains diagnostically useful in these circumstances (20).

3.13 Celiac Disease

Chronic diarrhea in infancy, especially with failure to thrive that presents some time after the introduction of gluten into the diet, should always suggest the diagnosis of celiac disease (see Chap. 21). In fact, this disorder is the most important cause of severe malnutrition accompanying chronic diarrhea in developed countries (21). Although this classical presentation has been reported to be less common in recent years, it still does occur. While small intestinal biopsy remains the ''gold standard'' for diagnosis combined with a response to a gluten-free diet, screening with antiendomysial antibody has proved to be diagnostically very

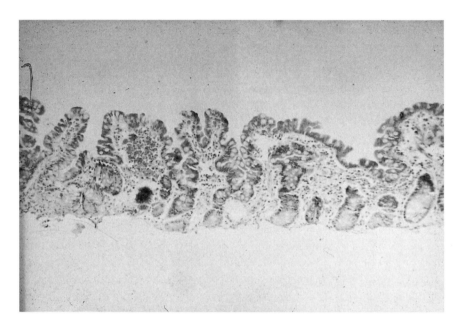

FIGURE 2 Cow's milk–sensitive enteropathy (histology).

useful. This is a permanent food intolerance unlike cow's milk–sensitive enteropathy and transient gluten intolerance; a gluten-free diet is required for life in patients with celiac disease. A further gluten challenge is required only in children who present at less than 2 years of age or who are atypical (12).

3.14 Intractable Diarrhea of Infancy

With the successful use of total parenteral nutrition and, indeed, of home parenteral nutrition, this group of disorders is emerging as a major management problem for pediatric gastroenterologists (22). It is a heterogenous disorder. A number of distinct syndromes have been recognized to cause it. These include microvillous atrophy and tufting enteropathy. There is frequently a genetic aspect, with first-cousin marriages being common in the families of such infants.

3.15 Autoimmune Enteropathy

This is a serious disorder (23) with a high mortality, but in recent times drugs such as cyclosporine and tacrolimus have immeasurably improved the outlook for this rare disorder (24).

3.16   Congenital Heparan Sulphate Deficiency

This rare cause of chronic diarrhea and enteric protein loss is associated with a normal small intestinal mucosa, but there is a congenital absence of the sulfated glycosaminoglycans, which leads to excessive protein leakage into the gut (25).

3.17   Intestinal Lymphangiectasia

This is another rare cause of chronic diarrhea with excess protein loss into the gut. There may be an enteropathy in these children, and dilated lacteals are highly characteristic. Circulating lymphopenia is a feature of the disorder.

3.18   Chronic Inflammatory Bowel Disease

Ulcerative colitis, Crohn's colitis (see Chap. 27), and cow's-milk colitis (see Chap. 25) typically present with chronic bloody diarrhea accompanied by mucus. Once infection with organisms such as *Shigella*, *Salmonella* and *Campylobacter* has been excluded, diagnosis should be successful. Circulating blood markers of inflammation, such as C-reactive protein, are important diagnostically, but ileocolonoscopy with barium studies is the cornerstone of diagnosis.

3.19   Pancreatic Disorders

Cystic fibrosis should always be considered when chronic diarrhea begins in early infancy, especially when accompanied by hypoalbuminemia and frequent chest infections (see Chap. 31). Swachmann's syndrome is a rare disorder involving exocrine pancreatic insufficiency and causing chronic diarrhea with cyclic neutropenia and metaphyseal dysostosis.

3.20   Motility Disorders

So-called toddler's diarrhea or "the peas and carrots" syndrome—better described as chronic nonspecific diarrhea or irritable bowel of infancy—is one of the commonest causes of chronic diarrhea in infancy and early childhood. It most often occurs, as this name implies, in the toddler age group but may occur in infants and persist into later childhood.

The nature of this common and self-limiting syndrome is not clear. The diarrhea is not associated with malabsorption but is related to a decreased mouth-to-anus transit time in an otherwise healthy child (26).

Small intestinal motility studies in such cases have shown that although fasting activity is normal, postprandial activity and its initiation is abnormal (27). Postprandial activity is weaker and short-lived, and MMCs are not disrupted by food—or, indeed, by glucose—as occurs normally. It is known that there is rapid gut transit time in this disorder. Milla (28), therefore, has proposed that this abnormality of migrating myoelectric complexes (MMCs) leads to rapid transit of small intestinal contents into the colon. This causes excess bile salts and partially digested food to enter the colon. It is suggested that further degradation by colonic bacteria might produce hydroxy fatty acids and unconjugated bile salts, which may act as secretogogues and so adversely affect absorption of water and electrolytes from the colon; they may also lead to increased production of prostaglandins. High levels of prostaglandin F in plasma have been found in children with this syndrome (29).

In a study of stool composition in such children, although the total quantities of stool bile acids did not differ from control values, the amount of water in the extractable water phase itself was increased (30). Double-lumen perfusion studies of the jejunum following a 12-hr fast in such children at Great Ormond Street Hospital for Children, London, have shown that the jejunum is not in a secretory state.

Cohen et al. (26) also reported that many of these children have had gastroenteritis or an acute illness immediately preceding or precipitating the onset of chronic diarrhea. This observation accords with that of Tripp et al. (31), who found enzymic changes similar to those observed in toddler's diarrhea in the small intestinal mucosa of children in the recovery phase of the postenteritis syndrome. This does, of course, raise the possibility that some cases are in fact induced by low-grade enteropathy, with the child maintaining weight by increasing intake. Cohen et al. (26) found that some children presenting with this syndrome have a low intake of dietary fat. They claimed that an increased fat intake in such children might lead to a complete resolution of their symptoms and suggested that the mechanism whereby fat consumption alters diarrhea is mediated via an effect on motility. An increased fluid intake has been proposed as a causative mechanism (32).

Burke and Anderson (33) have described this disorder as being responsible for the largest group of young children in developed communities referred for investigation because of persistent or intermittent looseness and frequency of stools. It is indeed the most common cause of chronic diarrhea without failure to thrive in early childhood.

Chronic nonspecific diarrhea usually has its onset between the ages of 6 and 20 months. Often, the child has previously been constipated, and sometimes has had infantile colic. In most children, the diarrhea ceases spontaneously between the ages of 2 and 4 years, sometimes earlier. The stool pattern is typically a large stool early in the day, formed or partly formed, followed by the passage of smaller, looser stools containing undigested vegetable material and mucus. The passage of undigested food is characteristic; indeed, one popular name for the syndrome stemming from this observation is the "peas and carrots syndrome." Despite the diarrhea, the child grows and develops completely normally. However, a severe perineal rash may accompany the diarrhea. Psychosomatic factors may also be important, as suggested by the higher proportion of children coming from families of the professional classes. Occasionally, the mother may become preoccupied with every stool the child passes, the loose stools causing severe anxiety despite the child's evident general well-being. This syndrome may be a cause of profound maternal distress, sometimes sufficient to cause family disharmony and even marital discord. One important social impact is that it may delay the child's ability to get out of diapers, which thus may prevent the child from being accepted for nursery education.

Small intestinal biopsy is indicated only when there is some doubt about the child's nutritional status or the presence of other symptoms (34). However, giardiais and sucrase-isomaltase deficiency can be confused with this disorder. The diagnosis is usually made on strictly clinical grounds.

It is important to differential toddler's diarrhea from cow's milk–sensitivity enteropathy, where the small intestinal mucosa is characteristically abnormal, and also from multiple food allergy. Small intestinal biopsy can be helpful, but it may not discriminate these children from those with multiple food allergy, as the small intestinal mucosa may also be normal in such children. Serum IgE is typically raised, specific radioallergosorbent (RAST) tests may be positive, and there is often eosinophilia in multiple food allergy but these are not features in children with chronic nonspecific diarrhea.

Treatment is usually reassurance and explanation. No specific treatment, either drug or dietetic, is of proven value. However, advice concerning reduction of fluid intake may be helpful when the infant has increased intake. An uncontrolled study of the use of psyllium, a dietary fiber derived from the seeds of the herbs *Plantago psyllium* and *P. indica* (*P. arenaria*), has claimed it to be therapeutically effective (34).

Loperamide has also been advocated and may be given to the child in those cases where maternal distress is severe in a dose of 0.1 mg/kg daily. Hamdi and Dodge (29) showed that loperamide gave symptomatic benefit to some children with this syndrome. The widespread use of antidiarrheal drugs in pediatrics is to be deplored, but occasionally a child with a severe form of this syndrome benefits from a course of loperamide.

3.21 Surgical Disorders

Massive small intestinal resection as a consequence of some surgical disaster, such as volvulus neonatorum occurring in early infancy, is an important cause of chronic diarrhea (see Chap. 29). Likewise, a blind loop syndrome as a sequel to surgery is another important cause.

3.22 Bile Salt Deficiency

This is a rare cause.

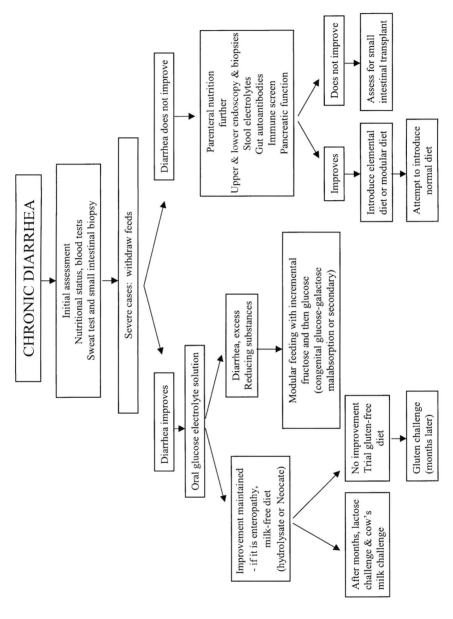

FIGURE 3 Algorithm for the diagnosis and management of chronic diarrhea.

3.23   Congenital Inborn Errors of Metabolism

These include congenital glucose-galactose malabsorption and sucrase-isomaltase deficiency (see Chap. 14). It is especially important to consider glucose-galactose malabsorption in differential diagnosis of chronic diarrhea in the newborn by testing the stools for excess reducing substances.

3.24   Referral to a Specialist

Whenever chronic diarrhea is associated with failure to thrive, referral to a specialist essential. In addition when chronic diarrhea is associated with the passage of blood and mucus. Suspected cow's-milk allergy can be treated by a short trial of a cow's milk–free diet; but if there is no response, again, specialist referral is required. Most cases of chronic nonspecific diarrhea can be managed without a referral.

4   CONCLUSION

Chronic diarrhea in infancy and childhood has many causes. The spectrum of etiology is geographically variable, with infection a more important cause in developing countries. Modern diagnostic techniques permit accurate diagnosis and effective therapy in most cases. There remains a residuum of children with intractable diarrhea where the prognosis is poor or uncertain. A practical approach to the diagnosis and management is presented in Figure 3.

REFERENCES

1. Soeparto P, Stobo EA, Walker-Smith JA. Role of chemical examination of the stool in diagnosis of sugar malabsorption in children. Arch Dis Child 1972; 47(251):56–61.
2. Soldan W, Henker J, Sprossig C. Sensitivity and specificity of quantitative determination of pancreatic elastase 1 in feces of children. J Pediatr Gastroenterol Nutr 1997; 24:53–55.
3. Durie P. Intestinal protein loss and fecal antitrypsin. J Pediatr Gastroenterol Nutr 1985; 4:345–347.
4. Huicho L, Campos M, Rivera J, Guerrant RL. Fecal screening tests in the approach to acute infectious diarrhea—a scientific overview. Pediatric Infect Dis J 1996; 15:486–494.
5. Tolboom JJM, Moteet M, Kabir H, Molatseli P, Fernandes J. Incomplete lactose absorption from breast milk during acute gastroenteritis. Acta Paediatr Scand 1986; 75:151–155.
6. Beattie RM, Walker-Smith JA, Murch SH. Indications for investigation of chronic gastrointestinal symptoms. Arch Dis Child 1995; 73:354–355.

7. Catassi C, Fabiani E. The spectrum of celiac disease in children. Baillieres Clin Gastroenterol 1997; 11(3):485–507.

8. Chan KN, Phillips AD, Mirakian R, Walker-Smith JA. Endomysial antibody screening in children. J Pediatr Gastroenterol Nutr 1994; 18:316–320.

9. Lipson A, Bartram CI, Williams CB, Slavin S, Walker-Smith JA. Barium studies and ileoscopy compared in children with suspected Crohn's disease. Clin Radiol 1990; 41:5–8.

10. Halligan S, Nicholls S, Bartram CI, Walker-Smith JA. The distribution of small bowel Crohn's disease in children compared to adults. Clin Radiol 1994; 49:314–316.

11. Thomson M, Kitching P, Jones A, Walker-Smith JA, Phillips A. Are endoscopic biopsies of small bowel as good as suction biopsies for diagnosis of enteropathy? J Pediatr Gastroenterol Nutr 1999; 29(4):438–441.

12. Walker-Smith JA, Guandalini S, Schmitz J, Shmerling DH, Visakorpi JK. Revised criteria for diagnosis of celiac disease. Arch Dis Child 1990; 65:909–911.

13. Chong SKF, Bartram C, Campbell CA, Williams CB, Blackshaw AJ, Walker-Smith JA. Chronic inflammatory bowel disease in childhood. BMJ 1982; 284:101–104.

14. Phillips AD. Mechanisms of mucosal injury: human studies in viruses and the gut. In: Farthing MJ, ed. Proceedings of 9th BSG and SK&F Workshop, 1988.

15. Hutchins P, Hindocha P, Phillips A, Walker-Smith JA. Traveler's diarrhea with a vengeance in children of UK immigrants visiting their parental homeland. Arch Dis Child 1982; 57:208–211.

16. Phillips AD, Thomas AG, Walker-Smith JA. Cryptosporidium, chronic diarrhea and the proximal small intestinal mucosa. Gut 1992; 33:1057–1062.

17. Walker-Smith JA. Pediatric problems in tropical gastroenterology. Gut 1994; 35:1687–1690.

18. Walker-Smith JA. Gastrointestinal food allergy in childhood: current problems. Nutr Res 1992; 12:123–135.

19. Walker-Smith JA. Cow's milk sensitive enteropathy: predisposing factors and treatment. J Pediatr 1992; (suppl):111–115.

20. Walker-Smith JA. Diagnostic criteria for gastrointestinal food allergy in childhood. Clin Exp Allergy 1995; 25(suppl 1):20–23.

21. Murch SH, Walker-Smith JA. The immunology of coeliac disease. Annales Nestlé 1993; 51:59–65.

22. Walker-Smith JA. Intractable diarrhea in infancy: a continuing challenge for the pediatric gastroenterologist. Acta Paediatrica Suppl 1994; 395:12–14.

23. Unsworth DJ, Hutchins P, Mitchell J, Phillips A, Hindocha P, Holborrow EJ, Walker-Smith JA. Flat small intestinal mucosa and autoantibodies against the gut epithelium. J Pediatr Gastroenterol Nutr 1982; 1:503–515.

24. Bousvaros A, Leichtner AM, Book L, Shigeoka A, Bildeu J, Samea F, Ruchee E, Mulberry A. Intestinal and pediatric autoimmune enteropathy with tacrolimus (FK506). Gastroenterology 1996; 111:237–240.

25. Murch SH, Winyard PJ, Koletzko S, Wehner B, Cheema HA, Risdon RA, Phillips AD, Meadows N, Klein NJ, Walker-Smith JA. Congenital enterocyte heparan sulphate deficiency with massive albumin loss, secretory diarrhea, and malnutrition. Lancet 1996; 347(9011):1299–301.

26. Cohen SA, Hendricks KM, Mathis RK, et al. Chronic non-specific diarrhea: dietary relationships. Pediatrics 1979; 64:402–407.
27. Fenton TR, Harries JT, Milla PJ. Disordered small intestinal motility: a rational basis for toddler's diarrhea. Gut 1983; 24:897–903.
28. Milla PJ. Motor disorders including pyloric stenosis. In: Walker WA, Durie PR, Hamilton JR, Walker-Smith JA, Watkins JR, eds. Pediatric Intestinal Disease, 2nd ed. St Louis: Mosby, 1996, pp 543–555.
29. Hamdi I, Dodge JA. Prostaglandins in non-specific diarrhea. Acta Paediatr Belg 1978; 31:106.
30. Jonas A, Diver-Haber A. Stool output and composition in the chronic non-specific diarrhea syndrome. Arch Dis Child 1982; 57:35–39.
31. Tripp JH, Muller DP, Harries JT. Mucosal (Na+-K+)-ATPase and adenylate cyclase activities in children with toddler diarrhea and the postenteritis syndrome. Pediatr Res 1980; 14(12):1382–1386.
32. Greene HL, Gishon FK. Excessive fluid intake as a cause of chronic diarrhea in young children. J Pediatr 1983; 102:836–840.
33. Burke V, Anderson CM. The irritable colon syndrome. In: Anderson CM, Burke V, eds. Pediatric Gastroenterology. Oxford: Blackwell, 1975; pp 469–489.
34. Smalley JR, Klish WJ, Campbell MA, Brown HR. Use of psyllium in the management of chronic non-specific diarrhea of childhood. J Pediatr Gastroenterol Nutr 1982; 361–363.

29

Short Bowel Syndrome

Jon A. Vanderhoof
University of Nebraska Medical Center, Omaha, Nebraska

Rosemary J. Young
Creighton University, Omaha, Nebraska

1 INTRODUCTION

Short bowel syndrome is not common in pediatrics; however, it presents those involved in the care of these patients with challenges that include alleviating symptoms, preventing nutritional deficiencies, and ensuring adequate growth and development. The pediatric patient with short bowel syndrome has numerous unique physical and psychological requirements above and beyond those of the adult patient. Short bowel syndrome is not anatomically defined. The generally accepted functional definition of short bowel syndrome implies malabsorption of nutrients, fluids, and/or electrolytes in the presence of a shortened small intestine (1). Numerous strides, both medically and surgically, have markedly improved the prognosis.

The small intestine is derived from the embryonic midgut and begins growing rapidly in length at the fifth week of gestation. The intestinal lengthening exceeds the rate of growth of the embryonic body; therefore it grows outside the abdomen until the 10th week (2). Term infants are thought to have a length of small bowel between 200 and 250 cm (3), with the mean adult length being approximately 620 cm (4). However, radiological measurement in adults undergoing small bowel enteroclysis have suggested a lesser mean length (5).

Massive small bowel resection most often occurs in the neonatal period. The ileum and the colon are the most frequently resected; however, varying degrees of jejunal removal occur as well. The remaining small bowel begins to adapt almost immediately. The length of bowel remaining correlates poorly with the development of malabsorptive diarrhea. The remaining length of intestine, therefore, cannot be relied upon solely for determining prognosis, as many other factors such as innervation, hormonal effects, and bacteria present in the bowel will affect adaptation.

Parenteral nutrition was previously the mainstay of therapy, permitting patients with shortened small intestine to live for extended periods of time beyond the functional capability of the remaining intestine. It has now been relegated to a supplementary role by improved enteral feeding techniques. Patients rarely suffer the complications of parenteral nutrition, but with the help of intense enteral nutrition techniques, they often attain near-normal eating patterns as therapy progresses. Intestinal and liver transplantation have also become options for those previously unable to adapt completely to enteral nutrition, allowing for discontinuation of total parenteral nutrition (TPN) and resolution of irreversible TPN-related liver disease.

Numerous controversial issues exist regarding the management of the pediatric patient with short bowel syndrome. Studies done in adults with short bowel syndrome do not easily translate into pediatric care; however, controlled trials in this group of children are often ethically difficult. Placebo-controlled trials are also limited by lack of adequate numbers of patients. Table 1 lists controversial issues in the care of the pediatric patient with short bowel syndrome.

This chapter reviews the causes of short bowel syndrome in pediatrics, the intestinal adaptation process, and interventions in both the initial and later phases of nutritional care. Complications and troubleshooting methods for both phases, as well as associated preventative techniques, are reviewed. Presentation of the rationale for interventions will clarify methods necessary to optimize adaptation.

TABLE 1 Controversial Issues

Method of enteral feeding (devices, route, timing)
Enteral formula type
Initiation of enteral feeding
Initiation of oral feedings (types, amount, timing)
Parenteral nutrition additives (i.e., carnitine)
Enteral formula additives (i.e., glutamine)
Dietary supplement additives (i.e., growth hormone)

2 ETIOLOGY

Short bowel syndrome in children may occur either congenitally or, more commonly, may follow intestinal resection in anatomically normal infants (Table 2). Congenital anomalies include congenital short bowel syndrome, atresias anywhere in the intestine, either isolated or multiple, and gastroschisis with associated intestinal shortening. Meconium ileus or plugging may result in necrosis due to mechanical distention of the bowel. Volvulus may also occur, especially in children with rotational anomalies. The largest number of patients, however, are those children who undergo resection due to necrotizing enterocolitis. The cause of necrotizing enterocolitis is not well understood; it affects mostly premature infants. Ischemic injury to the small intestine results in nonviable bowel, most often the ileum or proximal colon (6,7). Postulated causes include protein allergy, abnormal immunological response to bacteria, and ischemia. Conditions resulting in intestinal resection and short bowel syndrome in older children include Crohn's disease, tumors, radiation enteritis, and occasionally Hirschsprung's disease involving the small intestine.

Ideally, therapy for short bowel syndrome must be rooted in the knowledge of pathophysiological changes that result from resection of small intestine. The most obvious change is the overall loss of absorptive surface area; however, the inherent characteristics of the remaining small intestine are crucial in determining the functional ability of the bowel to adapt. Most commonly, the ileum and colon are resected, leaving a large portion of jejunum, often with only limited colon. The jejunal epithelium differs significantly from the ileum in that it is relatively porous, allowing free and rapid flux of water and electrolytes. It is a primary site of nutrient absorption, with characteristically long villi creating the large absorptive surface area. Most carbohydrate, protein, and water-soluble vitamins are absorbed in the upper 200 cm of jejunum. Fat absorption occurs over a larger area, with the distance increasing as intake is increased (8). The jejunum has a high concentration of enzymes and transport carrier proteins. Many small molecules and fluids are absorbed in the jejunum through the paracellular pathway,

TABLE 2 Etiology of Pediatric Short Bowel Syndrome

Congenital	Acquired
Short bowel	Necrotizing enterocolitis
Intestinal atresias	Volvulus
Gastroschisis	Tumors
Apple peel/Christmas tree deformity	Radiation enteritis
Hirschsprung's disease involving ileum	Crohn's disease
and colon	Mesenteric vascular occlusion
	Trauma

consisting of tight junctions or pores between the epithelial cells. The diameter of the pores is greatest in the jejunum and gradually decreases from proximal to distal small bowel. Therefore flux of fluid between the lumen and plasma can be relatively large, depending on the osmotic state of nutrients and fluid in the bowel. A rapid infusion of a hyperosmolar solution results in a flux of fluid from the plasma to the lumen to equalize the osmotic gradient (9,10). Normally, this fluid would be reabsorbed in the ileum and the colon via electrolyte transport, causing reabsorption of the fluid through solvent drag. In these areas, the porous structures between the cells are much smaller, significantly reducing the potential for back diffusion.

Retention of the colon generally improves prognosis. The colon efficiently absorbs sodium, so sodium depletion is unusual unless the colon is either resected or not utilized. The colon also absorbs short-chain fatty acids, which are an energy source, salvaging otherwise lost calories from malabsorbed carbohydrates. Unfortunately, the presence of malabsorbed long-chain fats and bile salts in the colon may result in watery diarrhea and increased oxalate absorption, with subsequent development of renal stones.

The ileum has less nutrient absorptive capacity but a much tighter epithelium with less porous junctions, thereby allowing more efficient absorption of fluid and electrolytes than the jejunum. The main nutrient absorbed from the ileum is the vitamin B_{12} intrinsic factor complex. Bile salts are also absorbed in the ileum through site-specific receptors. Therefore, loss of the ileum often results in vitamin B_{12} deficiency and chronic bile acid malabsorption with eventual bile-salt insufficiency with associated fat and fat-soluble vitamin malabsorption.

Peptides that regulate gastrointestinal motility are produced in the ileum. Peptide YY and enteroglucagon, thought to slow gut motility and reduce gastric emptying, are produced in the ileum (11). They are released when malabsorbed fat reaches the ileum. Loss of larger portions of the ileum results in a disruption of this mechanism and malabsorption is increased. Trophic gastrointestinal hormones such as neurotensin, epidermal growth factor, and insulin-like growth factor 1 (IGF-1) are also produced by the ileal mucosa, so ileal resection may decrease the potential for adaptation induced by these hormones (12).

The ileum has been shown to develop some jejunal functions of nutrient absorption. However, the jejunum cannot adapt to ileal functions. Therefore, deficiencies of bile acids and vitamin B_{12} will be lifelong problems in any patient with significant ileal resection. Although a primary resection of the ileum alone is associated with significant watery diarrhea, loss of the jejunum initially may result in more significant nutrient malabsorption until the ileum adapts.

The loss of the ileocecal valve results in greater flux of bacteria from the large to the small bowel. The valve also regulates the exit of fluid and malabsorbed nutrients from the small intestine, and, although this is thought to be a major factor in regulating bowel transit, other adaptive changes can often compensate for valve loss. Attempts to increase transit time with either medications or surgical procedures have often resulted in exacerbations of bacterial overgrowth. Small bowel bacterial overgrowth (SBBO) may become so serious that complications—including nutrient malabsorption, mucosal inflammation, and systemic inflammatory symptoms such as arthritis—occur. As bowel dilatation occurs during the adaptive process, gastrointestinal transit times from the stomach through the large bowel usually decrease over time.

3 CLINICAL MANAGEMENT

The most obvious problem to be dealt with in the treatment of short bowel syndrome is the diarrhea and subsequent dehydration and/or nutrient losses. A multistage process utilizing numerous therapies must be undertaken concurrently to provide the best circumstances for intestinal adaptation, allowing for eventual weaning of parenteral nutrition. Careful measures must also be followed to prevent complications associated with treatment. Table 3 summarizes the clinical management of pediatric short bowel syndrome.

3.1 Initial Phase

In most instances, parenteral nutrition is the primary source of nutrition early in therapy. The solution can often be a relatively standard mix providing nutrients and calories according to patient age and size (see Tables 4, 5, and 6). Depending on the location of the resection, the immediate postoperative period is characterized by aggressive need for monitoring fluid and electrolyte status with administration of appropriate replacement solution. Replacement fluids can be prescribed by monitoring stool or ostomy output for electrolyte content and replacing the amount of fluid loss milliliter for milliliter according to losses accrued in the

TABLE 3 Clinical Management of Short Bowel Syndrome

Parenteral nutrition	Enteral nutrition	Oral dietary therapy
Correct fluid and electrolyte imbalances	Begin as soon as possible	Initiate solids at age-appropriate time
Replete nutritional deficiency states	Initially use elemental diet containing adequate long-chain fats	Provide both macro- and micronutrient-containing foods
Wean as enteral nutrition is advanced	Administer feeding by continuous infusion	Provide low-glycemic-index foods
	Wean parenteral nutrition as enteral nutrition is advanced	

TABLE 4   Caloric Requirements—
Average Energy Requirements for
the Different Age Groups (kcal/kg/
day)

Age Group	Energy
Premature infants	120–150
Neonates	100–120
1–12 months	100
1–6 years	75–90
7–12 years	60–75
13–18 years	30–60
Adult	30–40

TABLE 5   Maintenance Pediatric Parenteral Nutrition Solution

Nutrient	Infants/toddlers	Children	Adolescents
Calories	80–120	60–90	30–75
Dextrose (mg/kg/day)	5–10	5–10	8–11
Protein (g/kg)	2.0–3.0	1.5–2.5	1.0–2.5
Fat (g/kg)	0.5–3.0	1.0–2.5	1.0–2.5
Sodium (mEq/kg)	2–5	2–5	60–150 mEq/day
Potassium (mEq/kg)	2–5	2–5	70–180 mEq/day
Chloride (mEq/kg)	2–5	2–5	60–150 mEq/day
Magnesium (mEq/kg) (125 mg/mEq)	0.25–1.0	0.25–1.0	8–32 mEq/day
Calcium (mEq/kg) (20 mg/mEq)	0.5–4.0	0.5–3.0	10–40 mEq/day
Phosphorus (mMol/kg) (31 mg/mMol)	0.5–2.0	0.5–2.0	9–30 mMol/day
Zinc (µg/kg)	50–250	50 (5 µg/day)	5000 µg/day (350 µg/kg/day)
Copper (µg/kg)	20	20 (300 µg/day)	300 µg/day (60 µg/kg/day)
Chromium (µg/kg/day)	0.20	0.20 (5 µg/day)	10–15 µg/day
Manganese (µg/kg/day)	1.0	1.0 (50 µg/day)	10–15 µg/day
Selenium (µg/kg/day)	2.0	2.0 (30 µg/day)	30–60 µg/day
Molybdenum (µg/kg/day)	0.25	.025 (5 µg/day)	20–120 µg/day
Iodide (µg/kg/day)	1.0	1.0 (50 µg/day)	150 µg/day
Pediatric multivitamin	1–3 kg:3.3 mL/day	3–39 kg:5 mL/day	>40 kg: use adult MVI
Iron	100 µg/kg/day	1.0 µg/day	1–3 µg/day

Key: MVI, multiple vitamin infusion.
Source: Modified from Ref. 42.

preceding 2 hr. Electrolytes of the secreted fluid assessed on a daily basis determine the type of replacement fluid to be ordered. It is not uncommon for high sodium losses to necessitate 80 to 100 mEq/L of sodium in this parenteral replacement solution to maintain fluid and electrolyte homeostasis. Replacing fluids with a solution separate from the parenteral nutrition solution and adjusting the rate of the replacement solution up and down as needed while concurrently giving the standard parenteral nutrition will ensure metabolic stability during the early phase of therapy. This will also be more economical than frequent alterations in parenteral nutrition.

Replacement of basic nutritional deficiency states, including proteins, vitamins, and minerals, is the initial role of the parenteral nutrition solution. Therefore, nutritional deficiency states at this time are relatively uncommon. The parenteral nutrition should replace nutrients and energy stores depleted during the stress of surgery and transient postoperative period of ileus (see Table 7). Parenteral nutrition should be carefully monitored via nutritional assessment, both clinically and via laboratory parameters, to ensure adequate nutritional rehabilitation during this time (see Tables 8 and 9).

When fluid and electrolyte losses have diminished, enteral feeding is begun. Most commonly, elemental diets delivered via continuous enteral infusion are utilized (1,13–14). Enteral nutrition is started very slowly. A dilute concentration is utilized initially and increased to .67 kcal/mL for infants less than 1 year of age or to 1.0 kcal/mL in older patients. Once the final concentration is achieved, the volume of enteral feeding is gradually increased. The initial advancement of concentration rather than rate in enteral feeding solution allows the transition from parenteral to enteral feeding without overloading the patient with fluid (14). Unless enteral feeding results in severe fluid depletion and loss of electrolytes, aggressive attempts at enteral delivery must be tested. Delivering even 0.25 cal/

TABLE 6 Standard Pediatric Total Parenteral Nutrition Solution

20%	Dextrose
2.5%	Amino acids
15 mEq/L	NaCl
15 mEq/L	Na acetate
20 mEq/L	K_3PO_4
10 mEq/L	Ca gluconate
5 mEq/L	Mg SO_4
2 mg/kg/day	PTE solution
5 mL/day	Pediatric vitamin solution

Key: PTE, pediatric trace elements.

TABLE 7 Metabolic Activity Factor
for Different Disease Conditions

Condition	Multiplication factor[a]
Fever	1.1–1.3
Failure to thrive	1.2–2.0
Elective surgery	1.0–1.1
Fractures	1.1–1.3
Severe infections	1.2–1.6
Burns	1.5–2.1
Cardiac disease	1.1–1.3
Crohn's disease	1.0–1.4
Short bowel syndrome	1.2–1.3

[a] Above basal energy requirements.

mL at 1 mL/hr may be beneficial to newborns in attempting to achieve intestinal adaptation.

Continuous enteral infusion may be a bit cumbersome, especially for patients in the home setting, but it has numerous advantages over bolus feeding. Continuous feeding is better tolerated in many respects and ultimately permits a greater percentage of total nutritional requirements to be delivered by the enteral route. Emesis is also reduced with continuous feeding (1,14). Use of continuous enteral infusion, given aggressively, results in stimulation of the enterocytes for adaptation and allows for carrier proteins to be continuously saturated, with max-

TABLE 8 Laboratory Monitoring of Pediatric Patients on Home Parenteral Nutrition

CBC with differential	Weekly × 2, then biweekly × 2, then monthly × 3, then every 3 months
Protime and PTT	Monthly
Electrolytes with pH and venous CO_2	Weekly × 2, then biweekly × 2, then monthly × 3, then every 3 months
Chemistry profile with magnesium and triglycerides	Weekly × 2, then biweekly × 2, then monthly × 3, then every 3 months
Fe, TIBC, ferritin	Monthly
D-lactate	Baseline first month, then PRN
Zinc	Baseline first month, then PRN
Selenium	Baseline first month, then PRN
B_{12} and folate	Baseline first month, then PRN

TABLE 9 Laboratory Monitoring of Pediatric Patients with Short Bowel Syndrome After TPN Is Discontinued

CBC with differential	Every 3 months × 1 year, then every 6 months
Electrolytes with pH and venous CO_2	Monthly × 3, then every 3 months
Chemistry profile with magnesium and triglycerides	Monthly × 3, then every 3 months
Fe, TIBC, ferritin, B_{12}, and folate[a]	Every 3 months × 2, then every 6 months
D-lactate	Every 3 months × 2, then every 6 months
Zinc, chromium, copper manganese and selenium[a]	Every 6 months
Vitamins A, E, and 25-hydroxy vitamin D	3 months after TPN discontinued, then every 6 months
Carnitine	Once a year

[a] Assuming baseline values were obtained on TPN.

imization of the overall functional workload of the intestine. As enteral nutrition reduces the demand for parenteral nutrition, the associated risk factors, which are the major causes of morbidity and mortality in patients with short bowel syndrome, are reduced.

Although continuous enteral feeding may be inconvenient, development of new portable enteral infusion pumps and backpacks permit children to have reasonable mobility as they grow and develop physically. Backpacking pumps on toddlers should not be utilized until they are walking independently. Caregivers can, however, utilize backpack devices attached to strollers and infant carriers.

Enteral feedings initially are given to enhance intestinal adaptation. The adaptation process begins within 24 to 48 hr after intestinal resection (12). The process begins with production of new enterocytes in the crypts, with gradual lengthening of the villi resulting in increased absorptive area. As the cells mature, absorptive capacity is increased. The ileum normally has shorter villi and reduced surface area relative to the jejunum when normally exposed to fewer nutrients in the physiological state. The ileum, however, has a greater capacity for adaptation than the jejunum and undergoes hyperplasia with greater nutrient exposure. Mucosal hyperplasia does not occur without enteral nutrition and, in fact, significant atrophy of the remaining small bowel mucosa may take place (15).

Nutrients stimulate adaptation via direct contact with the mucosal epithelium. When the workload of the epithelium is increased, greater autocrine and paracrine secretion of trophic substances occurs, which stimulates cell proliferation. Enteral nutrition also increases gastrointestinal secretions from the stomach, liver, pancreas, and small intestine, which themselves are trophic to the small bowel. Gastrointestinal hormones stimulated by enteral nutrition and secreted into the bloodstream also enhance adaptation. Numerous hormones such as enteroglucagon, neurotensin, epidermal growth factor, IGF-1, GLP-2, and even gastrin are likely involved (16,17). High levels of peptide YY may play a role in slowing gastric emptying as part of the "colonic brake" phenomenon (11).

Initially, patients with short bowel syndrome are given elemental or protein hydrolysate diets (18). Elemental (amino acid) formulas are available for pediatric use and have been formulated to deliver all necessary nutrients for infants. Well-balanced elemental formulas for the older child and adult also exist. Protein hydrolysate formulas may be tolerated, as most protein is absorbed in the form of di- and tripeptides. Elemental formulas are beneficial in reducing the risk of secondary protein intolerance (allergy), as many infants are intolerant of hydrolyzed cow's-milk protein. Carbohydrates in the enteral formulas are present, usually from one or more sources, including partially hydrolyzed starch and disaccharidases such as sucrose. Medium-chain fats are probably not beneficial despite their ease of absorption. They are only slightly better absorbed than long-chain fats. Their lower caloric density, greater osmotic load, and lack of positive effect on gut adaptation limits their usefulness. Since long-chain fats are more trophic to the small intestine than medium-chain fats, a mixture of both is most beneficial (18,19).

Commercially available elemental formulas such as Neocate, Neocate 1+, Pediatric Vivonex, or Elecare provide a balanced source of nutrition without potential allergic complications. These formulas are readily utilized and result in few complications due to the enteral nutrient choice. Commercially available protein hydrolysate formulas such as Alimentum (Ross Products) and Pregestimil and Nutramigen (Mead Johnson) have a relatively high fat content, reducing the osmotic load in the small intestine. The increased fat content of these formulas is also beneficial because of the stimulatory effect of fat on adaptation in the small intestine.

Low-fat, high-carbohydrate diets may be beneficial in decreasing oxalate absorption and decreasing calcium and magnesium losses, which are greater on a high-fat diet (20). In older infants and toddlers, fiber-supplemented complex formulas may be well tolerated, providing a firmer stool, along with the beneficial effects of the production of short-chain fatty acid, which provide additional calories and enhance intestinal adaptation. Formulas designed for adults may be used in older children. Pulmocare (Ross Products), originally designed for adults experiencing respiratory complications, is a high-fat, low-carbohydrate formula that may be beneficial in some children who are experiencing complications of bacterial overgrowth. Carbohydrates in any formula enhance bacterial growth, provide more substrate for bacterial fermentation, and increase the osmotic load in the bowel. Formula choices will vary as the child grows, but knowledge of the remaining intestinal anatomy will facilitate the decision.

Continuous enteral infusion is gradually advanced based on several parameters. A marked increase in stool loss by more than 50% is usually a contraindication to advancing enteral feedings. Likewise, stool losses greater than 40 to 50 mL/kg/day or ostomy output strongly positive for reducing substances suggest that enteral feeding advancement should be slowed. In patients with an intact large bowel, a decrease in stool pH below 5.5 is frequently indicative of carbohydrate malabsorption, and further advances in enteral feedings at this time will result in increases in osmotic diarrhea.

Even in the infant who has undergone extensive intestinal resection, bolus nipple feedings in very small volumes of the prescribed enteral formula are utilized to simulate normal developmental stages of feeding. Oral electrolyte solutions may be substituted for enteral formulas or used to dilute the selected formula if the infant has high-volume fluid losses. Ten to fifteen milliliters of solution two to three times a day may be beneficial in preventing feeding aversion at a later time. At any point, if stool losses are significant, nipple feeding may be discontinued. However, it also fosters infant/caregiver bonding, which often normally occurs during feeding time.

3.2 Later Phases

In most situations, parenteral nutrition at this stage is provided at home at significantly reduced cost savings with few complications, allowing the child to grow and develop in a more normal psychosocial environment (21). Parenteral feeding is weaned proportionately to advancement of enteral nutrition. Compensation for malabsorbed enteral calories will alter the parenteral calories required. Efforts to identify relative amounts of malabsorption (i.e., stool fat) are not helpful. Monitoring of the overall rate of weight gain is the most beneficial tool. At later stages, maintenance parenteral nutrition solutions are utilized, with infrequent monitoring of macro- and micronutrients. It is often tempting at this stage to rapidly wean parenteral nutrition in anticipation of discontinuing intravenous therapy as enteral nutrition is advanced. Often, a child may be successfully weaned from parenteral nutrition during the school-age years, only to require supplemental parenteral nutrition to maintain a normal rate of growth during puberty.

Parenteral nutrition can often be given intermittently in later stages, as enteral feedings are tolerated. At first, the parenteral nutrition infusion time per day is weaned. As the child gets older, higher total parenteral nutrition (TPN) infusion rates are tolerated and help to shorten infusion times. Monitoring of blood glucose levels and for symptoms associated with intravenous fluid under- and overloading is required. Once the total volume and/or the number of hours infused is low, intravenous infusions can be eliminated one or two nights per week. The subsequent number of days off can gradually be advanced as enteral nutrition continues to be tolerated. This entire process is very gradual and individualized and may take months or years to complete. There is an occasional child who is able to wean from parenteral nutrition but still suffers severe fluid and electrolyte losses, requiring intravenous fluid supplementation. These children do not require continuous infusion and can receive fluid replacement therapy overnight.

As a child approaches the toddler and school-age years, constant infusions of enteral feedings are difficult to maintain. While beneficial in enhancing adaptation and allowing the best absorption and utilization of nutrients, these often become somewhat cumbersome and esthetically unpleasant for the child. Additionally, due to improved control over gastric emptying and gut motility, the beneficial effects of continuous enteral infusion diminish with age.

Enteral feeding solutions at this stage should not be concentrated beyond 0.67 kcal/mL so as to avoid an excessive osmotic load in the small bowel, resulting in subsequent fluid losses. Attempts to advance enteral nutrition should be continuously tried as long as stool volumes do not increase excessively. Carbohydrate malabsorption is evidenced by glucose in the stool or, in those with an intact colon, a stool pH below 5. Lactose restriction is not necessary (22). Changes made in feedings should be isocaloric, as the caloric densities of parenteral and enteral nutrition often differ. Caloric requirements are gradually altered, based both on the child's rate of growth and estimated caloric needs, to ensure obtainment of appropriate growth percentiles for both height and weight. Excessive parenteral caloric administration may occur at this stage, as the child may be incapable of regulating his or her own nutrient intake. The medical team must carefully monitor growth to make certain that the child's height, weight, and height-for-weight ratio are appropriate. Use of a dedicated medical professional who is in constant contact with the child and caregivers is a key factor in the success of adequate progression through all phases of nutritional support.

Normal developmental stages of eating involving both chewing and swallowing should be initiated if the child is developmentally ready, even in those infants who may tolerate very few enteral calories or have enteral tubes in place. Pacifier use is not sufficient to meet these needs and, if normal feeding practices are delayed, may result in feeding refusal behaviors (see Chap. 13). While solid-food feedings are traditionally initiated with high-carbohydrate foods, children with short bowel syndrome do better with high-fat, high-protein foods. Meats are probably the best food group to initiate, as they provide less osmotic load to the small intestine and the fat provides an additional stimulant for intestinal adaptation. Ongoing monitoring of enteral tolerance continues during this time, and alterations in the amount or food type utilized are made as indicated. It may be more difficult to monitor stool-reducing substances of pH when solid foods

TABLE 10 Dietary Supplements

Supplement	Proposed mechanism/effect
Menhaden oil and/or arachidonic acid	Prostaglandin synthesis, trophic hormone secretion
Glutamine (nonessential amino acid)	Substrate for small bowel oxidative metabolism
	Mucosal hyperplasia
	Prevention of bacterial translocation by maintaining normal permeability
Growth hormone	Stimulates crypt cell production
	Mucosal hyperplasia
Short-chain fatty acids (acetate, propionate, and butyrate)	Butyrate production—a preferred substrate for energy metabolism in colonocytes
	Provision of 5–10% of daily energy requirements

are initiated. A certain level of malabsorption may be acceptable and tolerated as long as the child remains well hydrated, grows, and suffers no complications.

As enteral nutrition becomes the primary delivery mode, the child should be monitored more frequently for macro- and micronutrient deficiencies. This becomes particularly important as enteral tube feeding is weaned in exchange for oral nutrient intake. Additional nutrient supplements are often necessary during this time. These most often include zinc and vitamins A, D, E, and B_{12}.

During later phases of therapy, additional dietary supplements may be attempted in order to enhance enteral tolerance. Addition of fat (long- or medium-chain triglycerides—LCT or MCT) into the enteral formula at this stage may be beneficial in weaning the child from parenteral nutrition (22). Use of additives such as pectin, glutamine, growth hormone, and numerous others has been attempted with varying degrees of success. Table 10 lists some dietary supplements which have been utilized in pediatric short bowel syndrome.

4 COMPLICATIONS

Managing the complications that arise in pediatric patients with short bowel syndrome is an integral part in the care of these patients. While many of these complications arise from parenteral nutrition, others appear to be due to enteral nutrition advancement and subsequent malabsorption. Table 11 lists the most common complications, monitoring techniques, preventable interventions, and therapeutic measures in each situation.

Initially, fluid losses and electrolyte imbalance are common in patients undergoing massive intestinal resection. Frequent monitoring of electrolytes in both the serum and stool output is key to providing adequate replacement fluids. Avoidance of situations with potential to develop dehydration, such as environmental exposure to heat, is necessary in some children. Octreotide may be beneficial in the short term in reducing fluid losses in some patients with short bowel syndrome, although tachyphylaxis reduces its long-term usefulness. Keeping supplemental bags of intravenous fluid solution on hand for emergency situations may prevent rehospitalization.

Watery diarrhea is initially the most common complication of pediatric

TABLE 11 Complications

Potential complication	Monitoring techniques	Preventative methods	Therapeutic measures
Dehydration/ electrolyte loss	Lab	Salty snacks High-fat meals	Polycitra 1 mL/kg/ dose Bicitra 2 mL/kg/ dose
Sepsis	Lab	Sterile technique	Antibiotic
Diarrhea	Patient report	High-fat, low-carbo-hydrate diet	Loperamide 1–4 mg/day Cholestyramine
Small bowel bacterial overgrowth	D-lactate Breath hydrogen Urine indicans Duodenal aspirate	Low-carbohydrate diet Probiotics	Broad-spectrum antibiotics Avoid acid suppression
Nutritional deficiencies	Laboratory tests	Supplements	Supplements IV or PO
Acid peptic disease	Endoscopy		Receptor H_2 antagonist, PPI
TPN cholestasis/ gallstones	Ultrasound Laboratory tests	Actigal 15 mg/kg/ day tid	Gallbladder removal
Catheter complications	Laboratory tests	Meticulous technique	Line repair kits on hand Clot dissolver on hand
Renal calculi	Ultrasound	Low-oxalate diet ($\downarrow$ spinach, rhubarb, cocoa, and tea)	Surgery, lithotripsy

short bowel syndrome. Most often, excessive osmotic fluid load in the small intestine is the cause. Switching from bolus to continuous enteral feedings; altering enteral formula type to a low-carbohydrate, high-fat formula; or diluting enteral formulas may be beneficial in diminishing output. Use of somatostatin analogues, while beneficial in the short term, has not resulted in long-term benefits (24). Cholestyramine, which binds the malabsorbed bile acids that are increased in the colon following ileal resection, may help diminish the effects of secretory diarrhea due to bile acid malabsorption. This must be used judiciously, however, as some patients may have bile acid deficiency, which is exacerbated by cholestyramine through the binding of the few available bile salts needed for fat absorption (12). Loperamide has demonstrated safety in the pediatric age group and may be efficacious in slowing gut transit when taken one hour before meals.

Catheter complications early on primarily revolve around the occurrence of sepsis. Causes include intrinsic factors such as bacterial translocation, malnutrition, and immune suppression and extrinsic factors such as poor central line technique or lack of knowledge. If caregivers are adequately trained in the care of central lines, extrinsic factors are avoided. However, bacterial translocation from the gut, which occurs more frequently in infants less than 1 year of age, is more difficult to identify. As enteral feeding is advanced and/or bacterial overgrowth becomes a greater problem, subsequent seeding of the catheter of an older child with gut bacteria may also cause sepsis. Many times, it is difficult to identify whether the infection is related to poor catheter care or internal seeding, as both infections are usually caused by enteric organisms. Use of routine antibiotic flushes in the central line on a daily basis has been attempted with some success in preventing line infections (23). It is common to utilize nighttime TPN infusions with continuous enteral feeding. However, if watery diarrhea occurs at night, there may be a greater chance of extrinsic contamination. Use of daytime TPN infusions with small backpack pumps allows more attention to the infusion and may be helpful in recurrent line contamination.

In the later phases of clinical management, small bowel bacterial overgrowth (SBBO) often occurs. This is one of the least recognized but most common and treatable complications of pediatric short bowel syndrome. Whether aggressive enteral nutrition is utilized or not, this complication occurs in almost all children but does not necessarily cause symptoms. There are normally large numbers of bacteria in the bowel, with a progressive increase in numbers occurring along the length of the bowel. The diagnosis of SBBO based on bacterial counts is often not helpful, as the presence of symptoms cannot be correlated to bacterial count levels. Most bacteria in the intestinal tract are facultative organisms, with a variety of anaerobic organisms also present. These bacteria normally have a physiological role in deconjugating bile salts as well as producing some micronutrients, such as vitamin B_{12} and folate. Bacteria may be present in large enough numbers, however, to deplete the bile salt pool, which may contribute to fat malabsorption. Bacterial overgrowth can also cause mucosal inflammation due to toxins produced by the bacteria and by the breakdown of bacterial metabolites.

Symptoms of SBBO include bloating, abdominal cramping, exacerbation of diarrhea, and/or weight loss. Additionally, patients who were previously stable on their enteral nutrition regimen may present with failure to advance enteral feedings for an extended period of time. Because the diagnosis of SBBO is difficult, empirical treatment with broad-spectrum antibiotics may, in fact, be the most reliable method to identify its presence. The use of glucose or lactulose breath hydrogen tests may be helpful, but since not all bacteria are hydrogen-producing, other techniques may be needed. Measurement of urine indicans and/or serum D-lactate levels may be helpful. Endoscopy to obtain fluid for culture and sensitivity, once thought to be the "gold standard" for diagnosis, is rarely helpful, as obtaining pure samples from the duodenum is difficult and determining which of the cultured bacteria are causing symptoms is not possible.

Severe complications of bacterial overgrowth include D-lactic acidosis, colitis, and inflammatory arthritis. D-Lactic acidosis is a result of carbohydrate overload to the colon, which disturbs the normal pattern of colonic fermentation resulting in accumulation of D-lactate in the blood (25). A variety of neurological signs and symptoms culminating in seizures and coma may develop, especially in young children. D-Lactic acidosis should be suspected whenever there is acidosis with an unexplained anion gap. Colitis or ileitis may also occur due to SBBO. This may resemble Crohn's disease, although a diffuse inflammatory picture is more common (26). These symptoms may be so severe as to require not only antibiotic therapy but also the use of anti-inflammatory drugs such as corticosteroids and salicylates (27).

In the normal physiological state, prevention of bacterial overgrowth is maintained by gastric acid and bile, which kill the majority of pathogenic bacteria. Therefore, avoidance of potent gastric acid–suppressing medications such as proton-pump inhibitors may be helpful (28). Lowering the total carbohydrate component of the enteral diet reduces the substrate utilized by most bacteria for proliferation.

The most common treatment for SBBO involves using a rotating schedule of broad-spectrum antibiotics. Table 12 identifies some of the medications most commonly utilized. Creation of a surgical ileocecal valve in those who have had it removed has some theoretical promise; however, it has been associated with stasis which may enhance SBBO. As children with short bowel syndrome grow, they quickly learn to control stool frequency and often withhold large volumes of stool, which may exacerbate SBBO. Measures to enhance stooling, such as weekly flushing with polyethylene glycol solution via the enteral feeding tube

TABLE 12 Common Antibiotics to Treat Small Bowel Bacterial Overgrowth

Antibiotics	Doses
Gentamicin	5 mg/kg/day
Trimethoprim/sulfamethoxazole	8 mg/kg (trimethoprim)
	40 mg/kg (sulfamethoxazole)
Metronidazole	20 mg/kg/day
Ciprofloxin	
Amoxicillin/clavulanate potassium	30 mg/kg/day

or with other osmotic oral laxatives is particularly effective. Simple measures such as frequent toileting are also effective.

Nutritional deficiency states begin to occur when patients are free of parenteral nutrition (see Table 13). Normally, macronutrients such as carbohydrates, fats, and proteins can be absorbed in adequate quantities, but micronutrients—

TABLE 13 Nutrient Deficiencies

Nutrient	Signs/symptoms	Starting supplemental dose
Vitamin A	Night blindness, dry eyes	10,000 IU/day
Vitamin D	Demineralization of bones	20–50 µg/day
Vitamin E	Hemolytic anemia	400 IU/day
Vitamin K	Bruising	Mephyton 2.5–10 mg daily
Vitamin B_{12}	Weakness, megaloblastic anemia	500–1000/SQ/month Nascobal 1 application/week
Calcium	Depression, muscle spasm, arrhythmias	Infants—360 mg/day Children—540–800 mg/day Teenagers—1200 mg/day
Magnesium	Lethargy, tetanus	1–2.7 mEq/kg/day
Zinc	Alopecia, eczema-like lesions, diarrhea, anorexia	3–6 mg/kg elemental in TPN
Iron	Anemia	300 µg/kg/day IV 2 mg/kg/day PO
Essential fatty acids	Dermatitis, alopecia, thrombocytopenia, poor wound healing	Provision 2% of total calories
Selenium	Muscular complaints	50–100 µg/day
Carnitine	Cardiomyopathy, muscle weakness	50 mg/kg/day

including various trace elements and vitamins—are more likely to become deficient. Increased fat malabsorption from a prescribed high-fat diet may, however, facilitate oxalate absorption and result in hyperoxaluria and calcium oxalate stones (29). Dietary restriction of rhubarb, cocoa, and tea may be helpful. Malabsorption of fat-soluble vitamins—especially A, D, and E–is common and trace metal deficiencies, especially of iron and zinc, also occur. While monitoring of serum zinc levels is helpful, it inadequately reflects the patient's true zinc status. A low serum zinc level in association with a low serum alkaline phosphatase suggests deficiency to such a degree that it may result in poor growth and impaired intestinal adaptation. Patients with zinc deficiency typically have a crusting rash around the eyes, nose, mouth, and anus as well as loss of hair and appetite. Reduced bone mineral content may occur due to calcium malabsorption and can be assessed via bone densitometry (30). Low levels of phosphorus and calcium are easily corrected with supplements, and vitamin D can also be obtained by supplement or prescribing 15 to 20 min of daily sunshine. Magnesium deficiency commonly occurs and is often manifest by symptoms of fatigue, depression, muscle weakness, and excitability. Magnesium deficiency is difficult to treat, as oral enteral magnesium is poorly absorbed and causes an osmotic diarrhea. With ileal resection, careful monitoring of vitamin B_{12} levels is required. Selenium absorption may also be impaired. Both carnitine and choline deficiencies may be associated with the development of fatty liver associated with TPN administration; however, these do not appear to be factors in the development of TPN cholestasis (31).

Acid peptic disease often occurs in pediatric patients with short bowel syndrome. The volumes of both gastric secretion and acid production are increased, but the exact mechanism of this is not well known (32). However, alteration of normal gastrointestinal hormone production and metabolism may be a factor. Most pediatric patients with short bowel syndrome eventually become symptomatic and require intermittent use of acid-neutralizing solutions or acid-suppressant therapy on a long-term basis. This, of course, may complicate bacterial overgrowth. However, if symptoms of heartburn are present and contribute to a poor appetite, they must be treated. Elevated serum gastrin levels often present in short bowel syndrome may occasionally contribute to secretory diarrhea (18).

A major cause of death in children with short bowel syndrome is parenteral nutrition–related liver disease. This most commonly occurs in children on long-term parenteral nutrition, and the incidence increases inversely in proportion to age (33). The etiology is poorly understood. Toxicity of amino acids in parenteral nutrition solution, competition of amino acids with bile acids for transport across the hepatic canalicular membrane, production of toxins by unused bowel, excess nutrient administration, toxicity of unknown substances in the parenteral nutrition solution, and nonstimulation of gastrointestinal hormones that normally control biliary secretions have all been purported as possible mechanisms (1). It is well accepted that aggressive enteral nutrition providing at least 20 to 30% of total caloric needs, prevention of SBBO, and avoidance of catheter-related sepsis are all helpful in reducing parenteral nutrition–associated liver disease.

When parenteral nutrition–associated liver disease occurs, most often multifactoral situations are present, therefore necessitating a comprehensive treatment approach. Use of aggressive enteral nutrition early in the phases of treatment has been found to be protective. Use of ursodeoxycholic acid may also be helpful (34). Development of gallstones due to gallbladder stasis from lack of enteral feeding and cholesterol precipitation from the low concentration of bile salts in the bile may also occur. Although early cholecystectomy may be advocated for some patients on long-term parenteral nutrition, these patients may be also amenable to use of ursodeoxycholic acid therapy (35).

Catheter-associated complications in the later phases of the clinical management of the patient with short bowel syndrome include puncture, catheter deterioration, occlusion and thrombosis, and sepsis (see Chap. 17). The pediatric patient generally comes to see the central line as an inherent part of his or her body and keeps it well protected from accidental removal or injury. Catheter repair kits exist if inadvertent puncture or rupture of the tubing occurs. Use of medications to clear thrombosis have met with some success (36). Sepsis may occur at any time due to poor catheter care or bacterial translocation. However, situations such as Munchausen's syndrome and Munchausen by proxy should also be considered. Older patients unable to wean from parenteral nutrition and tolerate normal oral feeding may devise ingenious methods to experience alcohol via administration into a central line. Small household animals, such as hamsters and gerbils, may be attracted to the odors associated with intravenous or enteral formulas. Allowing a gerbil to crawl under a child's shirt may result in line puncture. Swimming in chlorinated pools is not a problem with proper care of a central line before and after swimming. However, swimming in ponds or rivers will often result in line-site or bloodstream infections. Life-threatening consequences such as these should be reviewed as the child becomes a teenager.

5   SURGICAL ISSUES

Patients with short bowel syndrome who have undergone previous intestinal resection may develop anastomotic ulcerations and strictures. These can occur at any time, from months to years after initial surgery (37). A sudden onset of anemia and either visible or occult positive stools should raise the suspicion of either the development of anastomotic ulcerations and/or small bowel bacterial overgrowth. Colonoscopy for visual assessment as well as obtainment of microscopic specimens for sampling may be required.

Bowel dilatation often occurs during the period of intestinal adaptation. This adaptive response, while beneficial in increasing surface area, may become so extreme as to exacerbate SBBO. Identified on upper GI/small bowel series, this problem may be alleviated using surgical tapering with or without concomitant lengthening (Bianchi procedure). These procedures may be beneficial in ameliorating symptoms without losing additional intestinal absorptive areas. Surgical procedures designed to slow intestinal transit via the creation of intestinal valve-like areas may be utilized. Surgical placement of enteral feeding tubes is often an ongoing situation. Use of reversed small bowel segments and colonic interposition have been used successfully in some adult patients with short bowel syndrome but are less successful in children (38). Fundoplication is rarely necessary.

Lillihei et al. (39) originally described small intestinal transplantation using a canine model. While this, theoretically, is an attractive option, complications have continued to make it a last resort. Problems with immune modulation and rejection are difficult. Pediatric small intestinal transplants are currently being done at several centers, the largest being at Pittsburgh, Pennsylvania; Omaha, Nebraska; Miami, Florida; and Paris, France. Results vary between centers. Preliminary experience has suggested that 1- to 2-year survival posttransplantation is better than 75%, decreasing to about 50% at 3–5 years (40). Centers with the most experience seem to have the best outcome. Combined liver/bowel transplantation is a potential option in patients with irreversible TPN liver disease and short bowel syndrome. However, because of the shortage of donors, this has become increasingly difficult. Isolated intestinal transplants may have a much lower complication rate and should be considered before irreversible liver disease occurs (41).

6 CONCLUSION

In many children with short bowel syndrome, adequate adaptation does not occur. These children are committed to a life on parenteral nutrition. If this is well monitored, development delays are relatively uncommon, school attendance is good, and children can be maintained in their home environment. Home-based parenteral nutrition permits an optimal psychosocial environment, and long-term survival in children on parenteral nutrition appears to be in the range of 80 to 85%, at least throughout early adulthood (21). Although 15 to 20% of these children will die, aggressive nutritional therapy by adequately trained medical staff often prevents this. Careful attention to details of nutrition support and monitoring for nutritional deficiency states after parenteral and enteral nutrition are important factors in ongoing success in adulthood. While modern nutritional support methods can provide excellent long-term survival and a reasonable quality of life, the pursuit for new treatment options should never be overlooked. While surgical procedures are sometimes indicated, primary medical management is the mainstay of therapy.

REFERENCES

1. Vanderhoof JA. Short bowel syndrome. In: Walker WA, Durie PR, Hamilton JR, Walker-Smith JA, Watkins JB, eds. Pediatric Gastrointestinal Disease, 2nd ed. St. Louis: Mosby, 1996, pp 830–840.

2. Gray SW, Skandalakis JE. Embryology for surgeons: The Embryological Basis for the Treatment of Congenital Defects. Philadelphia: Saunders, 1972, pp 129–133.

3. Raffensperger JG. Short gut syndrome. In: Raffensperger JG, ed. Swenson's Pediatric Surgery, 4th ed. New York: Appleton-Century-Crofts, 1980, p 502.

4. Underhill BML. Intestinal length in man. BMJ 1955; 2:1243–1246.

5. Fanucci A, Cerro P, Fanucci E. Normal small bowel measurements by enteroclysis. Scan J Gastroenterol 1988; 23:574–576.

6. Caniano DA, Starr J, Ginn-Pease ME. Extensive short bowel syndrome in neonates: outcome in the 1980s. Surgery 1989; 105:119–124.

7. Shulman R. Home parenteral nutrition. Paper presented at 6th International Symposium on Small Bowel Transplantation, October 7, 1999, Omaha, NE.

8. McIntyre PE, Fitchew M, Lennard-Jones JC. Patients with a high jejunostomy do not need a special diet. Gastroenterology 1986; 91:25–53.

9. Newton CR, Gonvers JJ, McIntyre PB, Preston DM, Lennard-Jones JE. Effect of different drinks on fluid and electrolyte losses from a jejunostomy. J R Soc Med 1985; 78:27–34.

10. Nightingale JM, Lennard-Jones JE, Walker ER, Farthing MJG. Jejunal efflux in short bowel syndrome. Lancet 1990; 336:765–768.

11. Nightingale JMD, Kamm MA, van der Sijp JRM, Ghatei MA, Bloom SR, Lennard-Jones JE. Gastrointestinal hormones in short bowel syndrome. Peptide YY may be the "colonic brake" to gastric emptying. Gut 1996; 39:267–272.

12. Vanderhoof JA. Short bowel syndrome: parenteral nutrition versus intestinal transplantation. Pediatr Nutr ISPEN 1999; 1(1):8–15.

13. Jeejeebhoy KN. Therapy of the short gut syndrome. Lancet 1983; 1:1427–1430.

14. Vanderhoof JA. Short bowel syndrome. In: Walker WA, Watkins JB, ed. Nutrition in Pediatrics 2nd ed. Hamilton, Ontario: Decker, 1996, pp 609–618.

15. Feldman EJ, Dowling RH, McNaughton J, Peters TS. Effects of oral versus intravenous nutrition on intestinal adaptation after small bowel resection on the dog. Gastroenterology 1976; 70:712–719.

16. Williamson RCN. Intestinal adaptation: mechanisms of control. N Engl J Med 1978; 298:1444–1450.

17. Williamson RCN. Intestinal adaptation and structural functional and cytokinetic changes. N Engl J Med 1978; 298:1393–1402.

18. Vanderhoof JA. Clinical management of the short bowel syndrome. In: Balistreri WJ, Vanderhoof JA, eds. Pediatric Gastroenterology and Nutrition. London: Chapman & Hall, 1990, pp 24–33.

19. Simko V, Lin WG. Absorption of different elemental diets in short bowel syndrome lasting 15 years. Dig Dis 1976; 21:419–425.

20. Lennard-Jones JE. Review article: practical management of the short bowel. Aliment Pharmacol Ther 1994; 8:563–577.

21. Vargas JH, Ament ME, Berquist WE. Long term home parenteral nutrition in pediat-

rics: 10 years of experience in 102 patients. J Pediatr Gastroenterol Nutr 1987; 6(1): 24–32.

22. Arrigoni E, Marteau P, Briet F, Pochart P, Rambaud JC, Messing B. Tolerance and absorption of lactose from milk and yogurt during short bowel syndrome in humans. Am J Clin Nutr 1994; 60:926–929.

23. Yao JCD, Arian CF, Karchmer AW. Vancomycin stability in heparin and total parenteral nutrition solutions: novel approach to therapy of central venous catheter related infections. J Pediatr Enter Nutr 1992; 6(3):268–274.

24. Nightingale JM, Walker ER, Burnham WR, Farthing MJ, Lennard-Jones JE. Short bowel syndrome. Digestion 1990; 45(1):77–83.

25. Buotos D, Pons S, Pernas JC, Gonzalez H, Caldarini MI, Ogawa K, DePaula JA. Fecal lactate and short bowel syndrome. Dig Dis Sci 1994; 39(11):2315–2319.

26. Taylor SF, Sondheimer JM, Sokol RJ, Silverman A, Wilson HL. Noninfectious colitis associated with short gut syndrome in infants. J Pediatr 1991; 119:24–28.

27. Vanderhoof JA, Young RJ, Murray N, Kaufman SS. Treatment strategies for small bowel bacterial overgrowth in short bowel syndrome. J Pediatr Gastroenterol Nutr 1998; 27:155–160.

28. Fried M, Siegrist H, Frei R, Frehlich F, Duroux P, Thorens J, Blum A, Bille J, Gonvers JJ, Gyr K. Duodenal bacterial overgrowth during treatment in outpatients with omeprazole. Gut 1994; 35:23–26.

29. Carter BS, Whitworth HS. Nephrolithiasis in an infant with short bowel syndrome. Clin Pediatr 1994; 33:741–742.

30. Dellert SF, Farell MK, Secker BL, Heubi JE. Bone mineral content in children with short bowel syndrome after discontinuation of parenteral nutrition. J Pediatr 1998; 132(3):516–519.

31. Moukarzel AA, Dahlstrom KA, Buchman AL, Ament ME. Carnitine status of children receiving long-term total parenteral nutrition: a longitudinal prospective study. J Pediatr 1992; 120:759–762.

32. Straus E, Gerson CD, Yalow RS. Hypersecretion of gastrin associated with short bowel syndrome. Gastroenterology 1974; 66:175–180.

33. Dorney SFA, et al. Improved survival in very short small bowel of infancy with use of long-term parenteral nutrition. J Pediatr 1985; 106:521.

34. Balistreri WF, A-Kader HH, Ryckman FC, et al. Biochemical and clinical response to UDCA administration in pediatric patients with chronic cholestasis. In: Paumgartner G, Stiehl A, Gerok W, eds. Bile Acids as Therapeutic Agents. Lancaster, UK: Kluwer, 1991, pp 323–333.

35. Roslyn JJ, Pitt HA, Mann L, Fonkalsrud EW, DenBensten L. Parenteral nutrition-induced gall bladder disease: a reason for early cholecystectomy. Am J Surg 1984; 148(1):58–63.

36. Brock-Cascanet PH. Treating occluded VAD. Infusion 1999; Jan:18–27.

37. Bhargawa SA, Putnam PE, Kocoshis SA. Gastrointestinal bleeding due to delayed perianastomotic ulceration in children. Am J Gastroenterol 1995; 90(5):807–809.

38. Warner BW, Ziegler MM. Management of the short bowel syndrome in the pediatric population. Pediatr Clin North Am 1993; 40(6):1335–1350.

39. Lillihei RC, Goott B, Miller FA. Surgery of the bowel: homografts of the small bowel. Surg Forum 1959; 10:197–201.

40. Langnas AN, et al. Human intestinal transplantation an effective treatment of intestinal failure. Paper presented at 6th International Symposium on Small Bowel Transplantation, Oct. 8, 1999, Omaha, NE.

41. Goulet O, Revillon Y, Jan D, De-Potter S, Colomb V, Sadoun E, Ben-Hariz M, Ricour C. Which patients need small bowel transplantation for neonatal short bowel syndrome? Transplant Proc 1992; 24(3):1058–1059.

42. Michail S, Vanderhoof JA. Parenteral nutrition in clinical practice. Ann Nestle 1996; 54:53–60.

30

Liver Disease

Deirdre Anne Kelly
Birmingham Children's Hospital, Birmingham, England

1 NEONATAL LIVER DISEASE

Almost two-thirds of children with liver disease present in the neonatal period with prolonged jaundice. Although physiological jaundice is common in neonates (Table 1), infants who have severe or persistent jaundice should be investigated to exclude hemolysis, sepsis, or underlying liver disease. Neonatal jaundice that persists beyond 14 or 21 days should always be investigated, even in breast-fed babies. The long-term prognosis of neonatal liver disease depends on its etiology (1).

1.1 Unconjugated Hyperbilirubinemia

The commonest causes of unconjugated hyperbilirubinemia are physiological jaundice or breast-milk jaundice (Tables 1 and 2), although systemic disease or hemolysis from any cause must be excluded.

Diagnosis and Management. It is important to establish Coombs positivity and glucose-6-phosphate dehydrogenase deficiency and to exclude red cell membrane defects such as spherocytosis. Systemic sepsis is an important cause of unconjugated hyperbilirubinemia in the early neonatal period and requires prompt treatment with antibiotics, fluids, phototherapy, and/or exchange transfusion.

TABLE 1   Physiological Neonatal Jaundice

Peak 2 to 5 days after birth
Normal stools and urine
More severe in premature babies
Clears within 2 weeks
May persist for 4 weeks in breast-fed infants
Can rarely lead to kernicterus
Diagnosis: 80% total bilirubin is unconjugated
Treatment includes fluids, reassurance, phototherapy

1.2   Inherited Disorders

1.2.1   Crigler-Najjar Types I and II

This rare autosomal recessive disease is secondary to a deficiency of the hepatic enzyme uridyl diglucuronyl transferase, which causes high levels of unconjugated hyperbilirubinemia in the postnatal period. In Crigler-Najjar type I, peak serum bilirubin levels vary between 250 and 850 umol/L (15–51 mg/dL), whereas in Crigler-Najjar type II, peak bilirubin levels are 200 to 300 μmol/L (12 to 18 mg/dL). Infants should be referred to a specialist center for diagnosis and initial management.

Diagnosis.   The diagnosis of Crigler-Najaar type I is made by aspiration of bile from the duodenum, as bilirubin diglucuronides are not present in Crigler-Najjar type I but small amounts are detected in type II. Liver biopsy to measure enzyme levels is not necessary.

TABLE 2   Causes of Unconjugated Hyperbilirubinemia

Physiological/breast-milk jaundice
Hemolysis
  Immune
  RBC membrane abnormality
Metabolic disorders
  Crigler-Najjar type I and II
  Gilbert's syndrome
  Galactosemia
  Fructosemia
Hypothyroidism
Sepsis
Hypoxia

Treatment.   Prompt treatment is required for Crigler-Najaar type I, with exchange transfusion and phototherapy to prevent kernicterus. There is no response to phenobarbitone. Long-term phototherapy is essential but becomes difficult when 12 to 16 hr per day of treatment is required for school-age children. Auxiliary liver transplantation is now the treatment of choice and effectively reduces bilirubin levels while retaining native liver for future gene therapy. Treatment for Crigler-Najaar type II is not required except for cosmetic reasons, but bilirubin levels reduce on phenobarbitone 5 to 15 mg/kg.

2   CHOLESTASIS IN THE NEWBORN

Clinical features suggesting liver disease include:

Conjugated hyperbilirubinemia
Pale stools and dark urine
Dysmorphic features
Bruising, petechiae, or bleeding
Hepatomegaly and/or splenomegaly
Slow weight gain or failure to thrive
Previous family history or consanguinity

The differential diagnosis is between extrahepatic biliary disease, the neonatal hepatitis syndrome, and intrahepatic biliary hypoplasia.

All children with persistent neonatal jaundice need thorough investigation (Fig. 1). If baseline tests are abnormal, referral to a specialized center may be required.

2.1   Extrahepatic Biliary Disease

Biliary atresia occurs in 1 per 14,000 live births worldwide. There is a slight female predominance. The etiology is unknown, although the association of biliary atresia with other extrahepatic anomalies suggests an abnormality of the embryological development of the biliary tree. There is no clear genetic basis or evidence of viral infection.

Pathogenesis.   Biliary atresia affects all parts of the biliary tree. There is gradual fibrosis and destruction of the extra and intra hepatic biliary ducts with progressive cholestasis.

Clinical Features.   Infants with biliary atresia are usually born at term with a normal birth weight. Jaundice is apparent on the second day of life but may be mistaken for physiological jaundice. Biliary obstruction, as evidenced by pale stools and dark yellow urine, gradually develops over the next 2 to 4 weeks

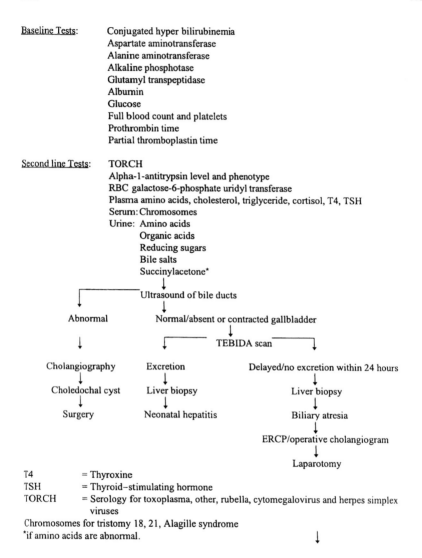

Baseline Tests: Conjugated hyper bilirubinemia
                  Aspartate aminotransferase
                  Alanine aminotransferase
                  Alkaline phosphotase
                  Glutamyl transpeptidase
                  Albumin
                  Glucose
                  Full blood count and platelets
                  Prothrombin time
                  Partial thromboplastin time

Second line Tests: TORCH
                     Alpha-1-antitrypsin level and phenotype
                     RBC galactose-6-phosphate uridyl transferase
                     Plasma amino acids, cholesterol, triglyceride, cortisol, T4, TSH
                     Serum: Chromosomes
                     Urine: Amino acids
                             Organic acids
                             Reducing sugars
                             Bile salts
                             Succinylacetone*

Ultrasound of bile ducts

Abnormal   Normal/absent or contracted gallbladder

                  TEBIDA scan

Cholangiography   Excretion   Delayed/no excretion within 24 hours
Choledochal cyst   Liver biopsy   Liver biopsy
Surgery   Neonatal hepatitis   Biliary atresia
                                        ERCP/operative cholangiogram
                                                Laparotomy

T4   = Thyroxine
TSH   = Thyroid–stimulating hormone
TORCH   = Serology for toxoplasma, other, rubella, cytomegalovirus and herpes simplex
            viruses
Chromosomes for tristomy 18, 21, Alagille syndrome
*if amino acids are abnormal.

FIGURE 1   Algorithm for investigation of neonatal liver disease.

and is associated with a gradual increase in liver size and failure to gain weight
despite a good appetite. Approximately 25% of babies have associated anomalies
such as dextrocardia, ventricular or atrial septal defects, polysplenia, and the hy-
povascular syndrome (HVS). The spleen is not enlarged unless there is significant
hepatic fibrosis. Ascites may occasionally be present.

Diagnosis.   The diagnosis of biliary atresia is dependent on:

1. Presence of conjugated hyperbilirubinemia.
2. Liver biochemistry indicating raised alkaline phosphatase (>600 IU/L) and gamma glutamyl transpeptidase (GGT) (>100 IU/L) and moderate elevation of alanine and aspartate transaminases (100 to 200 IU/L).
3. Abdominal ultrasound performed after a 4-hr fast will demonstrate either a contracted or absent gallbladder.
4. Radionuclide hepatobiliary imaging demonstrates no biliary excretion from the liver into the gut after 24 hr.
5. Histology demonstrates expansion of portal tracts, proliferation of bile ducts and ductules, with bile plugs, portal fibrosis, and portal edema. There may be an increase in inflammatory reaction at the porta hepatis and variable giant cell transformation of hepatocytes.

As none of these tests are pathognomonic for biliary atresia, the diagnosis should be confirmed by operative cholangiography with progression to a Kasai portoenterostomy if required (2).

Endoscopic retrograde cholangiography (ERCP) in this age group is now possible using prototype pediatric duodenoscopes. Biliary atresia can confidently be excluded if the biliary tree is visualized, but a failure to do so may be due to either technical failure or biliary atresia. Progression to operative cholangiography and laparotomy is then required.

Treatment.   Surgical treatment (the Kasai portoenterostomy) removes the obliterated biliary tract and creates a Roux loop that is anastomosed to the porta hepatis (see Chap. 33). Between 50 and 60% of cases achieve biliary drainage. The success of this operation depends on a number of factors including the timing of the operation, the expertise of the surgeon, the degree of hepatic fibrosis at operation, and the presence or absence of other congenital abnormalities (3).

Operations should be performed before 8 weeks of age if possible. Surgery is not recommended if there is advanced hepatic fibrosis with splenomegaly, ascites, or varices.

Complications.   Cholangitis presents with an increase in jaundice, pyrexia, acholic stools, and tenderness over the liver. It is prevented by oral prophylactic antibiotics given for 3 to 6 months. Broad-spectrum antibiotics (ceftazidime, amoxicillin, piperacillin, or ciprofloxacin) is usually effective.

Malabsorption is usually associated with a partially successful Kasai portoenterostomy and is an important factor in the development of malnutrition.

The development of cirrhosis and portal hypertension is inevitable even in those children who have had a successful Kasai portoenterostomy, although the need for transplantation varies with the rate of progression of liver disease and complications. Unsuccessful Kasai portoenterostomy is an immediate indication for liver transplantation, and these children should be referred early to specialized centers for follow-up (4).

2.2 Choledocal Cyst

Choledocal cysts are localized cystic dilatations of all or part of the common bile duct. Cysts are more common in Japan (1 in 100,000 live births) and in females in a ratio of 4 to 1. The cyst may present in infancy with prolonged jaundice and must be differentiated from biliary atresia or the neonatal hepatitis syndrome. In older children, a history of abdominal pain, jaundice, and abdominal mass is classic but a rare presentation in childhood. Jaundice may be intermittent and associated with ascending cholangitis and recurrent pancreatitis.

Diagnosis. Choledocal cysts are diagnosed by abdominal ultrasound (Fig. 2), which may detect the cysts antenatally. Confirmation of the anatomy is obtained by radioisotope scan, percutaneous transhepatic cholangiogram, or endoscopically by an endoscopic retrograde cholangiopancreatography. Histology of the liver usually indicates biliary fibrosis, cholestasis, and bile plugs in the portal tract. The histological features are completely reversible following successful surgery.

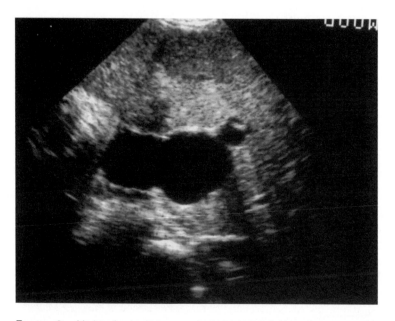

FIGURE 2 Abdominal ultrasound demonstrating a large cystic swelling, which was confirmed to be a choledochal cyst on endoscopic retrograde cholangiogram.

Management and Outcome. Surgical treatment includes excision of all the affected ducts and reestablishment of biliary drainage by forming a hepato-jejunostomy. Drainage of the cyst into adjacent duodenum or jejunum is now contraindicated because of the potential malignant transformation. The results of surgery are excellent, cholangitis is an occasional complication, and there is a 2.5% risk of malignancy in the residual biliary tree in adult life.

2.3 Spontaneous Perforation of the Bile Ducts

This is a rare complication in which perforation occurs at the junction of the cystic and common hepatic ducts, perhaps due to a congenital weakness, inspissated bile, or gallstones. Infants may present at any age from 2 to 24 weeks of age with abdominal distention, ascites, jaundice, and acholic stools. Biliary peritonitis—with bile in hydroceles, hernial sacs, and umbilicus—may be obvious.

The diagnosis may be confirmed by abdominal ultrasound, which may show free intraperitoneal fluid and dilated intrahepatic ducts. Hepatobiliary scanning will demonstrate isotope in the peritoneal cavity. Treatment includes peritoneal drainage followed by repair of the perforation.

2.4 Inspissated Bile Syndrome and Cholelithiasis

Bile duct obstruction secondary to inspissated bile syndrome may be secondary to total parenteral nutrition, prolonged hemolysis, and dehydration. It is more common in premature babies or those undergoing major surgery. The clinical picture is of biliary obstruction with pale stools, dark urine, and abnormal liver function tests. The diagnosis may be confirmed by ultrasound, which demonstrates a dilated intra- and extrahepatic duct system with biliary sludge. Percutaneous transhepatic cholangiography may be therapeutic with lavage of the biliary tree, but laparatomy and decompression of the biliary tree may be required. The use of ursodeoxycholic acid (20 mg/kg) may prevent the need for either surgical or radiological intervention.

Cholecystitis may occur in infants in association with gallstones from hemolysis or total parenteral nutrition (TPN) while acalculous cholecystitis may occur as part of generalized sepsis. In this young age group, operative cholecystectomy (rather than laparoscopic) is the treatment of choice for symptomatic cholecystitis in association with gallstones.

3 NEONATAL HEPATITIS SYNDROME

The neonatal hepatitis syndrome includes many different causes of neonatal liver disease (Table 3), which may have similar presentations. A unified approach is required for diagnosis (Fig. 1). The commonest causes are intrauterine infections

TABLE 3 Neonatal Hepatitis Syndrome

Disease	Diagnosis	Treatment
Intra-uterine infection		
Cytomegalovirus[a]	Urine for viral culture	Gancyclovir
Toxoplasmosis	IgM antibodies	Spiramycin
Rubella	IgM antibodies	Supportive
Herpes simplex	EM/viral culture of vesicle	Acyclovir
Syphilis	VDRL, FTA-ABS	Penicillin
Metabolic		
Alpha-1-antitrypsin[a] (AAT) deficiency	AAT level and phenotype	Supportive
Cystic fibrosis	Sweat chloride, immuno-reactive trypsin, $\Delta508$ mutation	Supportive
Galactosemia[b]	Galactose-1-6-phosphate uridyltransferase	Galactose-free diet
Tyrosinemia type I	Urine succinylacetone, serum amino acids, alpha-fetoprotein	NTBC
Niemann-Pick type C	Storage cells in bone aspirate and liver biopsy; fibroblast culture	Supportive
Wolman disease	Abdominal x-ray of adrenal glands	Supportive
Primary disorders of bile synthesis	Urinary bile acids by FAB-MS	Bile acids
Zellweger syndrome	Very long chain fatty acids	Supportive
Endocrine		
Hypopituitarism (septo-optic dysplasia)[b]	Cortisol, TSH, T4	Hormone replacement
Hypothyroidism	TSH, T4, free T4, T3	Hormone replacement

[a] Most common etiology.
[b] Less common but if missed may lead to growth failure, cataracts (galactosemia), or cirrhosis (hypopituitarism).

or inherited metabolic diseases. The diagnosis should be confirmed at a specialist center, but subsequent management is usually shared with the referral center. In contrast with children with extrahepatic biliary disease, babies with neonatal hepatitis syndrome have the following:

Small size for dates or with a history of intrauterine growth retardation
Pigment in the stools, although the urine is dark yellow
Dysmorphic features (Alagille's or Zellweger's syndrome)
Hepatosplenomegaly

Biochemical features include

Conjugated bilirubin >100 μmol/L (>6 mg/dL)
Alkaline phosphatase 600 to 800 IU/L
AST and ALT 200 to 300 IU/L
Hypoglycemia (glucose <2.5 μmol/L) (25 mg/dL)

Liver histology is nonspecific and demonstrates giant cell hepatitis with fibrosis of the portal tracts, extramedullary hematopoiesis, cholestasis, and biliary ductule proliferation. There may be histological overlap with biliary atresia (5).

3.1 Intrauterine Infection

The commonest cause of intrauterine infection causing neonatal hepatitis is cytomegalovirus (CMV) infection. Infants are small for date, with hepatosplenomegaly and may have thrombocytopenia, chorioretinitis, or microcephaly. The diagnosis (Table 3) is based on identification of IgM antibodies and viral culture. The outcome is variable. In most babies, the hepatitis resolves completely within 3 to 6 months, but neurological involvement with spasticity or sensorineural deafness and developmental delay may be present. Treatment with ganciclovir is rarely necessary.

Rubella hepatitis is almost unknown now, following universal vaccination, but it may present with neonatal hepatitis, cataracts, congenital heart disease, and deafness. Progressive liver disease has been reported.

Toxoplasmosis is rare but is associated with persistent neonatal jaundice, failure to thrive, hepatosplenomegaly, and central nervous system involvement with chorioretinitis, hydrocephaly, microcephaly, and intracranial calcifications. Treatment with spiramycin may be helpful. The long-term outcome is related to the neurological disease, as many children are blind or severely disabled by the time of diagnosis.

Herpes simplex in the newborn usually causes a multisystem disorder with encephalitis and acute liver failure. Antiviral treatment with acyclovir is successful if started early enough.

Congenital syphilis is now rare but may also cause a multisystem disease with intrauterine retardation, anemia, thrombocytopenia, nephrotic syndrome, skin rash, diffuse lymphadenopathy, and hepatomegaly. Diagnosis is based on serological testing (Table 3). Treatment with penicillin is usually curative.

Hepatitis A, B, and C and HIV are rare causes of persistent neonatal jaundice. Vertical transmission of hepatitis B or C leads to an asymptomatic carrier state.

3.2 Endocrine Disorders

3.2.1 Hypopituitarism

The neonatal hepatitis syndrome is associated with pituitary or adrenal dysfunction in approximately 30% of patients (6). Hypopituitarism may be due to hypothalamic dysfunction and is associated with septo-optic dysplasia, which includes absence of the septum pellucidum or malformation of the forebrain and hypoplasia of one or both optic nerves.

Clinical Presentation. Hypoglycemia is a prominent symptom, which is not associated with the severity of liver disease. Other signs of hypopituitarism include microgenitalia in boys, midline facial abnormalities, or nystagmus. A number of children may have severe cholestasis with acholic stools and dark urine; differentiation from biliary atresia may be difficult.

Diagnosis and Treatment. This is established by demonstrating abnormal thyroid function tests indicating hypothyroidism and a low random or 9 A.M. cortisol. A synacthen test is rarely required for confirmation. Treatment is with hormone replacement with thyroxine, hydrocortisone, and growth hormone. If diagnosed early enough, the liver disease will resolve completely, but hormone replacement is required lifelong.

4 INBORN ERRORS OF METABOLISM

The commonest inborn error of metabolism to present with persistent neonatal jaundice is α_1-antitrypsin deficiency, an autosomal recessive disorder with an incidence of 1 per 7000 live births worldwide. Infants may present with

    Intrauterine growth retardation
    Cholestasis
    Failure to thrive
    Hepatomegaly
    Vitamin K–responsive coagulopathy, which is more likely in those infants not given prophylactic vitamin K at birth and who are breast-fed

Diagnosis. Liver biochemistry is nonspecific, with elevated transaminases, alkaline phosphatase, and gamma glutamyl transpeptidase (GGT). Radiological investigations may be normal or suggest cholestasis, with a contracted gallbladder and delayed excretion of radioisotope on hepatobiliary scanning. The diagnosis is easily confirmed by detection of a low level of alpha$_1$-antitrypsin (<0.9 g/L). Liver disease is usually associated with phenotype protease inhibitor (PiZZ) but may occur with PISZ heterozygotes or other variants.

Liver histology demonstrates a giant cell hepatitis with characteristic periodic acid–Schiff (PAS) diastase-resistant positive granules of alpha-1-antitrypsin in hepatocytes, which may be detected by 6 to 8 weeks of age.

Management consists of nutritional support, fat-soluble vitamin supplementation, and treatment of pruritus and cholestasis (Table 4). The prognosis is varied. Jaundice disappears in most infants, of whom 30% have normal liver function, 30% develop cirrhosis, and 30% develop chronic liver failure requiring transplantation in childhood. Respiratory disease is rare in childhood, but long-term follow-up is essential to monitor growth, development, and the need for liver transplantation.

Genetic Counseling. Antenatal diagnosis by chorionic villus sampling is now available using synthetic oligonucleotide probes specific for the M and Z genes or by restriction fragment length polymorphism.

TABLE 4 Management of Neonatal Liver Disease

Nutritional support	
Formula feed	Energy intake 150–200 kcal/kg
Content	
Carbohydrate	Glucose polymers (8–10 g/kg/day)
Protein	Whey protein (2.5–3.5 g/kg/day)
Fat	50/50 MCT/LCT (8 g/kg/day)
Fat-soluble vitamins	A: 5–10,000 U/day
	E: 50–100 mg/day
	K: 1–5 mg/day
	D: 50 ng/kg/day
Pruritus/cholestasis	Phenobarbital 5–15 mg/kg
	Ursodeoxycholic acid 20 mg/kg
	Rifampicin 3 mg/kg
	Cholestyramine 1–2 g/day
	Topical skin care

4.1 Intrahepatic Biliary Hypoplasia

Intrahepatic biliary hypoplasia exists when there is an absence in, or reduction of, the number of bile ducts or ductules seen in portal tracts in association with normal-sized branches of portal vein and hepatic arteries. Biliary hypoplasia may occur in a wide spectrum of liver diseases, such as alpha-1-antitrypsin deficiency, chromosomal abnormality such as Down's syndrome, or intrauterine infection (cytomegalovirus). However, this condition is usually associated only with syndromic biliary hypoplasia or Alagille's syndrome or nonsyndromic biliary hypoplasia, which includes Byler's disease and progressive familial intrahepatic cholestasis (7).

4.2 Alagille's Syndrome

This is an autosomal dominant condition with an incidence of 1 in 100,000 live births worldwide. It is a multisystem disorder associated with cardiac, facial, renal, occular, and skeletal abnormalities. The genetic abnormality has been traced to a deletion on chromosome 20p which has now been identified as the *Jagged 1* gene (8).

Infants may present with persistent cholestasis, severe pruritus, hepatomegaly, and failure to thrive. The characteristic facial features are very difficult to identify in infancy but become more prominent later in childhood. They include a triangular face with high forehead and frontal bossing, deep-set, widely spaced eyes, saddle-shaped nasal bridge, and pointed chin (Fig. 3). Cardiac abnormalities include peripheral pulmonary stenosis, aortic valve stenosis, and tetralogy of Fallot. Skeletal abnormalities are widespread and include abnormal thoracic vertebrae, "butterfly" vertebrae, and curving of the proximal digits of the third and fourth fingers.

Posterior embryotoxon, which is detected on the inner aspects of the cornea near the junction of the iris, is demonstrated in 90% of patients by slit-lamp examination. Retinal pigmentation on fundoscopy and calcific deposits (optic drusen) in the optic nerve may be detected by ultrasound. Blindness may occur. Renal disease varies in severity from mild renal tubular acidosis to severe glomerulonephritis. One of the most difficult management problems is severe failure to thrive, which is complicated by gastroesophageal reflux and severe steatorrhea secondary to fat malabsorption or pancreatic insufficiency. Intracranial hemorrhage is also recognized in later life.

Diagnosis.   Liver biochemistry indicates severe cholestasis with

Conjugated bilirubin >100 mmol/L (>6 mg/dL)
Raised alkaline phosphatase >600 IU/L
Gamma glutamyl transpeptidase >200 IU/L
Raised transaminases
Plasma cholesterol >6 mmol/L (230 mg/dL)
Normal triglycerides 0.4 to 2 mmol/L

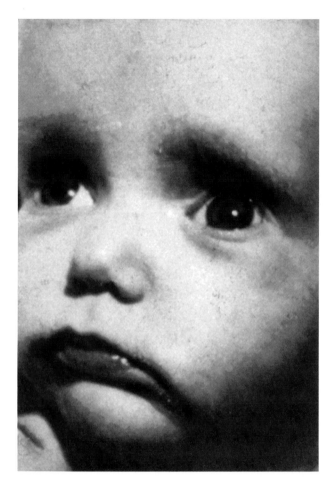

FIGURE 3 Alagille's syndrome is an autosomal dominant disorder in which the typical facies may be less obvious in infants. This boy demonstrates hypertelorism, widely spaced eyes, a depressed nasal bridge, and a pointed chin.

Tests of hepatic function such as albumin and coagulation are usually normal. Renal dysfunction may be identified by the presence of aminoaciduria or estimating urinary protein/creatinine ratio (normal <20 mg/L).

The skeletal abnormalities are easily identified by radiological examination of the chest and hands. Electrocardiography may demonstrate right bundle branch block or right ventricular hypertrophy in children with peripheral pulmonary stenosis. Echocardiography may be normal, but if cardiac abnormalities are suggested clinically, then cardiac catheterization should be performed for confirmation. Liver histology demonstrates a reduction in bile ducts.

Management and Outcome. Intensive nutritional support is essential (Table 4), and pancreatic supplements may be required. Pruritus may be intractable and an indication for liver transplantation.

Prognosis is varied and depends on the extent of liver, cardiac, or renal disease. Approximately 50% of children may regain normal liver function by adolescence, while others require liver transplantation in childhood. The indications for liver transplantation are the development of cirrhosis and portal hypertension, intractable pruritus, or severe decompensated growth failure.

Pretransplant cardiac surgery or balloon dilatation may be indicated for severe pulmonary stenosis.

4.3 Progressive Intrahepatic Cholestasis (Progressive Familial Intrahepatic Cholestasis, or PFIC)

This is the name given to a number of diseases in which there is persistent jaundice, cholestasis, hepatomegaly, pruritus, and failure to thrive (9). Many different variants and the genetic mutations for a number of these have been described (PFIC 1,2, and 3). Abnormalities in different bile acid transporters at the cellular level have been described.

4.4 Byler's Disease (PFIC I)

This severe form of familial idiopathic cholestasis was first described in an Amish family. In contrast to children with intrahepatic cholestasis of other causes, this group of children had a normal serum gamma glutamyl transpeptidase (GGT) and low or normal serum cholesterol. The clinical presentation is with persistent conjugated hyperbilirubinemia, severe pruritus, and growth retardation. Histology shows a lack of hepatic inflammation but a paucity of bile ducts and canalicular bile plugs. Cirrhosis develops in early childhood, requiring liver transplantation. PFIC 2 has a similar presentation to PFIC 1, while PFIC 3 is associated with a high GGT and less pruritus.

Treatment consists of nutritional support (Table 4) and palliation for pruritus, which includes biliary diversion, an operative technique in which the bile is diverted externally by an enterostomy. Most children have progressive fibrosis, with the development of cirrhosis and portal hypertension requiring liver transplantation in childhood.

4.5 Inherited Disorders of Bile Salt Metabolism

The development of new technology—fast atom bombardment ionization mass spectrometry (FAB MS)—has allowed many defects in primary bile acid synthesis to be identified.

Infants present with cholestasis, hepatomegaly, failure to thrive with or without pruritus, nonspecific biochemistry and liver histology. The diagnosis is made by identifying the specific abnormal bile acid metabolites in urine, which can be performed only at a specialized center.

It is essential to make the diagnosis, because without liver transplantation these diseases are fatal. However, treatment with a combination of oral bile acids, cholic acid, chenodeoxycholic acid, or ursodeoxycholic acid may prevent progression to cirrhosis if started early enough.

4.6 Zellweger's Syndrome (Cerebrohepatorenal Syndrome)

This is an autosomal recessive syndrome with multisystem disease, which is associated with absent or dysfunctional peroxisome biogenesis, leading to secondary defects of bile acid synthesis and abnormal beta oxidation of fatty acids. The incidence is 1 per 100,000 live births.

Infants present with severe hypotonia, feeding difficulties, and failure to thrive. Jaundice is present in only 50% of babies, but dysmorphic features— which include epicanthal folds, brush field spots, and a high forehead—are common in association with psychomotor retardation. There is multisystem involvement involving the brain, heart, liver, and kidneys. The diagnosis is confirmed by detecting very long chain fatty acids in serum.

Management and Outcome. Treatment is supportive, as death is inevitable. Liver transplantation is not indicated because of the progression of multisystem disease.

4.7 Cystic Fibrosis

Cystic fibrosis is an unusual cause of neonatal cholestasis, accounting for <1% of cases of persistent jaundice in children (see Chap. 31). It is an autosomal recessive disorder with an incidence of 1 per 2000 live births. The genetic defect has been localized to the long arm of chromosome 7, and more than 300 mutations have been identified in the gene coding for the cystic fibrosis transmembrane conductance regulator (CFTR). The commonest mutation is Δ 508, but no specific mutation is specific for liver disease.

Clinical Presentation and Diagnosis. Clinical symptoms include persistent cholestasis, meconium ileus, hepatomegaly, failure to thrive, and recurrent respiratory infections. Differentiation from biliary atresia may be difficult. Biochemical liver function tests reveal raised transaminases, alkaline phosphatase, and GGT. Immunoreactive trypsin may be higher than normal for age (>130 ng/mL). Serum cholesterol and triglycerides are usually normal. Although a sweat test is pathognomonic for this diagnosis, it is not worth doing in babies under 4 to 6 weeks of age (values of <50 mmol/L for <5 years). Liver histology is varied but usually demonstrates diffuse cholestasis with bile duct proliferation, focal biliary cirrhosis, and portal fibrosis.

Management and Outcome. Ursodeoxycholic acid (20 to 50 mg/kg/day) may be effective but is unproven. Nutritional support and fat-soluble vitamin supplementation are essential (Table 4).

Liver disease may resolve, but persistent jaundice with the development of cirrhosis, portal hypertension, and liver failure may occur. Ongoing malnutrition and respiratory disease may contribute to death in infancy.

4.8 Niemann Pick Disease Type C

This is a rare autosomal recessive disorder in which there is a defect in cholesterol esterification that results in a neurovisceral lipid storage disorder with an extremely varied spectrum of clinical findings (10). Sixty percent of children will present with prolonged cholestasis and hepatosplenomegaly in infancy; some will have fetal ascites. A number of children present later (3 to 5 years of age) with isolated splenomegaly and/or neurological signs and symptoms.

The diagnosis is determined by detecting PAS diastase-resistant storage material in Kupffer cells and hepatocytes in the liver or in the bone marrow. Neuronal storage indicating central nervous system involvement is present at birth and is demonstrated in the ganglion cells of a suction rectal biopsy. Skin fibroblast cultures will define the enzyme defect and enable antenatal diagnosis. Jaundice subsides in most children, although hepatosplenomegaly may persist. Sadly, all children develop neurological complications at a median age of 5 years, which include ataxia, convulsions, developmental delay, and dementia. Supranuclear ophthalmoplegia is pathognomonic for this condition. Most children die in late childhood or early adolescence from respiratory infections. Liver and bone marrow transplantation are not curative. Genetic counseling is essential and antenatal diagnosis may be performed by chorionic villus biopsy.

5 LIVER DISEASE IN OLDER CHILDREN

Liver disease in children older than 6 months may be acute or chronic. As in infancy, there is a predominance of inherited disorders (Table 5) and multisystem involvement.

5.1 Acute Liver Disease

Viral hepatitis, autoimmune hepatitis, and metabolic liver disease are the commonest causes of acute liver disease in childhood.

TABLE 5 Liver Diseases in Older Children

Disease	Diagnostic Investigations	Treatment
Hepatitis A, B, C, D, EBV, CMV	Serology	Supportive/ antivirals
Autoimmune hepatitis	IgG > 20 g/l C3, C4, LKM, ANA, SMA	Prednisone/ azathioprine
Wilson's disease	Serum Cu, ceruloplasmin, urinary Cu	Penicillamine
Alpha-1-antitrypsin deficiency	Alpha-1-AT level and phenotype	Supportive
Cystic fibrosis	Sweat test, liver biopsy	Supportive
Cryptogenic cirrhosis	Liver biopsy	Supportive
Primary sclerosing cholangitis	ERCP and liver biopsy	Ursodeoxycholic acid
Tyrosinemia type I	Urinary succinylacetone	NTBC
Hereditary fructose intolerance	Fructose 1-6-phosphate aldolase in liver	Fructose-free diet

Key: EBV, Epstein-Barr virus; CMV, cytomegalovirus; LKM, liver kidney microsomal antibodies; ANA, antinuclear antibodies; SMA, smooth muscle antibodies; C3, C4, complement; ERCP, endoscopic retrograde cholangiopancreatography; NTBC, 2(2 nitro-trifluoromethylbenzoyl)-1,3-cyclohexenedione.

5.1.1 Acute Viral Hepatitis

All forms of acute viral hepatitis may occur in children, including that caused by hepatitis A virus (HAV), hepatitis B virus (HBV), postransfusion hepatitis C virus (HCV), epidemic hepatitis E virus (HEV), Epstein-Barr virus (EBV), and cytomegalovirus (CMV).

Most cases of hepatitis are asymptomatic and anicteric. In symptomatic cases, a prodromal illness with vomiting, abdominal pain, lethargy, and jaundice is common. The diagnosis is confirmed by elevations of serum aminotransferases (ALT and AST 10 to 100 times normal), serum alkaline phosphatase (2.5 times normal), and specific viral serology.

Liver biopsy is not required for diagnosis unless the clinical course is complicated.

Management.   Uncomplicated acute hepatitis is managed at home. Hospital admission is required only if the child has severe vomiting leading to dehydration, abdominal pain, or lethargy, if coagulation parameters are prolonged, or if transaminase activity remains high. Fulminant hepatitis is a complication in less than 5% of pediatric cases. The main differential diagnoses are metabolic liver disease (e.g., Wilson's disease) and drug-induced liver disease.

5.1.2   Chronic Viral Hepatitis

Hepatitis B and C are the commonest causes of viral hepatitis in childhood but are unlikely to lead to serious liver disease until adolescence or adult life.

5.2   Hepatitis B

HBV is a hepatotropic DNA virus. Children are infected by vertical transmission from a carrier mother; horizontal transmission from parents and other family members; infected blood products; sexual abuse; or, in adolescents, drug abuse. There is an increased risk of environmental transmission in residential institutions and hemodialysis centers.

HBV carrier mothers, who are HB 'e' antigen positive, have the highest infectivity with 70–90% risk of transmission, HB 'e' antigen negative, but 'e' antibody positive mothers may also transmit infection, and their infants are particularly at risk of developing fulminant liver failure. Seventy percent of infants infected perinatally will become chronic carriers unless immunized at birth (11,12).

Most carrier children are asymptomatic, without signs of chronic liver disease. Biochemical parameters indicate mild elevation of transaminases (80 to 150 IU/L) with normal albumin, coagulation, and alkaline phosphatase. Liver histology indicates a chronic hepatitis in over 90% of the carriers.

Children with chronic HBV not only provide a continuing source of infection but also are at risk of developing cirrhosis and/or primary hepatocellular carcinoma. Chronic carriers should therefore remain under medical supervision in order to

1. Support and educate the family.
2. Screen and immunize family members.
3. Monitor seroconversion.
4. Detect progressive liver disease and/or hepatocellular carcinoma.
5. Consider antiviral therapy.

Annual review should include HBV serology and viral markers of HBV DNA, standard liver function tests, alpha-fetoprotein, and abdominal ultrasound. These reviews may be undertaken locally but referral for consideration of antiviral therapy should be to a specialized center.

Indications for treatment of chronic HBV are as follows:

Persistently raised serum aminotransferases
Presence of HBs antigen and 'e' antigen with detectable HBV DNA in
serum
Features of chronic hepatitis on liver biopsy

Interferon alpha (5 to 10 MU/m^2 three times a week) by subcutaneous injection for 6 months has a sustained clearance rate of 40 to 50% of those treated and is not recommended because of the side effects and poor results. Lamivudine, an oral antiviral agent, is a nucleoside analogue that has shown good short-term results in adults and is being evaluated in children.

5.2.1 Prevention of Hepatitis B

The most important strategy to prevent HBV transmission in childhood includes routine antenatal screening of all women during pregnancy, with immunization of at-risk infants or universal immunization of all infants.

5.3 Hepatitis C

The importance of HCV infection in children lies in its likelihood to develop into chronic liver disease. Children infected with HCV form three main groups: those who were parenterally infected prior to blood product and donor organ screening in 1990 (13), children who have been vertically infected (14), and a group of children who have been sporadically infected but the route of acquisition remains obscure.

Diagnosis. Diagnosis is made by screening children at risk. Serum aminotransferases are typically normal or very slightly elevated; HCV serology will indicate anti-HCV antibodies and the presence of HCV RNA by RT-PCR. Histology reveals classic features of chronic hepatitis C which include mild portal tract inflammation, lymphoid aggregates and mild periportal piecemeal necrosis with steatosis and apoptosis. In contrast to HBV infection, vertical transmission of HCV is unusual, ranging from 2 to 10% of offspring born to HCV RNA–positive mothers. The risk of transmission is increased to 48% by coexisting maternal HIV infection and in those with high HCV RNA titers. Breast-feeding is not contraindicated.

Management of Children with Chronic HCV. The first step is to establish the diagnosis not only by measuring anti-HCV antibody but also confirming that active infection is present by detecting HCV RNA by RT-PCR (Fig. 4). The natural history of chronic HCV in childhood is not known. The natural seroconversion rate appears to be approximately 20% in children who have received blood products. Long-term data on vertically infected infants are not available as yet.

Children with persistent positivity of HCV RNA and evidence of liver disease should be selected for therapy at a specialist center. Treatment with interferon alone is unsuccessful. The combination of interferon and ribavirin is being evaluated.

5.4 Autoimmune Hepatitis

Autoimmune hepatitis is a chronic inflammatory disorder that affects children of any age, from 6 months onward, although there is a 3-to-1 female preponderance (15). There are two forms of autoimmune hepatitis: type I, in which the nonspecific autoantibodies, antinuclear antibodies (ANA), and smooth muscle antibodies

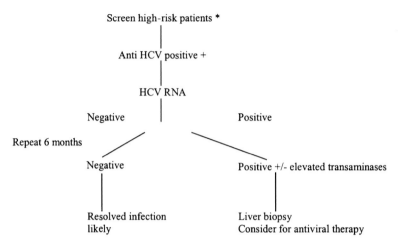

FIGURE 4   Algorithm for management of hepatitis C in childhood. *High-risk patients include: Recipients of multiple transfusions/pooled blood products. Infants of HCV positive mothers. +Anti-HCV by 3rd generation assay. May be positive in infants of HCV positive mothers up to 13 months by passive transfer.

(SMA) are positive, and type II, in which anti–liver, kidney, and mitochondrial (LKM) antibodies are positive.

In type I autoimmune hepatitis, the median age of onset is 10 years and the clinical presentation varies from acute hepatitis with autoimmune features to the slow development of cirrhosis, portal hypertension, and malnutrition. The association of multiorgan disease is higher in type I hepatitis, with autoimmune thyroiditis, celiac disease, inflammatory bowel disease, hemolytic anemia, and glomerulonephritis being the most common.

In type II autoimmune hepatitis, the age of onset is younger, median age of 7.4 years, and the clinical presentation is more likely to be acute, with fulminant hepatic failure. Multiorgan disease is less common. LKM II may develop in association with hepatitis C or be secondary to drugs such as antiepileptics. The diagnosis is made by the identification of

1. Elevated serum aminotransferases (10 times normal)
2. Increased total globulin or IgG concentrations greater than 1.5 times above the normal limit
3. Nonspecific autoantibodies (seropositivity for ANA, SMA, or LKM I antibodies—titers greater than 1:40). Up to 25% of children may not have detectable autoantibodies at presentation

4. Characteristic histological features of chronic hepatitis (increased portal inflammation)
5. Exclusion of hepatitis C and Wilson's disease

Management. Both forms of autoimmune hepatitis respond to immunosuppression with prednisone 2 mg/kg/day (maximum 60 mg) in association with azathioprine 0.5 to 2 mg/kg/day. Ninety percent of children will respond to the above regime, but cyclosporine (2 to 4 mg/kg/day) may be helpful in inducing or maintaining remission. It is usually impossible to discontinue corticosteroids and/or azathioprine.

Indications for liver transplantation include presentation with

1. Fulminant hepatic failure
2. Progression to end-stage liver failure
3. Intolerable side effects or failure of medical treatment

5.5 Sclerosing Cholangitis

The spectrum of sclerosing cholangitis in childhood includes neonatal sclerosing cholangitis and autoimmune sclerosing cholangitis in association with type I autoimmune hepatitis or immunodeficiency. Clinical features include abdominal pain, weight loss, intermittent jaundice resembling autoimmune hepatitis; cholestasis with cholangitis and pruritus or cirrhosis with portal hypertension. Laboratory investigation will indicate elevated alkaline phosphatase (>16 times normal), GGT (50 to 100 times normal). Bilirubin level may be normal or intermittently elevated in at least 50% of patients, serum transaminases are moderately elevated (50 times normal), prothrombin times and albumin levels are usually normal early in the disease. Elevated prothrombin time may be due to fat-soluble vitamin deficiency and is responsive to vitamin K. The diagnosis is confirmed by cholangiography [either operative, percutaneous, transhepatic, endoscopic, or magnetic resonance imaging (MRI)], which reveals typical lesions of irregular intrahepatic ducts, focal saccular dilatations, short annular strictures, an abnormally large gallbladder, and extrahepatic ductular irregularities (Fig. 5). Histology may demonstrate pathognomonic fibrous obliterative cholangitis with periductular fibrosis, but more often it indicates features of chronic hepatitis with cholestasis.

Treatment. Immunosuppression with predniso(lo)ne and azathioprine may be effective in sclerosing cholangitis associated with autoimmune hepatitis. Treatment of inflammatory bowel disease does not prevent progression of sclerosing cholangitis. Supportive therapy with fat-soluble vitamin supplementation, nutritional support, management of pruritus, and ursodeoxycholic acid (20 mg/kg/day) may be of benefit (16). Most children will progress to liver failure and require transplantation.

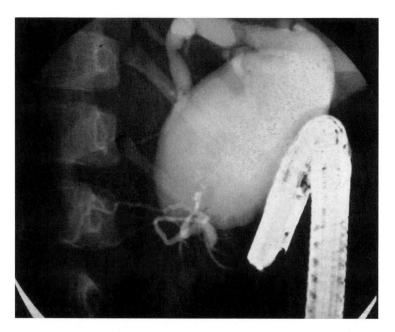

FIGURE 5   Sclerosing cholangitis may be diagnosed by endoscopic cholangio-pancreatography (ERCP). ERCP typically demonstrates lesions of irregular intrahepatic ducts, focal circular dilatations, short annular strictures, an abnormally large gallbladder, and extrahepatic ductular irregularities.

6   METABOLIC DISEASE IN OLDER CHILDREN

Metabolic disease in older children presents with hepatomegaly often without jaundice, with or without splenomegaly or neurological involvement. The main causes of metabolic liver disease in older children include alpha-1-antitrypsin deficiency, tyrosinemia type 1, glycogen storage diseases, hereditary fructose intolerance, Gaucher's disease, Wilson's disease, and cystic fibrosis.

6.1   Tyrosinemia Type 1

This rare autosomal disease more commonly presents with acute liver failure and is discussed in Section 10.7.

6.2   Glycogen Storage Disease

The hepatic glycogen storage disorders (GSD) are a group of inherited disorders affecting the metabolism of glycogen to glucose. Characteristic findings include hepatomegaly, growth failure, and hypoglycemia. The diagnosis is based on demonstrating the respective enzyme deficiency. All these diseases are autosomal recessive except for phosphorylase kinase deficiency, which is X-linked. They are best managed at a specialist unit.

6.3   Glucose-6-Phosphatase Deficiency Type 1a

Glucose-6-phosphatase is a microsomal enzyme found in hepatocytes, renal tubular epithelium, and pancreatic and intestinal mucosa, which is essential for hepatic glucose export. Deficiency of the enzyme results in complete dependency on dietary carbohydrate. The clinical and biochemical effects of the disease result from hypoglycemia and the body's response to it.

Clinical Presentation and Diagnosis.   Infants usually present with hypoglycemic seizures, hepatomegaly, and failure to thrive. Biochemical investigations reveal fasting hypoglycemia (<1.5 g/L) with lactic acidosis (>5 mmol/L) hyperlipidemia (cholesterol >6 mmol/L and triglycerides >3 mmol/L) and hyperuricemia. Hepatic transminases are usually normal or mildly elevated. Liver histology reveals fat and glycogen in liver cells. Histochemical stains for glucose-6-phosphatase are negative and the enzyme is not detected in liver.

Management and Prognosis.   The initial aim of dietary treatment is to provide a continuous supply of dietary glucose in order to maintain normal blood sugars. This is best achieved by frequent daytime feeding; use of oral uncooked cornstarch, which is hydrolyzed in the gut to release glucose slowly over hours; and continuous nocturnal enteral glucose feeds. If dietary control is strict in infancy, normal growth and development take place, although hepatomegaly and hyperlipidemia persist. Long-term complications include osteoporosis, renal dysfunction and calculi, and hepatic adenomata, which have the potential for malignant transformation. Liver transplantation will correct the hepatic metabolic defect but is not indicated for metabolic control.

Antenatal Diagnosis.   The gene for glucose-6-phosphatase has been isolated and many mutations described. Antenatal diagnosis by chorionic villus sampling is possible if a known mutation has been identified within the family.

6.4   GSD Types 1b and 1c

In these disorders, glucose-6-phosphatase is present but dysfunctional. Type 1b is due to a defect in glucose-6-phosphate transport into the microsome, while type 1c is due to abnormalities of phosphate transport out of the microsome. The clinical and biochemical features are similar to GSD type 1a. In GSD type 1b, neutropenia with recurrent infections, oral ulcers and inflammatory bowel disease have been reported. As the gene defect in GSD 1b and 1c has not yet been characterized, antenatal diagnosis is not possible.

6.5   GSD Type 3

In this disorder there is a deficiency in the debrancher enzyme or amylo-1-6-glucosidase deficiency. The metabolic defect is mild as other routes of gluconeogenesis are intact and there is no renal involvement. The defect is expressed in muscle in 85% of cases (type 3a).

Clinical Presentation and Diagnosis.   The clinical presentation is similar to GSD 1 without renal involvement. In time a peripheral myopathy and cardiomyopathy may develop. As the abnormally structured residual glycogen is fibrogenic, hepatic fibrosis, and cirrhosis are complicating features. Diagnosis is by identifying the deficient enzyme in leucocytes or liver tissue.

Management and Prognosis.   Dietary treatment is similar to GSD type 1 but a higher protein intake is recommended due to the demand of gluconeogenic amino acids. Most metabolic abnormalities diminish at puberty and long-term outcome is determined by the development of myopathy, cardiomyopathy, or cirrhosis.

Antenatal Diagnosis.   Antenatal diagnosis is possible by enzyme measurement or mutation analysis on chorionic villus samples.

6.6   GSD Type 4

This rare disease is due to a deficiency of the branching enzyme. It usually presents with evidence of severe liver disease in late infancy, but there may be cardiac, muscle, and neurological involvement. Hepatic histology demonstrates cirrhosis and accumulation of abnormally shaped glycogen, which is diastase-resistant.

Treatment and Prognosis.   Dietary treatment is as for other forms of glycogen storage disease. There is rapid development of cirrhosis, necessitating liver transplantation in the first 5 years of life. Progression of extrahepatic disease has been reported posttransplantation.

6.7   Hereditary Fructose Intolerance

This autosomal recessive disorder is due to the absence or reduction of fructose-1-phosphate aldolase B in liver, kidneys, and small intestine. The incidence has been estimate at 1 per 20,000 live births. The genetic mutation has been identified and is on chromosome 9.

Clinical Presentation and Diagnosis.   Clinical presentation is related to the introduction of fructose or sucrose in the diet, usually between 3 and 6 months of age. Vomiting is a prominent feature, with failure to thrive, hepatomegaly, and coagulopathy. Occasionally infants may present with acute liver failure with jaundice, encephalopathy, and renal failure. Renal tubular acidosis and hypophosphatemic rickets occur. Older children demonstrate aversion to fructose-containing food.

Biochemical liver function tests indicate raised hepatic transaminases, hypoalbuminemia, and hyperbilirubinemia. Plasma amino acids may be elevated secondary to liver dysfunction, and there may be hyperuricacidemia and hypoglycemia. Hematological abnormalities such as anemia, acanthocytosis, and thrombocytosis are associated. Urinary investigations will indicate fructosuria, proteinuria, amino aciduria, and organic aciduria in association with a reduction in the tubular reabsorption of phosphate. Diagnosis is suggested by reducing substances in the urine and confirmed by a reduction or absence of enymatic activity in liver or intestinal mucosal biopsy or by mutation analysis.

Hepatic pathology usually has excess fat in liver cells with fibrosis, which may progress to cirrhosis if fructose is continued.

Management and Prognosis.   Fructose elimination reverses hepatic and renal dysfunction. Antenatal diagnosis is possible by chorionic villus sampling.

6.8   Gaucher's Disease

Clinical Presentation and Diagnosis.   This autosomal recessive disorder is secondary to a deficiency of glucosyl-ceramide-beta-glucosidase, which is deficient in leukocytes, bone marrow, hepatocytes, and amniocytes. It may present in infancy with acute liver failure but is more usual in late childhood with hepatosplenomegaly and with respiratory, neurological, and bone disease.

The diagnosis is suggested by the identification of large, multinucleated Gaucher cells in bone marrow aspirate and liver confirmed by enzyme assay. Hepatic fibrosis may be severe, leading to cirrhosis.

Management and Outcome.   Recent therapy for Gaucher's disease includes enzyme replacement and bone marrow or liver transplantation.

6.9   Wilson's Disease

Wilson's disease is an autosomal recessive disorder with an incidence of 1 per 30,000 live births. The Wilson's disease gene is on chromosome 13 and encodes a copper-binding ATPase.

Clinical Features.   Clinical features in childhood include hepatic dysfunction (40%) and psychiatric symptoms (35%). Children under the age of 10 years usually present with hepatic symptoms. The hepatic presentation of Wilson's disease is with hepatomegaly, vague gastrointestinal symptoms, subacute or fulminant hepatitis, chronic hepatitis, or cirrhosis. Neurological symptoms are nonspecific. Children may present with deteriorating school performance, abnormal behavior, lack of coordination and dysarthria. Renal tubular abnormalities, renal calculi, and acute hemolytic anemia are associated features. The characteristic Kayser-Fleischer rings (demonstrating copper in the iris) are not usually detected before the age of 7 years and may be absent in up to 80% of older children.

Diagnosis. Biochemical liver function tests indicate chronic liver disease with low albumin (<35 g/L), minimal transaminitis, and a low alkaline phosphastase (<200 IU/L). There may be evidence of hemolysis on blood film.
The diagnosis is established by detecting

A low serum copper (<10 μmol/L)
A low serum ceuroloplasmin (<200 mg/L)
Excess urine copper (>1 μmol/24 hr) particularly after penicillamine treatment (20 mg/kg/day)
An elevated hepatic copper (>250 mg/g dry weight of liver)

Approximately 25% of children may have a normal or borderline ceruloplasmin, as it is an acute-phase protein.
Histological features of Wilson's disease depend on the clinical presentation. There may be microvesicular fatty infiltration of hepatocytes, chronic hepatitis, hepatocellular necrosis, hepatic fibrosis, and cirrhosis. In children with fulminant hepatitis, the histological features are those of severe hepatocellular necrosis with underlying cirrhosis.

Management and Prognosis. Current management includes a low-copper diet and penicillamine (20 mg/kg/day), which is effective if started before the development of significant hepatic fibrosis. If penicillamine toxicity is unacceptable, alternative therapy includes trientine (triethyline tetramine) 25 mg/kg/day in addition to oral zinc.
In asymptomatic children or those with minimal hepatic dysfunction, the outlook is excellent, although fulminant hepatic failure with hemolysis may occur if treatment is discontinued. Liver transplantation is essential therapy for children who present with subacute or fulminant hepatitis and in those with advanced cirrhosis and portal hypertension.

Family Screening. It is essential for the family to be screened in order to treat asymptomatic patients and to detect heterozygotes. The development of mutation analysis may be more reliable than measurement of serum copper and ceruloplasmin.

7 CYSTIC FIBROSIS LIVER DISEASE

The incidence of liver disease in children with cystic fibrosis (CF) varies from 4.5 to 20%, depending on age and the definition of significant liver disease (see Chap. 31).

Etiology. The etiology of CF liver disease has been only partially explained. Despite major advances in the understanding of the genetic defects in CF, no definite genetic mutation has been associated with the development of liver disease. The recent discovery of the CF transmembrane receptor (CFTR) in the apical membrane of biliary epithelial cells may be a major step in the understanding of the etiology. Bile acid malabsorption is a constant finding in untreated children with CF. It is possible that the abnormalities in bile salt concentration and the increase in hydrophobic and toxic bile acids may play an important role in the production of viscous bile and or biliary sludge, which may lead to partial biliary obstruction and focal biliary fibrosis.

Clinical Features. Most children with CF and liver disease are asymptomatic in the early stages. In infants, cholestatic neonatal hepatitis may be a presenting feature (see above), but more commonly the presentation is with asymptomatic hepatosplenomegaly or the complications of portal hypertension. Biliary disease includes asymptomatic gallstones in 20% and microgallbladder on ultrasound in 10 to 40%; biliary strictures are uncommon.

Diagnosis of Liver Disease. Early detection of liver disease using serum liver function tests is unsatisfactory. There are transient abnormalities of alkaline phosphatase in up to 50% of patients; increases in GGT in 30% of males, 60% of females; serum bilirubin levels and coagulation times remain normal until late in the disease. Ultrasonography may detect increased echogenicity of the liver with a microgallbladder with or without gallstones in 25% of patients.

Liver biopsy should be performed to establish the extent and severity of liver disease and is indicated when there is persistent transaminitis; hepatic echogenicity on ultrasound, hepatomegaly and/or splenomegaly, or evidence of hepatic dysfunction. Liver histology may indicate fatty infiltration, focal biliary cirrhosis, and multilobular cirrhosis.

Treatment. Treatment consists of nutritional support and the prevention and management of hepatic complications. Nutritional support is critically important in children with CF and is a major cause of malnutrition in these children, whether or not they have liver disease. If CF is complicated by clinically significant liver disease, then the following is recommended:

1. Increasing energy intake [150% of the estimated average requirement (EAR) by carbohydrate supplements, such as glucose polymers, or by increasing the percentage of fat]

2. Increasing the proportion of medium-chain triglyercides to 50% of the fat content
3. Supplementation with fat-soluble vitamins, including vitamin A (5000 to 15,000 IU daily); vitamin E (100 to 500 mg daily); vitamin D, given as alfa calcidol in the United Kingdom and calcitriol in the United States (50 ng/kg); and vitamin K (1 to 10 mg daily)

The use of ursodeoxycholic acid (UDCA) in the management of CF liver disease remains controversial. Administration of UDCA (10 to 20 mg/kg/day) improves the biochemical indices of liver function but may not affect the natural history of the disease unless prescribed prior to significant hepatic disease. The main hepatic complication of CF is the development of portal hypertension with esophageal varices, which should be diagnosed by endoscopy. Bleeding varices are treated with injection sclerotherapy band ligation, or transjugular intrahepatic shunts.

Prognosis and Liver Transplantation. CF liver disease is a progressive disease leading to cirrhosis and portal hypertension. Indications for liver transplantation include the development of end-stage liver failure with jaundice, ascites, and coagulopathy. Liver transplantation alone is indicated in children with CF liver disease prior to the development of significant pulmonary complication ($>$60% of normal function) in order to prevent the necessity for heart, lung, and liver transplantation.

Outcome following liver transplantation is similar to that of children transplanted for other causes of liver disease. Lung function may improve posttransplantation.

8 HEPATIC TUMORS

Liver tumors are relatively rare in childhood and occur in the region of 0.5 to 2.5 per million population.

8.1 Hepatoblastoma

Hepatoblastoma is most commonly seen in children under the age of 18 months and is rare after the age of 5 years. There is a male predominance of 3 to 2. The commonest presenting feature is of an abdominal mass and distention. Hepatoblastoma occurs with certain well-recognized associations, in particular familial adenomatous polyposis.

8.2 Hepatocellular Carcinoma

Hepatocellular carcinoma in childhood occurs at an older age than hepatoblastoma, usually as a complication of cirrhosis secondary to hepatitis B or C or alpha$_1$-antitrypsin deficiency. A rare tumor fibrolamellar hepatocellular carcinoma is occasionally seen in childhood and occurs in noncirrhotic livers. The clinical presentation is similar to that of hepatoblastoma.

Diagnosis in Both Tumors. Laboratory investigations will demonstrate

1. A normocytic normochromic anemia in 50% of children.
2. Thrombocytosis (greater than $1000 \times 10^9/L$) in 30% of children.
3. Liver function tests are normal in hepatoblastoma but may be abnormal in hepatocellular carcinoma due to underlying cirrhosis.
4. Alpha-fetoprotein may be a useful diagnostic and prognostic marker and is elevated in 90% of hepatoblastoma patients and 60% of hepatocellular carcinoma patients.
5. Transcobalamin-1 may be a useful marker in fibrolamellar hepatocellular carcinoma.

Radiological Imaging. Abdominal ultrasound, computed tomography (CT), or MRI will determine the site and extent of the lesion and establish the presence of any metastases while providing information as to suitability for surgical resection. Vascular structures are best identified on angiography or MRI and are an essential investigation prior to surgery. Chest x-ray and CT scanning are important baseline investigations to define the presence of pulmonary metastases. Liver biopsy is necessary for histological confirmation and selection of chemotherapy despite the risks of disseminating tumor.

Treatment and Outcome. With cisplatin and doxorubicin (PLADO), 90% of hepatoblastomas will respond to chemotherapy and surgery. A minority will require liver transplantation for unresectable tumors (17). An increasing number of patients have been successfully transplanted, with a similar 5-year survival of 80%.

Hepatocellular carcinomas are less responsive to treatment and only 50% will respond to PLADO chemotherapy. Surgical resection is less successful. The recent addition of carboplatin to PLADO may improve the response rate in these tumors.

Response to therapy may be monitored by serial measurement of alpha-fetoprotein levels. Patients with good responses to chemotherapy will have a rapid fall of serum AFP, while those children with persistent elevation of AFP are likely to have minimal residual disease or metastases.

9 MANAGEMENT OF CHRONIC LIVER DISEASE

The important principles of management of chronic liver disease are

Early and accurate diagnosis at a specialist center
Shared management with referral center

Nutritional support
Prevention and prompt management of hepatic complications
Early consideration for liver transplantation

Nutritional Support.   The key to effective nutritional support is the realization that an increased energy intake to overcome the hypercatabolic state is required. This is usually managed in infants by using a high-calorie protein feed providing between 150 and 200% of the EAR which may be given by a nocturnal nasogastric enteral feeding or continuous feeding (Table 4). It is usual to increase the medium-chain triglyceride content of the fat in order to reduce steatorrhea and to ensure adequate supplementation of fat-soluble vitamins (Table 4). In older children, supplements may be provided with high-calorie protein drinks. Parenteral nutrition may be required if enteral feeding is not tolerated due to ascites and variceal bleeding.

Hepatic Complications.   The commonest complications are the development of esophageal varices with bleeding, ascites, or encephalopathy.

Acute variceal bleeding should be managed in a standard way with resuscitation with blood products, endoscopic sclerotherapy, or esophageal banding for acute bleeding. Vasopressin or octreotide infusions may be necessary for prolonged or recurrent bleeding. The role of prophylactic propranolol is not established in children. In children with uncontrolled variceal bleeding, the insertion of a transjugular intrahepatic portosystemic shunt (TIPS—a shunt between hepatic and portal veins) has proved an effective management strategy in even quite small children.

Sepsis, particularly cholangitis and spontaneous bacterial peritonitis, should be appropriately treated with broad-spectrum antibiotics (cefuroxime 20 mg/kg/dose t.i.d., amoxicillin 25 mg/kg/dose t.i.d., and metronidazole 8 mg/kg/dose are useful first-line antibiotics).

Fluid retention, leading to ascites and cardiac failure, is inevitable in most children with liver failure. A combination of salt and fluid restriction (to two-thirds of maintenance fluids), diuretics (spironolactone 3 mg/kg/dose or furosemide 0.5 to 2 mg/kg/dose), and albumin infusions (either 4.5 or 20%) is often effective in establishing diuresis. Hemodialysis or hemofiltration are rarely required for children with chronic liver failure.

Encephalopathy is less common in children than in adults but may present with aggressive behavior or deterioration in school performance. It is associated with an elevated ammonia (>50 IU/L) and, electroencephalographic (EEG) findings of slow low-voltage waves. It is treated with a reduction in protein intake to approximately 1 g/kg/day.

Liver Transplantation.   Ultimately, all children with progressive liver disease will require liver transplantation. It is important to consider referral for transplantation early (see below), and close cooperation with a specialized center is essential.

10   ACUTE LIVER FAILURE IN INFANCY AND CHILDHOOD

The definition of acute liver failure or fulminant hepatic failure (FHF) is the development of hepatic necrosis with coagulopathy and encephalopathy occurring within 8 weeks of the onset of liver disease (18). This definition is hard to apply in pediatric practice, as many infants present with acute liver failure secondary to an inborn error of metabolism, implying preexisting disease. In addition, encephalopathy may be difficult to detect in infants and small children and be less severe than coagulopathy in the early stages. Thus, caution is required in defining fulminant hepatitis or acute liver failure in infancy. The etiology of acute liver failure is documented in Table 6.

10.1   Acute Liver Failure in Infancy

Acute liver failure in infancy usually presents with multisystem involvement (19). The diagnosis may initially be difficult, as jaundice may be a late feature. Infants are usually small for gestation date, with hypotonia, severe coagulopathy and encephalopathy. Neurological problems such as nystagmus and convulsions may be secondary to cerebral disease or encephalopathy. Renal tubular acidosis is

TABLE 6   Acute Liver Failure in Children

Fulminant hepatitis	Diagnostic investigations
Infection	
Viral hepatitis A, B, C; undefined, EBV, CMV	Viral serology
Poison/drugs	
Acetaminophen	Acetaminophen levels
Paracetamol	Paracetamol levels
Sodium valproate	Microvesicular fat in hepatocytes
Isoniazid, halothane	Helothane antibodies
Amanita phalloides	
Propylthiouracyl	
Autoimmune hepatitis	Autoimmune screen
Metabolic	
Wilson's disease	Cu, ceruloplasmin
Tyrosinemia	Urinary succinylacetone
Reye's syndrome	Microvesicular fat in liver
	Urinary dicarboxylic acids

common. Investigations include a search for multiorgan disease. These diseases are best diagnosed and managed at a specialized center (20,21).

10.2 Galactosemia

This rare autosomal disorder is secondary to a deficiency of galactose-1-phosphase uridyltransferase. Acute illness results from the accumulation of the substrate galactose-1-phosphate (gal-1-P) following the introduction of milk feeds.

Clinical Presentation and Diagnosis. Infants present with sepsis, hypoglycemia, and encephalopathy in the first few days of life or with progressive jaundice and liver failure. Cataracts are present. The disease may be complicated by gram-negative septicemia, which stimulates a severe, life-threatening bleeding diathesis. The diagnosis is established by the detection of urinary reducing substances in the absence of glycosuria and confirmed by reduced enzyme activity in erythrocytes. Hepatic pathology demonstrates fatty change, bile duct proliferation, and iron deposition with extramedullary hematopoiesis. Hepatic fibrosis and cirrhosis can be present at birth or develop if galactose ingestion persists.

Management and Prognosis. Liver function improves following exclusion of galactose from the diet unless liver failure or cirrhosis has developed. Galactose elimination is lifelong. The long-term outcome is disappointing. Learning difficulties and growth disturbance are described, and 75% of girls develop ovarian failure. Detection of galactosemia in a neonatal screening program will lead to early detection except for infants who present with fulminant hepatitis. Antenatal diagnosis is possible by chorionic villus sampling.

10.3 Neonatal Hemochromatosis

This presumed autosomal recessive disorder is the commonest cause of acute liver failure in the neonate. It is characterized by the prenatal accumulation of intrahepatic iron, due either to a primary disorder of fetoplacental iron handling or a secondary manifestation of fetal liver disease.

Clinical Presentation and Diagnosis. Intrauterine growth retardation and premature delivery is common. Clinical features include hypoglycemia, jaundice, and coagulopathy within the first 2 weeks with a fatal outcome without treatment.

Biochemical liver function tests demonstrate elevated bilirubin and transaminases and reduced albumin. Serum iron binding capacity is low and hypersaturated (90 to 100%), with a grossly elevated ferritin level ($>$1000 ng/L). Diagnostic liver biopsy is not feasible because of the coagulopathy, but extrahepatic siderosis is found in minor salivary glands obtained by lip biopsy. MRI may confirm excess hepatic or extrahepatic iron.

Management and Prognosis. Medical management includes supportive therapy for acute liver failure and an "antioxidant cocktail" that combines *N*-acetylcysteine (150 mg/kg/day), vitamin E (25 mg/kg/day), selenium (2 to 3 μg/kg/day), prostaglandin E1 (0.4–0.6 μg/kg/hr), and deferroxamine (30 mg/kg/day). Some children have responded to this regime, but the majority require liver transplantation. There is resolution of extrahepatic iron following successful liver transplantation.

Antenatal Diagnosis. Currently, early antenatal diagnosis is not possible.

10.4 Disorders of Mitochondrial Energy Metabolism

This group of disorders includes a wide range of clinical phenotypes with any mode of inheritance—autosomal recessive, autosomal dominant, or transmission through maternal DNA. A number of different defects involving the electron transport chain have been described. In the context of liver failure, two entities are relevant: isolated deficiencies of the electron chain enzymes and mDNA depletion syndromes

10.5 Deficiencies of the Electron Transport Chain Enzyme

The most common isolated defects are complexes 4 and 1, although multiple deficiencies have been reported. Infants present with multisystem involvement with hypotonia, cardiomyopathy, and proximal renal tubulopathy as well as a severe metabolic acidosis. Relevant diagnostic investigations include

Elevated blood lactate
Lactate/pyruvate ratio >20
Increased 3-OH-butyrate/acetoacetate ratio >2
Detection of specific organic acids, such as urinary 3-methyl-glutaconic acid

Coagulopathy is usually extreme and may prevent liver biopsy, muscle biopsy, or cerebrospinal fluid (CSF) examination. The definitive diagnosis is based on demonstrating biochemical dysfunction of electron chain function in liver or muscle by histochemistry or enzyme analysis in fresh tissue. Demonstration of an elevated CSF lactate compared to plasma lactate indicates neurological involvement.

Management and Prognosis. Supportive management is usually the only option. Liver transplantation is successful only if the defect is confined to the liver but is contraindicated if multisystem involvement is obvious, as neurological deterioration persists or may develop posttransplant. Antenatal diagnosis is rarely possible as the underlying gene defects are unknown.

10.6 Mitochondrial Depletion Syndrome

Mitochondria normally contain more than one copy of mDNA and replication is regulated by a number of factors encoded by nuclear genes. Mutations in these nuclear genes lead to a reduction in copy numbers of mDNA, resulting in mitochondrial depletion.

Clinical Presentation and Diagnosis.   The clinical presentation and biochemical findings are similar to those in infants presenting with isolated electron transport chain deficiencies. In most patients tissue measurement of electron chain activities show deficiencies in complexes 1, 3, and 4, although activity may be within the normal range. The diagnosis is confirmed by demonstrating an abnormally low ratio for mDNA/nuclear DNA in affected tissue.

Management and Prognosis.   Treatment is supportive, as liver transplantation is contraindicated (22). Antenatal diagnosis is not currently possible.

10.7 Tyrosinemia Type I

Tyrosinemia type I is an autosomal recessive disorder due to a defect of fumaryl acetoacetase (FAA), which is the last enzyme in tyrosine degradation. The gene for FAA is on the short arm of chromosome 15. Many mutations have been described. Toxic metabolites lead to liver, cardiac, renal, and neurological disease.

Clinical Presentation.   Clinical presentation is heterogeneous even within the same family. Acute liver failure is a common presentation in infants between 1 and 6 months of age that present with mild jaundice, coagulopathy, encephalopathy, and ascites. Hypoglycemia is common due either to liver dysfunction or to hyperinsulinism from pancreatic islet cell hyperplasia.

In older infants, failure to thrive, coagulopathy, hepatosplenomegaly, hypotonia, and rickets are common. Older children may present with chronic liver disease, a hypertrophic cardiomyopathy, renal failure, or a porphyria-like syndrome with self-mutilation. Renal tubular dysfunction and hypophosphatemic rickets may occur at any age. There is a high risk of hepatocellular carcinoma.

Diagnosis.   Biochemical liver function tests reveal elevated bilirubin, transaminases, and alkaline phosphatase and a reduced albumin. Plasma amino acids indicate a threefold increase in plasma tyrosine, phenylalanine, and methionine, with grossly elevated alpha-fetoprotein levels. Urinary succinyl acetone is a pathognomonic but not an invariable finding. The diagnosis is confirmed by measuring FAA activity in fibroblasts or lymphocytes.

Hepatic histology is nonspecific, with fatty change, siderosis, and cirrhosis, which may be present in infancy. Hepatocyte dysplasia is common and is associated with a risk of hepatocellular carcinoma.

Management. Initial management is with a phenylalanine- and tyrosine-restricted diet, which may improve overall nutritional status and renal tubular function but does not affect the progression of liver disease (23). The recent discovery of NTBC [2 (2 nitro-trifluoromethylbenzoyl)-1,3-cyclohexenedione], which prevents the formation of toxic metabolites, has altered the natural history of this disease in childhood. Worldwide, more than 100 children have been treated with NTBC. There is rapid reduction of toxic metabolites, normalization of tubular function, prevention of porphyria-like crises, and improvement in both nutritional status and liver function, particularly in those with acute liver failure.

The current indications for liver transplantation for this condition include the development of acute or chronic liver failure unresponsive to NTBC or suspicion of development of hepatocellular carcinoma.

Prognosis. The long-term outcome of children with tyrosinemia type I treated with NTBC is unknown. These children require long-term monitoring and follow-up with 6-monthly abdominal ultrasounds and CT scans or MRI and alpha-fetoprotein estimation for early detection of hepatocellular carcinoma.

Antenatal diagnosis is possible either by chorionic villus sampling, which measures FFA directly, from mutation analysis, or by measurement of succinyl acetone in the amniotic fluid. Prospective affected siblings may benefit from early NTBC therapy.

10.8 Familial Hemophagocytic Lymphohistiocytosis

This rare condition may be inherited as an autosomal recessive disorder or be secondary to a viral illness. There is progressive visceral, neurological, and bone marrow infiltration with lymphocytes and large erythrophagocytic histiocytes.

Clinical Presentation and Diagnosis. Children present with fever, hepatosplenomegaly, jaundice, skin rash, edema, and encephalopathy in the first year of life. There is a pancytopenia, coagulopathy, biochemical features of acute liver failure, hypofibroginemia, and hypotriglyceridemia. Diagnosis is established by identifying the characteristic erythrophagocytic histiocytes in bone marrow, liver, and CSF.

Treatment and Prognosis. The disease is usually fatal, although treatment with antimetabolites and steroids or bone marrow transplantation may be helpful. Liver transplantation is contraindicated if there is extensive bone marrow or neurological involvement.

11 ACUTE LIVER FAILURE IN OLDER CHILDREN

11.1 Fulminant Viral Hepatitis

All forms of acute viral hepatitis may present in childhood. In infants, infection with herpes simplex or other viruses (HSV1, HSV2, HSV6, varicella zoster, CMV) may cause particularly severe forms of hepatic failure.

Fulminant hepatitis in infants 3 months of age may develop secondary to vertical transmission from an HBS antigen–positive mother who has anti-HB 'e' antibody. The pathogenesis of this disease is unknown but may be related to the lack of protection of anti-E antibody in the neonate.

In older children hepatitis A and hepatitis non–A to G are the commonest causes of fulminant hepatitis, with an incidence ranging from 1.5 to 31%.

11.2 Drugs and Toxins

Liver injury due to drugs and toxins is the second most common cause of acute liver failure in older children (Table 6).

11.3 Sodium Valproate Toxicity

Sodium valproate is a branched medium-chain fatty acid with broad-spectrum antiepileptic activity. It has been associated with more than 150 cases of fatal hepatotoxicity worldwide, although the mechanism is unclear (24). Hepatotoxicity has occurred in patients with inborn errors of metabolism such as mitochondrial disorders, the urea cycle, and Alpers syndrome, suggesting that the normal response to valproate may precipitate hepatotoxicity in these conditions.

Clinical Features and Diagnosis. Hepatotoxicity may occur at any age but is more likely in children aged <2 years, those on multiple epileptic therapy, and who have previous neurological abnormalities or developmental delay. Clinical features include nausea, vomiting, increasing seizure frequency, jaundice, edema, and hypoglycemia, leading to drowsiness and coma usually within the first 6 months of treatment. Biochemical investigations reveal moderate increases in hepatic transaminases and bilirubin, hypoalbuminemia, and severe coagulopathy. Hepatic histology demonstrates severe microvesicular fatty change with hepatocellular necrosis and occasionally cirrhosis.

Treatment and Prognosis. Once liver disease is established, the outlook is poor unless valproate has been promptly discontinued. Liver transplantation is contraindicated, as neurological disease may progress.

11.4 Progressive Neuronal Degeneration of Childhood (Alpers Syndrome)

The etiology of this familial disorder is unknown. It is thought to be autosomal recessive and in some cases an electron chain transport defect has been identified.

Clinical Presentation and Diagnosis. Despite a normal neonatal period, there may be both physical and developmental delay followed by the sudden onset of intractable seizures between the ages of 1 and 3 years. Although biochemical evidence of liver dysfunction is often present at this stage, clinical liver involvement is a preterminal event. Hepatic disease presents as jaundice, hepatomegaly, and coagulopathy with rapidly progressive liver failure. There are no specific biochemical features. The EEG demonstrates high-amplitude polyspikes; CT or MRI scans show low-density areas in the occipital and posterior temporal areas. There is a gradual extinction of visual evoked responses.

Liver histology characteristically shows microvesicular fatty change, bile duct proliferation, and focal necrosis leading to bridging fibrosis and cirrhosis. Neuropathology reveals cortical involvement with neuronal cell loss and astrocyte replacement.

Management and Prognosis. The condition is uniformly fatal, with most children dying before 3 years of age, within a few months of developing overt liver disease. It is important to avoid the use of valproate, as it is likely to accelerate the development of liver disease. Liver transplantation is contraindicated, as neurological progression continues posttransplant.

Antenatal diagnosis is currently impossible.

Clinical Manifestations of Acute Liver Failure. The onset of liver disease varies according to etiology. There may be a prodromal illness with lethargy, fatigue, malaise, vomiting, diarrhea, and jaundice, with the subsequent development of coagulopathy and encephalopathy. Encephalopathy is difficult to detect in infants and may present with drowsiness, irritability, or day/night reversal of sleep rhythm. Older children become aggressive, which is misinterpreted as antisocial behavior. The later stages of encephalopathy and hepatic coma are similar in older children and adults. A poor prognosis is indicated if any of the following features are present:

Rise in bilirubin (greater than 300 umol/L; >6 mg/dL)
A fall in transaminases without clinical improvement and with increasing coagulopathy
Prothrombin time over 60 sec
Metabolic acidosis (pH less than 7.3)
Hypoglycemia (glucose less than 4 mmol/L 70 mg/dL)
A decrease in liver size (not usual in metabolic liver disease)
Increasing hepatic coma of grade II or III

Children developing these signs should be referred to a transplant unit immediately.

Supportive management for acute liver failure in childhood includes:

1. Maintaining blood glucose levels greater than 4 mmol/L (70 g/dL) with 10 to 50% dextrose
2. Fluid restriction, 50 to 75% of maintenance using colloid to maintain circulating volume

3. Prevention of gastrointestinal hemorrhage from stress erosions, using H$_2$ receptor antagonists (ranitidine 3 mg/kg IV bid) and sucralfate (2 to 4 g/day)
4. Prevention of sepsis with broad-spectrum antibiotics (amoxicillin, cefuroxime, and metronidazole)
5. Prophylactic antifungal therapy (fluconazole)
6. Treatment of coagulopathy, if required, with fresh frozen plasma and intravenous vitamin K (2 to 10 mg).
7. Management of hepatic encephalopathy is unsatisfactory. In the early stages, reduction of protein intake to 1 to 2 g/kg and provision of high-calorie feeds using glucose polymers (8 to 10 g/kg) and oral lactulose may be sufficient. Increasing encephalopathy unresponsive to conservative management requires elective ventilation.
8. The development of cerebral edema by clinical signs such as deepening coma, which may be detectable on CT scan, is an ominous sign. Conservative management includes fluid restriction (<50% or maintenance) and mannitol (0.5 g/kg IV every 6 to 8 hr) as well as elective hyperventilation. The role of intracranial pressure monitoring is controversial. Electrodes may be difficult to insert in children with severe coagulopathy, particularly as the blood product replacement may exacerbate cerebral edema. Intracranial pressure monitoring may improve selection for transplantation but does not affect overall survival.

Liver transplantation should be carefully considered in all children with acute liver failure, but difficulties arise in the selection of infants with inborn errors of metabolism because of the difficulty in excluding multisystem disease. Liver transplantation is indicated in those children who have poor prognostic factors—that is:

1. Non–A to G hepatitis
2. Rapid onset of coma with grade III or IV
3. Severe coagulopathy (may be more severe than encephalopathy in metabolic disease)
4. No evidence of irreversible brain damage on CT scan
5. No evidence of multisystem disease (normal muscle biopsy, normal EEG, normal CT scan)

Prognosis. The mortality without liver transplantation is greater than 70% for children who are in grade III or IV coma or who have persistently abnormal coagulation (prothrombin time >60 sec). Prognosis may be better in children with hepatitis A or those who have paracetamol or acetaminophen overdose (25).

There is a 50 to 70% survival following 1 year liver transplantation, which is less than that after transplantation for other indications.

12 LIVER TRANSPLANTATION

The success of pediatric liver transplantation has revolutionized the prognosis for many infants and children who would otherwise die of liver failure. The main factors in improving survival in this age group include advances in preoperative management, such as the treatment of hepatic complications, nutritional support, and selection for transplantation. The rapid development in innovative surgical techniques to expand the donor pool have extended liver transplantation to the neonatal age group, while improvements in postoperative management, including immunosuppression, have led not only to increased survival but also to an improved quality of life. The range of indications for liver transplantation in children now includes semielective liver replacement and transplantation for inborn errors of metabolism with extrahepatic disease and unresectable hepatic tumors.

12.1 Who and When to Refer for Transplantation

Liver transplantation is standard therapy for acute or chronic liver failure and certain inborn errors of metabolism. Biliary atresia is the commonest indication for children transplanted under the age of 2 years (Fig. 6).

12.2 Chronic Liver Failure

As many children with cirrhosis and portal hypertension have well compensated hepatic function, the timing of liver transplantation may be difficult to decide. In general, the most useful guide is a serial estimation of hepatic function, such as:

A persistent rise in total bilirubin ($>$100 umol/L) ($>$6 mg/dL)

Prolongation of prothrombin time [International Normalized Ratio (INR) $>$1.4]

Progressive fall in serum albumin ($<$35 g/L)

The development of protein energy malnutrition resistant to nutritional management (deterioration in measurements of triceps skin folds, midarm muscle area, negative growth velocity)

Hepatic complications such as chronic hepatic encephalopathy, refractory ascites, intractable pruritus, or recurrent variceal bleeding nonresponsive to optimal medical management

A significant reduction in developmental motor skills

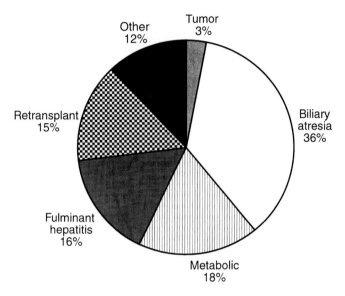

FIGURE 6 Indications for liver transplantation in children's Birmingham program, 1983–1999.

12.3 Acute Liver Failure

The indications for liver transplantation for children with acute liver failure depend on the etiology and the extent of the multisystem disease. In general children with fulminant hepatitis should be referred early to a specialist unit in the field of transplantation in order to provide time for stabilization and consideration for liver transplantation.

In children with a poor prognosis and therefore early listing for liver transplantation, criteria include

Non–A to G hepatitis
Rapid onset of coma with progression to grade III or IV hepatic coma
Diminishing liver size
A fall in serum transaminases associated with increasing bilirubin (>300 umol/L/18 mg/dL) and persistent coagulopathy (>50 sec)

Liver transplantation is contraindicated for children with evidence of multisystem involvement (e.g., mitochondrial disease) or irreversible brain damage from cerebral edema or hypoglycemia.

12.4   Inborn Errors of Metabolism

Liver transplantation is indicated for certain inborn errors of metabolism if the hepatic enzyme deficiency leads to:

1. Irreversible liver disease or liver failure (e.g., tyrosinemia type I, Wilson's disease)
2. Severe extrahepatic disease (e.g., renal disease in primary hyperoxaluria)

Selection of patients with severe extrahepatic disease is difficult as it is necessary to evaluate the child's quality of life on medical management and to compare the potential mortality and morbidity of the original disease with the risk complications and outcome following liver transplantation. The timing of transplantation in these disorders depends on:

The rate of progression of the disease
The affected child's quality of life on conservative management
The development of severe reversible extrahepatic disease

Evaluation for Transplantation. The aim of the evaluation process is to:

1. Assess the severity of liver disease and the extent of hepatic complications
2. Consider the technical aspects of the operation with regard to vascular anatomy and size
3. Exclude any significant contraindications to successful transplantation
4. Prepare the child and family psychologically

The histological diagnosis of the original disease should be reviewed and the severity and extent of hepatic function determined by evaluating:

Albumin (<35 g/L).
Coagulation time (INR >1.4).
Rise in bilirubin (>150 umol/L; >3 mg/dL) is usual is cholestatic patients, but may be a late feature in other diseases such as cystic fibrosis.
The extent of portal hypertension should be estimated by visualizing esophageal and gastric varices by gastrointestinal endoscopy.

It is normal to establish baseline renal function, hematological parameters, and background serology, which includes CMV status. The most important technical information required is the vascular anatomy and patency of the hepatic vessels. Most of this information may be obtained by color-flow Doppler ultrasound, although occasionally MRI or angiography may be required to clarify abnormal anatomy. Liver transplantation causes important hemodynamic changes during the operative and anhepatic phases; thus baseline information on cardiac and respiratory function is essential and may be obtained from an EKG, echocardiogram, or oxygen saturation study.

Neurodevelopmental Assessment.   One of the main aims of liver transplantation is to improve quality of life posttransplant; thus it is essential to exclude any neurological or psychological defects that may be irreversible posttransplant. The psychological and developmental assessment of children may be performed using the standard tests.

Dental Assessment.   Chronic liver disease has an adverse effect on the dentition of young children, which includes hypoplasia, staining of the teeth, and gingival hyperplasia. As gingival hyperplasia may be a significant problem posttransplant, good methods of dental hygiene should be established pretransplant.

Contraindications to Transplantation.   As medical and surgical expertise is improved, there are fewer contraindications to pediatric liver transplants based on technical restrictions of age and size. Increased experience has indicated that certain medical conditions are not curable by transplantation. These include

1.   The presence of severe systemic sepsis, particularly fungal sepsis
2.   HIV-positive children whose long-term prognosis is still unknown
3.   Malignant hepatic tumors with extrahepatic spread
4.   Severe extrahepatic disease that is not reversible posttransplant, including severe cardiopulmonary disease not amenable to corrective surgery or severe structural brain damage
5.   Mitochondrial disease with multisystem involvement

12.5   Preparation for Transplantation

12.5.1   Immunization

Most live vaccines are contraindicated posttransplant; thus it is essential to ensure that routine immunizations are complete (e.g., diphtheria, pertussis, tetanus and polio, pneumovax as protection from streptococcal pneumonia, and HIB for protection against *Haemophilus influenzae*). In children older than 6 months, measles, mumps, rubella, and varicella vaccination should be offered. Hepatitis A and B vaccinations may also be prescribed pretransplant.

12.5.2   Management of Hepatic Complications and Liver Failure

The treatment of specific hepatic complications is an important part of preoperative management (see Sec. 9). It is important that children be free of sepsis prior to transplantation; prophylactic antibiotics may be required. In children with acute liver failure, antifungal therapy should be started with either fluconazole or liposomal amphotericin while liver transplantation is being awaited. Fluid balance and treatment of ascites and before renal failure occurs is mandatory, but hemodialysis or hemofiltration is rarely required in chronic liver failure. However, these may be essential in managing fluid retention and cerebral edema in children with acute liver failure.

12.5.3 Nutritional Support

The development of effective nutritional strategies has been an important advance in the pre-operative management of children with chronic liver failure. These strategies may have improved morbidity and mortality posttransplant (see Table 4) (see Chaps. 16, 17).

12.5.4 Psychological Preparation

One of the most important aspects of the transplant assessment is the psychological counseling and preparation of both child and family. A skilled multidisciplinary team that includes a play therapist and psychologist is essential to the success of this preparation, which may be successfully achieved through innovative play therapy and toys and books suitable for children. Particularly careful counseling is required for parents of children referred for liver transplantation because of an inborn error of metabolism that has not led to liver failure. These parents may find it more difficult to accept the risks and complications of the operation, the potential mortality, and the necessity for long-term immunosuppression. Parents of children who require transplantation for fulminant hepatitis may be too distressed to fully appreciate the significance and implications of liver transplantation and may require ongoing counseling and education postoperatively.

12.5.5 Transplant Procedure

Liver grafts are selected on the basis of ABO compatibility and occasionally on CMV status.

12.5.6 Innovative Surgical Techniques

The traditional form of operation, orthotopic liver transplantation, is now a rare occurrence in pediatric liver transplantation due to the shortage of size-matched organs for young children (26). Most children receive either a reduction hepatectomy, in which left lateral segments of a larger liver are cut down to fit a child, or a split liver transplantation, in which a single donor liver is offered to two recipients. Of particular relevance for pediatric liver transplantation is the development of living-related transplantation, in which part of the parent's liver is given to the child. The main advantage of this technique is the ability to electively transplant children with end-stage liver failure because they have deteriorated significantly in terms of hepatic condition and nutritional status, the use of "good quality grafts," and the reduction in pressure on the organ donor pool.

Auxiliary liver transplantation is an alternative technique in which part of the donor liver is inserted beside or in continuity with the native liver, which is retained in case of graft failure or for future gene therapy (27). This is particularly appropriate for children with metabolic liver disease who have a functionally normal liver but severe extrahepatic disease (except for primary oxalosis, in which the enzyme deficiency causes overproduction of oxalate).

12.5.7 Posttransplant Management

The immediate postoperative period is concerned with

1. Monitoring graft function
2. Initiating immunosuppression
3. Prevention and management of complications

Graft function is evaluated by measuring

Acid-base status
Blood glucose levels
Coagulation times
Liver function, in particular bilirubin, transaminases, and alkaline phosphatase

Immunosuppression is initiated with corticosteroids (IV hydrocortisone or methylprednisolone, transferring to enteric coated prednisolone or prednisone once oral feeds are resumed), cyclosporine (Neoral) 5 mg/kg and azathioprine 2 mg/kg. Alternative first-line immunosuppression includes tacrolimus (0.15 mg/kg) with corticosteroids. Mycophenolate mofetil is a new immunosuppressant drug, which may be steroid-sparing and less nephrotoxic than cyclosporine and tacrolimus. It has not yet been fully evaluated in children.

Prophylactic antibiotics may be prescribed for 48 hr unless there is continuing infection. The incidence of stress ulcers and excess gastric acid secretion is reduced with ranitidine 3 mg/kg tid, sucralfate 2 to 4 g qid, and/or omeprazole 10 to 20 mg IV bid. Antiplatelet drugs such as aspirin and dipyridamole are prescribed to prevent vascular thrombosis, which is particularly common in children. These drugs are discontinued at 3 months. Most children require antihypertensive medication because of the effects of immunosuppressive therapy.

12.5.8 Early Postoperative Complications

1. Primary graft failure is a rare occurrence now, with improved medical and surgical management, but it may occur secondary to nonfunction (within 48 hr), hyperacute rejection (up to 4 days), or hepatic artery

thrombosis (0 to 10 days). The only successful treatment is retransplantation.

2. Hepatic artery thrombosis is more common in children than in adults because of the small size of the vessels, it occurs in 10% of children. The incidence has fallen following the introduction of reduction hepatectomy, with the use of larger donor blood vessels.

3. Oliguria may develop in association with poor graft function, hypovolemia, or immunosuppressive therapy. Most children improve with conservative management and less than 10% require dialysis for renal failure unless transplanted for acute liver failure.

4. Hypertension from cyclosporine, tacrolimus, or prednisolone therapy is common and responds to fluid restriction and standard therapy with nifedipine (5 to 10 mg per dose) and/or atenolol (25 to 50 mg per dose).

5. Acute cellular rejection responsive to increased immunosuppression occurs in 50 to 80% of children between 7 to 10 days. It is less common in infants (20%), which may be related to immune tolerance in this group. Most acute rejection episodes respond to pulse prednisolone (20 to 40 mg/kg/day) intravenously over 2 or 3 days. Conversion to a more potent immunosuppressive drug such as tacrolimus may be required in a minority of children.

6. Chronic rejection is less common (less than 10% of children) but may occur at any time posttransplant. There may be a response to an increase in immunosuppression or a change to tacrolimus immunosuppression, but many children require retransplantation.

7. Biliary complications occur in 18 to 20% of children and are more common in those receiving reduction hepatectomies. Biliary strictures may be secondary to anastomotic stricture, edema of the bile ducts, or hepatic artery ischemia, whereas biliary leaks may be secondary to leakage from the cut surface of the liver in reduction hepatectomy or from hepatic artery ischemia. Most biliary leaks will settle with conservative management, but large leaks leading to biliary peritonitis, biliary abscess, or sepsis will require surgical drainage and reconstruction. Many biliary strictures may now be managed medically with ursodeoxycholic acid (20 mg/kg/day) or radiologically using percutaneous transhepatic cholangiography dilatation of the stricture, and placement of a biliary stent.

8. Bacterial sepsis remains the commonest complication following liver transplantation and may be related to central line insertion.

9. Fungal infections (*Candida albicans* or *Aspergillus*) have been documented in up to 20% of patients, particularly those receiving liver transplantation for fulminant hepatitis.

12.5.9 Late Complications After Liver Transplant

Complications after 3 weeks may occur at any time posttransplant and include

1. Side effects of immunosuppression
2. CMV or EBV infection
3. Posttransplant lymphoproliferative disease
4. Late biliary strictures
5. Late hepatic artery or portal vein thrombosis
6. Growth failure

12.5.10 Immunosuppressive Therapy

There are numerous side effects of immunosuppressive therapy (Table 7), which include the effect of corticosteroids on growth and ultimate height. Hirsutism and gingival hyperplasia, which are well known side effects of cyclosporine, have an important effect on quality of life, particularly in adolescents. Nephrotoxicity, which is common to both cyclosporine and tacrolimus, needs careful monitoring of immunosuppressive levels to minimize this long-term effect.

12.5.11 CMV and EBV Infection

The majority of children undergoing liver transplantation are negative for both CMV or EBV. CMV infection is a particular problem posttransplantation because the majority of donor livers (particularly reduction hepatectomies from adults) are likely to be CMV-positive. CMV infection is inevitable between 5 and 6 weeks posttransplant despite prophylaxis with acyclovir or gancyclovir. CMV disease is treated effectively with high-dose gancyclovir (5 mg/kg) and hyper-immune CMV globulin.

The development of primary EBV infections is a significant long-term

TABLE 7 Immunosuppressive Complications After Transplantation

Steroids	Stunting
	Hypertension
	Cushingoid facies
Cyclosporine	Hirsutism
	Gingival hyperplasia
Cyclosporine/tacrolimus	Nephritis
	Hypertension
	Nephrotoxicity
	Posttransplant lymphoproliferative disease
Tacrolimus	Hyperglycemia
	? Cardiomyopathy

problem. Sixty five percent of children undergoing liver transplantation will be EBV-negative and will have a primary infection within 6 months of transplantation. It is important to diagnose primary EBV infection as early as possible (EBV early capsid antigen and PCR) so that immunosuppression may be reduced to prevent further progression to posttransplant lymphoproliferative disease.

12.5.12 Posttransplant Lymphoproliferative Disease (PTLD)

There is a close relationship between primary EBV infection and the development of lymphoproliferative disease, which ranges from benign hyperplasia to malignant lymphomas (28). In the majority of children, the clinical features represent infectious mononucleosis, with a minority developing isolated lymphoid involvement or malignant lymphoma. The diagnosis is based on identifying the characteristic histology from the affected tissue. Although almost every organ in the body may be affected, the liver and gut are most usually involved. It is clear that PTLD is more likely if immunosuppression is intense.

Treatment includes reduction of immunosuppression and acyclovir (3 mg/ m^2), which is effective in the majority. If the PTLD becomes overtly malignant, chemotherapy with standard lymphoma treatment is required.

12.5.13 Growth Posttransplant

The majority of children will achieve normal growth posttransplant, but approximately 20% will have continuing problems which nutrition and growth.

The most important factors related to growth failure postransplant are:

Excessive corticosteroid dosage
Recurrent hepatic complications and cholestasis
Intercurrent illnesses, such as EBV and CMV
Behavioral problems that interfere with calorie intake

Successful management of growth failure involves a skilled multidisciplinary team, including a dietician and a psychologist, ensuring adequate calorie intake (by nasogastric tube if necessary), and early reduction or discontinuation of corticosteroid therapy.

12.5.14 Recurrent Disease Posttransplant

Liver transplantation is rarely required for children with hepatitis B or C, but recurrence is inevitable for both viruses. Recent data indicate that up to 25% of children transplanted for autoimmune hepatitis will have a recurrence, both immunologically and histologically.

The outcome for children transplanted for malignant hepatic tumors is related to the rate of recurrence, which is low if there are no extrahepatic metastases at the time of surgery.

12.5.15 Survival

Current results from international units indicate that 1-year survival after pediatric liver transplantation may be as high as 90%, while long-term survival rates (5 to 8 years) range from 60 to 80% (29). Patients receiving elective living-related transplantation may have a higher 1-year survival (94%) compared to those receiving cadaveric grafts (78%), whereas children transplanted for acute liver failure or fulminant hepatitis have 1-year survival rates of only 60 to 70%.

12.5.16 Outcome Following Metabolic Liver Transplantation

In alpha$_1$-antitrypsin deficiency, Byler's disease, and Wilson's disease, there are both phenotypic and functional cures of the original disease. In tyrosinemia type I, liver transplantation corrects hepatic enzyme deficiency and prevents the development of liver cancer, although the kidney continues to produce toxic metabolites. Long-term nephrotoxicity from immunosuppressive agents is therefore a problem in this group of children.

In Criglar-Najjar type I, urea cycle defects, and primary oxalosis, the metabolic defect is completely corrected and rehabilitation depends on the extent of extrahepatic disease pretransplant.

12.5.17 Quality of Life Posttransplant

Children who survive the initial 3-month posttransplant period without major complications should achieve a normal lifestyle, despite the necessity for continuous immunosuppressive monitoring. Prospective studies have indicated the rapid return to normal nutritional status in over 80% of children within 1 year posttransplant. Linear growth may be delayed between 6 and 24 months posttransplant, which is directly related to steroid dosage and to malnutrition and preoperative stunting.

Prospective studies have shown that there is an initial deterioration in psychosocial development posttransplant, which may be related to the hospitalization and stress from the transplant operation. Following the resumption of normal life, there is a return to pretransplant psychosocial scores within 1 to 2 years. Most children return to nursery or normal school within 3 months of transplantation. Long-term studies have shown that children surviving liver transplantation enter puberty normally; girls will develop menarche and both boys and girls will have pubertal growth spurts. Successful pregnancies have been reported.

12.5.18 Long-Term Monitoring Posttransplant

The essential requisites of posttransplant monitoring include:

> Maintenance of normal growth and development
> Maintenance of normal liver function
> Regular assessment of liver function, hematology, and coagulation

Prevention of nephrotoxicity secondary to immunosuppressive drugs
Regular urea, creatinine, annual glomerular filtration rate
Regular trough levels of neoral/tacrolimus
Change to less nephrotoxic drugs (e.g., mycophenolate mofetil) if necessary
Prevention of PTLD
Evaluation of EBV PCR with reduction in immunosuppression if necessary
Monitoring blood pressure
Detection of hepatic complications posttransplant
Annual abdominal ultrasound for vascular patency and biliary dilatation
Liver biopsy to detect rejection, cholangitis, or hepatitis
Prevention of intercurrent viral infections—e.g., varicella and measles immunoglobulin
Encouragement of normal life with resumption of schooling/nursery

13 SUMMARY

Liver transplantation is now the accepted treatment for acute or chronic liver failure, with the expectation of long-term survival and good quality of life.

REFERENCES

1. Deutsch J, Smith AL, Danks DM, Campbell PE. Long term prognosis for babies with neonatal liver disease. Arch Dis Child 1985; 60:447–451.
2. Mowat AP, Psacharopoulos HT, Williams R. Extrahepatic biliary atresia versus neonatal hepatitis: review of 137 prospectively investigated infants. Arch Dis Child 1976; 51:763–770.
3. McClement JW, Hard ER, Mowat AP. Results of surgical treatment for extrahepatic biliary atresia in the United Kingdom. BMJ 1985; 290:345–347.
4. Nio M, Ohi R, Hayashi Y, Endo N, Ibrahim M, Iwani D. Current status of 21 patients who have survived more than 20 years since undergoing surgery for biliary atresia. J Pediatr Surg 1996; 31:381–384.
5. Chang MH, Hsu HC, Lee CY, Wang TR, Kao CL. Neonatal hepatitis: a follow-up study. J Pediatr Gastroenterol Nutr 1997; 6:203–207.
6. Ellaway CJ, Silinik M, Cowell CT, Gaskin KJ, Kamath KR, Dorney S, Donaghue KC. Cholestatic jaundice and congenital hypopituitarism. J Paediatr Child Health 1995; 31:51–53.
7. Alagille D, Odiévre M, Gautier M, Dommergues JP. Hepatic ductular hypoplasia associated with characteristic facies, vertebral malformations, retarded physical, mental and sexual development, and cardiac murmur. J Pediatr 1986; 86:63–71.
8. Li L, Krantz ID, Deng Y, Genin A, Banta AB, Collins CC, Qi M, Trask BJ, Kuo WL, Cochran J, Costa T, Pierpont ME, Rand EB, Piccoli DA, Hood L, Spinner NB. Alagille syndrome is caused by mutations in the human Jagged 1, which encodes a ligand for Notch 1. Nature Genet 1997; 16:243–251.

9. Bull LN, Carlton VE, Stricker NL, Baharloo S, DeYoung JA, Freimer NB, Magid MS, Kahn E, Markowitz J, DiCarlo FJ, McLoughlin L, Boyle JT, Dahms BB, Faught PR, Fitzgerald JF, Piccoli DA, Witzleben CL, O'Connell NC, Setchell K, Agostini RM Jr, Kocoshis SA, Reyes J, Knisely AS. Genetic and morphological findings in progressive familial intrahepatic cholestasis (Byler disease [PFIC-1] and Byler syndrome): evidence for heterogeneity. Hepatology 1997; 26:155–164.

10. Kelly DA, Portmann B, Mowat AP, Sherlock S, Lake BD. Niemann-Pick disease type C: diagnosis and outcome in children, with particular reference to liver disease. J Pediatr 1993; 123:242–247.

11. Delaplane D, Yogev R, Crussi F, Shulman ST. Fatal hepatitis B in early infancy: the importance of identifying HBsAg positive pregnant women and providing immunoprophylaxis to their newborns. Pediatrics 1983; 72:176–180.

12. Beath SV, Boxall EH, Watson RM, Tarlow MJ, Kelly DA. Fulminant hepatitis B in infants born to anti-HBe hepatitis B carrier mothers. BMJ 1992; 304:1169–1170.

13. Bortolotti F, Jara P, Diaz C, Vajro P, Hierro L, Giacchino R, de la Vega A, Crivellaro C, Camarena C, Barbera C, et al. Post-transfusion and community-acquired hepatitis C in childhood. J Pediatr Gastroenterol Nutr 1994; 18(3):279–283.

14. Ohto H, Terazawa S, Sasaki N, Hino K, Ishiwata C, Kako M, Ujiie N, Endo C, Matsui A, et al. Transmission of hepatitis C virus from mothers to infants. N Engl J Med 1994; 330:744–750.

15. Gregorio GV, Portmann B, Reid F, Donaldson PT, Doherty DG, McCartney M, Mowatt AP, Vergani D, Mieli-Vergani G. Autoimmune hepatitis in childhood: a 20-year experience. Hepatology 1997; 25:541–547.

16. Balistreri WF. Bile acid therapy in pediatric hepatobiliary disease: the role of urseodeoxycholic acid. J Pediatr Gastroenterol Nutr 1997; 24:573–589.

17. Achilleos QA, Buist LJ, Kelly DA, McMaster P, Mayer AD, Buckels JAC. Unresectable hepatic tumours in childhood and the role in liver transplantation. J Paediatr Surg 1996; 11:1563–1567.

18. Bhaduri BR, Mieli-Vergani G. Fulminant hepatic failure: pediatric aspects. Semin Liver Dis 1996; 16:349–355.

19. Devictor D, Tahiri C, Rousset A, Massenavette B, Russo M, Huault G. Management of fulminant hepatic failure in children—an analysis of 56 cases. Crit Care Med 1993; 21:348–349.

20. Beath SV, Brook GD, Kelly DA, Cash AJ, McMaster P, Mayer AD, Buckels JAC. Successful liver transplantation in babies under 1 year. BMJ 1993; 307:825–828.

21. Bonatti H, Muiesan P, Connolly S, Vilca-Melendez H, Nagral S, Baker A, Mieli-Vergani G, Gibbs P, Rela M, Heaton ND. Liver transplantation for acute liver failure in children under 1 year of age. Transplant Proc 1997; 29:434–435.

22. Thomsom M, McKiernan P, Buckels J, Mayer D, Kelly D. Generalised mitochondrial cytopathy is an absolute contraindication to orthotopic liver transplantation in childhood. J Pediatr Gastroenterol Nutr 1998; 26:478–481.

23. Lindstedt S, Holme E, Lock E, Hjalmarson O, Strandvik B. Treatment of hereditary tyrosinaemia type I by inhibition of 4-hydroxphenyl pyruvate dioxygenase. Lancet 1992; 340:813–817.

24. Bryant AE 3rd, Dreifuss FE. Valproic acid hepatic fatalities: III. US experience since 1986. Neurology 1996; 46:465–469.

25. Rivera-Penera T, Gugig R, Davis J, McDiarmid S, Vargas J, Rosenthal P, Berquist W, Heyman MB, Ament ME. Outcome of acetaminophen overdose in pediatric patients and factors contributing to hepatotoxicity. J Pediatr 1997; 130:300–304.

26. Newell KA, Alonso EM, Whitington PF, Bruce DS, Millis JM, Piper JB, Woodle ES, Kelly SM, Koeppen H, Hart J, Rubin CM, Thistlethwaite JR Jr. Posttransplant lymphoproliferative disease in pediatric liver transplantation: interplay between primary Epstein-Barr virus infection and immunosuppression. Transplantation 1996; 62:370–375.

27. De Ville de Goyet J, Hausleithner V, Reding R, Lerut J, Janssen M, Otte JB. Impact of innovative techniques on the waiting list and results in paediatric liver transplantation. Transplantation 1993; 56:1130–1136.

28. Rela M, Muiesan P, Andreani P, Gibbs P, Mieli-Vergani G, Mowat AP, Heaton N. Auxiliary liver transplantation for metabolic diseases. Transplant Proc 1997; 29: 444–445.

29. Yandza T, Gauthier F, Valayer J. Lessons from the first 1000 liver transplantation in children at Bicetre Hospital. J Pediatr Surg 1994; 29:905–911.

31

Diseases of the Pancreas

Kevin J. Gaskin

Royal Alexandra Hospital for Children, Sydney, New South Wales, Australia

1   INTRODUCTION

As an introduction to this chapter some aspects of pancreatic physiology, particularly in regard to the secretion and action of pancreatic enzymes, are reviewed below.

Pancreatic digestive enzymes, as listed in Table 1, are produced in pancreatic acinar cells and secreted into the duodenum in response to gut hormones, neural mechanisms, neurotransmitters, and other peptides—a process that may be modulated by circulating regulatory proteins, including somatostatin and the insulin, epidermal, and fibroblast growth factors (1).

Classically, enzyme secretion is thought to occur in response to cholecystokinin released from the small intestinal enterochromaffin cells into the circulation, directly as a result of the stimulatory effects of fat and protein entering the duodenum during a meal. Likewise, the gut hormone secretin is released as a direct result of acid entering the duodenum; it stimulates the production and release of pancreatic HCO_3^-, the anion that contributes most to pancreatic fluid secretion. In the process of acinar cell enzyme production, enzymes are produced as inactive or zymogen forms and are packaged into zymogen granules prior to release from the acinar cell. The inactive proteases (zymogens) released into the duodenum

TABLE 1   Pancreatic Digestive
Enzymes

Proteases
  Trypsin
  Chymotrypsin
  Carboxypeptidases
  Elastase
Lipolytic enzymes
  Lipase + cofactor colipase
  Phospholipases
  Carboxyl ester hydrolase
Glycolytic enzymes
  Amylase

---

during a meal require activation. This process is initiated by enteropeptidase, the small intestinal brush-border enzyme, a specific serine protease that hydrolyzes the N-terminal hexapeptide from trypsinogen to form active trypsin (2). Trypsin itself can then hydrolyze further molecules of trypsinogen to generate more trypsin and, as such, trypsinogen activation is autocatalytic, with a cascade effect in trypsin production. Trypsin will also activate the other zymogens, chymotrypsinogen, procarboxypeptidases, proelastase, prophospholipase, and procolipase by similar cleavage of an N-terminal polypeptide from the precursor molecule. The multiple proteases thus produced in the small intestinal lumen have specific actions in hydrolyzing proteins and polypeptides. The two major exopeptidases, carboxypeptidases A and B, hydrolyze the carboxyl group from proteins. In contrast to A, carboxypeptidase B prefers to cleave peptide bonds after arginine or lysine residues. Of the endopeptidases, trypsin specifically hydrolyzes peptide bonds on the C side of the positively charged residues, arginine and lysine, if the next residue is not proline. Chymotrypsin hydrolyzes proteins on the carboxyl side of the aromatic side chains—tryptophan, phenylalanine, and tyrosine—and large hydrophobic molecules like methionine. Elastase has a broad specificity, preferring small neutral residues like alanine, glycine, and serine where the next residue is not proline.

Lipase is secreted in its active form into the duodenum; but in the presence of bile acids in the small intestine, it is completely inhibited. When emulsified triglyceride droplets enter the duodenum, bile salt micelles occupy the oil and water interface, preventing access of lipase to the surface of the oil droplet and thus inhibiting its activity (3,4). The cofactor colipase can attach itself to lipase molecules and also to bile acids, displacing them from the lipid surface and thus giving access of lipase molecules to the surface of the lipid droplet, allowing lipolysis to occur. Phospholipases A1 and A2 have an important role in hydrolyzing phosphatidylcholine (lecithin) to the water-soluble lysolecithin. The latter may be absorbed and detoxified in the enterocyte to glycerophosphorylcholine. There is also evidence that the pancreatic enzyme carboxyl ester hydrolase (CEH) will hydrolyze lysolecithin to GPC within the intestinal lumen. CEH is remarkable, as its gene sequence in pancreatic tissue appears identical to that of the bile salt–stimulated lipase in breast tissue and human milk. Why, from a physiological point of view, this should be the case is uncertain, but it may well be that pancreatic CEH production is limited in the neonatal period and that the lack thereof is compensated by CEH in human milk.

Pancreatic zymogen production is evident during early fetal life (5). Trypsin, chymotrypsin, phospholipase A, and lipase are present in the 14-week-old human fetal pancreas, and they increase steadily with gestational age. Amylase has been detected from as early as 16 weeks' gestation. Postnatally in premature infants, Zoppi et al. (6) demonstrated—during pancreatic stimulation tests—that duodenal trypsin, lipase, and amylase were considerably lower than in full-term infants. By 6 months of age, secretion of trypsin and lipase is commensurate with that in older children, but there is debate regarding amylase secretion, which may not be fully developed till 2 years of age.

Functionally, there is a large reserve of exocrine pancreatic function. This is evident in infants undergoing subtotal pancreatectomy for nesidioblastoma, where in excess of 95% of the pancreas is removed, yet in most cases normal absorption is retained. Furthermore, in a large study of exocrine pancreatic function using a quantitative pancreatic stimulation technique and fat balance studies in children with either cystic fibrosis (CF) or Shwachman syndrome (SS), patients with fat malabsorption were demonstrated to have less than 2% of the average lipase/colipase output evident in the controls (7). Of those CF or SS patients with normal fat absorption, lipase/colipase output ranged from 2% up to values within the control range. In a later study using the same techniques, some CF infants with normal absorption at the time of neonatal screening diagnosis at 2 months demonstrated lipase/colipase outputs within the adult normal range, suggesting that lipase and colipase outputs are well developed even in early childhood (8).

These studies have also led to a better definition of pancreatic dysfunction. Previously, patients with pancreatic disease and normal fat absorption were described as having varying degrees of pancreatic insufficiency or as being partially pancreatic deficient. Currently the accepted terminology is that patients with *pancreatic insufficiency* (PI) have fat malabsorption (i.e., insufficient enzyme output to prevent malabsorption), and those with normal absorption are *pancreatic sufficient* (PS), as they have sufficient endogenous enzyme output to prevent malabsorption.

2 PANCREATIC DISEASES

The spectrum of pancreatic disease in children is outlined in Table 2. The disorders range from inherited disorders (e.g., CF and SS) and congenital structural

TABLE 2   Pancreatic Diseases in Childhood

Inherited disorder
  Cystic fibrosis
  Shwachman syndrome
  Pearson's marrow-pancreas syndrome
  Johansson-Blizzard syndrome
  Pancreatic agenesis
  Isolated enzyme deficiencies
    Trypsinogen
    Enteropeptidase
    Lipase
    Colipase
  Inherited recurrent pancreatitis
Congenital structural anomalies
  Annular pancreas
  Ectopic pancreas
  Pancreas divisum
Acquired anomalies
Pancreatitis
  Viral infections
  Mumps
  Adenovirus
  Coxsackie
  Hepatitis A and B
  Trauma
  Drugs
    Diuretics
    Cytotoxic agents: L-asparaginase
    Structural anomalies: choledochal cyst, gall-
      stones
  Systemic disease:
    Reye's syndrome
    Hemolytic uremic syndrome
    Systemic lupus
    Metabolic diseases
      Hypertryglyceridemias
      Organic acidurias—e.g., methylmalonic aci-
        dosis
      Cystic fibrosis
Primary protein energy malnutrition
Tumors
  Benign
    Cystadenoma
    Lymphangioma
    Hemangioendothelioma
  Malignant
    Adenocarcinoma
    Pancreatoblastoma

anomalies such as annular pancreas to acquired problems, including pancreatic dysfunction associated with primary protein energy malnutrition and pancreatitis. Pancreatic tumors are rare in childhood but are described briefly at the end of the chapter.

2.1 Cystic Fibrosis

CF is inherited as an autosomal recessive disorder and classically is characterized by suppurative lung disease, pancreatic insufficiency, and an elevated sweat chloride concentration greater than 60 mmol/L. It is caused by mutations of the CF fibrosis transport regulator (CFTR) gene located at 7q31 (9). The CFTR gene controls the production of the CFTR protein, which has been demonstrated to function as a cell-membrane cAMP-dependent Cl^- channel (10). Mutations of the CFTR gene produce a protein that either cannot locate in the cell membrane or, if it does, the channel function and chloride transport are impaired. Loss of cAMP-dependent chloride channel function is associated with increased sodium reabsorption in airway epithelium, activation of alternate chloride channels, and interference with intracellular organelle pH and macromolecular production. Secretory epithelium in airways, pancreatic ducts, small intestinal enterocytes, and cholangioles exhibits poor secretion of electrolytes and fluid, with subsequent production of viscous secretions and, pathophysiologically, obstruction to the ducts of the organs involved. In absorptive epithelium, namely the sweat duct, poor chloride reabsorption leads to elevation of the sweat chloride concentration.

Pancreatic disease in CF can be directly attributed to impaired electrolyte and fluid secretion (11). Ductal cells demonstrate impaired cAMP-dependent Cl^- channel function with poor chloride secretion into the ductal lumen. As a consequence, Cl^-/HCO_3^- exchange and HCO_3^- secretion is also impaired (12). Poor Cl^-/HCO_3^- exchange, however, does not account entirely for low HCO_3^- secretion; it is likely that the latter is also contributed to by poor HCO_3^- secretion through cAMP-dependent channels and alternate chloride channels. The impaired alkalinization of pancreatic fluid may cause protein precipitation, as evident with the zymogen membrane–associated glycoprotein-2, which in acidic conditions can form a tridimensional fibrillar network as a nidus for protein plug formation. Poor fluid secretion can further enhance the likelihood that protein plugs will obstruct the smaller pancreatic ducts.

Obstruction of the pancreatic ducts and ductules leads directly to damage of pancreatic acinar cells. Although the exact mechanism of this damage is unknown, newborn CF patients demonstrate elevations of serum trypsinogen and lipase, suggesting that they have a "subclinical" form of pancreatitis. Whether the acinar changes result from obstruction or inflammation or can be directly attributed to chloride channel dysfunction of the acinar cell, the pancreatic disease is probably progressive at least during the last trimester, as indicated by the occurrence of pancreatic insufficiency in premature CF infants. Full-term CF neonates born with meconium ileus demonstrate pancreatic insufficiency, as evident by fat malabsorption when tested near birth. Pathological studies of infants dying from meconium ileus have demonstrated some preservation of acinar tissue, but over time, within the first 5 years of life, the acinar tissue is destroyed and replaced by fibrofatty tissue and cyst formation (11). The relative preservation of acinar tissue in the first 3 to 6 months of life is consistent with the high serum trypsinogen levels. Subsequently, trypsinogen declines to very low levels through the first 2 to 5 years of life, consistent with progressive destruction of functioning acinar tissue (13).

The above findings are of importance with reference to the evolution of clinical pancreatic disease. At diagnosis in a neonatal screening program 60% of infants will have fat malabsorption, and quantitative pancreatic stimulation tests demonstrate that such infants have less than 1% of average normal enzyme secretion (8). Thus, although acinar tissue is still present at this age, enzyme output into the duodenum is nearly absent. Of the other 40% of infants who are pancreatic sufficient with normal absorption at neonatal diagnosis approximately one-third will experience a decline in pancreatic function over a 5-year period. With this decline in function the infants become pancreatic insufficient, which accounts for the patients in unscreened populations who present with fat malabsorption during later childhood after having had clinically normal absorption prior to this time. Variably, 10 to 20% of patients remain pancreatic sufficient into adolescence/early adulthood and demonstrate normal or raised serum trypsinogens (13). Some of these persistently PS patients are in fact at risk of developing pancreatitis. PS patients undergoing quantitative pancreatic function tests have varying enzyme secretion from as low as 2% to within the normal adult range. Those with less than 10% function at neonatal diagnosis are more predisposed to develop PI with age, but not exclusively so, as certainly patients with high function have become insufficient at older ages with or without developing clinical pancreatitis.

Following the discovery of the "cystic fibrosis gene," there have been considerable efforts to correlate specific combinations of mutations with the two pancreatic phenotypes—i.e., PI and PS. The first large study in this regard, assessing only the major CF mutation ΔF508, compared the patient's pancreatic status according to three major genotype groupings, ΔF508 homozygotes, ΔF508 compound heterozygotes, and non-ΔF508 compound heterozygotes, as per Table 3 (14). In this older group of CF patients, virtually all ΔF508 homozygotes and 70% of ΔF508 compound heterozygotes were PI. In contrast, over 60% of the non-ΔF508 patients were PS. Further insight into this association was provided when certain non-ΔF508 mutations—including R117H, A455E, 3849 + 10kbC → T, and R347P—were shown to be associated with PS even if in combination with a known PI mutation, e.g., ΔF508 (15). This work suggested that certain

TABLE 3 Genotype/Pancreatic
Phenotype Relations in Cystic
Fibrosis

Genotype	PI	PS
ΔF508/ΔF508	99	01
ΔF508/other	70	30
Other/other	34	66

Key: PI, % of patients with pancreatic insufficiency; PS, % of patients with pancreatic sufficiency.
Source: Adapted from Ref. 14.

non-ΔF508 mutations conferred the PS status, and the effect of these mutations
was dominant. These findings have been further expanded by an assessment of
the function of the CFTR protein in regard to five classes of mutations (16). PI
is predominant in mutation classes I, II, and III, where the CFTR protein fails
to localize in the cell membrane (classes I and II) or, if it does localize, fails to
demonstrate chloride secretion (class III). In contrast, PS patients have class IV
and V mutations, where the CFTR protein localizes to the cell membrane and
demonstrates partial function.

Among infants and young children, as indicated above, there is a much
higher proportion who have some residual pancreatic function (8); that is, a higher
proportion (up to 30%) of ΔF508 homozygous patients are PS at diagnosis, but
it is among this group that one sees a decline in function as they become PI at
a later age. Still unclear is why these patients experience a slower decline in their
pancreatic function compared to those who are PI at diagnosis and why, in fact,
some ΔF508 homozygotes retain their pancreatic function into adulthood. It must
be emphasized these correlations are not only of scientific/academic interest—
as, clearly, patients with PS not only have a milder pancreatic disease but also
experience less lung, liver, and gut problems. Epidemiological data have further
indicated that PS patients have a median survival of over 50 years compared with
PI patients, with a median survival of near 30 years of age.

Except for the occurrence of pancreatitis in a small proportion, PS patients
are generally asymptomatic from a gastrointestinal point of view. PI patients, on
the other hand, have maldigestion and malabsorption of both macronutrients and
micronutrients and are thus at considerable risk for malnutrition, growth failure,
hypoproteinemia, and the consequences of deficiencies of fat-soluble vitamins,
as outlined in Table 4. Symptomatically untreated PI patients will have bulky,
malodorous, loose, oily stools. Parents occasionally give graphic descriptions of
"bacon fat" or "melted cheese" stools, indicating that the patient has both mal-

TABLE 4 Complications of Pancreatic Insufficiency

Maldigestion and malabsorption of macronutrients
  Consequences:
    Growth failure
    Failure to gain weight, or weight loss with wasting of muscle and subcutaneous fat
    Hypoproteinemia and edema
    Oily, malodorous bowel movements
    Excess fecal bile acid losses and development of lithogenic bile
Malabsorption of micronutrients
  Fat-soluble vitamins:
    A: Night blindness
      Xerophthalmia
      Benign intracranial hypertension
    E: Peripheral neuropathy
      Ataxia
      Spinocerebellar tract degeneration
      External ophthalmoplegia
    D: Rickets
      Osteomalacia

digestion and malabsorption of ingested triglyceride. This observation can be confirmed by simple stool microscopy demonstrating an abundance of undigested fat droplets in the specimen. Formal 3- to 5-day fat and nitrogen-balance studies—where dietary intake of these nutrients is estimated from a weighed food intake and fecal fat and nitrogen are measured chemically—indicate that PI patients, on average, malabsorb near 40% of their fat intake and 30% of their nitrogen intake (17). Fat malabsorption (fecal fat >7% of fat intake) is the accepted "gold standard" marker indicating the presence of pancreatic insufficiency and the necessity for oral enzyme replacement therapy (OERT).

Patients who are older at diagnosis may complain of night blindness, excessive bruising, or ankle swelling related to edema and hypoproteinemia in addition to their lung symptomatology. A key feature in undiagnosed patients is growth failure with either wasting, stunting, or decreased linear growth velocity due to chronic undernutrition. Among both the screened and unscreened group of infants, hypoalbuminemia and edema may be present, indicating the severe degree of protein maldigestion and malabsorption.

In addition to the direct consequences of pancreatic insufficiency, CF patients can experience a number of gut and biliary complications, as shown in Table 5. The reader is referred to detailed descriptions of these entities elsewhere (11,18). Briefly, neonatal meconium ileus affects some 10 to 20% of CF infants.

TABLE 5 Gastrointestinal, Liver, and Biliary Tract
Complications of Cystic Fibrosis

Gastrointestinal
  Esophagus
    Gastroesophageal reflux
    Esophagitis
    Esophageal varices with portal hypertension
  Small intestinal
    Neonatal
      Meconium ileus
      Intestinal atresia
      Volvulus
      Intestinal perforation
      Meconium peritonitis
    Postneonatal
      Distal intestinal obstruction syndrome
      Intussusception
      Appendicitis
      Appendiceal abscess
      Appendiceal mucocele
      Crohn's disease
      Celiac disease
      Giardiasis
    Colonic
      Fecal impaction
      Megacolon
      Rectal prolapse
      Fibrosing colonopathy
      Crohn's disease
Biliary tract disease
  Microgallbladder
  Cystic duct atresia
  Gallstones
  Distal common duct stenosis
  Sclerosing cholangitis
Liver disease
  Hepatosteatosis
  Focal biliary cirrhosis
  Multilobular cirrhosis

While its etiology is uncertain, it likely relates to the underlying gut secretion deficit and may be compounded by the presence of pancreatic insufficiency. Infants with meconium ileus present with neonatal gut obstruction and may have associated anomalies, including malrotation with volvulus or intestinal atresia. Infants with uncomplicated meconium ileus may respond to medical treatment with hyperosmotic radiopaque enemas (Gastrografin) or, if unresponsive, will need surgical intervention. Some will present with meconium peritonitis heralded by peritoneal and intra-abdominal calcification and require immediate surgery. Currently, with intravenous nutrition, the vast majority of these infants survive this early insult complicating their disease. In later life 10 to 20% of children and young adults will experience inspissation of fecal contents into the ileum, cecum, and ascending colon, an entity described as distal intestinal obstruction syndrome (DIOS). Again, the etiology of DIOS is unclear but has been related to lack of compliance to OERT, to the underlying intestinal secretion deficit, and to impaired intestinal motility. It may be associated with intussusception or appendiceal fecal masses. Usually, uncomplicated DIOS responds to lavage regimens either orally, via nasogastric tubes, or per rectum. Failure to respond should initiate further investigation with ultrasound to determine if an intussusception or appendiceal mass is present and a diagnostic enema using water-soluble contrast agents to determine the presence of intraluminal masses or mucosal pathology. Fortunately, most cases of fecal impaction are mild; in the absence of obstruction, they respond well to liquid mineral oil regimens. This entity must be distinguished from other intestinal complications, including Crohn's disease and the recently described problem of fibrosing colonopathy. The latter has been associated with the ingestion of high-dose lipase OERT preparations and the ingestion of lipase doses in excess of 20,000 U/kg/day. Following the recommendations for patients not to exceed 10,000 U/kg/day and the withdrawal of high-dose OERT from the market, this entity has substantially declined.

Liver and biliary tract disease are relatively common complications of CF and contribute considerably to morbidity and, to a lesser extent, even mortality (18) (see Chap. 30). Hepatosteatosis is the most common liver problem, affecting over 60% of patients. Its etiology is unknown and it appears not to cause significant problems. The classical entity is focal biliary fibrosis or cirrhosis, a patchy fibrosis pathognomonic of cystic fibrosis (Fig. 1). It appears to be associated with intracholangiolar eosinophilic plugging with subsequent obstruction, inflammation, and scarring proximal to the obstruction. CFTR protein has been localized to bile duct epithelium and dysfunction thereof is considered a major contributor/precursor to the occurrence of bile duct plugging. What is not clear is why ductal plugging/obstruction is of a patchy distribution and why a large number of patients with severe underlying mutations and secretion deficits do not develop liver disease. Distal obstruction of the common bile duct may contribute to this process

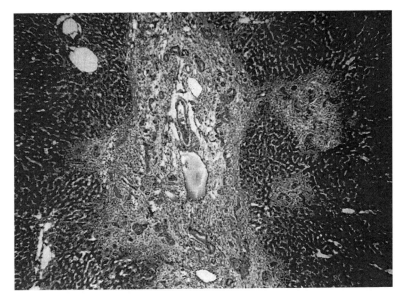

FIGURE 1 Focal biliary fibrosis. Photomicrograph showing expanded portal triad with fibrosis, bile duct proliferation, and a cholangiole (center of picture) with eosinophilic plug.

as may the occurrence of lithogenic bile as a result of bile acid malabsorption. In the progression of the liver disease, coalescence of focally scarred areas is considered to contribute to the development of multilobular biliary cirrhosis (Fig. 2) the more severe liver problem, which is associated with portal hypertension. Management of the latter is complex, particularly if it occurs in association with severe lung disease. In this circumstance, bleeding esophageal varices are best managed with less invasive, nonsurgical regimens, including esophageal variceal sclerotherapy or banding procedures. In some, such interventions fail, a likelihood increased by the concurrence of hypersplenism with thrombocytopenia and coagulation defects. Patients in this category may have to undergo portal shunt procedures but are at high risk in the presence of a coagulopathy and hypoproteinemia. Although it is unusual for CF patients to develop liver failure with synthetic protein and coagulation factor defects, the occurrence of liver failure is now well recognized in some patients. These patients can undergo successful liver transplantation when they have only mild to moderate lung disease, but in the presence of severe pulmonary disease, fungal colonization of the lung, and diabetes, the procedure is contraindicated. Clearly, it is ideal to prevent liver failure, and in

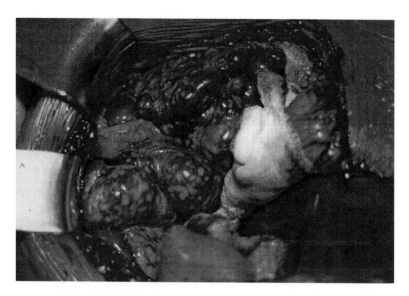

FIGURE 2   Severe multilobular cirrhosis in a patient with cystic fibrosis. Focal scarring is evident within the lobules.

this regard the advent of ursodeoxycholate therapy to encourage bile secretion was a distinct possible treatment. However, results to date are equivocal and the Cochrane analysis of the studies performed did not favor this treatment (19).

Biliary tract disease, including cholelithiasis and bile duct stenosis, has been described with varying frequency (18). The occurrence of cholelithiasis has declined markedly since the introduction of microspheric OERT, with the concomitant marked improvement in fat absorption and prevention of fecal bile acid losses. However, in the presence of right-upper-quadrant pain, both ultrasonography and hepatobiliary scintigraphy should be used to search for bile duct stenosis and/or gallstones. Persistent pain may necessitate surgical intervention, depending on pulmonary status.

Appendiceal disease in cystic fibrosis is considered an unusual or even rare occurrence affecting approximately 1% of the population (11). This entity is often overlooked, with delayed diagnosis a frequent event, and is associated with either perforation or abscess formation. The delay or confusion is related to the common presentation with a tender mass lesion in the right iliac fossa, most often attributed to the occurrence of DIOS. Appendicitis may also be masked by the intercurrent administration of antibiotics, both in terms of systemic symptoms (e.g., fever) and localized tenderness. Although the hallmark feature of rebound tenderness should alert the physician to localized inflammation and the possibility of appendicitis, the more frequent occurrence of DIOS often sways the diagnosis. If any doubt exists, it is important to obtain an ultrasound or computed tomography (CT) examination to localize the appendix and determine whether there are inflammatory features, including abscess formation. Certainly, if symptoms and tenderness persist despite lavage and colonic evacuation, surgical intervention is required.

Finally, rectal prolapse is worthy of mention. It occurs in 10 to 15% of younger children with CF and may be the presenting feature at diagnosis in unscreened populations. It can occur in PI or PS patients and thus it is not necessarily dependent on the presence of malabsorption. As it occurs in PS patients who, at a younger age, can be relatively asymptomatic, a sweat chloride is mandatory in patients presenting with isolated rectal prolapse. Frequent recurrence may well necessitate intervention with pararectal triple saline injections under anesthesia.

2.2 Shwachman Syndrome

This unusual disorder consists of a spectrum of problems including pancreatic hypoplasia; bone marrow depression with neutropenia, thrombocytopenia, and/ or red cell aplasia; metaphyseal dysostosis; and, clinically, short stature (20,21). A summary of the findings is presented in Table 6. Most commonly, it presents as an autosomal recessive disease, though there are some families where consecutive generations are involved. Its incidence is generally unknown but may be as high as 1 per 10,000 live births.

Infants usually present with pancreatic insufficiency manifest by malabsorption from birth, with or without associated sepsis due to neutropenia. Pancreatic insufficiency is associated with undernutrition and fat-soluble vitamin deficiencies, as in CF. Longitudinal studies of pancreatic function have demonstrated that malabsorption may improve with age, with over 50% of the patients maintaining normal absorption without OERT over 5 years of age. Histologically, SS patients have replacement of pancreatic acinar tissue by fatty infiltration but preservation of ductal structures. These findings are consistent with quantitative pancreatic stimulation test data demonstrating impaired enzyme secretion (poor acinar function) but normal water and electrolyte secretion consistent with the preservation of the ductal system. Given that some patients who become PS at an older age and thus would be relatively asymptomatic, this entity must be considered in older children presenting with short stature but a normal linear growth velocity. Hematologic abnormalities are very common in this disorder, including intermittent and persistent neutropenia, anemia, thrombocytopenia, and pancytopenia. These complications are a direct result of bone marrow dysfunction, characterized by a hypocellular marrow, maturation delay, or arrests and myelodysplasia. Clonal cytogenetic abnormalities have included monosomy 7 and 5 and complex abnormalities with isochromosome 7 and deletion of 20q. Myelodys-

TABLE 6   Features of Shwachman Syndrome

Clinical
  Short stature
  Oily stools
  Recurrent infections
    Ear infections
    Systemic sepsis
    Skin boils
    Perianal disease
  Bruising
Pancreatic hypoplasia (with pancreatic insufficiency)
Bone marrow arrest
  Neutropenia
  Thrombocytopenia
  Red cell aplasia
  Pancytopenia
  Leukemia
Bone
  Metaphyseal dysplasia
  Retarded bone age
  Flared ribs
  Thoracic dystrophy
Miscellaneous
  Skin: ichthyosis
  Renal: renal tubular acidosis
  Liver: steatohepatitis
  Developmental impairment

---

plasia and clonal cytogenetic abnormalities are specific risk factors for the development of leukemia. Although the latter has been described in up to 33% of some groups with SS, the complication was not recognized in a recent large study (21). Leukemia is usually of the acute myelogenous type, and there is a strong male predominance despite near equivalent male/female occurrence of myelodysplasia. Patients with bone marrow abnormalities obviously need to be followed carefully, particularly those with myelodysplasia and clonal cytogenetic problems. However, as yet there is sparse evidence to indicate that regular bone marrow examination lessens morbidity or mortality or improves their quality of life.

Neutropenia and neutrophil migration defects are associated with sepsis, which can be severe, causing considerable morbidity and mortality. Fortunately, mortality from sepsis these days is unusual, probably related to the recognition of the underlying disease and the heightened awareness that SS patients, with their associated neutropenia, are predisposed to sepsis.

Metaphyseal dysplasia is a radiological diagnosis affecting nearly 50% of patients. It is characterized by lesions at the ends of long bones but is rarely present before 12 months of age. In contrast, rib flaring and thoracic dystrophy can occur from birth. Rarely are these problems associated with major clinical dysfunction. The bone dysplasias likely contribute to short stature, as the latter, given lack of growth in response to OERT, does not appear nutritional in origin.

2.3 Pearson's Marrow-Pancreas Syndrome

This syndrome is characterized by severe macrocytic anemia, neutropenia, and variable thrombocytopenia (22,23). Classically, the bone marrow shows evidence of ringed sideroblasts and vacuolization of erythroid and myeloid precursors. The patients appear transfusion-dependent, at least in the first years of life. They exhibit diarrhea with malabsorption and are all PI, requiring OERT. At autopsy, features include extensive pancreatic fibrosis with acinar atrophy, partial small intestinal villous atrophy, and hepatosteatosis with or without cirrhosis, which may be complicated by liver failure. Other manifestations have included a Fanconi type of renal tubular dysfunction, photosensitivity, diabetes mellitus, hydrops fetalis, and—in some who survive into later childhood—a Kearns-Sayre type of syndrome with a pigmentary retinopathy, ataxia, proximal muscle weakness, and external ophthalmoplegia. Over 75% of patients with Pearson's syndrome demonstrate a large 4000 to 5000–base pair deletion in mitochondrial DNA, and complex 1 of the respiratory chain enzymes is most affected by the deletion. The deletions are found in 80 to 90% of the most severely affected cells, and part of the variable phenotype is related to the proportion of affected cells.

2.4 Johansson-Blizzard Syndrome

This rare disorder presents with pancreatic insufficiency, imperforate anus, nasal cartilage agenesis, hair anomalies, absent permanent teeth, deafness, mental retardation, hypothyroidism, and growth hormone deficiency (24).

2.5 Pancreatic Agenesis

Pancreatic agenesis is a rare disorder characterized by the occurrence of pancreatic insufficiency and diabetes mellitus in the neonatal period and low birth weight associated with intrauterine growth retardation. In transgenic mice, pancreatic agenesis has been induced by targeted disruption of the insulin promotor factor-1 gene (IPF-1), and one human case of pancreatic agenesis was associated with a single nucleotide deletion within codon 63 of the IPF-1 gene at 13q 12.1, producing a truncated IPF-1 protein (25). There have been long-term survivors, but patients require both OERT and insulin and appear at risk from candidal sepsis.

2.6 Isolated Enzyme Deficiencies

The best-described defects include trypsinogen, lipase, colipase, and enteropeptidase (enterokinase) deficiency. They are probably inherited as autosomal recessive disorders and would appear to be extremely rare. However, they are of importance, as they demonstrate the significance of each enzyme and coenzyme in protein or fat digestion. Enteropeptidase and trypsinogen deficiency are associated with severe, watery, oily diarrhea and hypoalbuminemia from birth. Unless these deficiencies are recognized, the infant will die of malnutrition. Enteropeptidase deficiency can be recognized by the absence of trypsin activity in duodenal juice and then normal activity when the same juice is incubated with enteropeptidase or minute amounts of trypsin. In trypsinogen deficiency, the latter step does not result in trypsin activity. Both of these disorders present with watery diarrhea, protein maldigestion and malabsorption, and associated hypoproteinemia and edema. In enterokinase deficiency, procolipase is not activated, and thus these patients also have fat malabsorption. OERT corrects the digestive anomalies in both disorders. In lipase and colipase deficiency, patients present with severe oily diarrhea, graphically described by parents as bacon fat, melted butter or cheese, or cooking-oil stools. Again, these isolated enzyme defects respond dramatically to OERT, but to date long-term follow-up data are not available to determine the prognosis of patients so affected.

2.7 Annular Pancreas

The pancreas develops as early as the fourth week of gestation from two endodermal buds outpouching from either side of the duodenum. On the right of the duodenum the ventral bud has two parts, right and left, on either side of the common bile duct. While the left part atrophies, the right part migrates posterior to the duodenum and, with duodenum rotation, ends up to the left of the duodenum inferior to the dorsal pancreatic bud, to which it fuses. The duct of the ventral bud enters the common bile duct distally and fuses to the dorsal bud duct proximally. This new duct (the duct of Wirsung) forms the main pancreatic duct, and the minor duct remaining in the dorsal bud (the duct of Santorini), which may atrophy. In annular pancreas, the right ventral bud adheres to the surface of the duodenum and, as the latter rotates, forms a ring around the duodenum.

The true incidence of this anomaly is unknown. Approximately 50% of cases present in childhood and 80% of these have neonatal duodenal obstruction. The anomaly is commonly associated with Down's syndrome. Surgical intervention is required for those with obstruction, but complications—including biliary tract obstruction, gut dysmotility, and failure to thrive—are common (26).

2.8 Pancreas Divisum

As indicated above, there are a number of anomalies that can occur during the development of the pancreas. On occasions, the dorsal and ventral buds of the pancreas fail to fuse, thus creating a true pancreatic divisum. Various degrees of fusion occur and in each case the minor duct in the dorsal bud (the duct of Santorini) may undergo involution and closure, effectively obstructing pancreatic outflow from the dorsal bud. Therefore this condition can be associated with the development of pancreatitis.

2.9 Pancreatitis

2.9.1 Acute Pancreatitis

Acute pancreatitis in children is generally caused by viral infections, trauma, or drugs, but it can also be related to systemic disease, including Reye's syndrome, hemolytic uremic syndrome, systemic lupus erythematosus, or as a complication of metabolic diseases, as per Table 2.

Clinically, children with pancreatitis present with vomiting and epigastric pain, the latter radiating directly through to the back. Typically, the pain is aggravated by food or drink and may restrict movement. The patient may adopt abnormal postures (e.g., knee-chest position) either laterally or prone and maintain these positions for prolonged periods because of the constancy of the pain. Very occasionally, patients will present with ascites with or without pain, and some with hemorrhagic pancreatitis may experience retroperitoneal bleeding and tracking of blood between muscle layers to the flanks of the abdomen. Traumatic injuries may be obvious, as with seat-belt injuries in motor vehicle accidents or bicycle handlebar injuries. However, nonaccidental trauma may not be clinically evident. In the absence of a history of a specific trauma incident, one should be alerted to this entity if other inexplicable injuries are present (noncontemporaneous fractures) or there is duodenal trauma (e.g., duodenal hematoma).

Diagnosis is dependent on the demonstration of raised serum pancreatic enzymes (e.g., elevated amylase, lipase or trypsinogen). The patient may demonstrate hypocalcemia or hyperglycemia in severe pancreatitis and anemia in hemorrhagic pancreatitis. Imaging of the pancreas with ultrasound, computed tomography (CT), and magnetic resonance imaging (MRI) is essential in establishing the diagnosis, looking for complications (e.g., pancreatic pseudocysts), or eliciting associated injuries, duodenal hematoma or rupture, and pancreatic/bile duct trauma or rupture. The recently developed noninvasive magnetic resonance cholangiopancratography (MRCP) technique can be used to demonstrate ductal obstruction or rupture.

Currently, treatment consists of gut rest, intravenous fluids, and analgesia. Adjunctive therapy—including gastric acid suppression, circulation support, treatment of hypocalcemia and use of antibiotics as required—depends on the patient's progress. Pancreatic pseudocysts are common after trauma, and such patients will require prolonged intravenous nutrition and surgical intervention, such as a cystgastrostomy. Duct rupture will usually require surgical intervention—either removal of the distal segment or a Peustow procedure.

2.9.2 Recurrent Acute and Chronic Pancreatitis

There are multiple causes of recurrent pancreatitis in children, as per Table 2. In general, they are either structural problems associated with choledochal cyst, pancreatic divisum, or annular pancreas or occur as part of an underlying metabolic disease, including CF, hyperlipidemia, organic aciduria, or hypercalcemia. The most common form of inherited recurrent acute or chronic pancreatitis is caused by mutations in the cationic trypsinogen gene at 7q35 (27). Patients with these mutations can often present in early childhood with pancreatitis and may progress to pancreatic calcification, pancreatic insufficiency, and pseudocyst formation and may later have a higher risk of pancreatic cancer. Recent data suggests that patients with the R117H mutation in exon 3 have an earlier (childhood onset) compared to the later adolescent/adult onset in patients with the N21I mutation in exon 2.

Investigation of patients with recurrent pancreatitis depends to some extent on the clinical presentation. Patients with a family history of demonstrated calcific pancreatic disease are likely to have hereditary pancreatitis, an entity that can be confirmed by genotyping for mutations of the cationic trypsinogen gene. Likewise, patients with a personal or family history suggestive CF or inherited metabolic disease can be screened for such disorders. Often the clinical presentation does not reveal the etiology and patients should then undergo investigation to determine the presence of surgically correctable diseases, such as choledochal cyst or gallstones, or investigations for CF (sweat chloride) or hyperlipidemia (cholesterol, triglycerides). Patients with CF with pancreatitis will have pancreatic sufficiency.

In assessing for anatomical surgical problems, basic noninvasive investigations include abdominal ultrasound, hepatobiliary scintigraphy (HBS), abdominal CT scan, and the more recently developed MRCP technique. The ultrasound, CT, and HBS imaging procedures can screen for biliary tract disease, including stones and choledochal cysts, and also determine the presence of pancreatic complications, including pseudocyst formation. The MRCP technique can image both the biliary and pancreatic ductal system, but either PTC or ERCP may be required to provide a definitive diagnosis.

Surgery is indicated for cases of pancreatitis associated with gallstones or cysts or in cases with pancreatic duct obstruction.

2.10 Tumors of the Pancreas

Benign tumors of the pancreas in children include cystadenoma, lymphangioma, and hemangioendothelioma, which usually present as mass lesions compressing and obstructing the biliary tree, thus causing liver dysfunction with cholestasis. The rare malignant tumors of the head of the pancreas, in contrast to those in adults, are more likely to present with pain and pancreatitis rather than obstruction to the biliary tree. Pancreatoblastoma, a peculiar tumor, is a dense fibrous mass and, although malignant, has a comparatively good prognosis following surgical resection.

Abdominal ultrasound, CT and MRI scanning can readily define the tumors and can also be used for guiding needle biopsies to determine a histological diagnosis.

3 TESTS OF PANCREATIC FUNCTION

A variety of tests are available to determine the presence or absence of pancreatic insufficiency and the degree of residual function in patients with pancreatic sufficiency.

3.1 Stool Analysis

Although of questionable sensitivity, the presence of fat droplets on fecal microscopy—confirmed by staining with oil red O—is highly suggestive of pancreatic insufficiency. Malabsorption is best demonstrated by a 5 day fat-balance study where weighed dietary intake data are recorded for 5 days and fecal fat output is measured over the final 3 days and then expressed as a percentage of the daily dietary fat intake.

3.2 Other Tests

Other noninvasive tests—including serum trypsinogen, fecal chymotrypsin, or elastase—are reasonable alternatives in detecting the presence of PI and/or PS but cannot determine the degree of preservation of pancreatic function in PS patients. In this regard the only available test capable of measuring residual function is the quantitative marker perfusion pancreatic stimulation test using the hormonal stimulants cholecystokinin (pancreozymin) and secretin (8). However, this is an invasive test that is not well tolerated by younger children without sedation, and it is available in only a few centers worldwide as an investigative technique (8).

4 ENZYME REPLACEMENT THERAPY

Oral enzyme replacement therapy (OERT) using the recently developed microspheric preparations has contributed markedly to the management of pancreatic insufficiency in childhood pancreatic disease. Prior to the marketing of these preparations in the early 1980s, patients received enzyme powder produced in either tablet or capsule form. With such preparations the enzymes were mainly inactivated in the stomach as a result of acid pepsin digestion. PI patients averaging a fecal fat of 40% off OERT would minimally improve their malabsorption to 30% of fat intake, despite often consuming massive doses of enzyme (50 to 100 capsules per meal) (17). The new microspheric preparations were designed to prevent gastric inactivation of the enzyme by incorporating the enzyme into microspheres with a pH sensitive coating, the latter resisting acid dissolution and dissolving only at a pH above 6, which is present in the upper duodenum. Several studies in older children and adolescents have demonstrated that by increasing the dose from 6 to 25 to 30 standard 5000-IU lipase capsules, a plateau effect is observed, with fecal fats averaging 10 to 15% of fat intakes, with up to 50% of patients achieving fat excretions of less than 10% of fat intake. These results were clearly better than those achieved with the older preparations.

Notwithstanding these excellent overall results, a small number of patients (up to 5%) have failed to respond to these regimens. Some have been demonstrated to have a consistently low duodenal pH and have been helped by adjuvant gastric acid suppression therapy using H_2 receptor antagonists or proton blocking agents. Still others do not respond to the adjuvant medication; in such cases, other causes of malabsorption, including celiac disease, giardiasis, small bowel bacterial overgrowth, and biliary tract disease should be sought and treated appropriately.

Many clinics have allowed patients to self-regulate their dose of OERT. As a result, patients often consume doses of enzymes well in excess of recommendations. Unfortunately, stool consistency does not necessarily correlate with fecal fat measurements; thus, in most cases, these excessive doses have not been justified (28). Of equal concern, as many patients consumed large numbers of capsules, high-dose lipase preparations (>20,000 IU/capsule) were marketed in order to decrease the number of capsules consumed per meal. Again, in clinics where patients self-regulated their dose, excessive amounts of enzyme, in some instances >60,000 IU/kg/day, were consumed. The latter was linked epidemiologically with the occurrence of a new intestinal complication, fibrosing colonopathy. This entity that has substantially decreased following withdrawal or more stringent regulation of the use of enzyme preparations (29,30). As a result of the occurrence of fibrosing colonopathy the U.S. Cystic Fibrosis Foundation recommended that enzyme doses should not exceed 2500 IU/kg per meal or 10,000 U/kg/day. In this regard it is worth noting that normal growth in CF patients has been achieved in some clinics using a dose of 5000 IU/kg/day (8), and there would appear to be little justification for exceeding this dose unless individual patients were clearly shown by fecal fat testing to require higher dose regimens (i.e., to maintain a fecal fat <20% of fat intake).

Whether one uses the standard preparations; i.e., 5000 to 10,000 IU/capsule, or higher-dose lipase preparations up to 20,000 IU/capsule will often depend on patient preference. Dividing a high-dose lipase capsule for young children, for instance, is unnecessary when one can provide a whole capsule or multiples of whole capsules of standard preparations to arrive at the appropriate dose. One also has to consider the effect of having multiple brands and doses available, as patients often perceive that there is a benefit from the higher-dose preparations when in fact this premise has not been proven.

REFERENCES

1. Solomon TE. Control of exocrine pancreatic secretion. In: Johnson LR ed. Physiology of the Gastrointestinal Tract, New York; Raven Press, 1994, pp 1499–1529.
2. Voet D, Voet JG. Biochemistry, 2nd ed. New York: Wiley, 1995.
3. Hofmann AF. Lipase, colipase amphipathic dietary proteins and bile acids: new interactions at an old interface. Gastroenterology 1978; 75:530–532.
4. Gaskin KJ, Durie PR, Hill RE, Lee LM, Forstner GG. Colipase and maximally activated pancreatic lipase in normal subjects and patients with steatorrhea. J Clin Invest 1982; 69:427–434.
5. Track NS, Creutzfeldt C, Bokermann M. Enzymatic, functional and ultrastructural development of the exocrine pancreas: II. The human pancreas. Comp Biochem Physiol 1975; 51A:95–100.
6. Zoppi G, Andreotti G, Payno-Ferrara F, Njai DM, Guburro D. Exocrine pancreatic function in premature and full term infants. Pediatr Res 1972; 6:880–886.
7. Gaskin KJ, Durie PR, Lee L, Hill R, Forstner GG. Colipase and lipase secretion in childhood onset pancreatic insufficiency. Gastroenterology 1984; 86:1–7.
8. Waters DL, Dorney SFA, Gaskin KJ, Gruca MA, O'Halloran M, Wilcken B. Pancreatic function in infants identified as having cystic fibrosis in a neonatal screening program. N Engl J Med 1990; 322:303–308.
9. Riordan JR, Rommens JM, Kerem B, Alon N, Rozmahel R, Grzelczak Z, Zielenski J, Lok S, Plavsic N, Chou JL, Drumm ML, Iannuzzi MC, Collins FS, Tsui L-C. Identification of the cystic fibrosis gene:. cloning and characterisation of complementary DNA. Science 1989:245:1066–1073.
10. Bear CE, Li CH, Kartner N, Bridges RJ, Jensen TJ, Ramjeesingh M, Riordan JR. Purification and functional reconstitution of the cystic fibrosis transmembrane conductance regulator (CFTR). Cell 1992; 68:809–818.
11. Forstner GG, Durie PR. Cystic fibrosis. In: Walker A, Durie P, Hamilton JR, Walker-Smith J, Watkins J, eds. Pediatric Gastrointestinal Disease, 2nd ed. Philadelphia: Decker 1996, pp 1466–1487.
12. Marino CR, Gorelick FS. Scientific advances in cystic fibrosis. Gastroenterology 1992; 103:681–693.
13. Durie PR, Forstner GG, Gaskin KJ, Moore DJ, Cleghorn GJ, Wong SS, Corey ML. Age-related alterations of immunoreactive pancreatic cationic trypsinogen in sera from cystic fibrosis patients with and without pancreatic insufficiency. Pediatr Res 1986; 20:209–213.
14. Kerem E, Corey M, Kerem B, Rommens J, Markiewicz D, Levison H, Tsui L-C, Durie PR. The relationship between genotype and phenotype in cystic fibrosis—analysis of the most common mutation (ΔF508). N Engl J Med 1990; 323:1517–1522.
15. Kristidis P, Bozon D, Corey M, Markitwicz D, Rommens J, Tsui L-C, Durie P.

Genetic determination of exocrine pancreatic function in cystic fibrosis. Am J Hum Genet 1992; 50:1178–1184.

16. Wilschanski M, Zielenski J, Markiewicz D, Tsui L-C, Corey M, Levison H, Durie PR. Correlation of sweat chloride concentration with classes of cystic fibrosis transmembrane conductance regulator gene mutations. J Pediatr 1995; 127:705–710.

17. Forstner G, Gall G, Corey M, Durie P, Hill RE, Gaskin K. Digestion and absorption of nutrients in cystic fibrosis. In: Sturgess J ed. Perspectives in Cystic Fibrosis: Proceedings of the 8th International Congress on Cystic Fibrosis. Mississauga, Ontario: Imperial Press, 1980, pp 137–148.

18. Gaskin KJ. Liver and biliary tract disease in cystic fibrosis. In: Suchy FJ, ed. Liver Disease in Children. St Louis: Mosby, 1994, pp 705–719.

19. Cheng K, Ashby D, Smyth R. Ursodeoxycholic acid for cystic fibrosis-related liver disease. Cochrane Library 1999; 2:1–11.

20. Aggett PJ, Cavanagh NPC, Mathew DJ, Pincott JR, Sutcliffe J, Harries JT. Shwachman's syndrome. Arch Dis Child 1980; 55:331–347.

21. Ginzberg H, Shin J, Ellis L, Morrison J, Ip W, Dror Y, Freedman M, Heitlinger LA, Belt MA, Corey M, Rommens JM, Durie PP. Shwachman syndrome: phenotypic manifestations of sibling sets and isolated cases in a large patient cohort are similar. J Pediatr 1999; 135:81–88.

22. Pearson HA, Lobel JS, Kocoshis SA, Naiman JL, Windmiller J, Lammi AT, Hoffman R, Marsh JC. A new syndrome of refractory anaemia with vacuolisation of marrow precursors and exocrine pancreatic dysfunction. J Pediatr 1979; 95:976–984.

23. Sokol RJ, Treem WR. Mitochondria and childhood liver diseases. J Pediatr Gastroenterol Nutr 1999; 28:4–16.

24. Johanson A, Blizzard R. A syndrome of congenital aplasia of the alae nasi, deafness, hypothyroidism, dwarfism, absent permanent teeth and malabsorption. J Pediatr 1971; 79:982–987.

25. Stoffers DA, Zinkin NT, Stanojevic V, Clarke WL, Habener JF. Pancreatic agenesis attributable to single nucleotide deletion in the human IPF1 gene coding sequence. Nature Genet 1997; 15:106–110.

26. Bailey PV, Tracy TF, Connors RH, Mooney DP, Lewis JE, Weber TR. Congenital duodenal obstruction: a 32-year review. J Pediatr Surg 1993; 28:92–95.

27. Gorry MC, Gabbaizedeh D, Furey W, Gates LK, Preston RA, Aston CE, Zhang Y, Ulrich C, Ehrlich GD, Whitcomb DC. Mutations in the cationic trypsinogen gene are associated with recurrent acute and chronic pancreatitis. Gastroenterology 1997; 113:1063–1068.

28. Lebenthal E. High strength pancreatic exocrine enzyme capsules associated with colonic strictures in patients with cystic fibrosis: "more is not necessarily better." J Pediatr Gastroenterol Nutr 1994; 18:423–425.

29. Smyth RL, Ashby D, O'Hea U, Burrows E, Lewis P, van Velzen R, Dodge JA. Fibrosing colonopathy in cystic fibrosis: results of a case control study. Lancet 1995; 346:1247–1251.

30. Fitzsimmons SC, Burkhart GA, Borowitz D, Grand RJ, Hammerstrom T, Durie PR, Lloyd-Still JD, Lowenfels AB. High-dose pancreatic enzyme supplements and fibrosing colonopathy in children with cystic fibrosis. N Engl J Med 1997; 336:1283–1289.

32

Pediatric Upper Gastrointestinal Endoscopy, Endoscopic Retrograde Cholangiopancreatography, and Colonoscopy

George Gershman

Harbor-UCLA Medical Center, Torrance, California

Marvin E. Ament

Mattel Children's Hospital at UCLA, UCLA School of Medicine, Los Angeles, California

1   UPPER ENDOSCOPY

1.1   Introduction

In the late 1960s and early 1970s, sporadic attempts were made to perform eso-phagogastroduodenoscopy (EGD) in children using fiberscopes designed for adults (1–3). However, the actual "birth" of pediatric EGD occurred only when prototypes of pediatric flexible gastro- and panendoscopes became commercially available. Subsequently, the pediatric community received unequivocal evidence of very low rates of complications related to upper-gastrointestinal (GI) endos-copy, high diagnostic yields, cost-effectiveness (due to the safe use of the proce-dure in outpatient settings), and the ability to perform a variety of therapeutic procedures successfully adopted from adult GI practice. All of these led to a widespread use of EGD in pediatrics (4–8).

1.2   Preparation

The patient should receive an explanation of the events that will take place the day of the procedure in terminology that he or she is capable of understanding. Patients should be fasted for at least 4 to 6 hr prior to the procedure. Children who take medications for seizure disorders should be allowed to take the medications as usual. Children who are very frightened may benefit from a low dose of diazepam orally 30 min prior to their arrival at the procedure suite.

1.2.1   Antibiotic Prophylaxis for Patients with Heart Disease

Recommendations from the American Heart Association for prophylactic antibiotics in susceptible patients indicate that they should only be used for those patients at high risk for endocarditis and brain abscess and for those undergoing a procedure with a high risk of bacteremia.

1.3   Instrumentation

The wide variety of pediatric fiberscopes and videoendoscopes currently available makes it feasible to perform EGD in neonates and even in preterm babies weighing more than 2000 g. Over the last decade there has been a tendency to replace fiberscopes with videoendoscopes, which provide better-quality images as well as mucosal details. The other important advantages of videoendoscopes are supplementation of medical records with photodocumentation, electronic storage, and transmission/exchange of visual information necessary for second opinions or teaching purposes.

Endoscopes 5.3 to 8.0 mm in diameter should be used in neonates and infants below 6 months of age in order to avoid compression of the trachea and/ or overstretching of the greater curvature of the stomach. This will effectively decrease the risk of vagal reactions, diminish respiratory or cardiovascular distress (especially in small-for-gestational-age neonates or infants or patients with preexisting cardiovascular or respiratory diseases), and facilitate intubation of the distal duodenum. Endoscopes with an outer diameter of 8.0 to 9.0 mm are appropriate for use in infants over 6 months of age and in toddlers. School-age children may be examined by either 9 or 9.8 mm endoscopes, depending upon the goal of the procedure. It is also important to note that endoscopes with a 2.8-mm biopsy channel can accommodate the majority of the existing therapeutic accessories and the larger-volume forceps.

1.4   Sedation

In the early and mid 1970s, most pediatric endoscopies were performed using general anesthesia. In the late 1970s and early 1980s there was a trend toward deep or conscious sedation using combinations of intravenous (IV) meperidine, diazepam, promethazine, and/or chlorpromazine with or without topical pharyngeal anesthesia. Currently, there is no consensus regarding the choice of anesthesia or sedation for endoscopic procedures in children. Available data suggests that EGD could be effectively and safely performed under conscious or deep sedation in the majority of pediatric patients who meet the criteria of the American Society of Anesthesiologists (ASA) physical status classification class 1 or 2 (Table 1) (9–12). Most pediatric sedation protocols for EGD include meperedine, fentanyl, midazolam, and/or promethazine. This method of sedation is easily reversible by naloxone and flumazenil, provides antegrade amnesia, and is also substantially less expensive as compared with general anesthesia. However, narcotics in combination with benzodiazepines significantly increase the risk of respiratory depression (13). Oxygen desaturation may occur even before endoscopy and does not necessarily present with irritability or other changes in a patient's behavior. That is why objective parameters such as respiratory rate, pulse, and oxygen saturation must be monitored during sedation, the procedure itself, and recovery. This is especially important for neonates and infants, who are more sensitive to esophageal intubation and gastric distention. The current recommendation for maximum doses of fentanyl are 4 $\mu g/kg$ and for midazolam, 0.3 mg/kg. The initial dose of fentanyl (1.0 $\mu g/kg$) and midazolam (0.1 mg/kg) must be injected through a well-secured IV line, followed by a repeat dose every 2 to 3 min. Each subsequent dose may be given if no significant depression in respiration, oxygen desaturation, significant tachycardia, or decrease in blood pressure occurs. If an adequate level of sedation has not been achieved with approximately three-quarters of the estimated dose of fentanyl and midazolam, the first dose of promethazine (0.5 mg/kg) may be administered. The rest of the fentanyl and midazolam and repeat doses of promethazine are reserved for patients who will not tolerate insertion of the mouthpiece or endoscope itself. Special attention must be paid to the correct size and placement of the pulse oximeter sensor because detachment from the skin, displacement of the two diodes more than 2 to 3 mm, or exposure to ambient light may lead to optical shunt and falsely high or low

TABLE 1 American Society of Anesthesiologists Physical Status Classification for Anesthesia Risk

1	Healthy patient
2	Mild systemic disease (absent or only slight functional limitation, gross obesity)
3	Severe systemic disease (definite functional limitation)
4	Severe systemic disease (constant threat to life)
5	Moribund patient (unlikely to survive 24 hr)

Source: Ref. 13.

readings (14). A low oxygen saturation reading on the monitor must be correlated with the plethysmographic waveform as well as the skin color and pulse before any decisions regarding intervention are made. If the skin is pink and the patient is not bradycardic, partial or complete detachment of the sensors must be suspected and resolved.

Although cardiac arrest has not been described as a complication of EGD in children, cardiac arrhythmias (typically sinus tachycardia) secondary to oxygen desaturation or vagal reactions may develop. Oxygen supplementation or withdrawal of the instrument usually reverses the arrhythmia. In case of conscious or deep sedation, the pediatric gastroenterologist must be familiar with resuscitation of apnea and/or cardiac arrest.

General anesthesia with or without tracheal intubation is indicated for children considered ASA class 3 to 5. It is also reserved for patients who failed conscious or deep sedation, children with morbid obesity or sleep apnea, certain procedures such as esophageal dilatation, or percutaneous endoscopic gastrostomy (PEG) in children with seizure disorders.

1.5 Technique of Passing an Endoscope

The sedated patient is placed in the left lateral position with the head slightly extended to decrease the angle between the oral and esophageal axis. The endoscope must be inspected for proper functioning and lubricated prior to insertion. A good indicator of adequate sedation is if the mouthpiece can be placed without the child's resistance. Once this is achieved, there are two different techniques for performing EGD: either two endoscopists or one endoscopist and an assistant respectively manipulate the shaft and the control block of the endoscope or one endoscopist performs the entire procedure. The latter method is more difficult, but in skillful hands it provides many benefits in orientation and in quick response to changes in observation and feeling of resistance. Following lubrication and downward deflection, the endoscope is inserted into the mouth and gently advanced toward the root of the tongue. The instrument should never be advanced using force. To facilitate esophageal intubation, the endoscopist can either wait until there is spontaneous opening of the upper esophageal sphincter and then gently twist the shaft of the instrument or slightly insufflate the pharynx with air. After the upper esophageal sphincter has been passed, the endoscope is advanced along the lumen. The border between the esophageal and gastric mucosa, the so-called Z line, appears as a junction between the slightly pale esophageal and the pink gastric mucosa.

Upon entry into the stomach (recognizable by the characteristic folds of the greater curvature and a pool of mucus), the endoscope is rotated clockwise and turned down until a clear picture of the upper body appears. At that point, three to four slightly outlined folds of the lesser curvature can be recognized at 1 to 2 o'clock. These folds quickly disappear during insufflation. The greater curvature is seen as prominent waving folds between 6 and 8 o'clock. To provide good tolerance of the procedure, we recommend minimal insufflation of the stomach, especially in infants, in whom overinflation may induce irritability, retching, and increased respiratory distress.

The normal pylorus looks like a small ring that disappears during peristalsis, but even at that moment it is not difficult to find if the endoscopist follows the prepyloric folds and guides the endoscope slightly down to avoid flipping into the U position. As soon as the pylorus is passed through, the endoscope may be advanced forward very quickly. At that moment an endoscopist must be careful to avoid blind trauma to the duodenal wall.

The hallmark of the second portion of the duodenum is the papilla of Vater, which is located at 9 to 10 o'clock or 11 to 12 o'clock, depending upon how the duodenum is approached. The minor duodenal papilla is located about 2 or 3 cm proximal to the major duodenal papilla. It looks like a small (4- to 5-mm) sessile polyp. Moving distally from the area of the major papilla, the endoscopist may easily recognize the prominent pulsation of the superior mesenteric artery, which is a hallmark of the third portion of the duodenum. The lumen of the fourth portion of the duodenum narrows toward the ligament of Treitz.

Careful observation is necessary during insertion and withdrawal of the endoscope. When the endoscope is pulled back to the gastric body, a retrograde observation (U turn) of the proximal portion of the stomach (including cardia, subcardia, gastric fundus, and proximal body) may be performed.

In case of bleeding (especially variceal bleeding), it is reasonable to make a U-turn maneuver at the beginning of the gastroscopy. To make this maneuver, the fibroscope is bent up, turned toward the anterior wall (10 o'clock), and slowly advanced until the panorama of the proximal stomach appears. Then the fiberscope is pulled back and rotated either clockwise or counterclockwise.

At the end of the gastroscopy, it is necessary to deflate the stomach. Finally, the entire esophagus is assessed a second time. This is especially important in infants with possible congenital anomalies such as tracheoesophageal fistula (Fig. 1).

1.6 Biopsy Technique

Histological verification of many diseases involving the upper GI tract (e.g., esophagitis, gastritis, celiac disease, etc.) is crucial for a definitive diagnosis. In this respect, sufficient tissue samples and proper orientation are the keys to correct interpretation of the biopsy. It is always possible to obtain an adequate tissue sample (even with a small forceps) if an endoscopist is familiar with the appropriate technique. There are certain universal rules:

1. Endoscopic biopsy is not a blind procedure.
2. The forceps should not be advanced more than 2 cm beyond the tip of the endoscope.

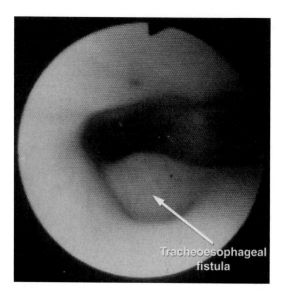

FIGURE 1 Tracheoesophageal fistula: a prominent "dimple" on the anterior wall of the upper esophagus.

3. Forceful pushing of the forceps against a wall is a dangerous and ineffective way to obtain more tissue.

Technically, an esophageal biopsy is more difficult than either a gastric or duodenal biopsy. The most common indication for esophageal biopsy in pediatrics is to rule out esophagitis. For correct interpretation, each biopsy should be located using the Z line as the reference point. To avoid confusing results, at least two biopsies must be taken from 2 cm above the gastroesophageal junction. The suspected disease determines the number and the site of the gastric and duodenal biopsies. For example, to rule out *Helicobacter pylori* gastritis, four biopsies must be obtained: two samples must be taken from the prepyloric antrum (one sample is necessary for the CLO test), one from the lesser curvature of the antrum, and one from the greater curvature of the distal body (15).

In case of an ulcer or erosion, biopsies should be taken from their margins. Special attention should be paid to the first biopsy performed. This is important because the lesion may be covered with blood and subsequent target biopsies could be difficult to make.

The best site for a duodenal biopsy is the edge of the valvulae conniventes. A perpendicular orientation of the forceps to the mucosal folds eliminates excessive pressure on the tissue, prevents mucosal trauma and artifacts of the biopsy, and augments the size of the sample. Comparison of endoscopic and blind duodenal biopsy has shown that the former could substitute for a blind capsule biopsy for diagnosis of celiac sprue and other mucosal diseases (16–18). If celiac sprue is suspected, at least four samples of tissue must be obtained from the second or third portion of the duodenum.

1.7 Indications

The broad spectrum of indications for upper-GI endoscopy in children may be subdivided into three categories (Table 2):

1. Indications for emergency endoscopy
2. Indications for elective diagnostic endoscopy
3. Indications for therapeutic endoscopy

Chronic recurrent abdominal pain (RAP) is the most common indication for EGD simply because it exists in 10 to 17% of children between 5 and 14 years of age (19) (see Chap. 22). According to current knowledge, more than 90% of children with this complaint have "functional" abdominal pain. If the clinical scenario is indicative of organic causes of pain, EGD with biopsy is the best tool for the diagnosis of peptic ulcer, gastritis, duodenitis, and other mucosal diseases.

TABLE 2 Indications for Upper-GI Endoscopy

Urgent endoscopy	Elective diagnostic endoscopy	Therapeutic endoscopy
GI bleeding	Recurrent upper abdominal pain	Foreign-body removal
Caustic ingestion	Dysphagia/odynophagia	Sclerotherapy
Foreign-body ingestion	Vomiting	Placement of gastrostomy tube
	Weight loss	Electrophotocoagulation
	Anemia/occult blood loss	Polypectomy
	Malabsorptive chronic diarrhea	Dilation of esophageal stricture
	Radiographic evidence of mucosal lesions	Pneumodilation of achalasia
	Evidence of mass lesion by upper-GI series	Botox injection
	Familial polyposis or Peutz-Jegher syndrome	

1.8 Bleeding

Upper-GI bleeding in children is probably the most serious condition requiring endoscopy (see Chap. 26). The goal of the upper-GI endoscopy in children with melena or hematemesis is to define the source of bleeding and to perform therapeutic procedures such as sclerotherapy, electro/photocoagulation, and injection of vasoconstrictive agents if necessary. The same questions are always raised in such circumstances. Is the patient stable? Is the source of bleeding within the upper GI tract or is it simply epistaxis? What is the optimal time for endoscopy?

In case of bleeding from an ulcer, endoscopy may predict the risk of recurrence based upon location and appearance: pigmented spots (Fig. 2), an adherent clot (Fig. 3), a visible vessel or blood spurting, and location of an ulcer on the posterior wall of the duodenum are important prognostic factors. EGD also helps to make the best choice of treatment based upon the detected source of bleeding (e.g., gastritis versus primary or secondary ulcer; variceal bleeding versus hypertensive gastropathy).

The frequency of aspirin-induced gastric and duodenal lesions is substantially less now than in the past because acetaminophen is used more commonly. However, they still do occur because many over-the-counter "cold medications" contain salicylates. Two types of lesions are often observed. Type 1 is acute gastritis involving multiple separate or confluent red dots with or without erosions

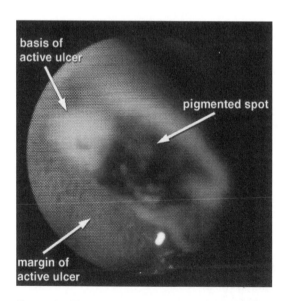

FIGURE 2   Pigmented spot at the base of the active ulcer of the gastroentero-anastomosis. There is a minimal risk of recurrent bleeding from such an ulcer.

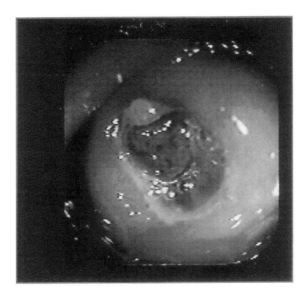

FIGURE 3 Duodenal ulcer with adherent clot. This type of ulcer is associated with an increased risk of recurrent bleeding and requires endoscopic treatment with a heater probe.

and with a white center and red rim. Type 2 is a large ulcer (usually gastric) with flat, smooth margins surrounded by pink or patchy erythematous mucosa without evidence of chronic inflammation. Nonsteroidal anti-inflammatory drugs (NSAIDs) may cause similar lesions.

The other type of drug-induced lesion is hemorrhagic gastritis. The hallmark of hemorrhagic gastritis is subepithelial hemorrhages with or without mucosal edema. It may be either localized or widespread. In severe lesions, a large area of gastric surface may be actively bleeding.

Although peptic ulcer disease is a relatively rare problem in pediatric patients, it comprises at least half of the cases of bleeding from the upper GI tract in school-age children. The majority of bleeding ulcers are located in the duodenal bulb. In general, at least 80% of bleeding episodes cease spontaneously; but if the bleeding is arterial, the incidence of recurrent episodes will be increased and may potentially become life-threatening. If spurting blood or a visible vessel has been found, the risk of recurrent bleeding is high even after initially successful endoscopic hemostasis. These patients require careful observation and aggressive treatment. Most often, recurrence of bleeding is seen within 3 days of the initial episode. If an ulcer has a clear base or pigmented spot, the risk of further bleeding is minimal and therapeutic endoscopy is not indicated.

The two therapeutic methods most commonly used in pediatric patients with a nonvariceal upper-GI bleed are bipolar electrocoagulation and treatment by heater probe. This probe is now commercially available for pediatric (9.8-mm) endoscopes. Both methods provide enough heat for coagulation of mesenteric arteries up to 2 mm, as demonstrated in experimental models. Advantages of the heater probe include no direct contact of electricity with the tissue, adjustable depth of coagulation, and no adherence to the tissue. The use of laser photocoagulation in pediatric patients has been quite limited because of potential transmural tissue damage and the high cost of the equipment. This could change with the availability of the argon plasma coagulation technique.

Chronic Peptic Ulcers. Peptic ulcer disease tends to occur in school-age children and is more common in boys (see Chap. 20). In most cases, primary ulcers are located in the duodenal bulb. The active stage of peptic ulcer disease usually manifests by significant spasm and rigidity of the duodenal bulb. These conditions may be aggravated by scarring from previous relapses or by manipulations with the endoscope per se. In such circumstances maximal attention must be paid to indirect endoscopic signs such as convergence of mucosal folds, severe erythema, or edema of the duodenal mucosa. If necessary, glucagon may be used to reduce spasm of the duodenum. It is not unusual to find multiple or "kissing" duodenal ulcers in children with peptic ulcer disease. That is why a thorough examination of the opposite wall has to be carried out whenever an ulcer or a scar is detected.

1.9 Gastroesophageal Reflux Disease (GERD)

In children with GERD, upper-GI endoscopy is indicated if symptoms persist in spite of standard therapy or if esophagitis or its complication is suspected (see Chap. 19). Reflux esophagitis in children presents endoscopically with characteristics that are used to grade the findings on a scale of 0 to 5 (20).

> Grade 0 represents esophageal mucosa that is normal in appearance.
> Grades 1 and 2 are subjective mucosal changes such as patchy or linear erythema, edema, and vertical lines.
> Grade 3 is defined by the presence of erosion (Fig. 4).
> Grades 4 and 5 manifest by the presence of ulcer and stricture, respectively.

This classification reflects the fact that EGD alone has low sensitivity and specificity for diagnosis of reflux esophagitis in children. This is particularly true regarding normal-appearing esophageal mucosa and subjective endoscopic criteria (grades 0 to 2). Thus, it is imperative to obtain esophageal biopsies for histological confirmation of esophagitis. A big advantage of EGD is the ability to assess the severity and extent of the esophageal lesions and to perform a target

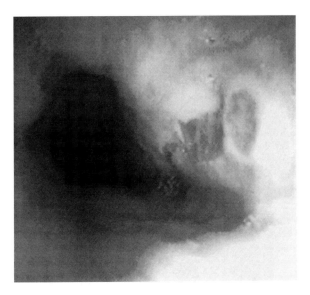

FIGURE 4 Erosion of the esophageal mucosa in a patient with reflux esophagitis. According to the Los Angeles classification of reflux esophagitis in adults, similar lesions have been called mucosal brakes.

biopsy as well as a thorough assessment of entire upper GI tract, which permits the diagnosis of synchronous lesions in the stomach and duodenum.

A stricture due to reflux esophagitis in children is usually short and located in the distal esophagus. The exceptions are the patients with repaired esophageal atresia and long segment Barrett's esophagus (BE). Uncomplicated esophageal stricture appears as a white, annular, or rarely crescent-shaped infundibular narrowing with a central lumen surrounded by actively inflammed or pale mucosa (Fig. 5). An esophageal stricture becomes asymmetrical if it is complicated by a coexisting ulcer. If the narrowing is short, located just above the Z line, and surrounded by normal-appearing esophageal mucosa, a Schatzki ring should be considered. On rare occasions, a severe stenosis of the middle esophagus may be caused by tracheobronchial remnants. This type of stenosis is usually symmetrical but more elongated than a stricture secondary to esophagitis. Translucent cartilages and absence of inflammation assist with the diagnosis.

Barrett's esophagus (BE) is rare in children. However, it must be kept in mind due to its malignant potential. Ten cases of esophageal cancer related to BE in children have already been described (21). By definition, BE is an extension of columnar epithelium with specialized goblet cells that undergo metaplasia and grow into the tubular esophagus. An esophagogram does not have diagnostic

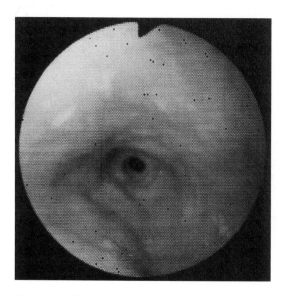

FIGURE 5   Esophageal stricture secondary to chronic gastroesophageal reflux.

value because there is no specific radiological sign of BE. Blind suction biopsy
directed by esophageal manometry has been used in the past, but it had significant
sampling error and could not be used for correct histological mapping. Currently,
endoscopy with multiple biopsies is the "gold standard" for the diagnosis of
BE. The role of endoscopy is to identify abnormal areas of esophageal mucosa,
such as tongue-like protrusions from the Z line toward the thoracic esophagus
(Fig. 6) or, in rare cases, separate islands of pink mucosa or ulcers surrounded
by patches of esophageal mucosa. Endoscopy also helps to distinguish between
the displacements of the columnar epithelium toward the tubular esophagus from
a hiatal hernia. The endoscopic sign of hiatal hernia is cephalad displacement of
the proximal margin of the gastric cardia mucosal folds by 2 cm or more above
the diaphragmatic notch. The diagnosis of BE requires esophageal biopsies from
different levels above the Z line. At least two samples should be taken from each
level. The tissue samples should be stained with Alcian blue at pH 2.5 to identify
goblet-cell metaplasia, which is diagnostic. If only cardiac gland metaplasia is
found, BE must be suspected and endoscopy with biopsy should be repeated in
1 year. Endoscopic surveillance at 3- to 4-year intervals has been proposed for
children over 10 years of age with diagnosed BE but no evidence of dysphagia.

    Infectious esophagitis is a frequent cause of dysphagia and odynophagia
in immunocompromised children. The most common types of infectious esopha-

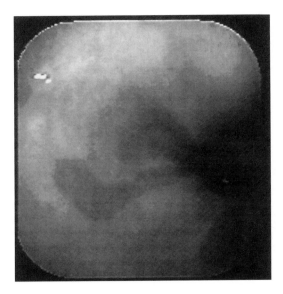

FIGURE 6   Barrett's esophagus with the long red "tongues" of metaplastic epithelium of the distal esophagus.

gitis are due to *Candida*, cytomegalovirus (CMV), or herpes simplex virus (HSV). Endoscopy with brush cytology and biopsy are the most reliable diagnostic methods. Candida esophagitis may present with erythematous mucosa covered by scattered or confluent white, cream-colored, thick plaques with greatest density in the distal esophagus (Fig. 7). Shallow serpiginous ulcerations surrounded by normal mucosa are often seen in CMV esophagitis. Histological marks of CMV are basophilic, intracellular inclusions, a clear halo surrounding the nucleus and the presence of multiple smaller intracytoplasmic inclusions that are positive on periodic acid–Schiff staining.

Herpes simplex virus is the most common cause of herpetic esophagitis. The disease may start with herpetic lesions on the lips or buccal mucosa, followed by odynophagia or dysphagia. The endosopic hallmark of herpetic esophagitis is aphthoid-like ulcers with a raised erythematous margin and gray or yellowish base. These ulcers are typically seen in the middle or upper esophagus. In advanced disease, diffuse involvement of mucosa with confluent ulcers, exudate, or friability may occur (Fig. 8).

To obtain adequate tissue samples with the replicating virus, the biopsy should be taken from the margin of the ulcer. Multinucleated giant cells and ballooning of the cells, prominent eosinophilic intranucleic "ground glass" inclusions, and chromatin margination are diagnostic.

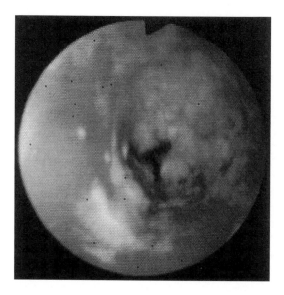

FIGURE 7 Candidal esophagitis: erythematous esophageal mucosa covered by scattered, cream-colored, thick plaques.

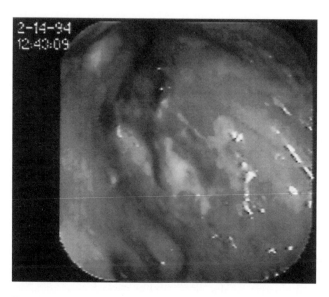

FIGURE 8 Herpetic esophagitis: patchy erythema and confluent shallow ulcers and exudate.

1.10 Caustic Ingestion

Despite precautions, corrosive injuries still occur, usually as tragic accidents. These incidents take place mostly in young children under 5 years of age or during suicide attempts by teenagers. Lye ingestion induces severe injuries, primarily to the esophagus, although strong acid may create more diffuse lesions including the stomach or duodenum. Sodium hydroxide in different preparations induces rapid liquefaction necrosis with deep (even full-thickness) injuries. Respiratory distress, esophageal perforation, or periesophageal inflammation with subsequent mediastinitis and peritonitis are the most serious short-term complications of caustic ingestion. Immediate and long-term outcomes are directly related to the degree of burn. The absence of visible lesions on the lips or the oral or pharyngeal mucosa does not correlate with the absence of esophageal or gastric injuries. As soon as the patient is stable, upper-GI endoscopy must be done under general anesthesia, especially if the patient is agitated, drooling, tachypneic, or hemodynamically unstable. In superficial involvement, the esophageal mucosa appears erythematous or edematous with minimal or no mucosal peeling. If the injury is more extensive, the sloughing of the mucosa is more expansive and leaves behind hemorrhagic exudate, islands of mucosal debris, or ulcerations. The hallmark of severe esophageal burns is the presence of an eschar or deep ulcers. It is not uncommon that in severe burns the esophagus is difficult to assess due to obliteration of the lumen as the result of severe spasm and edema of a deeply injured wall. Any attempt at forceful maneuvers or insufflation must be avoided. Patients with no visible mucosal lesions may be discharged home. The rest of the patients with caustic ingestions must be hospitalized for at least 24 to 48 hr if the injury is mild. Withholding of oral feedings, parenteral nutritional support, broad-spectrum antibiotics, and steroids are the conventional therapies for patients with the moderate or severe burns. Nasogastric intubation has also been used with apparent success.

1.11 Sclerotherapy

Endoscopic injection sclerotherapy (ES) is a highly effective alternative to the shunting procedure in patients with portal hypertension. It has increasingly been used in pediatric patients for rapid hemostasis and to reduce frequency of recurrent bleeding (22–25).

Elevated pressure of the portal system due to either extra- or intrahepatic origin may appear as a dilatation of the esophageal and gastric submucosal veins with or without varices, hypertensive gastropathy, and—less often—with plethoric veins or varices of the small and large intestine. The indications for sclerotherapy are active bleeding from esophageal varices, history of upper-GI bleeding, and a failed shunting procedure. The goal of sclerotherapy varies from temporary hemostasis in children waiting for liver transplantation to complete obliteration of varices in children with an extrahepatic block of portal flow.

As mentioned above, the patient must be stabilized hemodynamically before the procedure. The pressure in the portal system may be lowered by administration of either vasopressin or somatostatin or its synthetic analogue, octreotide (the latter two substances have less systemic side effects). Placement of an Ewald tube is necessary for gastric lavage and assessment of bleeding activity in these cases.

If the intensity of hematemesis excludes emergency endoscopy, the Sengstaken-Blakemore tube is indicated. After establishment of initial hemostasis, the patient must be appropriately sedated. Usually intravenous sedation is adequate. Indications for general anesthesia must be considered individually. Prior to sclerotherapy, panendoscopy is required to rule out coexistent sources of bleeding. Many different sclerosants—including ethanol, sodium morrhuate, ethanolamine, and tetradecyl—have been used. In general, lipid-soluble sclerosants have more systemic side effects (fever, pleural effusion, chest pain, or adult respiratory distress syndrome). The incidence of complications is directly related to the total amount of sclerosant utilized. Injection of sclerosants can be done intra- or paravariceally (or both), starting from the Z line and moving cephalad in a circumferential fashion along the lowest 5 cm of the distal esophagus. If there is no sign of active bleeding, the tortuous varices with cherry red spots, red wale markings, or hematocytic spots must be sclerosed first, as they have a higher risk of rupture. In our practice we use an intravariceal injection of up to 1 mL sclerosant per spot and not more than 5 to 6 mL per session unless we are dealing with an adolescent. In this case, the volume of sclerosant depends on the size of the patient. Control of oozing from a site of injection may be achieved by applying pressure with the endoscope to the varix or via additional paravariceal injection of a sclerosant. Decompression of the stomach after each injection is necessary to prevent aspiration.

After initial endoscopic hemostasis (which is successful in more than 80% of cases), repeat sessions of sclerotherapy are necessary for complete obliteration of varices. Usually the procedure is performed once a week in the first month, followed by a monthly schedule as indicated. In case of deep esophageal ulcers, the scheduled session of sclerotherapy must be postponed. The incidence of recurrent variceal bleeding fluctuates between 8 and 31%. The bleeding may be severe but is usually controllable endoscopically. Most uncontrolled bleeding is related to gastric varices or severe hypertensive gastropathy. An average of four to six sessions of sclerotherapy are necessary to achieve complete obliteration of esophageal varices. Several complications of sclerotherapy have been described. The most common is transient chest pain and low-grade fever, followed by esophageal ulceration (3 to 33%), bleeding from the site of injection, and esophageal stricture (4.5 to 20%).

As a rule, the small, shallow esophageal ulcers do not have any medical significance and heal spontaneously or with treatment with sucralfate or H_2 blockers. Deep ulcers may be the source of bleeding or esophageal stricture and must be treated aggressively. An esophageal stricture due to sclerotherapy is easily managed by dilatation. Transient changes of esophageal motility and gastroesophageal reflux have been described in adults, but the real incidence of these complications in children is unknown.

1.12 Endoscopic Variceal Ligation

Endoscopic variceal ligation (EVL) has been successfully used in adults for more than a decade (26–30). The technique of EVL is relatively simple and can be very effective for hemostasis of bleeding varices. Available data support at least an equal efficacy of EVL and ES in terms of eradication of varices and/or frequency of rebleeding. Moreover, recent publications have challenged a concept of ES as the treatment of choice of esophageal varices. EVL decreases the number of endoscopic sessions necessary to eradicate esophageal varices. It also reduces the frequency of local complications such as deep ulcerations and stricture. The device consists of two cylinders. The inner cylinder has ''O'' rings (up to 10 rings in the latest models), which can be released by a trigger unit attached to the biopsy channel and connected to the inner cylinder through the trip wire. The varix to be ligated is suctioned up into the cylinder. When the varix is inside the inner cylinder, the ''O'' ring released from the inner cylinder by the trip wire strangulates it. Several factors have slowed the use of EVL in pediatrics. The major one is the size of the ligation device. It is designed for an endoscope at least 10 mm in diameter. According to our experience and published data, EVL can be safely performed in children over 1 year of age (31).

Repeat EVL is necessary within 3 to 4 weeks and then continuously on a monthly basis until complete eradication of the varices is achieved. The most common complication of EVL is esophageal ulceration. Unlike ulcers after ES, EVL-induced ulcers are usually more superficial. The long-term efficacy of EVL to prevent rebleeding after variceal eradication in children is unknown. Preliminary results of short-term follow-up data are compatible with the outcome of ES. However, long-term follow-up studies are necessary. An absence of systemic complications along with further modifications of the ligator device suitable for the smaller pediatric endoscopes could make EVL a treatment of choice of variceal bleeding in children.

1.13 Gastritis

During endoscopic examination of the stomach, several mucosal patterns may be found: normal-appearing gastric mucosa, which is pink and smooth with visible vessels more prominent in proximal areas; focal or diffuse erythema; edema;

erosions; nodularity; and petechiae. The clinical scenario and histological data determine the value of these findings.

For instance, if the clinical history is positive for salicylates or ingestion of other NSAIDs, the finding of mucosal edema, petechiae, or erosions is diagnostic, although gastric erosions have been found in asymptomatic volunteers. Because there is no strong correlation between endoscopic and histological changes of gastric mucosa in terms of chronic gastritis, any endoscopically suspicious areas must be verified by target biopsies. This is especially important for the detection of *Helicobacter pylori* (HP), as it may substantially change the approach to therapy (see Chap. 20). Although nodularity of the antral mucosa has been found in about 50% of HP-colonized children (32–34), this endoscopic sign cannot substitute for histological identification of S-shaped bacteria on the surface of the gastric mucosa (stained by the Warthin-Starry or Giemsa technique). A finding of gastric erosions also has a different diagnostic value. In immunocompromised children, it could be the sign of viral gastritis. In CMV gastritis, the inflammation usually involves a submucosal layer of the stomach. Endoscopically, it may appear as an irregular, nodular gastric surface with shallow ulcerations or apparent gastric ulcer. If an inflammation occurs in the antrum or prepyloric area, it may cause gastric outlet obstruction and occasionally mimic a submucosal tumor (Fig. 9). The intranuclear inclusions and positive tissue culture are diagnostic. Herpetic

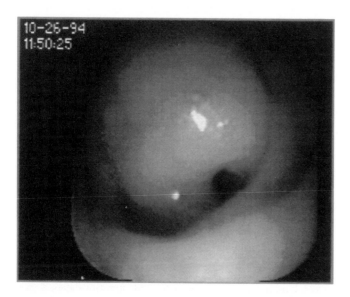

FIGURE 9   A submucosal mass in the prepyloric antrum due to cytomegalovirus gastritis in a patient after liver transplantation.

gastritis may be found in children with HIV infection or after bone marrow or liver transplantation. EGD shows small, shallow ulcers with a whitish exudate at the base. Ulcers may coalesce and be surrounded by erythematous mucosa. Biopsy from the margin of the ulcer and a tissue culture are necessary to confirm herpetic infection.

1.14 Pediatric Hypertrophic Gastropathy or Ménétrier's Disease

Ménétrier's disease is a rare cause of protein-losing enteropathy in children, but over the last decade the number of published cases has doubled. The exact etiology of the disease is unknown, but currently the role of CMV infection is the focus of investigation (35–37).

In Ménétrier's disease, EGD shows an enormous amount of gelatinous mucus in the stomach, giant gastric rugae in the fundus or gastric body that remain unchanged despite vigorous insufflation, and edematous mucosa often with shallow ulceration. Histological signs of Ménétrier's disease are hypertrophic and dilated gastric glands filled with mucus, basilar cystic changes, and mixed infiltration of the lamina propria with neutrophils, lymphocytes, eosinophils, and occasional plasma cells. Unique features of Ménétrier's disease in children are reversible endoscopic and histological changes in the gastric mucosa and the disappearance of clinical symptoms with adequate therapy in the majority of patients.

1.15 Crohn's Disease

Current data suggests that involvement of the upper GI tract in pediatric patients with Crohn's disease occurs more often than previously thought (see Chap. 27) (38–40). The rate of positive findings of a noncaseating granuloma in the stomach or duodenum in unselected patients who underwent EGD was higher than in selected patients with presumptive symptoms of upper GI tract involvement: dysphagia, aphthoid lesions in the mouth, epigastric pain, weight loss, nausea, vomiting, or blood loss (41). In addition, 11.4 to 29% of patients with onset of Crohn's disease may have an isolated inflammation of the stomach and duodenum (42,43). Thus, routine use of EGD in patients with suspected Crohn's disease is indicated. Endoscopic findings of skipped lesions—such as aphthous ulcers, nodularity, thickening of mucosal folds, rigidity or narrowing of the antral portion of the stomach or proximal duodenum—are suggestive of Crohn's disease. The serpiginous or longitudinal ulcers are rarely seen in children. But if they are found, they may help to distinguish this condition from peptic ulcer disease.

The goal of histological evaluation of the stomach and the duodenum in children with suspected Crohn's disease is finding noncaseating granulomas, which occur in 30 to 40% of cases. There is no significant difference in the detection of granulomas in biopsies taken from endoscopically normal or abnormal areas of gastric or duodenal mucosa. That is why multiple samples of endoscopically normal or altered mucosa must be obtained to increase the diagnostic value of the procedure. The absence of noncaseating granulomas, however, does not rule out Crohn's disease. The presence of focal inflammation with "crypt abscess," focal lymphoid aggregates, and fibrosis may be diagnostic in children with a suggestive history and confirmed Crohn's disease in the small or large intestine.

1.16   Gastric Tumors

Gastric tumors in children are rare and usually benign. In the majority of cases they are either ectopic pancreas or hyperplastic polyps (44–46). Ectopic pancreas is often asymptomatic and, in most children, is an incidental finding during an endoscopy or upper gastrointestinal series. The true prevalence of this finding in children is unknown. In the stomach, ectopic pancreas is located on the greater curvature of the antrum and appears as a dome-shaped excavation with a central depression. It is usually covered by unchanged gastric mucosa. Sometimes the lesions may protrude less toward the gastric lumen and remind one of a bagel or doughnut. A biopsy is not indicated, as an ectopic tissue arises from the submucosal or subserosal layers.

A small hyperplastic gastric polyp is usually asymptomatic unless it is located near the pylorus and causes gastric outlet obstruction or anemia (47,48). More often, a hyperplastic polyp in a child is single, sessile, smaller than 1 cm, and located in the antrum. It is not considered premalignant. Endoscopic polypectomy is indicated only if the patient is symptomatic or the polyp is big, erythematous, or ulcerated. Endoscopic surveillance after polypectomy is unnecessary if the diagnosis of hyperplastic polyps is confirmed histologically.

In generalized juvenile polyposis or Peutz-Jegher syndrome, gastric polyps may occur throughout the stomach (Fig. 10). These may be removed endoscopically in one or several sessions, but sometimes their number precludes total eradication. In these cases, the largest polyps should be removed.

Malignant tumors of the stomach account for only 5% or less of all malignant neoplasms in children. Most often such a tumor is a non-Hodgkin's type of lymphoma or leiomyosarcoma (49,50). Gastric bezoars must be included in the differential diagnosis because their clinical symptoms may simulate malignancy, especially if a palpable mass or anemia is present. Usually these symptoms are related to trichobezoars, which have indolent courses and may occupy virtually the whole stomach and proximal duodenum, causing irritation of the gastric mucosa, secondary gastric ulcers, and anemia. Such a bezoar must be removed surgically, although an alternative treatment by extracorporeal shock-wave lithotripsy in an 8-year-old child has been described (51). Phytobezoars may easily be cut down into small fragments able to pass through the gut with an endoscopic snare.

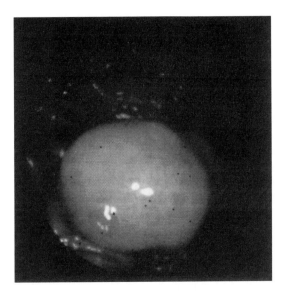

FIGURE 10   Gastric polyp in a patient with Peutz-Jegher syndrome.

1.17   Foreign Bodies

The approach to foreign bodies in the upper GI tract could require either conservative observation or urgent care. Fortunately, more than 90% of swallowed objects spontaneously pass through the GI tract: these include coins less than 2 cm in diameter [e.g., dimes (17 mm) or pennies (18 mm)] or an elongated object less than 2 cm in width or 5 cm in length (3 cm for infants) (52,53). If such as object is retained in the stomach for more than 4 weeks or the patient becomes symptomatic, an endoscopic removal should be performed. The most commonly used retrieval device for coins is the "rat-tooth jaws" forceps. A more aggressive approach is necessary if a child has swallowed a disk battery, which may induce low-voltage burns and tissue damage due to the corrosive action of the leaking concentrated alkaline solution. If a battery remains in the stomach after 48 hr, it should be removed endoscopically. In the past, grasping devices were not available to secure a smooth foreign body without a risk of losing it in the stomach, esophagus, or pharynx. Currently, a disposable 2.5-mm retrieval net (U.S. Endoscopy Group Inc., Mentor, Ohio) can be used.

A foreign body retained in the esophagus is a medical emergency. Clinical manifestations vary from no symptoms to, in infants and children, irritability, respiratory distress, chest-pain, drooling, wheezing or gagging. Anteroposterior

(AP) and lateral chest films are very useful to distinguish esophageal from tracheal localization and to estimate the size and nature of the object. An esophageal foreign body usually lodges in the crycopharyngeal sphincter or the distal esophagus (in case of preexistent strictures). In the latter case, a piece of meat or other solid food is the most common source of obstruction. Different endoscopic techniques and devices have been elaborated to remove certain types of foreign bodies. Any V-shaped object in the esophagus, such as an open safety pin with the sharp edge pointing cephalad (Fig. 11), must be gently brought into the stomach, reversed, and removed in a retrograde fashion.

All sharp foreign bodies—such as pins, toothpicks, and chicken bones—should be removed endoscopically from the stomach or duodenum immediately because of the high risk of intestinal perforation, usually in the area of the ileocecal valve. A latex protector hood (Medical Innovations Corporation, Draper, Utah) minimizes the risk of mucosal trauma.

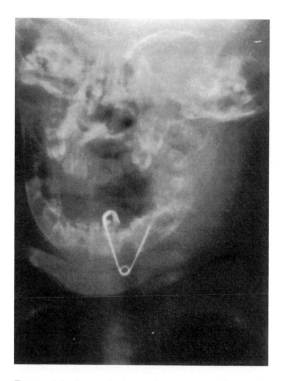

FIGURE 11 Lateral view of an open safety pin in the cervical esophagus of an 8-month-old infant. The foreign body was removed endoscopically under general anesthesia.

The key to a successful procedure is adequate anesthesia and appropriate instrumentation. Careful endoscopic examination immediately after removal of a foreign body must be performed to exclude any esophageal or pharyngeal trauma. If these areas appear normal and the patient is asymptomatic, same-day discharge is reasonable. If an initial roentgenogram revealed a sharp foreign body in the small intestine, careful observation and daily radiographs are necessary. Symptoms of nausea, vomiting, abdominal pain, or fever suggest a complication. If the sharp object fails to progress for 3 consecutive days, surgery should be considered.

1.18 Celiac Sprue

Partial or total atrophy of the small bowel mucosa may be the endpoint of different pathological processes, including celiac sprue, giardiasis, cow's-milk allergy, postinfectious inflammation, and immunodeficiency (see Chaps. 16, 21, and 25). It is not uncommon for the clinical symptoms of these conditions to overlap. Moreover, even celiac sprue has a variety of presentations, including monosymptomatic ones such as anemia, short stature, constipation, etc. (54,55).

For more than three decades, jejunal capsule biopsy was the cornerstone for the diagnosis of celiac sprue. But it is time-consuming, requires fluoroscopy, and has a certain failure rate. Recently, it has gradually been replaced in adults and children by endoscopic biopsy (56–58). Moreover, EGD may provide additional information about concomitant lesions in the upper GI tract or accidentally discover mucosal changes suggestive of celiac sprue in children with equivocal clinical scenarios. The major endoscopic finding of celiac sprue in children is notched duodenal folds or ''scalloping'' of the valvulae conniventes (Fig. 12). In the active phase of celiac disease, the duodenal mucosa appears grayish, edematous, and mosaic, with an increased vascular pattern in the proximal duodenum. Duodenal folds are coarse, with a scalloped appearance more prominent on their edges. Mucosa between the duodenal folds has a cobblestone or honeycomb pattern. These endoscopic signs are usually more prominent in the distal duodenum or proximal jejunum. Although duodenal or jejunal mucosa in celiac sprue patients is not friable, it bleeds more intensively after the biopsy than in nonspecific duodenitis, albeit not to the degree of a significant hemorrhage. The endoscopic signs of celiac sprue are not highly specific. At least four biopsies from the distal portion of duodenum are required. All specimens must be properly oriented for correct assessment of villous architecture. In patients on a strict gluten-free diet, a full normalization of small bowel mucosa is the general rule. In noncompliant children, especially adolescents, a flat mucosa may be clinically silent.

1.19 Intestinal Lymphangiectasia

It is not uncommon to find scattered whitish spots in the second or third portion of the duodenum during routine upper-GI endoscopy in children. These lesions

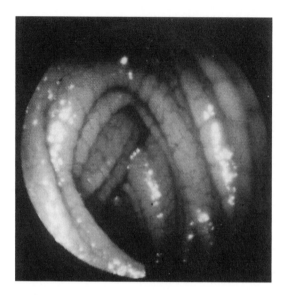

FIGURE 12 Scalloping of the valvulae conniventes in a patient with celiac sprue.

represent dilated lacteals extending up into the small bowel villi. They may or may not be clinically relevant. Since the original description of these lesions as a sign of intestinal lymphangiectasia (59), it has been established that the same endoscopic and histological picture might represent functional lymphangiectasia or even the early stage of fat absorption (60,61). Thus, an endoscopic finding of white, scattered spots in the distal duodenum or proximal jejunum that are not flushed out, white villi, or chylous material covering the mucosa should be correlated to the clinical picture to establish their clinical significance.

In intestinal lymphangiectasia, the majority of patients suffer from chronic diarrhea, edema, lymphocytopenia, and abnormal fecal fat excretion. Additional signs such as failure to thrive, susceptibility to infection due to intestinal losses of immunoglobulins and intestinal sequestration of lymphocytes, chylous effusion (both pleural and/or peritoneal), abdominal swelling, and hypocalcemia have been described (62,63). Although endoscopic and histological findings are present in most patients, in some cases they could be absent at initial endoscopy and biopsy. If primary or secondary intestinal lymphangiectasia is suspected clinically but EGD with small bowel biopsy is normal or equivocal, a repeat EGD with multiple target biopsies after a fat-loading meal has been found to be very effective in confirming the diagnosis (64). The other reason to perform multiple biopsies is to avoid false-negative results due to possible patchy distribution of the disease in the duodenum or jejunum.

2 ENDOSCOPIC RETROGRADE CHOLANGIOPANCREATOGRAPHY (ERCP)

Since the first report of successful ERCP in three children in 1976 (65), dozens of these procedures have been performed (66–69). It was clearly shown that it is technically feasible to perform cannulation and filling of the pancreatic and biliary ducts with more than 90% success even in neonates. Of course, the aspect of sedation or general anesthesia, the right choice of endoscopes, and technique of cannulation are very important, but even more important is a reasonable approach to the indications for this invasive and expensive procedure. There are four major categories of indications for ERCP:

1. Neonatal cholestasis of unclear etiology to rule out biliary atresia to avoid unnecessary surgery
2. Known causes of cholestasis that require verification of ductal anatomy or therapeutic procedures, such as sphincterotomy or placement of a stent
3. Recurrent pancreatitis
4. Recurrent abdominal pain similar to biliary-type colic with abnormal liver function tests, which could not be explained by findings obtained from ultrasound, HIDA scans, or abdominal computed tomography (CT)

The role of ERCP in the diagnosis of biliary atresia is controversial. Clinical judgment combined with the results of laboratory tests, ultrasound, HIDA scan, and a liver biopsy are not 100% definitive and leave behind about 5 to 10% of infants in whom the correct diagnosis may be established by exploratory laparotomy and a surgical cholangiogram. The major input of ERCP in such cases is to avoid unnecessary surgery that may accelerate a deterioration of an already compromised liver function and create additional difficulties for liver transplantation in the future. The reasonable counterargument is possible false-positive results of ERCP in neonates and infants due to technical failure of cannulation of the common bile duct. This question was addressed in two large series of ERCP in neonatal cholestasis: there was only one false-positive diagnosis of biliary atresia (3%) (67,68)

The diagnosis of abnormal anatomical connections between the distal common bile duct and pancreatic duct is another area where ERCP is very useful. In the majority of children with a choledochal cyst, there is a joint area of the common bile duct and pancreatic duct, longer than 15 mm, that is referred to as a common channel (Fig. 13).

Pancreas divisum is a relatively common anomaly of fusion of the dorsal and ventral portions of the pancreas. It may be the cause of pancreatitis in case of stenosis of a minor pancreatic duct. Successful treatment of pancreas divisum in children with recurrent pancreatitis by endoscopic sphincterotomy of a minor duodenal papilla and a stent procedure has been reported (69,70).

ERCP is also useful for the diagnosis of chronic pancreatitis in children. Irregularities of the main pancreatic duct with areas of dilatation and narrowing are diagnostic.

ERCP is the procedure of choice in children with suspected primary sclerosing cholangitis (Fig. 14) or choledocholithiasis with dilatation of the common bile duct and cholestasis. Conversely, the yield of ERCP is very low in patients with idiopathic biliary colic.

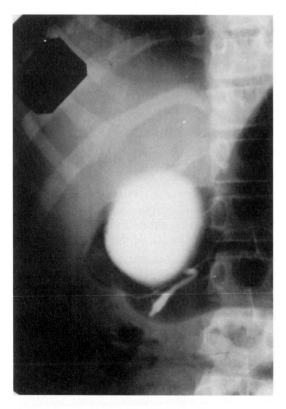

FIGURE 13 Choledochal cyst with a long common channel.

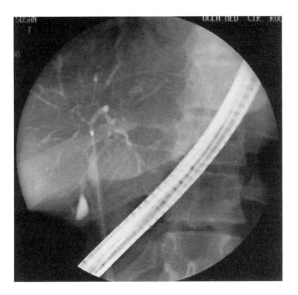

FIGURE 14   Endoscopic retrograde cholangiopancreatography demonstrating multiple strictures of the intrahepatic ducts in a patient with primary sclerosing cholangitis.

3   COLONOSCOPY

Flexible colonoscopy is a diagnostic technique that was developed for direct inspection of the rectosigmoid and colonic mucosa as well as for histological confirmation of mucosal abnormalities as well as for therapeutic procedures to treat lower gastrointestinal bleeding due to polyps or arteriovenous malformations (71,72). Pediatric and adult patients may have similar symptoms indicating the need for a colonoscopy: diarrhea, hematochezia, change in stool caliber, rectal pain, and/or lower abdominal pain. They differ in that adult patients far more commonly undergo a colonoscopy to look for malignancy, polyps, arteriovenous malformations, and diverticula.

3.1   Indications for Colonoscopy

There are eight indications for diagnostic colonoscopy; these are listed in Table 3. In addition, colonoscopy and biopsy are indicated for surveillance for detection of malignancy in patients with long-standing inflammatory bowel disease, those who have undergone ureterosigmoidostomy, and patients with polyposis syndromes.

Tᴀʙʟᴇ 3   Indications for Colonoscopy

Lower gastrointestinal bleeding
  Hematochezia
  Melena
  Fecal occult blood
Inflammatory bowel disease
  Diagnosis
  Management
      Extent and severity
      Unclear response to treatment
      Surveillance for colorectal cancer
Unexplained chronic diarrhea
Evaluation of anatomic abnormalities seen on barium
      enema
Family history of a familial polyposis syndrome
Cancer surveillance
  Ulcerative colitis
  Polyposis syndrome
  Adenomatous or mixed polyp
Intraoperatively
  Detection of lesions that cannot be detected on palpa-
      tion and/or inspection
Therapeutic colonoscopy
  Polypectomy
  Treatment of bleeding, angiodysplasia
  Removal of foreign body
  Decompression of toxic megacolon or colonic vol-
      vulus
  Dilation with balloon of stenotic lesions

Patients who have undergone small intestinal transplantation may need to undergo ileoscopy and/or colonoscopy to obtain specimens from transplanted bowel, looking for rejection and evidence of lymphoproliferative disease.

3.2   When Diagnostic Colonoscopy Is Not Indicated

Colonoscopy is not indicated in patients with:

1. Acute self-limited diarrhea
2. Gl bleeding with a demonstrated upper-Gl source
3. Stable recognized irritable bowel syndrome
4. Chronic nonspecific abdominal pain

5. Constipation with or without fecal impaction
6. Inflammatory bowel disease that is responding to treatment

Diagnostic colonoscopy is absolutely contraindicated in anyone with fulminant colitis or toxic megacolon, suspected perforated viscus, or recent intestinal resection (Table 4). However, patients with acute severe colitis in whom cultures are negative for bacterial pathogens and parasites, such as *Entamoeba histolytica* and *Trichuris trichiura*, should have an examination of the rectum and distal sigmoid colon to help establish whether they have a specific type of colitis. In such cases, limiting the area viewed as indicated does not pose an undue risk. There are times when direct visualization of the mucosa gives a specific diagnosis, as when pseudomembranes are seen.

Physicians should not consider colonoscopy in patients who have chronic or recurrent abdominal pain without other signs and symptoms such as weight loss, failure to grow, loss of appetite, perianal disease, and positive indicators for inflammatory bowel disease, such as an elevated sedimentation rate, increased C-reactive protein, and positive screening panel for inflammatory bowel disease.

3.3 Preparation of the Patient for Colonoscopy

A successful colonoscopy requires a series of factors, as listed in Table 5. Preparing infants and children for colonoscopy can be difficult. Young children may be satisfied with an explanation such as ''You are going to have a test to look at where your 'poop' comes from, and it has to be clean inside to take a good look.'' In school-age children and adolescents, more complete explanations may be provided depending on the child's level of sophistication. It is useful to show

TABLE 4 Contraindications to Colonoscopy

Contraindications to colonoscopy
  Peritonitis
  Bowel perforation
Possible contraindications to colonoscopy
  Acute severe colitis
  Intestinal obstruction
  Recent surgical anastomoses
Inability to visualize mucosa
  Poor bowel preparation
  Acute massive gastrointestinal bleeding
Associated abnormalities or medical problems
  Coagulopathy (no biopsies)
  Severe underlying medical problems

TABLE 5 Fifteen Steps to Ensure Complete and Successful Colonoscopy

1. Good bowel preparation to allow for optimal visualization.
2. Superior sedation and patient monitoring (responds to calling name but resumes sleeping when not aroused).
3. Continuous patient monitoring with pulse oximeter.
4. Vital signs, BP every 5 min.
5. Respirations every 5 min.
6. Cardiac rate every 5 min.
7. Check videocolonoscope for function before starting procedure.
8. Proceed gently.
9. Keep the colonoscope as straight as possible; try to keep lumen in view.
10. Inflate with as little air as possible.
11. Suction with lumen in view to aid in telescoping of colonoscope.
12. Pull back and move forward to telescope bowel into instrument.
13. Use passage of mucosa over tip with visualization of vascular pattern as best clue that tip is passing along mucosal wall.
14. Palpate for loops; have nursing assistant check for them; reduce them when they develop.
15. Look for anatomic landmarks, bluish discoloration of splenic flexure, bluish coloration of hepatic flexure, Crow's foot in cecum and appendix.

the children and parents diagrams of the rectum and colon and the distal small bowel to make them aware of what is going to be examined, and providing such knowledge ahead of time may make the child or adolescent more amenable to the procedure and more cooperative in preparing for the examination. Children should be shown pictures of the instruments used and a simple diagram of what may be normally seen.

The most difficult thing to do is to prepare the bowel so that it can be adequately visualized. A number of different regimens based either on washout of the bowel (lavage) or cathartics are available. Both methods are subject to failure because they rely upon the cooperation of the child; thus the best efforts to get the colon adequately cleaned out may be fruitless. In the case of infants, the best technique is usually one involving clear liquids and milk of magnesia. Milk of magnesia should be given two nights before the procedure and at midday the day before the procedure in a dose of 1.0 mL/kg of body weight. Magnesium citrate may also be used in children above 1 year of age. This may be divided into two doses and given 24 hr and 12 hr before the colonoscopy. It is best given cold and over ice or mixed with lemon- or lime-type soft drinks. Some individuals become nauseated by this and other cathartics. It is often best to give the dose of magnesium citrate in four fractions over a 4-hr period. The night before the colonoscopy, a glycerin suppository should be administered to enhance evacuation of the colon. This technique is probably the most benign of the methods available and less likely to meet resistance. In the lavage method, the patient is allowed to eat and drink until the afternoon before the procedure. The patient is then asked to fast for 4 hr. A lavage solution contains osmotically active substances such as polyethylene glycol or mannitol. Currently, mannitol is rarely used because it can be utilized by colonic bacteria and produce flammable gas, which increases the risk of complication during electrocoagulation or endoscopic polypectomy. The solutions are available flavored. The patient is given 5 to 10 mL/kg up to 250 mL by mouth every 10 min until the rectal effluent is clear. Some adolescents will take this solution readily. In the younger child, success is less assured. In uncooperative patients, hospitalization 24 to 48 hr prior to the procedure may be necessary to cleanse the colon. A nasogastric tube is placed and the solution is administered through it. The patient can be given metoclopramide 0.1 mg/kg to a maximum of 10 mg 20 min before the lavage is begun to enhance or speed up gastric emptying. Some patients may develop vomiting in response to the lavage. In these instances, the rate of infusion may have to be curtailed. We have found that by infusing the solution continuously over a period of 12 hr, we may be able to overcome the problem of vomiting. If one uses the lavage technique, there should be some concern if stool is not passed within the first 4 hr, in which case the infusion should be stopped. The rate of infusion is usually in the order of 100 to 200 mL/hr up to a full volume of 4L. Simultaneously, we often administer an intravenous solution to provide maintenance fluids and electrolytes. Enemas are not useful if the purpose of the colonoscopy is to look for evidence of inflammatory bowel disease in the rectum and sigmoid colon, as enemas usually cause erythema of the colonic mucosa and petechiae, giving a false-positive macroscopic image. Normal rectal mucosa is shown in Figure 15.

For recommendations on sedation and antibiotic prophylaxis for patients with heart disease, see Section 1, above.

3.4 Equipment

Virtually all fiberoptic colonoscopies today are done with videocolonoscopes. With these, the image is captured by a computer chip at the end of the instrument and transported to a video screen. Videocolonoscopes are available in sizes that range from 11.3 to 13.7 mm in diameter and 130 cm in length. The working channel through which accessories can be passed (i.e., biopsy and retrieving forceps, snares and baskets) can range from 2.8 to 4.2 mm. The fields of view and angulation capabilities are similar for most colonoscopes. The larger channel allows for better accessories to be used. The size and the character of the endo-

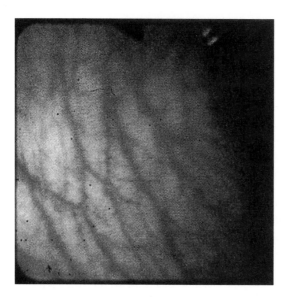

FIGURE 15 Normal rectal mucosa.

scopes are selected to be appropriate for the age and size of the patient. For infants and toddlers, pediatric upper-GI videoendoscopes with an external diameter of 9.7 mm are used. Endoscopes used to examine the upper GI tract in infants and toddlers are less stiff and have a smaller suction channel than colonoscopes which makes them more technically difficult to use. However, their greater flexibility may be an advantage. Adult-size colonoscopes may be used effectively in most school-age children.

3.5 Technique for Colonoscopy

The purpose of deep, continuous sedation is to provide the patient with maximal comfort and amnesia while allowing him or her to communicate with the physician. Colonoscopy should be nearly painless. When pain or discomfort is voiced or observed, a change in the technique or position can usually relieve symptoms and is a sign that tension on the colonic wall has been relieved. This interaction between the patient and physician is lost if the patient is under general anesthesia. If a patient is under general anesthesia, significant tension may be placed on the bowel, which increases the risk of colonic perforation. When the patient indicates discomfort, it is a sign for the endoscopist to either withdraw the instrument or decompress the bowel. After adequate sedation is achieved, the patient is placed on his or her left side. The endoscopist advances the colonoscope as quickly but as gently as possible to the cecum or to the area where the suspected pathology appears.

The principal points in performing an effective colonoscopy are to minimize pain and discomfort. It is critical to try to keep the lumen of the bowel in sight, knowing where the tip of the colonoscope is and trying to keep the colonoscope straight, with avoidance of loops. Transillumination of the bowel with the tip of the endoscope through the abdominal wall helps determine its localization. If the tip of the scope is in the left lower quadrant and most of the endoscope is within the colon, you should suspect that a loop has been created. Certain areas of the colon are characteristic and allow the endoscopist to identify the location of the instrument. Such is the case of the triangular folds of the transverse colon (Fig. 16). Increased tension on the sigmoid colon with the presence of a large loop can result in sufficient discomfort to the patient to make the procedure impossible to complete. If a loop develops within the sigmoid or other segments of the colon, the endoscope can be flexed to hook a catch around a fold so as to anchor the tip while the insertion tube is drawn back in a clockwise loop. This can straighten the sigmoid loop. Another common technique that we use to advance the scope is to telescope the bowel on the endoscope by advancing and withdrawing it repetitively. Suction of air and fluid from the colon can also be used to advance the tip of the scope. This is probably one the most useful techniques. Positioning the patient to be prone or on the right side may also help

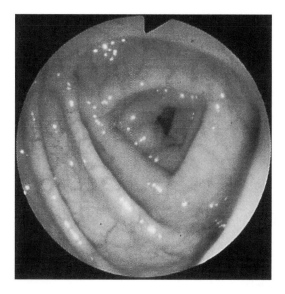

FIGURE 16 Transverse colon: note the triangular appearance of the folds.

to maneuver the instruments through a difficult colon. Gentle but continuous pressure on the abdomen at the apex or the top of the loop while the insertion tube is withdrawn can help to straighten a loop and advance the tip of the instrument. Intubation of the terminal ileum is perhaps not achieved in 20% of cases. This is because the ileocecal valve is tucked behind a fold and special techniques must be used to enter the terminal ileum. These techniques include suctioning air and fluid to partially collapse the cecum and open the valve, placing the patient in a prone position to bring the ileocecal valve into view of the endoscope, and retroflexing the tip and withdrawing the colonoscope a few centimeters to better visualize and approach the terminal ileum (Fig. 17). The colonoscope must be as straight as possible, without loops, to enter the terminal ileum. The mucosal pattern of the colon is best evaluated as the instrument is slowly withdrawn. However, we think it is important to carefully look at the mucosa as one is advancing forward, since trauma can sometimes occur with the passage of the instrument. If abnormalities are not identified beforehand, one is always left wondering whether what one sees is due to colonoscopy or to the underlying pathology.

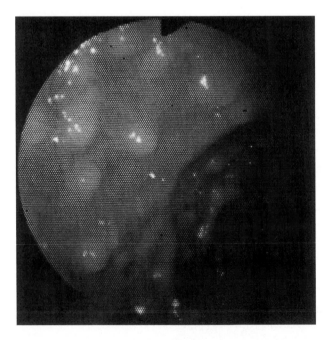

FIGURE 17 Normal terminal ileum.

3.6 Risk and Complications of Colonoscopy

The potential risk and complications of colonoscopy include bleeding, perforation, infection, and difficulties with sedation (such as paradoxical reaction to the agent used) (Table 6). A higher dose of analgesic medication may be required for colonoscopy versus upper intestinal endoscopy because procedures involving the colon may produce more intensive pain and or require a longer procedure time. One must be very vigilant when endoscoping children because there may be a small margin between inadequate sedation and oversedation.

Bowel perforation and hemorrhage are serious but rare complications of colonoscopy. During diagnostic colonoscopy, the estimated frequency of colonic perforation is in the range of 0.2 to 0.8%. This is an extremely low risk of perforation. The frequency is higher with therapeutic colonoscopy procedures such as polypectomy but still comparatively rare, ranging from 0.5 to 3%. Mortality is extremely low and should be substantially less than 0.2%. Although perforations commonly occur in the rectosigmoid area, they can occur anywhere along the colon. The reasons they occur most frequently in this region is because of the semifixed position of the rectosigmoid and because inexperienced colonoscopists often try to push ahead when they cannot clearly see where the lumen is going. Damage to the colonic mucosa can occur from mechanical forces, by forceful insertion of the colonoscope, and laceration and tears with the biopsy forceps.

Therapeutic procedures such as polypectomy, electrocoagulation, and dilatation of a rectal or colonic stricture may also have complications. Significant hemorrhage following colonoscopy is extremely rare. Colonic perforations in most instances involve exploration or conservative management, which means stopping all feedings and prescribing intravenous antibiotics for 7 to 14 days.

Bacteremia in colonoscopy with or without biopsy is said to occur in up to 4% of patients. Despite these recommendations, antibiotic prophylaxis is often

TABLE 6 Common Complications of Colonoscopy

Sedation-related
Oversedation—hypotension, apnea and bradycardia, transient hypoxemia
Paradoxical reaction to agents
Procedure-related
Hemorrhage
Perforation
  Complete
  Incomplete
Fever and bacteremia
Abdominal distention (excessive use of air insufflation)

used inappropriately. Pathogens transmitted to the patient by contaminated endo-scopes consist mainly of bowel-type flora—i.e., gram-negative flora as well as Staphylococci and streptococci. The transmission of infection to the colonoscopes is due to poor or inadequate cleaning techniques and inability to adequately de-contaminate the endoscope because of its complex design (73).

3.7 Specific Indications

3.7.1 Rectal Bleeding

Not every child with hematochezia requires colonoscopy. Careful history and physical examination may identify diagnoses such as recent exposure to antibiot-ics to suggest antibiotic-associated colitis, perianal streptococcal cellulitis, or an anal fissure. Stool studies on a patient who has rectal bleeding should include a smear for polymorphonuclear leukocytes. Bacterial culture (for *Shigella*, *Salmo-nella*, *Campylobacter*, *Escherichia coli*, and *Yersinia enterocolitica*) should be done if leukocytes are present. If antibiotics have been taken in the previous 3 months, *Clostridium difficile* toxin titers (A and B) should be obtained. Stools should be examined for *E. histolytica* and *T. trichiura*. Stools should also be tested for the presence of eosinophils and Charcot-Leyden crystals, since their presence indicates allergic colitis.

In the pediatric patient with persistent or recurrent hematochezia and no identifiable cause, colonoscopy or flexible sigmoidoscopy is the procedure of choice to search for mucosal changes or other lesions associated with bleeding. Several causes of bleeding are shown in Figures 18 to 25. Ulcerative colitis is characterized endoscopically by obscuration of submucosal blood vessels, spon-taneous or induced mucosal friability, and microulceration. Ulcerative colitis may and typically does begin in the rectum and spreads proximally. It may be mild or intense and involve all or part of the rectum and colon. Colitis of Crohn's disease may be patchy, mild or intense, and may involve all or just a part of the colon. Fifty percent of patients with Crohn's colitis have rectal sparing, while in ulcerative colitis the inflammation tends to be contiguous. Patients who have gross ulcerations at colonoscopy are much more likely to have Crohn's disease (Figs. 19 and 26) than ulcerative colitis (Fig. 20). The ulcerations typically have serpiginous borders. Aphtha-like lesions may occur in isolated patches in Crohn's disease. Twenty five percent of patients who at colonoscopy have evidence of colitis will have changes that cannot be classified microscopically (74). The im-portance of the colonoscopy in patients with inflammatory bowel disease is to define the extent of the inflammation, obtain sample tissues to look at microscopi-cally to establish the specific diagnosis, and as an aid in planning therapy.

Clostridium difficile may produce a characteristic pseudomembrane; how-ever, this is not pathognomic for this bacterium and may also be seen in shigello-sis. Allergic colitis, which is more typically seen in young infants, may be nonspe-

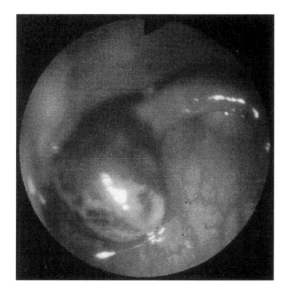

FIGURE 18 Juvenile rectal polyp with a long stalk.

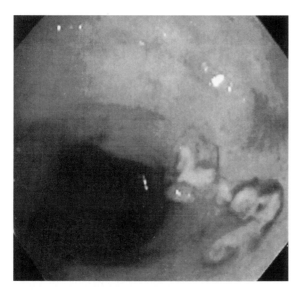

FIGURE 19 Crohn's disease: note multiple longitudinal ulcers and focal inflammation in the colonic mucosa.

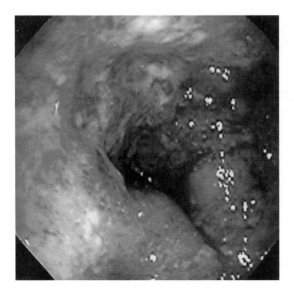

FIGURE 20   Severe ulcerative colitis.

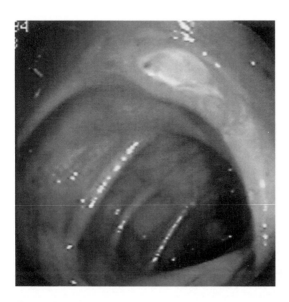

FIGURE 21   Colonic ulcer in a 15-year-old patient with posttransplant lymphoproliferative disease.

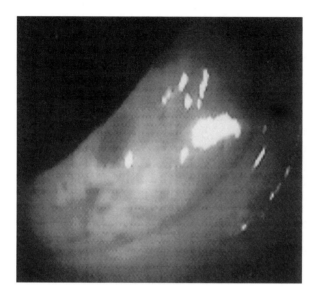

FIGURE 22   Multiple arteriovenous malformations.

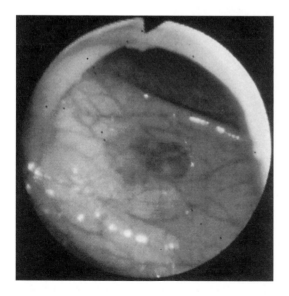

FIGURE 23   Flat hemangioma of the colon.

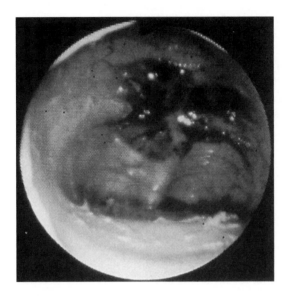

FIGURE 24 Excavated hemangioma of the colon.

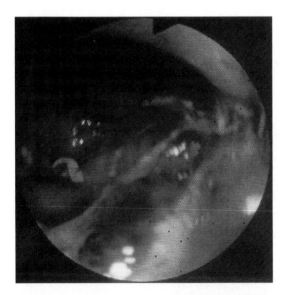

FIGURE 25 Prominent edema and hemorrhages at the sigmoid colon in a 4-year-old boy with Henoch-Schkonlein purpura.

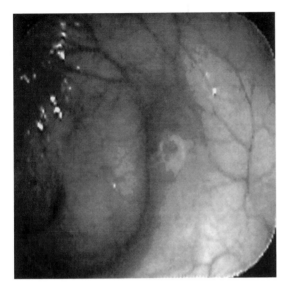

FIGURE 26   Aphthoid colonic ulcer in a patient with Crohn's disease.

cific. Polyps, foreign bodies, and internal trauma from sexual abuse may all be identified at colonoscopy. Also, rare lesions such as arteriovenous (AV) malformations (Figs. 22 and 23) or rectal varices may also be visualized. Abuse of cathartics may also be recognized by the typical tigroid stripes seen in the mucosa.

3.7.2   Chronic Diarrhea

Chronic nonbloody diarrhea is an uncommon indication for colonoscopy; however, if it has been chronic in nature and the stool cultures and ova/parasites have been nondiagnostic, we recommend it (see Chap. 28). Approximately 5% of patients who have colitis will not have polymorphonuclear leukocytes present in their stool. Microscopic colitis has been described in children presenting with chronic diarrhea, abdominal pain, loss of appetite, and weight loss.

3.7.3   Cancer Surveillance

Adenocarcinoma of the Colon in Ulcerative Colitis.   Development of adenocarcinoma of the colon in children is extremely rare but does occur even in those who never had ulcerative colitis (75). It typically presents with intermittent rectal bleeding and no diarrhea or with a progressive change in stool caliber. This is why children with either persistent or recurrent painless rectal bleeding should undergo a colonoscopy.

The determining factor in who develops cancer in ulcerative colitis seems to be the severity of the original attack as well as the extent of mucosal involvement. The cancer risk for patients with universal colitis involving the entire colon is 3% in the first decade of disease and 1 to 2% per year after this. Patients with universal colitis should begin biyearly colonoscopy 8 years after onset of disease. However, it is a substantially lower risk. The risk is greatest in those with strictures similar to those patients with ulcerative colitis.

Familial Polyposis.   Children of patients with inherited polyposis syndromes should have a surveillance colonoscopy to identify the presence of polyps; this is recommended to begin at 11 years of age (Fig. 27). Once the patient is recognized to have inherited the condition, a decision must be made with regard to when to perform a colectomy and ileal anal pull-through. The dilemma in some of these patients is that these polyps may develop in the stomach and small intestine.

3.7.4   Therapeutic Colonoscopy

Polypectomy.   Nodular lymphoid hyperplasia of the colon, typically seen in early infancy, is characterized by umbilicated lesions in the rectum, sigmoid,

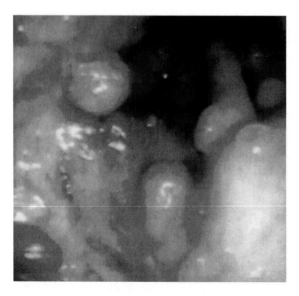

FIGURE 27 Multiple tubular adenomas of the colon in a 6-year-old boy with Gardner's syndrome.

and/or colon. These require no intervention. Juvenile or inflammatory polyps are most common in the 4- to 6-year-old age group, but they may be present as early as age 1 (Fig. 18). They are uncommon after age 18. Although autoamputation may occur in these cases, many such polyps will not disappear spontaneously (Fig. 28). This is the reason why, when patients present with rectal bleeding and polyps are suspected, we endoscope the colon and snare the polyp.

Hereditary polyposis syndromes are often confirmed by colonoscopy and polypectomy. The purpose of the colonoscopy in these patients is to snare the polyp by passing a snare wire over the polyp and tightening the loop around the base like a lasso. Electrocautery current is passed through the wire snare to desiccate the stalk and coagulate the blood vessels feeding the polyp. The wire loop is then closed around the stalk, mechanically cutting the cauterized tissue. The polyp is then usually retrieved with a snare forceps.

Stricturectomy. Strictures of transmural lesions of the colon can result from Crohn's disease and from necrotizing enterocolitis. The traditional method of treating this has been surgical exploration, resection, and stricturoplasty. Recently, balloon dilators passed through the colonoscope have been used to dilate lesions without surgery.

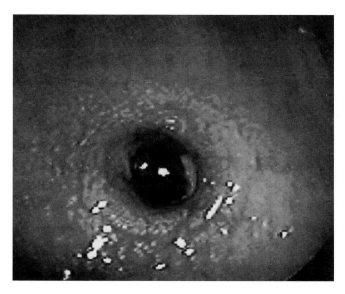

FIGURE 28   Colonic ulcer covered by a thrombus due to a recent spontaneous amputation of a juvenile polyp.

Vascular Lesions. Special instruments are needed to treat vascular lesions such as an AV malformations and hemorrhoids. Electrocoagulation with a heater probe has been useful in treating AV malformations in the colon that bleed.

REFERENCES

1. Freeman NV. Pediatric gastroscopy. Lancet 1971; 1(7713):1351.
2. Cotton PB, Rosenberg MT, Waldram RPL, Axon ATR. Early endoscopy of esophagus, stomach, and duodenal bulb in patients with haematemesis and melena. BMJ 1973; 2:505–509.
3. Cremer M, Peeters JP, Emonts P, Rodesch P, Cadranel S. Fiberendoscopy of the gastrointestinal tract in children—experience with newly designed fiberscopes. Endoscopy 1974; 6:186–189.
4. Mougenot JF, Montagne JP, Faure C. Gastrointestinal fibro-endoscopy in infants and children: Radio-fibroscopic correlations. Ann Radiol 1976; 19(1):23–34.
5. Ament ME, Christie DL. Upper gastrointestinal fiberoptic endoscopy in pediatric patients. Gastroenterology 1977; 72:1244–1248.
6. Candranel S, Rodesh P, Peeters JP, Cremer M. Fiberendoscopy of the gastrointestinal tract in children. Am J Dis Child 1977; 131:41–45.
7. Graham DY, Klish WJ, Ferry GD, Sabel JS. Value of fiberoptic gastrointestinal endoscopy in infants and children. South Med J 1978; 71(5):558–560.
8. Liebman WM. Fiberoptic endoscopy of gastrointestinal tract in infants and children. Am J Gastroenterol 1977; 68:362–366.
9. Ament ME, Brill JE. Pediatric endoscopy, deep sedation, conscious sedation, and general anesthesia—what is best? Gastrointest Endosc 1995; 41(2):173–175.
10. Balsells FB, Wyllie R, Kay M, Steffen R. Use of conscious sedation for low and upper gastrointestinal endoscopic examinations in children, adolescents and young adults: A twelve year review. Gastointest Endosc 1997; 45:375–380.
11. Tolia V, Peters JM, Gilger MA. Sedation for pediatric endoscopic procedures. J Pediatr Gastroenterol Nutr 2000; 30:477–485.
12. Schneider AJL. Assessment of risk factors and surgical outcome. Surg Clin North Am 1983; 63:1113–1116.
13. Zeltzer LK, Jay S M, Fisher DM. The management of pain associated with pediatric procedures. Pediatr Clin North Am 1989; 36:941–964.
14. Poets CF, Southall DP. Noninvasive monitoring of oxygenation in infants and children: practical considerations and areas of concern. Pediatrics 1994; 93(5):737–746.
15. Genta RM, Graham DY. Comparison of biopsy sites for the histological diagnosis of Helicobacter pylori: a topographic study of *H. pylori* density and distribution. Gastrointest Endosc 1994; 40(3):342–345.
16. Gillberg R, Ahren C. Coeliac disease diagnosed by means of duodenoscopy and endoscopic duodenal biopsy. Scand J Gastroenterol 1977; 12:911–916.
17. Barakat MH, Ali SM, Badawi AR, Khuffash FA, Fernando N, Majeed HA, Tungaker MF. Peroral endoscopic duodenal biopsy in infants and children. Acta Paediatr Scand 1983; 72:563–569.

18. Oderda G, Ansaldi N. Comparison of suction capsule and endoscopic biopsy of small bowel mucosa. Gastrointest Endosc 1987; 33(3):265–266.

19. Wyllie R, Hyams JS. Pediatric Gastrointestinal Disease. Philadelphia: Saunders, 1999, pp 3–4.

20. Boyle JT. Gastroesophageal reflux in the pediatric patients. Gastroenterol Clin North Am 1989; 18:315–337.

21. Hassall E, Dimmick JE, Magee JF. Adenocarcinoma in childhood Barrett's esophagus: case documentation and need for surveillance in children. Am J Gastroenterol 1993; 88:282–288.

22. Hassall E, Berquist WE, Ament ME, Vargas J, Dorney S. Sclerotherapy for extrahepatic portal hypertension in childhood. J Pediatr 1989; 115(1):69–74.

23. Paquet KJ, Lazar A. Current therapeutic strategy in bleeding esophageal varices in babies and children and long-term results of endoscopic paravariceal sclerotherapy over twenty years. Eur J Pediatr Surg 1994; 4:165–172.

24. Howard ER, Stringer MD, Mowat AP. Assessment of injection sclerotherapy in management of 152 children with oesophageal varices. Br J Surg 1988; 75:404–408.

25. Stringer MD, Howard ER. Long-term outcome after injection sclerotherapy for esophageal varices in children with extrahepatic portal hypertension. Gut 1994; 35: 257–259.

26. Stiegmann GV, Goff JS. Endoscopic esophageal varix ligation: preliminary clinical experience. Gastrointest Endosc 1988, 34(2):113–117.

27. Stiegmann GV, Goff JS, Sun JH, Wilborn S. Endoscopic elastic band ligation for active variceal hemorrhage. Am Surg 1989; 55(2):124–128.

28. Saeed ZA, Michaletz PA, Winchester CB, Woods KL, Dixon WB, Hieser MC, Gentry KR, Ramirez FC. Endoscopic variceal ligation in patients who have failed endoscopic sclerotherapy. Gastrointest Endosc 1990; 36(6):572–574.

29. Laine L, Cook D. Endoscopic ligation compared with sclerotherapy for treatment of esophageal variceal bleeding: a meta-analysis. Ann Intern Med 1995, 123:280–287.

30. Baroncini D, Milaudri G, Borioni D, Piemontese A, Cennamo V, Billi P, Dal Monte PP, D'Imperio N. A prospective randomized trial of sclerotherapy versus ligation in the elective treatment of bleeding esophageal varices. Endoscopy 1997; 29:235–240.

31. Price MR, Sartorelli KH, Karrer FM, Karrer FM, Narkewicz MR, Sokol RJ, Lilly JR. Management of esophageal varices in children by endoscopic variceal ligation. J Pediatr Surg 1996; 31(8):1056–1059.

32. Prieto G, Polanco I, Larrauri J, Rota L, Lama R, Carrasco S. Helicobacter pylori infection in children: clinical, endoscopic and histological correlations. J Pediatr Gastroenterol Nutr 1993; 14(4):420–425.

33. Bujanover Y, Konikoff F, Baratz M. Nodular gastritis and Helicobacter pylori. J Pediatr Gastroenterol Nutr 1993; 16(2):120–124.

34. Hassall E, Dimmick J. Unique features of helicobacter pylori disease in children. Dig Dis Sci 1991; 36(4):417–423.

35. Leonidas JC, Beathy EC, Wenner MA. Menetrier's disease and cytomegalovirus infection in childhood. Am J Dis Child 1973; 126:806–808.

36. Coad NAG, Shah KJ. Menetrier's disease in childhood associated with cytomegalo-

virus infection: a case report and review of literature. Br J Radiol 1986; 59:615–620.

37. Kovacs AA, Churchill MA, Wood D, Mascola L, Zaia JA. Molecular and epidemiologic evaluations of cluster of cases of Menetrier's disease associated with cytomegalovirus. Pediatr Infect Dis J 1993; 12(12):1011–1014.

38. Lenaerts C, Roy CC, Vaillancourt M, Weber AM, Morin CL, Seidman E. High incidence of upper gastrointestinal tract involvement in children with Crohn's disease. Pediatrics 1989; 83(5):777–781.

39. Mashako MNL, Cezard JP, Navarro J, Mougenot JF, Sonsino E, Gargouri A, Maherzi A. Crohn's disease lesions in the upper gastrointestinal tract: correlation between clinical, radiological, endoscopic and histological features in adolescents and children. J Pediatr Gastroenterol Nutr 1989; 8:442–446.

40. Ruuska T, Vaajalahti P, Arajarvi P, Maki M. Prospective evaluation of upper gastrointestinal mucosal lesions in children with ulcerative colitis and Crohn's disease. J Pediatr Gastroenterol 1994; 19:181–186.

41. Griffiths AM, Alemayehu E, Sherman P. Clinical features of gastroduodenal Crohn's disease in adolescents. J Pediatr Gastroenterol Nutr 1989; 8:166–171.

42. Danzi JT, Farmer RG, Sullivan BH, Rankin GB. Endoscopic features of gastroduodenal Crohn's disease. Gastroenterology 1976; 70:9–13.

43. Nugent FW, Richmond M, Park SK. Crohn's disease of the duodenum. Gut 1977; 18:115–120.

44. Lucaya J, Ochoa J. B. Ectopic pancreas in the stomach. J Pediatr Surg 1976; 11:101–102.

45. Strobel CT, Smith LE, Fonkalsrud EW, Isenberg JN. Ectopic pancreas tissue in the gastric antrum. J Pediatr 1978; 92(4):586–588.

46. Buts JP, Gosseye S, Claus D, de Montpellier C, Nyakabasa M. Solitary hyperplastic polyp of the stomach. Am J Dis Child 1981; 135:846–847.

47. Sanna CM, Loriga P, Dessi E, Frau G, Congiu G, Corrias A, Corda R. Hyperplastic polyp of the stomach simulating hypertrophic pyloric stenosis. J Pediatr Gastroenterol Nutr 1991; 13:204–208.

48. Brooks GS, Frost ES, Wesselhoeft C. Prolapsed hyperplastic gastric polyp causing gastric outlet obstruction, hypergastrinemia, and hematemesis in an infant. J Pediatr Surg 1992; 27:1537–1538.

49. Harris GJ, Laszewski MJ. Pediatric primary gastric lymphoma. South Med J 1992; 85(4):432–434.

50. Mahour GH, Isaacs H, Chang L. Primary malignant tumors of the stomach in children. J Pediatr Surg 1980; 15(5):603–608.

51. Benes J, Chumel J, Jodl J. Stuka C, Nevoral J. Treatment of a gastric bezoar by extracorporeal shock wave lithotripsy. Endoscopy 1991; 23:346–348.

52. Byrne WJ. Foreign bodies, bezoars and caustic ingestion. Gastrointest Endosc Clin North Am 1994; 4(1):99–119.

53. Berggreen PJ, Harrison E, Sanowski RA, Ingebo K, Noland B, Zierer S. Techniques and complications of esophageal foreign body extraction in children and adults. Gastrointest Endosc 1993; 39(5):626–630.

54. Anderson CH. Malabsorption in childhood. Arch Dis Child 1966; 41:571–596.

55. Cacciari E, Salardi S, Gicognani A, Cicognani A, Collina A, Pirazzoli P, Tassoni

P, Biasco G, Corazza GR, Cassio A. Short stature and celiac disease: a relationship to consider even in patients with no gastrointestinal tract symptoms. J Pediatr 1983; 103:708–711.

56. Gillberg, Ahren C. Coeliac disease diagnosed by means of duodenoscopy and endoscopic biopsy. Scand J Gastroenterol 1977; 12:911–916.

57. Mee AS, Burke M, Vallow AG, Newman J, Cotton PB. Small bowel biopsy for malabsorption: comparison of the diagnostic accuracy of endoscopic forceps and capsule biopsy specimens. BMJ 1985; 291:769–772.

58. Barakat MH, Ali SM, Badawi AR, Khuffash FA, Fernando N, Majeed HA, Tungaker MF. Peroral endoscopic duodenal biopsy in infants and children. Acta Pediatr Scand 1983; 72:563–569.

59. Waldman TA, Steinfeld JL, Dutcher TF, Davidson JD, Gordon RS. The role of gastrointestinal system in ''idiopathic hypoproteinemia.'' Gastroenterology 1961; 41:197–207.

60. Femppel J, Lux G, Kaduk B, Roesh W. Functional lymphangiectasia of the duodenal mucosa. Endoscopy 1978; 10:44–46.

61. Patel AS, De Ridder PH. Endoscopic appearance and significance of functional lymphangiectasia of the duodenal mucosa. Gastrointest Endosc 1990; 36:376–378.

62. Vardy PA, Lebenthal E, Shwachman H. Intestinal lymphangiectasia: a reappraisal. Pediatrics 1975; 55(6):842–851.

63. Abramowsky C, Hupertz V, Kilbridge P, Czinn S. Intestinal lymphangiectasia in children: a study of upper gastrointestinal endoscopic biopsies. Pediatr Pathol 1989; 9:289–297.

64. Veldhuyzen van Zanten SJO, Bartelsman IFWM, Tytgat GNJ. Endoscopic diagnosis of primary intestinal lymphangiectasia using a high fat meal. Endoscopy 1986; 18:108–110.

65. Waye JD. Endoscopic retrograde cholangiopancreatography in infant. Am J Gastroenterol 1976; 65:461–463.

66. Urakami Y, Seki H, Kishi S. Endoscopic retrograde cholangiopancreatography (ERCP) performed in children. Endoscopy 1977; 9:86–91.

67. Wilkinson ML, Mieli-Vergani G, Ball C, Portman B, Mowat A. Endoscopic retrograde cholangiopancreatography in infantile cholestasis. Arch Dis Child 1991; 66(1):121–123.

68. Guelrud M, Jaen D, Mendoza S, Plaz J, Torres P. ERCP in the diagnosis of extrahepatic biliary atresia. Gastrointest Endosc 1991; 37(5):522–526.

69. Guelrud M, Mujica C, Jaen D, Plaz J, Arias J. The role of ERCP in the diagnosis and treatment of idiopathic recurrent pancreatitis in children and adolescents. Gastrointest Endosc 1994; 40(4):428–436.

70. Brown CW, Werlin SL, Geenen JE, Schmalz M. The diagnostic and therapeutic role of endoscopic retrograde cholangiopancreatography in children. J Pediatr Gastroenterol Nutr 1993; 17(1):19–23.

71. Hassall E, Barclay GN, Ament ME. Colonoscopy in childhood. Pediatrics 1984; 73:594–599.

72. Fox VL. Colonoscopy. In:Walker WA, Durie PR, Hamilton JR, et al. eds. Pediatric Gastrointestinal Disease, 2nd ed. St. Louis, Mosby, 1996, pp 1533–1541.

73. Spach DH, Silverman FE, Stamm WE. Transmission of infection by gastrointestinal endoscopy and bronchoscopy. Ann Intern Med 1993; 118:117–128.
74. Surawicz CM, Haggitt RC, Hussemann M, McFarland LV. Mucosal biopsy diagnosis of colitis: acute self limited colitis and idiopathic inflammatory bowel disease. Gastroenterology 1994; 107:755–763.
75. Nugent FW, Haggitt RC, Gilpin PA. Cancer surveillance in ulcerative colitis. Gastroenterology 1991; 110:1241–1248.

33

Surgical Operations of the Gastrointestinal Tract

Akira Okada

Osaka University Medical School, Suita, Osaka, Japan

Akio Kubota

Osaka Medical Center and Research Institute for Maternal and Child Health, Izumi, Osaka, Japan

1 FUNDOPLICATION FOR GASTROESOPHAGEAL REFLUX

The Working Group of the European Society of Paediatric Gastroenterology and Nutrition (ESPGEN) on gastroesophageal reflux disease (GERD) has proposed guidelines for its treatment of GERD (1) (see Chap. 19). According to those guidelines, the therapeutic approach consists of four phases: phases 1 to 3 include positional treatment, dietary advice, and drug therapy, while phase 4 consists of surgical therapy. In young infants without associated central nervous system injury, GERD tends to improve spontaneously. In these patients, surgery should be avoided as long as medical therapy remains effective. However, in children with neurodevelopmental impairment, medical therapy may be less likely to be successful and surgery may be indicated at an earlier time than in normal children because natural resolution is less likely to occur (2). This is also true for infants with other significant associated illnesses, such as cardiovascular malformations, severe pulmonary insufficiency, and musculoskeletal abnormalities. A Nissen fundoplication with gastrostomy is the most commonly performed procedure to treat GERD in infants and children (3). Most patients experience marked clinical improvement, as demonstrated by no further evidence of reflux, significant weight gain, and improvement of other symptoms. Ramachandran and colleagues recommend a Thal fundoplication (partial wrap) because it preserves the ability to vomit, is easier to perform, and is less invasive (4). Another option is the procedure described by Boix-Ochoa. Whether a fundoplication should be performed every time a gastrostomy is placed is a very controversial issue. In some instances, particularly in neuromuscularly impaired children, a gastrostomy may aggravate GERD. On the other hand, children with severe neurodevelopmental delays who undergo a fundoplication may benefit from a gastrostomy for gastric decompression and feeding. Delayed gastric emptying may also be responsible for increased risk of recurrent reflux. There is no agreement as to what preoperative tests may be helpful in predicting which children will also need a fundoplication when a gastrostomy is placed. A 24-hr pH probe and an upper-GI barium exam may be helpful.

A fundoplication may result in gagging, retching, and gas bloating in the early postoperative period. This usually subsides in 4 to 6 weeks in the majority of patients. One of the most common troublesome late complications is mechanical small bowel obstruction. In neurologically impaired patients, this may be fatal because of the delay in recognizing the condition. Wrap herniation, or "slipped Nissen," is another possible complication, which accounts for the largest cause of recurrence of reflux and reoperation. Especially in neurologically impaired children, the recurrence rate is as high as 25%, and relapse of symptoms is noted in 71% of patients (5). Various factors play a role in predisposing neurologically impaired children to have reflux. External factors include scoliosis, chronic recumbency, and aerophagia with increased intra-abdominal pressure. Internal factors include gut dysmotility with gastric stasis and constipation. Recently, laparoscopic fundoplication has become a common surgical procedure for treating GERD in children (6).

2 PYLOROPLASTY FOR HYPERTROPHIC PYLORIC STENOSIS

Nowadays, most of the babies with hypertrophic pyloric stenosis are operated on within 24 hr of admission to the hospital. Medical treatment of hypertrophic pyloric stenosis (HPS) with intravenous atropine, as used in Japan, has received reappraisal (7). Extramucosal pyloromyotomy (Ramstedt-Fredet) is the surgical treatment of choice for HPS. Some modifications have been introduced in recent years to lessen the surgical stress and minimize the surgical scar. In 1991, Alain and colleagues described the first two cases of HPS treated by laparoscopic pyloroplasty; since then, the laparoscopic approach has become more accepted (8). To avoid a large incision, the circumumbilical or intraumbilical arcuate incision has been developed for intra-abdominal pyloromyotomy (9,10). The postoperative management of uncomplicated pyloromyotomy is routine. Oral feedings can be resumed as early as 6 hr postoperatively with a small volume of glucose solution, increasing the volume and concentration every 3 to 4 hr until the infant can take milk (11). Other surgeons refeed rapidly without diluting the formula. It is common for occasional vomiting to occur the first few days after a pyloromyotomy.

In Japan, Nagita and colleagues reported that 22 of 23 infants with HPS became free of vomiting after treatment with intravenous atropine sulfate for 1 to 8 days, and adverse effects were negligible (12). According to those authors, only a small number of patients with HPS who were resistant to atropine therapy required pyloromyotomy. However, there is no strong argument against surgical treatment, as it results in prompt recovery as well as a shorter hospital stay.

3 SURGICAL TREATMENT OF HIRSCHSPRUNG'S DISEASE

Regardless of the length of the aganglionic segment, Hirschsprung's disease (HD) requires surgical treatment. If an infant presents with abdominal distention and episodes of severe diarrhea as well as failure to thrive, enterocolitis secondary to Hirschsprung's disease must be considered. This condition requires nil per os, intravenous fluids and antibiotics, and decompression of the rectum by irrigation. If intestinal dilatation still persists or if the infant is physiologically unstable, an urgent enterostomy should be performed. Frozen-section biopsies are indispensable to determine the site for the enterostomy, which should be made in the area of ganglionic bowel immediately above the transition zone.

Many definitive procedures and their modifications have been performed over the past four decades. The Swenson procedure was the first to address the resection of the distal aganglionic segment (13). Three other main modifications by Duhamel (14), Rehbein (14), and Soave (16) were reported thereafter and satisfactory results were obtained with all three procedures. Generally, the choice of procedure is determined by the surgeon's training and personal preference. Swenson's procedure consists of a full-thickness resection of the aganglionic segment with a subsequent coloanal anastomosis and pull-through abdominal anastomosis (13). Careful dissection of the muscle coat as low as the internal sphincter is the crucial point of this procedure. This operation requires a meticulous technique and is associated with a high risk of anastomotic leakage. The Soave procedure also resects the full-thickness bowel to the level of the peritoneal reflection and then removes only the mucosa, leaving the muscular wall behind. The full-thickness normal bowel is then pulled through the muscular sleeve (hence the name *endorectal pull-through*) and sewn to the anus (16). To avoid the difficulty of mucosectomy in a small pelvic cavity, extra-anal mucosectomy using a prolapsing technique was recently introduced. The Duhamel procedure is a retrorectal transanal pull-through that leaves a rectal blind pouch, which leads to fecal retention and subsequent anastomotic stenosis (14). To avoid this crucial disadvantage, several modifications have been devised. Among them is a Z-shaped anastomosis described by Ikeda (17), using a crushing clamp or GIA stapler (U.S. Surgical Co., Norwalk, Connecticut) (18). For those with total-colon aganglionosis or extensive aganglionosis, Martin applied the procedure adding an extended side-to-side anastomosis between normal pull-through intestine and an aganglionic colon patch to provide additional absorptive surface and an additional fecal reservoir (19). Recently, a laparoscopically assisted pull-through technique was described that can be used in neonates as a single-stage procedure (20).

Postoperative death is attributed solely to persistent enterocolitis. Although rare, the most frequent and troublesome but not fatal complication is anastomotic leakage with abscess formation or peritonitis and subsequent anastomotic stenosis. Although severe fecal soiling is rare, minor soiling may persist for years postoperatively but usually resolves gradually. Residual constipation may sometimes occur.

4 TOTAL COLONIC RESECTION WITH ILEOANAL ANASTOMOSIS

Familial polyposis, ulcerative colitis, and total colonic aganglionosis are absolute indications for total colectomy followed by ileoanal anastomosis. If ulcerative colitis is refractory to intensive medical therapy including steroid therapy, total colectomy should be performed as the next step. If an anal fistula or abscess is diagnosed, Crohn's disease should be strongly suspected and a pull-through procedure not performed because it could lead to malfunction of the pouch from the development of Crohn's disease in the area.

Total colectomy with mucosal proctectomy and a straight ileoanal anastomosis is used in many pediatric patients with ulcerative colitis because children tolerate straight ileoanal anastomosis well and there have been less complications compared with the procedures with a reservoir (21). This, however, is a controversial issue, as many surgeons prefer the J-pouch. In inflammatory bowel disease, a complete diverting ileostomy is mandatory. The most frequent and troublesome complication of an endorectal pull-through is an anastomotic leak and infection of the rectal muscle cuff, leading to pelvic abscess and sometimes more annoying vaginal or urethral fistula formation. Pouchitis is also a possible complication.

Fecal staining or occasional soiling may persist for a long time; however, in most patients this will improve with time.

5 FISTULECTOMY FOR FISTULA-IN-ANO

Fistula-in-ano invariably follows a perianal abscess and is most commonly seen in infants, particularly in males. Eighty percent of cases of fistula-in-ano heal spontaneously within the first year of life, and 94% disappear within 2 years (22). Surgical treatment is performed by curettage or opening the sinus tract throughout its length. The operative wound is left open. Postoperative warm baths (sitz baths) and cleansing usually result in prompt healing.

6 KASAI HEPATIC PORTOENTEROSTOMY FOR BILIARY ATRESIA

Biliary atresia is considered to be the result of various obliterative processes of the biliary system during fetal period. In correctable biliary atresia, the proximal hepatic duct (see Chap. 30) is patent and the obstruction to bile flow lies outside the liver, whereas in noncorrectable biliary atresia, there are no grossly patent ducts outside the liver. In the latter type, which comprise 80% of total cases of biliary atresia, a microscopically patent channel is mostly found in the fibrous remnants of the biliary tree. Dissection of the proximal fibrous remnants followed by bile duct (Kasai) reconstruction improves the chances of successful bile drainage if adequately performed in the early period of life (23). Laparotomy for infants with suspected biliary atresia should be performed as early as possible so as to limit the progression of hepatic injury. The aim of surgery in biliary atresia is to achieve continued and adequate bile flow. Bile duct reconstruction is usually performed by creating a Roux-en-Y hepatic portojejunostomy (23). Insufficient bile flow following hepatic portoenterostomy indicates that a duct of adequate size had not been reached or that the operation was delayed too long. Recurrent cholangitis is the most frequent and serious postoperative complication, occurring in about 40 to 100% of infants. This is not only a debilitating condition for patients but also contributes to ongoing liver fibrosis/cirrhosis. In the series of Ohi, the 10-year survival rate was 72% for those operated on before 60 days of age, whereas it was only 15% for those operated on after 90 days (24). With the development of an improved operative technique, there are an increasing number of jaundice-free postoperative patients. At present, unfortunately, a certain number of patients develop severe liver cirrhosis and portal hypertension and finally succumb to liver failure unless a transplant is performed. In Japan, a huge series of living-related partial liver transplantations have been successfully performed, specially by Tanaka and associates in Kyoto (25).

7   SURGICAL TREATMENT OF CHOLEDOCHAL CYST (CONGENITAL DILATATION OF BILE DUCT)

Since the concept of pancreaticobiliary maljunction was introduced by Babbitt (26), there has been considerable progress in the study of the pathophysiology and surgical treatment of choledochal cysts (congenital dilatation of the bile duct). The choledochal cysts are excised and a hepatojejunostomy is created. Simple drainage of the cyst without resection, or cystoenterostomy, predisposes to recurrent pancreatitis, high risk for calculus formation, and even carcinogenesis (27). The 155 cases of congenital dilatation of the bile ducts treated at Osaka University Medical School during a 40-year period can be classified into two types according to the morphological features of dilatation of the bile duct: 113 cases of cystic type and 42 of cylindrical type. Of interest is that, in all patients less than 1 year of age, the disease was of the cystic type and presented with either a palpable mass or jaundice as the main symptom, whereas in patients above 1 year of age the disease was of either the cystic or cylindrical type and was associated with a history of episodes of abdominal pain accompanied by an elevated level of serum amylase (28). This suggests the existence of maljunction-inducing pancreatitis. Histological sections of the resected cysts from patients under 1 year of age showed severe changes, possibly as a result of refluxed activated pancreatic juice; in contrast, histological sections from the remaining patients of all ages showed only thickening of the fibrous layer. Thus, such variable morphological features and clinical signs and symptoms in congenital dilation of the bile ducts are highly dependent on two factors: age of onset and reflux of pancreatic juice into the bile duct through the maljunction.

8   CHOLECYSTECTOMY FOR CHOLELITHIASIS

In general, cholelithiasis can be seen in patients with or without hemolytic disease. Regardless of the origin, the major clinical problems related to the gallbladder result from the development of gallstones. Andrassy and colleagues reported that children under 15 years of age accounted for only 0.72% of all cholecystectomies at their medical center (29). Ordinarily, cholelithiasis in children is rare; however, under certain pathological conditions, the incidence of lithogenesis is increased. Common hemolytic disorders associated with the development of cholelithiasis include sickle cell anemia (SC), hereditary spherocytosis (HS), and thalassemia. Among these, gallstones are most frequently encountered in children with HS (30 to 60%) (30,31). However, cholelithiasis is more often encountered in patients without hemolytic disease. Cholelithiasis occurs even in the newborn and is found in increasing numbers with each decade of life. There is a predominantly female prevalence with the reported female-to-male ratio being 11:3. Pellerin has suggested that a disturbance of the enterohepatic cycle of bile salts results in gallstone formation, as 20% of his patients with cholelithiasis had undergone resection of the small intestine (32). Furthermore, cholelithiasis is also known to develop following cardiac replacement (33), repair of duodenal atresia or stenosis (34), gastrectomy, and surgery for hypertrophic pyloric stenosis and gastroesophageal reflux. A number of cases of parenteral nutrition (PN)–associated cholestasis and ensuing development of gallstones have been reported (35,36). The most important factor contributing to gallbladder stasis may be lack of gallbladder emptying or impaired enterohepatic circulation of bile acids secondary to fasting. It has also been reported that sludge formation occurs at a high incidence as early as 10 days after initiation of PN (37). When the diagnosis of cholelithiasis is made and the patient presents with clinical symptoms, cholecystectomy is indicated in the early stage. Asymptomatic stones should be treated by elective cholecystectomy. In patients with spherocytosis, cholecystectomy should be performed simultaneously with splenectomy if the patient is older than 5 years of age. Spontaneous resolution of cholelithiasis occurs in idiopathic cholelithiasis or transient hemolysis of infants (38,39) and in PN-associated cholelithiasis (37). Spontaneous resolution of gallbladder sludge may occur with resumption of enteral feeding. Therefore, for cholelithiasis in infants without definite hemolytic disease and in patients receiving PN, conservative management with serial monitoring by ultrasound is recommended. There is a report that cholecystokinin-octapeptide prevented sludge formation (40).

Laparoscopic procedures are nowadays becoming common for many kinds of abdominal surgery. Among them, cholecystectomy is recognized as one of the best indications (41). Compared with open procedures, laparoscopic procedures are less invasive and are excellent from the cosmetic point of view. Although the safety of laparoscopic cholecystectomy has been established, complications such as injury to a bile duct, a blood vessel, and other structures may occur with a somewhat higher incidence with the laparoscopic procedure than with the open method if the surgeon is not very skilled.

9 OPERATION FOR PANCREATIC PSEUDOCYST

In children, most pancreatic pseudocysts are caused by abdominal injury, particularly abdominal compression. It develops when compression of the body of the pancreas across the vertebral column causes laceration of the pancreatic duct and parenchyma. Roughly one-half of the cases resolve spontaneously with conservative treatment. Smaller cysts, less than 5 cm in diameter, are more likely to resolve. It has been proposed that the criteria for operative drainage should be restricted to cases with a cyst not resolving after 6 weeks of observation or increasing in size or a cyst with signs of infection or worsening of clinical symptoms (e.g., increasing abdominal pain) (42). An additional benefit of expectant management of pancreatic pseudocysts is that the more mature and thickened the cyst wall is, the easier it is to drain. There is abundant literature on percutaneous drainage of pseudocysts in children, particularly in pseudocysts of traumatic origin.

Pseudocysts occur in about 20% of chronic relapsing pancreatitis and only 20% of them resolve spontaneously. There is a potential for infection, hemorrhage or rupture; therefore, for persistent cysts, surgical treatment is required. In persistent pancreatic pseudocysts, percutaneous drainage with the aid of ultrasonography is a safe and effective procedure, but it is less effective than in traumatic pseudocysts. Pancreatic fistula formation may occur with percutaneous catheter insertion. After a surrounding capsule has formed following conservative management, internal drainage by cystojejunostomy or cystogastrostomy can be performed effectively.

10 LAPAROSCOPIC SURGERY

In 1973, Gans performed the first laparoscopy in pediatric patients, mainly for diagnostic use (43). Since Holcomb and others reported laparoscopic procedure (cholecystectomy) for therapeutic use in 1990 (41), an exponentially increasing number of cases of laparoscopic surgery have been reported in pediatric patients, and these procedures have involved various devices with special instruments and techniques. Most of the reports say that hospital stays after laparoscopic surgery are considerably shorter, patients have fewer complaints, and that they return to school and regular activities sooner than with open surgery. Nowadays, laparoscopic surgery has become an attractive alternative to a variety of operative procedures conventionally performed by open surgical techniques— i.e., appendectomy, pyloroplasty, cholecystectomy, splenectomy, fundoplication, and pull-through for Hirschsprug's disease. Laparoscopy is contraindicated in patients who are at risk of puncture of the abdominal wall—e.g., those with peritonitis, intestinal obstruction, extensive adhesions, or scarring.

ACKNOWLEDGMENT

The editor wishes to thank Dr. Mary Brandt for her comments.

REFERENCES

1. Vandenplas Y, Ashkenazi A, Belli D, Boige N, Bouquet J, Cadranel S, Cezard JP, Cucchiara S, Dupont C, Geboes K, et al. A proposition for the diagnosis and treatment of gastro-oesophageal reflex disease in children: a report from a working group on gastro-oesophageal reflex disease. Eur J Pediatr 1993; 152:704–711.
2. Vane DW, Harmel RP, King DR, Boles ET Jr. The effectiveness of Nissen fundoplication in neurologically impaired children with gastroesophageal reflux. Surgery 1985; 98:662–667.
3. Fonkalsrud EW, Ellis DG, Shaw A, Mann CM Jr, Black TL, Miller JP, Snyder CL.

A combined hospital experience with fundoplication and gastric emptying procedure for gastroesophageal reflux in children. J Am Coll Surg 1995; 180:449–455.

4. Ramachandran V, Ashcraft KW, Sharp RJ, Murphy PJ, Snyder CL, Gittes GK, Bickler SW. Thal fundoplication in neurologically impaired children. J Pediatr Surg 1996; 31:819–822.

5. Martinez DA, Ginn-Pease, Caniano DA. Sequelae of antireflux surgery in profoundly disabled children. J Pediatr Surg 1992; 27:267–273.

6. Meekan JJ, Georgeson KE. Laparoscopic fundoplication in infants and children. Surg Endosc 1996; 10:1154–1157.

7. Swift PG, Prossor JE. Modern management of pyloric stenosis—must it always be surgical? Arch Dis Child 1991; 66:667.

8. Alain JL, Grousseau D, Terrier G. Extramucosal pylorotomy by laparoscopy. J Pediatr Surg 1991; 26:1191–1192.

9. Tan KC, Bianchi A. Circumumbilical incision for pyloromyotomy. Br J Surg 1986; 73:399.

10. Donnellan WL, Cobb LM. Intraabdominal pyloromyotomy. J Pediatr Surg 1991; 26:174–175.

11. Carpenter RO, Schaffer RL, Maeso CE, Sasan F, Nuchtern JG, Jaksic T, Harberg FJ, Wesson DE, Brandt ML. Post-operative ad lib feeding for hypertrophic pyloric stenosis. J Pediatr Surg: 1999; 34:959–961.

12. Nagita A, Yamaguchi J, Amemoto K, Yoden A, Yamazaki T, Mino M. Management and ultrasonographic appearance of infantile hypertrophic pyloric stenosis with intravenous atropine sulfate. J Pediatr Gastroenterol Nutr 1996; 23:172–177.

13. Swenson O, Bill AH. Resection of rectum and rectosigmoid with preservation of the sphincter for benign spastic lesions producing megacolon. Surgery 1948; 24: 212–220.

14. Duhamel B: Une nouvelle opération pour le mégacôlon congénital: L'abaissement rétro-rectal et trans-anal du côlon et son application possible au traitement de quelques autres malformations. Presse Med 1956; 64:2249–2250.

15. Rehbein F, von Zimmerman VH. Ergebnisse der intraabdominalen Resektion bei der Hirschsprung Krankheit. Zentralb Chir 1959; 84:1744–1752.

16. Soave F: Die nahlose Colon-Anastomose nach extramucoser Mobilienung und Herabziehung des Rectosigmoides zur chirurgischen Behandlung des Morbus Hirschsprung. Zentrelbl Chir 1963; 88:1241–1249.

17. Ikeda K. New techniques in the surgical treatment of Hirschsprung's disease. Surgery 1967; 61:503–508.

18. Ravitch HM, Rivarola A. Enteroanastomosis with an automatic instrument. Surgery 1966; 59:270–277.

19. Martin LW. Total colonic aganglionosis: preservation and utilization of the entire colon. J Pediatr Surg 1982; 13:635–637.

20. Morikawa Y, Hoshino K, Matsumura K, Yoshioka S, Yokoyama J, Kitajima M. Extra-anal mucosectomy: laparoscopic-assisted endorectal pull-through using prolapsing technique. J Pediatr Surg 1998; 33:1679–1681.

21. Coran AG. The surgical management of ulcerative colitis, familial polyposis and total colonic aganglionosis in infants and children. J Jpn Soc Pediatr Surg 1996; 32:863–871.

22. Watanabe Y, Todani T, Yamamoto S. Conservative management of fistula in ano in infants. Pediatr Surg Int 1998; 13:274–276.

23. Kasai M, Kimura S, Asakura S, et al. A new operation for "non-correctable" biliary atresia: hepatic portoenterostomy. Shujutsu 1959; 13:733–739.

24. Ohi R, Ibrahim M. Biliary atresia. Semin Pediatr Surg 1992; 1:115–124.

25. Tanaka K, Tanaka K, Uemoto S, Tokunaga Y, Fujita S, Sano K, Nishizawa T, Sawada H, Shirahase I, Kim HJ, Yamaoka Y, et al. Surgical techniques and innovations in living related liver transplantation. Ann Surg 1993; 217:82–91.

26. Babbitt DP: Congenital choledochal cysts. New etiological concept based on anomalous relationship of the common bile and pancreatic bulb. Ann Radiol 1969; 12:231–240.

27. Okada A, Oguchi Y, Kamata S, Ikeda Y, Kawashima Y, Saito R. Common channel syndrome: diagnosis with endoscopic retrograde cholangiopancreatography and surgical management. Surgery 1983; 93:634–642.

28. Okada A, Nakamura T, Higaki J, Okumura K, Kamata S and Oguchi Y. Congenital dilatation of the bile duct in 100 instances and its relationship with anomalous function. Surg Gynecol Obstet 1990; 171:291–298.

29. Andrassy RJ, Treadwell TA, Ratner IA, et al. Gallbladder disease in children and adolescents. Am J Surg 1976; 132:19–21.

30. Barker K, Martin FRR. Splenectomy in congenital microspherocytosis. Br J Surg 1969; 56:561–564.

31. Lawrie GM, Ham J. The surgical treatment of hereditary spherocytosis. Surg Gynecol Obstet 1974; 139:208–210.

32. Pellerin D, Bertin P, Nihoul-Fekete CI, et al. Cholelithiasis and ileal pathology in childhood. J Pediatr Surg 1975; 10:35–41.

33. Williams HJ, Johnson KW. Cholelithiasis: a complication of cardiac valve surgery in children. Pediatr Radiol 1984; 14:146–147.

34. Tchirkow G, Highman LM, Shafer AD. Cholelithiasis and cholecystitis in children after repair of congenital duodenal anomalies. Arch Surg 1980; 115:85–86.

35. Peden VH, Witzleben CI, Skelton MA. Total parenteral nutrition. J Pediatr 1971; 78:180–181.

36. Kubota A, Okada A, Nezu R, et al. Hyperbilirubinemia in neonates associated with total parenteral nutrition. J Parenter Enter Nutr 1988; 12:602–606.

37. Matos C, Avni EF, Gansbeke DV, et al. Total parenteral nutrion (TPN) and gallbladder diseases in neonates. J Ultrasound 1987; 6:243–248.

38. Keller MS, Markle BM, Laffey PA, et al. Spontaneous resolution of cholelithiasis in infants. Radiology 1985; 157:345–348.

39. Jacir NN, Anderson KD, Eichelberger M, et al. Cholelithiasis in infancy: resolution of gallstones in three of four infants. J Pediatr Surg 1986; 21:567–569.

40. Sitzmann JV, Pitt HA, Steinborn PA, Pasha ZR, Sanders RC. Cholecystokinin prevents parenteral nutrition induced biliary sludge in humans. Surg Gynecol Obstet 1990; 170:25–31.

41. Holcomb III GW, Olsen DO, Sharp KW: Laparoscopic cholecystectomy in the pediatric patient. J Pediatr Surg 1991; 26:1186–1190.

42. Archives MS, Garcia V. Pancreatic trauma. In: Balistreri WF, Ohi R, Todani T, et al, eds. Hepatobiliary, Pancreatic and Splenic Disease in Children: Medical and Surgical Management. Amsterdam: Elsevier, 1997; pp 495–509.

43. Gans SL, Berci G. Peritoneoscopy in infants and children. J Pediatr Surg 1973; 8: 399–405.

Index